Maternal Mortality
A Global Factbook

Compiled by

Carla AbouZahr and Erica Royston

Division of Family Health
World Health Organization, Geneva

D1208428

World Health Organization
Geneva, 1991

Cover design: Marilyn Langfeld
Cover illustration: Farida Zaman
Book design and pagesetting: Marilyn Langfeld
Maps and figures: WHO Graphics

CONTENTS

ACKNOWLEDGMENTS

W̲e would like to thank the many people who have made the publication of this book possible: Sundari Ravindran who worked on the first draft of the country profiles; Sue Armstrong for her assistance with the introductory chapters which draw heavily on Preventing Maternal Deaths, a book which she co-edited with one of us; and Mark Belsey and Angèle Petros-Barvazian for their unswerving support, guidance and encouragement. Last but not least we are indebted to the hundreds of researchers whose work we have analyzed, abstracted and reproduced.

Financial assistance for the preparation and printing of this book was provided by the United Nations Population Fund (UNFPA) and the United Nations Children's Fund (UNICEF).

FOREWORD

Every minute of every day a woman dies as a result of pregnancy or childbirth somewhere in the world. She may be a teenage bride, physically not yet sufficiently developed for childbirth, struggling to give birth to a first baby, far from professional help. She may be a woman who has delivered in hospital who dies for want of blood or drugs that are in short supply. Or she may be an older woman already struggling to feed a large family who tries secretly and in desperation to terminate an unwanted pregnancy.

Such statistics tend to numb the mind, leaving most people feeling hopeless and helpless in the face of so huge and pervasive a problem. But unlike the global figures, the statistics in this book are revealing rather than stunning. They show the number of maternal deaths, their causes and the circumstances surrounding them in each particular setting, they detail the avoidable factors involved and thus provide the basis for the measures that need to be undertaken to ensure that they do not recur. The background statistics shed light on women's lives in each country, their chances of going to school, eating well, and receiving health care; the age at which they are likely to get married, their chances of planning their families and the number of children they are likely to bear. These details are vital to the analysis, for the death of a woman in pregnancy or childbirth is rarely totally unpredictable. Usually it is the outcome of a chain of events and disadvantages throughout her life, not least of which is her lack of access to skilled obstetric care. Only by understanding this and possessing the basic data can effective action be taken to halt this silent and unnecessary toll of lives.

This factbook has been compiled in order to share with everyone working for safe motherhood the rich and highly instructive collection of materials which the World Health Organization, as part of its Maternal Health and Safe Motherhood Programme, has assembled in the course of its work. We hope that it will provide a useful factual basis for action for all those concerned with preventing maternal mortality and disability and the suffering resulting therefrom; the national and international development community, policy makers and health planners, managers of maternal health and family planning services, hospital administrators, trainers of health workers, professional associations, women's organizations and all groups and individuals striving to meet the 1990s challenge of improved health for women throughout the world.

Angèle Petros-Barvazian
Director
Division of Family Health
World Health Organization

12 July 1991

1.
INTRODUCTION

Worldwide an estimated 500,000 women die as a result of pregnancy each year. The vast majority of these deaths need never have happened. We have, for several decades, had the knowledge and means to remove much of the risk and uncertainty associated with childbearing. In the industrialised countries maternal deaths are now rare events. But the benefits of modern maternity care have been largely denied to women in poor countries, where risks of pregnancy and childbirth up to 200 times higher than those of Europe and North America are commonplace. All but 1% of the annual half million maternal deaths occur in the developing world.

But maternal death is only the tip of the iceberg. Because they lack skilled maternity care millions of women are in a state of constant and debilitating ill-health, which they often accept fatalistically as the normal and unavoidable price of childbearing.

This situation is not new, but until recently few people were aware of the enormity of the problem. In the parts of the world where maternal mortality is high, deaths are rarely recorded, and even if they are, the cause of death is usually not given. This tragic picture has only gradually become clearer, largely as a result of a growing number of good community surveys conducted since the mid 1970s which drew attention to the unacceptably high rates of maternal mortality and serious morbidity for the first time. These studies, many of which were supported by WHO and funded by UNFPA, were undertaken in a range of countries and became instrumental in drawing attention to the underlying epidemiology of maternal mortality.

When these studies were formally reviewed at an Inter-Regional Meeting on the Prevention of Maternal Mortality, held at WHO, Geneva in November 1985, the documents produced represented the scientific basis and the broad directions for a call to action. In effect, they laid the ground work for the second major development in the prevention of maternal mortality and morbidity.

In February 1987, the Safe Motherhood Conference held in Nairobi, Kenya served as a watershed for the recognition of the pressing need for action to counteract the enormous inequities in the health of women. It also gave rise to the launch of the Safe Motherhood Initiative which has led to a new level of international activity to reduce maternal mortality by half by the year 2000.

With the growing motivation and political will the need for better information has become more acute. Knowledge and understanding are a precondition for action at all levels of the health care and other systems. Those able to bring about change in women's reproductive health, in particular maternal health, including those able to influence change makers, have to be motivated and informed. They need sound information not only on how the needed changes can be brought about, but also on the nature and extent of the problems they are faced with. In most countries reliable information is not readily available. Researchers and decision makers have to piece together a picture from whatever is available; be it the rare community studies, hospital studies or descriptive accounts.

These are not always easy to come by and much interesting and useful information on women's reproductive experiences is hidden away in obscure journals and reports, in doctoral theses and in consultant briefings. This book is an attempt to bring together information from all such disparate sources, as well as that more readily available in government reports and scientific journals, in order to give as complete a picture as possible of maternal mortality in all the countries of the world.

Suggesting solutions to the problem is not the purpose of this book; those looking for ways to combat maternal mortality should refer to other WHO publications and in particular to "Preventing Maternal Deaths" edited by Erica Royston and Sue Armstrong, WHO, Geneva, 1989, to which this forms a companion volume.

2.
THE GLOBAL PICTURE

2.1 DIMENSIONS OF THE PROBLEM

Today's rates of maternal mortality show a far greater disparity between countries than even the infant mortality rate, which is most often taken as the measure of comparative disadvantage. Every time a woman in the world's poorest communities becomes pregnant she runs a risk of dying as a result of pregnancy and childbirth that is up to 200 times higher than the risk run by a woman in, say, Western Europe. And not only does she run a greater risk, she also undergoes that risk more often.

No one knows precisely how many women die as a result of pregnancy and childbirth each year. Only 29 governments of developing countries were able to provide the United Nations with estimates of their national maternal mortality for the year 1988.[0337] And studies in countries as diverse as Bangladesh, Egypt, Jamaica, Papua New Guinea and the USA have shown that less than half the maternal deaths which occur are actually reported.[1528]

On the basis of available data – such as those contained in this factbook – it is, however, possible to estimate that at least half a million women die from causes related to pregnancy and childbirth each year. 99% of these deaths occur in developing countries, which account for 88% of the world's births, see Table 2.1 and Figure 2.1. These are based on regional estimates as calculated by WHO and do not imply that all countries within each region have similar rates. The highest number of maternal deaths – about a third of a million annually – occurs in Asia, with the countries of Southern Asia being worst affected. Three countries – India, Pakistan and Bangladesh – between them account for 28% of the world's births and 46% of its maternal deaths. The second worst affected conti-

nent is Africa, where around 150 000 women die each year. The figure for Latin America is 34 000 maternal deaths annually, compared with just 6 000 for the developed countries combined.

Though the largest number of maternal deaths occurs in Asia, the risks of pregnancy are highest in sub-Saharan Africa. A study in one rural area of the Gambia between 1981 and 1983 recorded a rate of

Table 2.1 Estimates of maternal mortality
(about 1983)

UN Region	Live births (millions)	Maternal mortality rate (per 100,000 live births)	Maternal deaths (thousands)
World	128.3	390	500
Developed countries	18.2	30	6
Developing countries	110.1	450	494
Africa	23.4	640	150
Northern Africa	4.8	500	24
Western Africa	7.6	700	54
Eastern Africa	7.0	660	46
Middle Africa	2.6	690	18
Southern Africa	1.4	570	8
Asia	73.9	420	308
Western Asia	4.1	340	14
Southern Asia	35.6	650	230
Southeastern Asia	12.4	420	52
East Asia	21.8	55	12
Latin America	12.6	270	34
Middle America	3.7	240	9
Caribbean	0.9	220	2
Tropical South America	7.1	310	22
Temperate South America	0.9	110	1
Oceania	0.2	–	2

Estimates of the number of births are for 1980-85 from UN Demographic indicators of countries: Estimates and projections as assessed in 1980. New York, Department of International Economic and Social Affairs, United Nations, 1982. Maternal mortality rates are WHO estimates.

2 420 maternal deaths per 100 000 live births.[1131] This is exceptionally high, though community rates of up to 1 000 per 100 000 live births have been reported from rural areas elsewhere in Africa, and rates of over 500 from several cities. A study in Addis Ababa, for example, reported a rate of 566.[1120]

Everywhere rates tend to be lower in urban areas than in rural, which reflects the easier access of the city-dweller to medical services. In Andhra Pradesh, India, for example, the urban rate is 545 compared with a rural rate of 874.[1259] Similarly a survey of 30 provinces of China revealed average rates of 115 in the countryside and 50 in towns.[3014]

Asia is the continent with the greatest disparity in maternal mortality rates between countries. At one extreme are Hong Kong, Singapore and Japan whose national maternal mortality rates – 4, 7 and 11 per 100 000 live births respectively – are comparable with the lowest in Europe. At the other extreme are countries like Yemen, where the rate is 1 000, and Bali, Indonesia, where a recent study found a rate of 718 per 100 000 live births.[0258]

On average, maternal mortality rates are higher in Southern Asia than in other regions of the continent. Community studies in the early 1980s reported rates of over 500 per 100 000 live births in Bangladesh,[0554,0830] for example, and in 1978 the government of Pakistan

estimated the national rate at between 600 and 800.[0518] Sri Lanka is an exception in the region. Through a concerted effort to make maternity more safe, it succeeded in reducing maternal mortality from 522 between 1950-55, to 80 in 1987.[1445]

Most of the data pertaining to Latin America are based on civil registration and tend to be underestimates, (see also Chapter 3). Recent studies in Argentina, Brazil and Jamaica [2316,1992,1343] have shown maternal mortality rates to be up to 100% higher than those from civil registers.

The highest rates based on vital registration are to be found in Ecuador and Paraguay and high rates have been reported by government sources in Peru and Haiti. Rates can vary considerably within a country. Thus in Manaus, North East Brazil, a rate of 310 is reported, compared to 99 in rural Sao Paulo State.[0555]

Maternal mortality rates in Latin America are increased by high levels of abortion in many places. Overall the lowest levels of maternal mortality are to be found in the temperate areas, and the highest in the tropical areas.

In Asia and Africa maternal deaths account for between 21% and 46% of all deaths of women of reproductive age, compared with less than 1% in the United States.[1528]

Figure 2.1 Maternal mortality rates in developing countries by UN region
(maternal deaths per 100 000 live births)

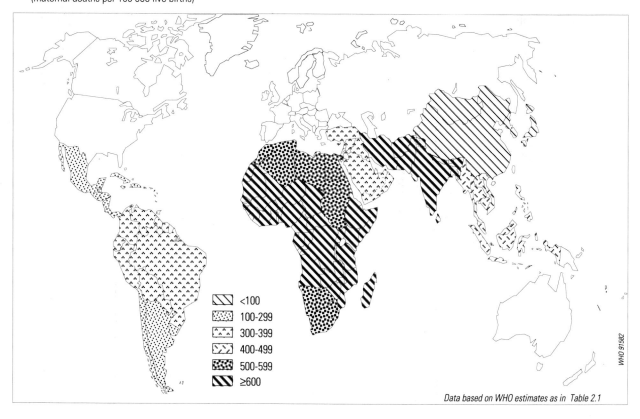

⬚⬚⬚	<100
⬚⬚⬚	100-299
⬚⬚⬚	300-399
⬚⬚⬚	400-499
⬚⬚⬚	500-599
⬚⬚⬚	≥600

Data based on WHO estimates as in Table 2.1

WHO 91582

Maternal mortality rates in Western and Northern Europe are mostly around 10 per 100 000 live births, with the exception of the Scandinavian countries where rates are around half this. Rates in Southern and Eastern Europe are slightly higher but, with the exception of Romania (149 in 1984) where abortion, until recently, took an unusually high toll, are still rarely above 30.[1445] With rates in Canada, the USA, New Zealand and Australia in line with those in Europe, it is estimated that the average maternal mortality rate in the developed world as a whole is about 30.

2.1.1 A historic view of maternal mortality

A look back into history reveals that pregnancy and childbirth were once as hazardous for women in Europe as they are for many women in the developing world today. In eighteenth century rural France, for example, the maternal mortality rate was well over 1 000 [0270] as it was also in Sweden.[1253] Before the discovery of antibiotics and the perfection of such techniques as caesarean delivery and blood transfusion, rich and poor were equally affected: a study of the ruling families of Europe showed a rate of about 2 000 per 100 000 births between the years 1500 and 1850.[0270]

In fact, the rarity of maternal deaths in the developed world is a relatively new phenomenon. In 1920 the United States had a maternal mortality rate of 800 per 100,000 live births.[0337] Until 1935 the registered rate for England and Wales remained constant at about 400 per 100,000.[0587] Rates started to decline dramatically thereafter, coinciding with the development of obstetric techniques and improvements in the general health status of women (Figure 2.2).

Figure 2.2 Trends in maternal mortality, England & Wales, 1911–1981

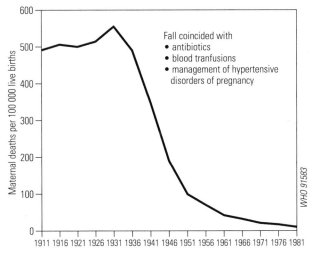

Adapted from: Macfarlane, A. and Mugford, M. Birth counts: statistics of pregnancy and childbirth, HMSO, London, 1984

The last twenty-five years alone have seen significant declines in maternal mortality in almost all developed countries, and the following table is an indication of the downward trend:

Table 2.2 Changes in maternal mortality in selected countries [0834]

Country	1965	1975	Change	Latest
USA	32	13	-59%	8 (1988)
France	23	20	-13%	9 (1988)
FRG	69	40	-42%	5 (1989)
Czechoslovakia	35	18	-49%	10 (1989)
Greece	46	19	-59%	5 (1987)
Portugal	85	43	-48%	10 (1989)
Japan	88	29	-67%	11 (1989)
Romania	86	121	+41%	149 (1984)
Romania excluding abortion	65	31	-52%	21 (1984)

With a few exceptions the trends in developing countries have been more difficult to follow. As a general rule, however, in countries where the rates were already below 100 further progress has been made, whereas in most countries with very high rates there is little evidence of any progress.

2.1.2 A woman's risk of dying

The ratio of maternal deaths to live births measures the risk of dying as a result of a given pregnancy. Thus a rate of 700 per 100 000 live births means that a woman's chance of dying each time she becomes pregnant is about one in 140. This is not uncommon in the developing countries; by contrast the risk of dying for a woman in Scandinavia who becomes pregnant is about one in 25 000.

These figures represent the risk faced by a woman at each pregnancy; her *lifetime* chance of maternal death will also depend on the number of times she becomes pregnant. If a woman with a one in 140 chance of dying as a result of each pregnancy becomes pregnant six times, her lifetime risk is one in 23.

Overall, women in Africa have the highest lifetime risk of maternal death because the effect of high mortality rates is compounded by high fertility. The average number of live births per woman is 6.4, (the number of pregnancies will be even higher). Taking this figure in conjunction with an average maternal mortality rate for Africa of 640, the average lifetime risk has been estimated at one in 25. But in rural Africa it is not uncommon for women to have eight children and to have been pregnant several more times. Thus, for many African women the lifetime risk of dying from pregnancy-related causes may be as high as one in 15.

By contrast the average in the industrialized countries is between one in 1 750 and one in ten thousand.

High risk pregnancies

Undoubtedly the major factor which determines a pregnant woman's risk of maternal death is the lack of access to well equipped health care services. (see section 2.3 below) Nevertheless, some women run additional risks.

The risk of dying is not spread evenly between pregnancies. The age of the woman and the number of her previous pregnancies have a bearing on the outcome. The safest age for childbearing is from 20 to 24 years. Women become fertile several years before their bodies are really able to cope with pregnancy and childbirth. At menarche they have approximately 4% more height and 12-18% more pelvic growth ahead of them.[0582] Thus, women who become pregnant during their teens are at greater risk of complications, such as obstructed labour, and death.

A study in Matlab, Bangladesh showed that girls aged 10-14 years had a maternal mortality rate five times that of women aged 20-24 years. And for teenagers of 15-19 years the rate was still twice that of the 20-24 year olds.[0131] Similarly, a study in Nigeria found the maternal mortality rate for girls under 15 years to be seven times that of women aged 20-24 years, while for 16 year olds it was 2.5 times higher.[1356]

Teenage pregnancy is common in the developing world where the age of marriage remains low. An estimated 28% of women in Africa give birth by the age of 18 years, compared with 18% in Asia and 21% in Latin America.[1711]

Even in developed countries where women have access to high quality maternity care the excess risk associated with extreme youth persists. In the United States, for example, girls under the age of 15 have a maternal mortality rate three times higher than women of 20-24 years,[0608] even though the degree of risk faced by a privileged woman is not comparable with that faced by an underprivileged one under any circumstances. A 15-year old girl in the United States is, for example, still far less likely to die as a result of pregnancy than a 22-year old woman living in a remote area of the Gambia.

Older women who become pregnant also face an increased risk of death compared with women in the prime childbearing years, and research shows that the risk begins to rise from about the age of 30. Studies from six developing countries that allowed comparisons of maternal mortality rates between different age groups showed that women aged 35-39 were between 85% and 460% more likely to die from a given pregnancy than women aged 20-23.[1547] In Jamaica, women of 30-34 had a maternal mortality rate twice as high as women of 20-24, and for those over 40 the rate was increased five-fold.[1343] And in the United States the maternal mortality rate for women aged 40-44 was ten times that of women aged 24 and 25 years.[0608]

The excess risk to older women is particularly significant because in many parts of the world births to women over 35 years make up a sizeable proportion of all births. For example, in Bangladesh the proportion is 25%, in Nigeria 15%, in Senegal 17%, in Sri Lanka 11% and in the USA 21%.

As far as parity is concerned, studies from many countries show that, whatever the age of the mother, the second and third births are most trouble-free, and that the risk of serious complications and death increases steadily thereafter. In Jamaica, for example, a woman giving birth to a fifth or subsequent child was 43% more likely to die than a woman giving birth to a second child. And in Portugal women giving birth for the fifth time were three times more likely to die than women undergoing their second births, while women having their sixth or later births were at even greater risk.[1547]

Lack of adequate spacing between pregnancies also increases the risk to the mother because she does not have time to recover from the extra physical demands made upon her by pregnancy and lactation. But though a woman's general health is obviously undermined by such a pattern of childbearing – particularly where poverty denies her adequate food, rest and medical care – the extra risk has seldom been quantified. In one rare example from Honduras, women with a birth interval of less than a year faced twice the risk of death compared with those with longer birth intervals.[2776]

Besides age, parity and the spacing of pregnancies, the mother's stature is also of significance to childbearing. There is a correlation between height and pelvic size, and women of small stature are particularly susceptible to obstructed labour. This is well illustrated by a study from Nigeria: of a sample of women having their first babies and who received prenatal care, 40% of those under 1.45 metres required operative delivery because of a small pelvis, whereas the proportion was 14% for women 1.50 metres and less than 1% for women who were 1.60 metres and taller.[1356]

Women's stature, their growth during adolescence, and their ability to recover from the physical demands of pregnancy and breastfeeding are all related to their general health and nutritional status – both of which are determined by health care and food intake since early childhood and through adolescence. In societies where, by tradition, women eat last and eat least, their bodies will be ill-equipped to cope with their reproductive roles.

2.2 THE CAUSES OF MATERNAL DEATH

Maternal mortality in the developing world is not a chance event. It is the endpoint of a process that begins at birth and develops over a woman's entire reproductive lifetime. As with most such processes, it has its origins in many intertwined factors, starting with the social status and position of women, greatly affected by the economic resources and infrastructure of the country, and immediately dependent on the accessibility and availability of skills, materials and facilities for family planning and maternity care.

It is customary to classify the causes of maternal deaths under three headings: direct, indirect and coincidental. Direct causes refer to those diseases or complications which occur only during pregnancy and they include abortion, ectopic pregnancy (pregnancy which develops outside the uterus), hypertensive diseases of pregnancy, antepartum and postpartum haemorrhage, obstructed labour, and puerperal sepsis. Indirect causes are those diseases which may be present even before pregnancy but are aggravated by pregnancy; examples include heart disease, anaemia, essential hypertension (high blood pressure of unknown origin), diabetes mellitus and haemoglobinopathies (diseases of the red blood cells). Coincidental causes are fortuitous in nature, and deaths from road traffic accidents are a typical example.

In fact the reasons why women die in pregnancy and childbirth are many layered. Behind the medical causes there are logistic causes – failures in the health-care system, lack of transport, etc. And behind these are all the social, cultural and political factors which together determine the status of women, their health, fertility and health-seeking behaviour.

2.2.1 Direct medical causes

The direct causes together with anaemia are responsible for more than 80% of all maternal deaths reported from the developing countries and the picture is remarkably similar wherever rates of maternal mortality are high.

Haemorrhage

Obstetric haemorrhages can be divided into those that occur during pregnancy (antepartum) and those that occur after delivery (postpartum). Antepartum haemorrhages before the 28th week of pregnancy may be caused by abortion (spontaneous or induced) or by ectopic pregnancy (when the fertilised ovum implants itself outside the uterus, most commonly in the fallopian tube). Those that occur after the 28th week of pregnancy are generally caused by premature separation of the placenta from the wall of the uterus, or by placenta praevia – a condition in which the placenta's position is abnormal, being attached to the lower rather than the upper part of the uterus.

The commonest causes of postpartum haemorrhage are retention of the placenta after delivery (normally the placenta is expelled within 30 minutes of the infant's birth), and failure of the uterus to contract and close down the blood vessels after delivery. Postpartum haemorrhage is most common among multiparous women who are particularly vulnerable because their uteri tend to be stretched and scarred from numerous pregnancies.

Obstetric haemorrhage is the leading cause of maternal death in the developing world, accounting for 30% of the total. More than half these deaths occur in the countries of South Asia, and a further 19% in countries of South East Asia.

Because haemorrhage is difficult to predict and swift to kill, rates for this cause of death are slow to decline even when the overall rate of maternal mortality declines. Reducing deaths from haemorrhage requires relatively sophisticated skills and facilities, as well as ready access to them when emergencies occur.

These points are well illustrated by studies in China which show that, though the country has been generally successful in reducing maternal mortality, haemorrhage still accounts for 50% of maternal deaths in rural areas remote from hospitals compared to 25% in urban areas where hospitals are accessible. [1419] In Cuba, however, a steep decline in haemorrhage deaths was responsible for much of the overall decline in maternal mortality between 1962 and 1988. [0834]

Puerperal sepsis (infection)

A major cause of infection is the entry of germs into the genital tract through the use of unwashed hands and unsterilised instruments during delivery. Sepsis is one of the most frequent complications of illegal abortion. The introduction of foreign objects such as leaves, earth or cow-dung into the birth canal by traditional birth attendants who believe these things are beneficial is also a common cause of infection in developing countries.

Women who remain undelivered many hours after their membranes have ruptured are particularly susceptible to infection. Without the benefit of antibiotics a woman still in labour 12 hours after rupture of her membranes is at serious risk of infection, and the proportion rises to almost 100 percent of women who remain undelivered after 24 hours.[1528]

Sepsis is, in fact, very rare if delivery is straightforward, normal and spontaneous and so long as nothing is introduced into the vagina during labour. Yet this is the second most important cause of maternal death in developing countries, accounting for up to 20% of the total.

Sepsis is usually the first cause of death to decline as the overall rate of maternal mortality falls, particularly where the overall rate was originally very high. In Sri Lanka the proportion of deaths due to puerperal sepsis declined from 25% to 3% (excluding abortion) in about 30 years.[1526] In England and Wales the maternal mortality rate from sepsis alone fell from 104 to 32 in the quinquennium 1935-40 (Figure 2.3).

Reduction in deaths from sepsis generally reflects both improvements in the standard of delivery care, such as for example the emphasis on "The Three Cleans" in China, and the lower case fatality resulting from the wider use of antibiotics.

Figure 2.3 Maternal mortality rates by cause, England and Wales, 1935–1980

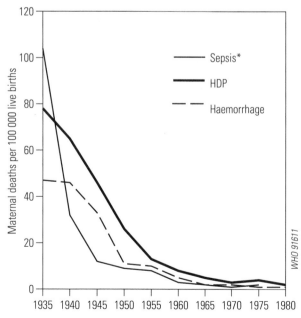

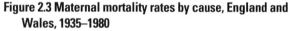

* excluding abortions
Adapted from: Macfarlane, A. and Mugford, M. Birth counts: statistics of pregnancy and childbirth, London HMSO, 1984.

Hypertensive disorders of pregnancy

The symptoms of hypertensive disorders of pregnancy (HDP) are a rise in blood pressure, swelling of the hands, feet and face, and protein in the urine. If left untreated HDP can rapidly lead to eclampsia, or convulsions, which may result in brain damage, or death from heart failure, kidney failure or brain haemorrhage. In tropical Africa the disease tends to progress from the first to the last stage particularly rapidly, often within 24 hours, whereas elsewhere the time between onset of symptoms and death (if untreated) is more usually two days.

In developing countries HDP is most often seen in very young women and those pregnant for the first time. It is rare in subsequent pregnancies except in certain circumstances such as when the mother is extremely obese, diabetic, already suffers from hypertension or is expecting a multiple birth. The causes are unknown. The disease is more common in black and Indian women than in white women, and it affects all social classes equally though it tends to kill the poor more often than the rich because they are less likely to receive essential health care.

HDP is the third most important cause of maternal death in developing countries, accounting for 10-15% of the total and considerably more in many Latin American countries. As with haemorrhage, HDP as a cause of death is relatively slow to decline as overall maternal mortality falls because it too depends on the availability of high quality professional healthcare (Figure 2.3). This is well illustrated by the case of Sweden, a country which now has an extremely low maternal mortality rate (around 4 per 100 000), where the decline in eclampsia deaths was not due to a reduction in the incidence but rather to a reduction in the case fatality rate from 14% in 1950-55 to 3% in 1971-80.[1253]

Obstructed labour

Obstructed labour is commonly caused by disproportion between the size of the baby's head and the space in the bony birth canal (cephalo-pelvic disproportion) as a result of physical immaturity or stunting in the mother, or distortion of her pelvis through disease or malnutrition. Alternatively it may be caused by an abnormal position of the fetus when the mother goes into labour, or by obstruction of the birth canal by the placenta.

Without professional treatment a woman with obstructed labour will eventually die of haemorrhage, rupture of the uterus, infection or sheer exhaustion.

Obstructed labour is most prevalent in conditions of poverty and underdevelopment. The women most at risk are the very young, women of small stature, and those who have suffered previous pregnancy complications. Rupture of the uterus is rare in first deliveries, but a common consequence of obstructed labour in those who have borne many children.

Information on the incidence of and mortality from obstructed labour is patchy, probably because in many countries deaths as a result of this condition are classified under the final cause of death, which may be sepsis, haemorrhage, uterine rupture or obstetric shock. Obstructed labour and its consequences are the most important reported cause of maternal death in Sub-Saharan Africa.[0422]

In addition, obstructed labour is the direct cause of one of the most distressing forms of long term morbidity resulting from poor pregnancy care, namely obstetric fistula.[2301,2923]

Preventing deaths from obstructed labour requires professional expertise and sophisticated facilities, but because it can, in many cases, be predicted, prenatal care has a vital role to play in referring those women at particular risk to hospital. The incidence of this condition also declines as a result of socio-economic measures such as raising the age of marriage and combatting poverty.

Abortion

In many parts of the world abortion is illegal or severely restricted by law. Elsewhere, though abortion may be legal, governments have yet to provide adequate services to meet demand. As a result, a large proportion of the world's women are without access to safe termination of pregnancy carried out by qualified personnel under aseptic conditions.

However, neither lack of access to safe procedures nor its illegal status seem to deter women from having the abortions they want. There can be no accurate figures for an activity that most participants wish to keep secret; besides, many abortion deaths will appear in the statistics under the final cause of death, which may be sepsis or haemorrhage. Nevertheless it is apparent that unsafe abortion is both widespread and a major cause of maternal death in developing countries.

On the basis of informed guesswork it has been estimated that between 40 million and 60 million women a year seek terminations of an unwanted pregnancy,[1475] making the the rate of abortion worldwide 30-45 per 1 000 women of reproductive age. Generally speaking abortion is more prevalent in urban areas than rural.

Abortion mortality worldwide is estimated to be between 100 000 and 200 000 women per year. Complications of unsafe abortion are among the leading causes of maternal death in Latin America. Reports from many other developing countries cite abortion as being one of the main underlying causes of maternal death, if not the main one. For example, in community studies it was found to account for 17% of maternal deaths in Cordoba, Argentina,[2316] 18% in Bangladesh,[0597] 29% in Addis Ababa, Ethiopia,[1120] and 7% in Indonesia.[0258]

2.2.2 Indirect medical causes of death

There are several diseases which, though not caused by pregnancy, are aggravated by the condition and render the pregnant woman more susceptible to death. Examples include heart disease, essential hypertension, diabetes mellitus, malaria and viral hepatitis. The effect of such diseases on maternal mortality generally is overshadowed by the major direct causes. However, indirect causes including anaemia are responsible for about 20% of maternal deaths in the developing world.

Anaemia

A pregnant woman is considered to be anaemic when the concentration of haemoglobin in her bloodstream is below 110g/l. Anaemia is widespread in developing countries, affecting an estimated two-thirds of pregnant women (excluding China), compared with 14% of pregnant women in developed countries. The highest rates for anaemia are found in Asia, followed by Oceania and Africa.

The condition plays an important part in maternal mortality, both directly and indirectly. Death from anaemia is the result of heart failure, shock or infection that has taken advantage of the patient's impaired resistance to disease.

While less severe anaemia may not cause death directly, it frequently contributes to maternal deaths from other causes. For example, anaemic women do not tolerate blood loss as well as healthy women and are therefore more likely to die if they start to haemorrhage. And because anaemia lowers resistance to disease, such women are more susceptible to puerperal infection. They are also poor anaesthetic and operative risks.

A twelve-hospital study in Indonesia between 1977 and 1980 found the maternal mortality rate for anaemic women to be 700 per 100 000 live births as against 197 per 100 000 for non-anaemic women.[0138]

Malaria

For reasons that are not yet known, resistance to malaria built up during childhood begins to break down in the pregnant woman from about the 14th week, the process being most marked in first pregnancies.

The disease is mentioned as a cause of maternal death in several African and Asian countries and is thought to be a contributing factor in many deaths.

Viral hepatitis

Viral hepatitis is a disease in which the liver is invaded and damaged by certain viruses to which pregnant women seem particularly vulnerable. It is associated with poverty and insanitary living conditions and, as well as being more common in pregnant than non-pregnant women, it is also more serious, with case-fatality rates up to 3.5 times higher. In studies from Ethiopia and Iran incidence rates for pregnant women were twice as high as those for non-pregnant women. [1451,1452]

Malnutrition increases the chances of contracting the disease and also of dying from it. Of pregnant women in an Indian hospital who had viral hepatitis, 15% of the 156 women who were adequately nourished died, while 25% of the 76 women who were malnourished died. [1848]

Death is the result of liver failure or haemorrhage and, according to selected studies, hepatitis deaths are significant in India, Nigeria, Malawi and Senegal. In Addis Ababa in 1983 viral hepatitis was reported to be the third most important cause of maternal death. [1803] And in India the disease has gained prominence in recent years: whereas 50 years ago it accounted for only 0.5-3% of maternal deaths in Madras and Bombay, today it accounts for around 10-12% of such deaths.

2.2.3 Non-medical causes

The medical causes of maternal death represent only the most visible dimension of a multi-layered problem. In reality it is often logistical or health service factors that determine whether a woman with pregnancy or labour complications lives or dies.

Questions of logistics

In many countries maternal mortality rates are significantly higher in the rural areas than in the urban, and this underlines a crucial point: that lack of access to hospital for complicated delivery or in emergencies is often a root cause of death.

It has been estimated that 10% of all pregnancies develop complications; and a woman who lives far from medical help is obviously more vulnerable to dying as a result. In many places health facilities are concentrated in urban areas. For example, of 200 obstetricians working in Nigeria in 1980, 90% were based in the national or state capital cities. The situation is similar in other parts of Africa, where 50-75% of physicians may be based in urban areas that account for only 10% of the population.

Rural women wanting to reach hospital often face a multitude of obstacles. Roads from the villages or remote homesteads may be rough, or even impassable at certain times of the year; transport may be nonexistent or unreliable because there are no spare parts or fuel to keep vehicles on the road; or people may simply be too poor to pay for fares. Some of the highest maternal mortality rates have been reported from the Gambia, where a 1982-3 study in the Farafeni area revealed that women faced a 200km journey, including a ferry crossing of the river Gambia, to the capital city, Banjul, for specialist treatment. [1462]

Sometimes treatment itself costs money, or there are tips or bribes to pay along the way which may constitute barriers as formidable as lack of transport to very poor people. A certain reluctance among rural women to venture into the alien world of city and hospital, where they may not be treated with respect, may also tip the balance against their survival.

Shortcomings in the health service

A hospital study in Africa found that of a series of 81 maternal deaths, failures in the health service were implicated in over half the cases. This is a common phenomenon in developing countries, many of which are struggling with inadequate resources and overwhelming health problems.

Health service factors that may affect maternal mortality include shortages of drugs and equipment, lack of blood for transfusion, shortages of trained personnel, and careless treatment such as neglect of symptoms. In one country shortages of personnel were so acute that six out of the nine provinces do not have the services of a specialist obstetrician at their disposal. Overcrowding is such that the bed occupancy rate was 130%. Drugs were in such short supply in hospital that treatment was delayed until a patient's family bought drugs from the pharmacy.

Studies from four countries identified staff shortcomings as contributory factors in 11%-47% of maternal deaths. [1547] And an enquiry in Jamaica into all maternal deaths between 1981 and 1984 concluded that avoidable health service factors were involved in 68%. [1343]

Sometimes the cause of a maternal death is iatrogenic – i.e. a direct result of medical treatment, and some deaths following caesarean delivery may be an example. By their very nature operative deliveries, which require anaesthesia, carry more risk than normal deliveries. And to the risks inherent in surgery is added the risk associated with the complication that made the caesarean necessary. The risks of each will vary from one situation to another. In the Sudan, for example, a study of all deaths following caesarean deliveries carried out in the Khartoum hospital between 1978-82 found that only 6 of the 24 could be attributed to the original pregnancy complication. The other 18 were directly attributable to the operation.[0004] Similarly a study in Cuba covering the period 1980-84, found that 41 of 54 deaths from sepsis followed caesarean delivery. In the same study there were thirteen deaths associated with anaesthesia during caesarean delivery.[1547]

Questions of social status

The status of women in the community also strongly affects maternal mortality for a number of reasons, amongst others, because it influences the pattern of childbearing. In many societies a woman's only path to personal fulfillment and social status is through marriage and motherhood. Early marriage followed swiftly and frequently by pregnancy and childbirth – a pattern carrying many risks – is therefore encouraged.

Poverty and underdevelopment are major factors in maternal mortality, too, but to these are added the effects of sex discrimination which makes women the poorest of the poor. Many of the health problems that affect women in their childbearing years have their roots in childhood. Typically where women's status is low, girl children are under-valued from birth. Their needs always take second place to those of the male members in the family: they are likely to eat last and get less of the nutritious foods than their brothers, to get less health care and education, and to be expected to help with household duties at an earlier age.

In Zaria, northern Nigeria, it is estimated that 25% of childbearing women are physically stunted by malnutrition. Here teenage marriage is the custom, and this serves to compound the risk of obstructed labour already conferred by poor physical growth.[1356]

There are links between educational status and maternal mortality too. One study in Zaire, for example, found that the maternal mortality rate for women with no education was 720 as against 130 for women with some education.[0924] Moreover, studies from many countries reveal that the number of children a woman bears is in inverse proportion to the number of years she has attended school, and that educated women are less likely than their uneducated sisters to marry young.

As well as limiting the opportunities a woman has of finding fulfillment outside marriage, lack of education often limits the power she has even within the family. As has been seen, uneducated women have typically little say in matters of fertility and family planning, but in some communities they are not even allowed to decide for themselves whether to seek health care. That is the prerogative of their menfolk, and there are cases where women have died of childbirth complications simply because their husbands were away from the village and no one was prepared to take the unfortunate woman to hospital without his permission.

For these and many other related reasons, high rates of maternal mortality are invariably found in communities where the status of women is low.

2.3 COVERAGE OF MATERNITY CARE

As the preceding sections make clear, the causes of maternal death are complex and may be rooted in poverty and sex discrimination since a woman's own childhood. Thus maternal mortality can be (indirectly) reduced by measures to combat poverty and discrimination generally. But experience shows that good quality maternity care – and particularly access to life-saving treatment for high risk women and in emergencies – coupled with family planning care, is essential in reducing maternal mortality. Such care is always present and functioning in places where the maternal mortality rate is low, and absent, inaccessible or malfunctioning in places where the rate is high.

Because some 10% of pregnancies develop complications, (the figure is probably much higher among deprived populations where the general level of health is extremely poor), even in ideal circumstances there will always be some women who will require highly skilled assistance – such as caeserean delivery, blood transfusion, anti-convulsant therapy – without which they will die. This is well demonstrated by a study [1498] between 1975 and 1982 of a religious group in the USA who accepted no medical intervention whatsoever during pregnancy and childbirth, which recorded a maternal mortality rate of 870, though the women were well nourished and in good health generally. This rate was almost 100 times higher than that for the rest of the population in the state in which the religious group lived, whose health status was comparable but who accepted maternal health care.

2.3.1 Care during delivery

It is estimated that only around 52% of births in the developing world are attended by trained personnel. This means that nearly half the world's infants are delivered with the help of untrained traditional birth attendants, family members or by the mother alone. When complications arise they have no adequate way of dealing with them and although medical assistance may be sought it is often only after considerable hesitation. Moreover, the difficulties of reaching help are frequently insurmountable. All too often, the mother reaches skilled care when she is already past the point at which intervention can be successful. The presence of a skilled person during delivery, even outside an institutional setting, can substantially reduce delays in reaching life-saving intervention.

The highest proportion of births attended by a trained attendant in the developing world is in East Asia where coverage levels are uniformly high in all countries except in the rural areas of the Republic of Korea. By contrast some of the world's lowest coverage levels are in South Asia, where rates below 10% are common and urban/rural differentials particularly marked. Coverage levels in urban areas five times those of the levels in rural areas are not unusual. Among countries with the lowest rural coverage are Afghanistan, Bangladesh, Nepal and Yemen.

In Africa urban/rural differences, while not so marked as in Asia, are still significant, with rates of coverage in urban areas commonly twice those of rural areas. Countries of this region tend to have a uniformly low level of maternity care coverage, starting from 2% in Somalia.

There are wide variations in coverage in Latin America, ranging from 35% to more than 90%. Generally coverage is higher in the richer states of temperate South America. Here, too, urban coverage may be twice that of the rural areas.

In the developed countries, by contrast, there is almost complete maternity care coverage, with the average for the developed world as a whole being 99%; see Table 2.3 and Figure 2.4. It should be noted that the data on coverage, like those on maternal mortality rates shown earlier, are regional estimates and there are a number of country exceptions within regions. For example, although coverage in Southern Asia as a whole is only 25%, in Sri Lanka around 90% of deliveries take place in the presence of a trained attendant.

2.3.2 Prenatal care

The fact that a woman delivers at home without the help of a trained attendant does not necessarily mean she has received no health care during pregnancy. She may well have been seen by health staff at the prenatal clinic but delivered at home because the maternity hospital was inaccessible or because home deliveries and traditional birth attendants are more culturally acceptable.

Rates of coverage for prenatal care vary widely, ranging from 2-99% in Africa, from 8-98% in Asia, and

Table 2.3 Coverage of maternity care [3139]

(about 1985)

UN region	Percent of births with trained attendant
World	58
Developed countries	99
Developing countries	52
Africa	38
Northern Africa	30
Eastern Africa	37
Middle Africa	22
Western Africa	38
Southern Africa	64
Asia*	49
Southern Asia	25
Western Asia	63
Southeastern Asia	45
East Asia*	94
Latin America	86
Middle America	80
Caribbean	78
Tropical South America	73
Temperate South America	93
Oceania*	42

*   Japan, Australia and New Zealand have been excluded from the regional estimates, but are included in the total for developed countries. No data are available for the USSR.

WHO estimates.

from 23-98% in Latin America. As well as promoting general health during pregnancy, the main objectives of prenatal care are to screen pregnant women for risk factors that make hospital delivery advisable, to treat problems that arise during pregnancy, and to refer problems such as bleeding, that require special care. Thus, the effectiveness of prenatal care in saving lives depends to a large extent on an efficient referral system to higher levels of care where necessary. This is well demonstrated by the Gambia where some of the highest rates of maternal mortality have been recorded and yet which has levels of prenatal care coverage of between 80% and 90%. For women in rural areas with poor transport systems, the benefits of such care in screening for risk factors and detecting complications are often dissipated by the fact that they are beyond the reach of blood transfusion and surgical facilities.

Another factor which is often ignored is that the simple existence of prenatal care tells very little about the quality of that care. Facilities may lack even the most basic resources; drugs, the means to measure blood pressure or haemoglobin, or even water and electricity. Or often, routine monitoring is carried out with no follow-up of abnormal findings.

2.3.3 Under-utilization of facilities

Sometimes lack of care is the result of under-utilization of the facilities that have been provided for pregnant women. Besides the fact that such facilities may be too far from people's homes or too costly to make them accessible, there are other factors that cause women to stay away from clinics and hospitals.

Firstly, women may lack awareness of the seriousness of a problem. In Anantapur, India, when family members of women who died were asked if they had been aware of the seriousness of the patient's condition, over 20% said they had not. Of those who said they had been aware, the vast majority took steps to call a health worker or get the patient to hospital.[1547]

Women may be intimidated by the staff and atmosphere in health institutions: those facilities which get a reputation for not treating women with respect are particularly likely to be under-used. A study in Malaysia found that women's refusal to go to hospital for one reason or another contributed to 10% of maternal deaths.[0380,0838]

Studies in Zaire and Ethiopia offer further interesting insights into why women might stay away from maternity facilities. In the Zaire study 13 of 20 maternal deaths occurred during the first five months of planting and harvest seasons when women are par-

ticularly busy in the fields and reluctant to take time off.[0924] Researchers in Ethiopia found that 60% of those who did not receive prenatal care had unwanted pregnancies, and that women with unwanted pregnancies who did seek prenatal care tended to visit MCH clinics that were free of cost.[0596]

It is frequently the case that those who design health services do not take enough care to make them convenient or culturally acceptable to women. Thus, for example, busy women who attend a prenatal clinic may not be able to collect medicines on the same premises but have to spend time, and perhaps money, going elsewhere. Or clinics in rural areas where sexual taboos are strong may be staffed predominantly by men.

2.3.4 Family Planning

Family planning has a major role to play in saving maternal lives because many deaths are the result of unregulated fertility and unwanted pregnancy. However in many parts of the developing world family planning coverage is extremely low. In Africa as a whole, the percentage of married women of reproductive age who are practicing contraception is estimated to be about 17%, while the comparable figures for East and South Asia are 70% and 40% respectively, and 60% in Latin America.

Figure 2.4 Coverage of maternity care in developing countries by UN region
(% of births with trained attendant)

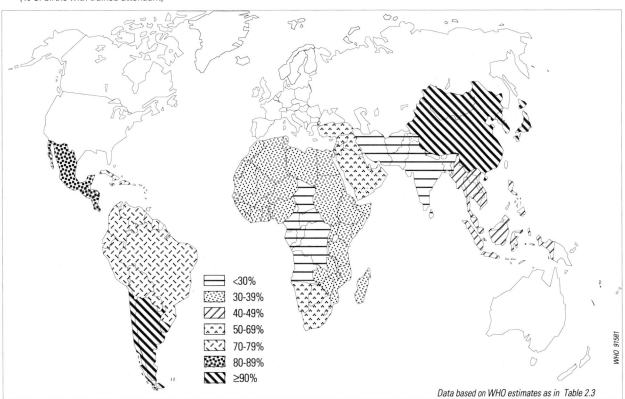

Data based on WHO estimates as in Table 2.3

Low rates of contraceptive use may be the result of lack of services; alternatively services that are provided may be culturally inappropriate or give people insufficient choice to meet their needs. Whatever the reason, the unmet need for family planning remains high. A recent analysis of "wanted" fertility compared with actual fertility in 48 populations showed that around 22% of all births were "unwanted".[3125]

If all women who said they wanted no more children were actually able to stop childbearing, the number of births would be reduced by an average of 35% (4.4 million) in Latin America, 33% (24.4 million) in Asia and 17% (4 million) in Africa.[1528] Maternal mortality would fall by even higher proportions since the births that would be averted would tend to be the high parity/high risk births and the unwanted pregnancies which so often lead to unsafe abortion.

2.4 REFERENCES

WHE 0004   Abbo, A.H. Preventable factors in maternal mortality in Khartoum Teaching Hospital. *Arab Medical Journal*, 1982; 4(11,12): 23-28.

WHE 0131   Chen, L.C. et. al. Maternal mortality in rural Bangladesh. *Studies in Family Planning*, 1974; 5(11): 334-341.

WHE 0138   Chi, L.C. et. al. Maternal mortality at twelve teaching hospitals in Indonesia: an epidemiologic analysis. *International Journal of Gynaecology and Obstetrics*, 1981; 19(4) 259-266.

WHE 0258   Fortney, J.A. et. al. Reproductive mortality in two developing countries. *American Journal of Public Health*, 1986; 76(2): 134-136.

WHE 0270   Gutierrez, H. & Houdaille, J. La mortalité maternelle en France au XVIIIe siècle. *Population*, 1983; 6: 975-994.

WHE 0337   Maine D. Mothers in peril: the heavy toll of needless deaths. *People*, 1985; Vol.12, No.2.

WHE 0380   Karim, R. *Priorities for MCH/FP/HSR in Malaysia: application of the risk approach*. Paper presented to the Meeting of the Steering Committee of the Task Force on the Risk Approach and Programme Research in MCH/FP Care, Geneva, 1983.

WHE 0422   Mafiamba, P.C. *Problems in human reproduction in Cameroon*. In: WHO Regional Multidisciplinary Consultative Meeting on Human Reproduction, Yaoundé, 4-7 December, 1978. Unpublished WHO document HRP/RMC/78.4. 1978.

WHE 0518   Pakistan, Planning Commission, Planning and Development Division. *Health and health-related statistics in Pakistan*. 2nd ed. Islamabad, Printing Corporation of Pakistan Press, 1978.

WHE 0554   Islam, K. & Bachman, S. PHC in Bangladesh — too much to ask? *Social Science and Medicine*, 1983; 17(19): 1463-1466.

WHE 0555   Lacreta, O. and Maretti, M. Mortalidade materna. *Revista Brasileira de Medicina*, 1982; 39(3): 89-106.

WHE 0582   Moerman, M.L. Growth of the birth canal in adolescent girls. *American Journal of Obstetrics and Gynaecology*, 1982; *143(5): 523-528.*

WHE 0587   Macfarlane A. & Mugford, M. *Birth Counts: statistics of pregnancy and childbirth*. Vol. 1. London, Her Majesty's Stationery Office, 1984

WHE 0596   Kwast, B.E. et al. *Report on maternal health in Addis Ababa*. Addis Ababa, Swedish Save the Children Federation, 1984.

WHE 0597   Lindpainter, L.S. et. al. *Maternity-related mortality in Matlab Thana, Bangladesh, 1982*. Final Report for the Community Services Research Working Group, International Centre for Diarrheal Diseases Research, Bangladesh, Undated.

WHE 0608   Rochat, R.W. Maternal mortality in the United States of America. *World Health Statistics Quarterly*, 1981; 34: 2-13.

WHE 0830   World Health Organization. Southeast Asia Regional Office. *Maternal mortality*. (WHO internal memorandum), 1983

WHE 0834   World Health Organization. *World health statistics annual – vital statistics and causes of death*, Geneva. (various years)

WHE 0838   Yadav H. Study of maternal deaths in Kerian (1976-80). *Medical Journal of Malaysia*, 1982; 37(2): 165-169.

WHE 0924   Smith, J.B. et. al. *Hospital deaths in a high risk obstetric population: Karawa, Zaire*. (Unpublished document from Family Health International), 1985. 0924. Sundari.

WHE 1120   Kwast, B.E. et al. Epidemiology of maternal mortality in Addis Ababa: a community-based study. *Ethiopian medical journal*, 1985; 23(7): 7-16.

WHE 1131   Lamb, W.H. et al. Changes in maternal and child mortality rates in three isolated villages over ten years. *Lancet*, October 20, 1984.

WHE 1253   Hogberg, U. *Maternal mortality in Sweden*. Umea, Sweden, Umea University, 1985

WHE 1259   Bhatia, J.C. *A study of maternal mortality in Anantapur district, Andhra Pradesh, India*. Bangalore, Indian Institute of Management, 1986

WHE 1322   Justesen, A. An analysis of maternal mortality in Muhimbili Medical Centre, Dar es Salaam, July 1983 – June 1984, preliminary report. *Journal of Obstetrics and Gynaecology of Eastern and Central Africa*, 1985; 4: 5-8.

WHE 1343   Walker, G.J. et al. Maternal mortality in Jamaica. *Lancet*, 1986; 1 (8479); 486-488.

WHE 1356   Harrison, K.A. Childbearing, health and social priorities. A survey of 22,774 consecutive births in Zaria, Northern Nigeria. *British Journal of Obstetrics and Gynaecology*, 1985, Supplement No.5.

WHE 1419   Zhang, L. and Ding, H. Analysis of the causes of maternal death in China. *Bulletin of the World Health Organization*, 1988; 66(3): 387-389.

WHE 1445   *World Health Organization*. Data reported by Member States and retained on WHO Data Bank.

WHE 1451   Tsega, E. Viral hepatitis during pregnancy in Ethiopia. *East African Medical Journal*, 1976; 53(5): 270-277.

WHE 1452   Borhanmanesh, F. et. al. Viral hepatitis during pregnancy. *Gastroenterology*, 1973; 64: 304-312.

WHE 1462   Greenwood, A. et. al. A prospective study of pregnancy in a rural area of the Gambia, West Africa. *Bulletin of the World Health Organization*, 1987; 65(5): 635-644.

WHE 1475   Henshaw, S.K. Induced abortion: a worldwide perspective. *Family Planning Perspectives*, 1986; 18(6) 250-254.

WHE 1498   Kaunitz, A.M. et al. *Perinatal and maternal mortality in a religious group avoiding obstetric care*. American Journal of Obstetrics and Gynecology, 1984; 150(7): 826-831.

WHE 1526   Vidyasagara, N.W. *Maternal services in Sri Lanka*. Paper presented to the Tenth Asian and Oceanic Congress of Obstetrics and Gynaecology, Colombo, 1985.

WHE 1528   Maine, D. et. al. *Prevention of maternal deaths in developing countries: program options and practical considerations*. World Bank paper prepared for the International "Safe Motherhood" Conference, Nairobi, February 10-13, 1987.

WHE 1547   World Health Organization. *WHO Interregional Meeting on Prevention of Maternal Mortality, Geneva, 11-15 November 1985*. Unpublished report WHE/86.1.

WHE 1711   UN Population Division. *Contraceptive practice: Selected findings from the World Fertility Survey Data*. New York, 1986.

WHE 1803   Kwast, B.E. & Stevens, J.A. Viral hepatitis as a major cause of maternal mortality in Addis Ababa, Ethiopia, *International Journal of Gynecology and Obstetrics*, 1987; 25: 99-106.

WHE 1848   Bhalerao, V.P. et. al. Viral hepatitis in pregnancy. *Indian Journal of Public Health*, 1971; 18(4): 165-170.

WHE 1904   Nlome-Nze, R. et al. *La mortalité maternelle au Centre Hospitalière de Libreville (Gabon), 1986*. Unpublished document.

WHE 1992   Laurenti, R. *Mortalidade de mulheres de 10 a 49 anos no município de Sao Paulo (com enfase a mortalidade materna): alguns resultados de una investigacao*. Paper presented at WHO/PAHO Workshop on Maternal Mortality, 12 – 15 April, 1988, Sao Paulo, Brazil.

WHE 2301   Zacharin, R. *Obstetric fistula*. Vienna, Springer-Verlag, 1988

WHE 2316   Molina Morey de Illia, M. et al. *Resumen de la metodologia y resultados de la investigacion sobre mortalidad materna en la Provincia de Cordoba, Argentina*. Unpublished, 1989.

WHE 2776   Castellanos, M. et al. *Mortalidad materna,* Investigación sobre mortalidad de mujeres en edad reproductiva con énfasis en mortalidad materna, Honduras, 1990.

WHE 2923   Waaldijk, K. *The surgical management of bladder fistula in 775 women in Northern Nigeria*. Doctoral thesis, University of Utrecht, 1989.

WHE 3014   Zhang, Lingmei. *Analysis of surveillance results on maternal death in 30 provinces, municipalities and autonomous regions of China*. Beijing Municipal Maternal Health Institute, Beijing, 1991.

WHE 3125   United Nations Population Fund. *The State of the World Population, 1991,* UNFPA, New York, 1991.

WHE 3139   World Health Organization. *Coverage of maternity care*. WHO document no. WHO/FHE/89.2.

3.
MEASURING
MATERNAL MORTALITY

Measuring the extent and causes of maternal mortality in a given country or community is extremely difficult. Different approaches have been used over the years with varying degrees of success. Each method of measurement has both advantages and shortcomings. Some methods, successfully used by experts in related fields such as infant mortality, are unsuited to the study of maternal mortality. As a result researchers, insufficiently familiar with previous work on maternal mortality, have wasted a great deal of time, effort and money only to obtain information of questionable scientific value.

The studies described in the country profiles cover a wide spectrum of research methods. In order to enable the reader to better judge the value of the information presented in the profiles and to be aware of its limitations, this chapter of the factbook provides an overview of the issues involved.

3.1 DEFINITIONS

3.1.1 Maternal death

Intuitively one would expect the definition of a maternal death to be a simple matter. Childbirth is a memorable event and death in childbirth even more so. In practice, however, matters are not that clear cut. If the definition of a maternal death is to include all deaths due to pregnancy and childbirth it must include deaths taking place before childbirth (e.g. abortion, ectopic pregnancy), those taking place during childbirth (e.g. antepartum, intra-partum and postpartum haemorrhage), as well as deaths taking place some time after the actual event of childbirth (e.g. sepsis). Moreover, not all maternal deaths are directly due to conditions resulting solely from pregnancy. Some are caused by pre-existing conditions which have been aggravated by pregnancy (e.g. hepatitis). This distinc-

tion is clearly made in the Ninth and Tenth Revisions of the International Classification of Diseases (ICD 9 and 10) which define a maternal death as follows:[(0881)]

A maternal death is defined as the death of a women while pregnant or within 42 days of termination of pregnancy, irrespective of the duration and the site of the pregnancy, from any cause related to or aggravated by the pregnancy or its management but not from accidental or incidental causes.

Maternal deaths should be subdivided into two groups:

1) Direct obstetric deaths: those resulting from obstetric complications of the pregnant state (pregnancy, labour and puerperium), from interventions, omissions, incorrect treatment, or from a chain of events resulting from any of the above.

2) Indirect obstetric deaths: those resulting from previous existing disease that developed during pregnancy and which was not due to direct causes, but which was aggravated by physiologic effects of pregnancy.

Whilst scientifically incontrovertible, the drawback of this ICD definition is that maternal deaths can, and indeed do escape being classified as maternal because the precise cause of death cannot be given even though the fact of the woman having been pregnant is known. In developing countries such under-registration is extremely common, but it also frequently occurs in developed countries. An annotation on the death certificate of a woman in the reproductive age group known to be pregnant at the time of her death or known to have been pregnant at any time within the previous 42 days, would go some way to correcting this.

To facilitate the identification of 'maternal' deaths under such circumstances, the ICD 10 has introduced a new category, that of *pregnancy-related death* which is defined as:

the death of a woman while pregnant or within 42 days of termination of pregnancy, irrespective of the cause of death and is intended for use *in countries that wish to identify deaths occurring in pregnancy, childbirth and up to 6 weeks after the end of pregnancy but where the cause of death cannot be identified precisely.*

A significant feature of the new definition is that it is a time-of-death measure, analogous to infant mortality which can, where such information is available, also be analyzed by cause, i.e. into direct and indirect, obstetric and fortuitous or external causes.

The ratio between the three components of maternal mortality thus defined depends critically on the level of maternal mortality. Fortunately countries where the level is low and the inclusion of external causes might render an estimate of maternal mortality including such causes less useful for monitoring and planning, are usually those with good cause of death registration where the separation into the three components should not pose insurmountable difficulties. In countries were the maternal mortality rate is high the bias introduced into estimates of maternal mortality by the inclusion of external causes is usually very low and well worth the overall improvement in the total estimate. In rural Bangladesh (MMR = 570) it was found, for example, that 90% of the deaths of women who were pregnant or had been pregnant within the preceding 90 days, were due to maternal causes.[0131] An Egyptian inquiry (MMR = 263) found 87% of such deaths to be due to maternal causes.[0226]

Modern life-sustaining procedures can prolong dying and delay death. This means that in developed countries a growing proportion of maternal deaths are taking place after 42 days. For this reason ICD 10 has introduced another new category, namely the *late maternal death,* defined as:

> *the death of a woman from direct and indirect obstetric causes more than 42 days but less than 1 year after termination of pregnancy.*

3.1.2 Rates and ratios

Whilst the number of maternal deaths occurring in a given locality (or country) is a useful measure of magnitude that can be used for the analysis of causes and for planning MCH services, it cannot be used as an indicator to measure change or to make comparisons between locations. Moreover, the total number of maternal deaths is a function of two variables – fertility, i.e. the probability of becoming pregnant and, once pregnant, the risk of dying therefrom. A reduction in either component can effect a reduction in the numbers of women dying from maternal causes.

The best measure of this compound risk is expressed by the relationship between the number of maternal deaths and the number of women of reproductive age. This is a true maternal mortality rate, in

the same way as relating all deaths from malaria to the total population is the malaria mortality rate.

Considerable confusion has arisen because the term *maternal mortality rate* has traditionally been used to measure only one component of this compound risk, namely the chance of dying from a given pregnancy. This latter risk is correctly measured by relating maternal deaths to pregnancies. In practice, however, it is impossible to identify the exact number of pregnancies occurring in a given period of time. Even in countries with the most advanced and efficient vital registration systems, women whose pregnancy ends in a spontaneous abortion any time during the first 28 weeks are not registered and hence are automatically excluded from the population at risk of dying from a maternal death (although they may appear in the numerator if the cause of death is diagnosed as such). Similarly, the recording of pregnancies which result in a late fetal death is often far from complete. As a result, the population at risk of a maternal death is generally taken to be the number of live births which is assumed to be a good proxy indicator of the number of pregnancies. Typically, in countries with low induced abortion rates, the former is within 10 per cent of the latter which is unlikely to markedly affect the overall rate. Statistically speaking, this measure is therefore not a true maternal mortality rate, but rather a *maternal mortality ratio*. The ICD 10 definition iterates the ICD 9 definition, however, and calls this the *maternal mortality rate*, and defines it as:

> *The number of maternal deaths per 100 000 live births.*

The rate can also be expressed per 1 000 or 10 000 live births.

Because of conflicting usage by the writers of the sources used and the (theoretically incorrect) ICD definitions, this book uses the term *maternal mortality rate* for both measures, but always specifies the denominator, i.e. live births or the number of women of reproductive age.

3.2 HOW RELIABLE ARE "OFFICIAL" RATES?

Most official maternal mortality rates, with the notable exception of hospital rates (see below) are underestimates. The reasons for this will vary according to certification practices, the degree of sophistication of the vital registration system or whether indeed a vital registration system exists at all. Cause of death is routinely reported in only 78 countries or areas covering a total population of 1.8 billion, or 35% of the world's population.[3147]

Where good vital registration does exist, the biases are usually due to incorrect classification of the cause of death. There may be many social, religious, emotional or practical reasons for not classifying a maternal death as such. Deaths of unmarried women or those resulting from the complications of abortion, for example, may often be attributed to another cause to avoid embarrassing the surviving family; this would be all the more likely if the abortion was illegal. The extent of this type of underreporting can be considerable. Another common cause for underreporting is a wish to avoid blame.

In most developed countries and in most hospital settings all over the world there is usually an inquiry following a maternal death. It is, therefore, not difficult to imagine that in many cultures this constitutes a strong incentive to attribute a maternal death to a less blameworthy cause. Such misrepresentation may not be very common in countries with a tradition of "no name, no blame" confidential inquiries, but seems to be quite common elsewhere.

In countries with very low rates of maternal mortality very few maternal deaths actually take place in obstetric departments of large hospitals because, when life-threatening conditions such as acute renal failure arise the patient is usually transferred to another specialist department. If she dies there the death will be certified by a non-obstetric specialist and the cause of death appearing on the certificate may well not mention the obstetric condition which triggered the fatal sequence of events.

Evidently, even in countries where all or most deaths are medically certified, maternity-related mortality can still be grossly underestimated. A study conducted in the USA by the New Jersey Health Department identified an additional 26 maternal deaths in that State during 1974-75 over and above the 30 deaths reported in the vital statistics.[0846] A Centre for Disease Control study found that the incidence of maternal mortality in the USA in 1974-8 was 12.1 per 100 000 live births rather than the reported rate of 9.6.[0891] Intensive surveillance through a review of death certificates and selected medical records in Puerto Rico in 1978 and 1979 revealed that only about 27 per cent of pregnancy-related deaths had been recorded through the registration system.[0757] By linking death certificates of women in the childbearing ages with birth certificates of their offspring, researchers reported a 50 per cent increase in the number of known maternal deaths in Georgia in 1975 and 1976 compared with the figure obtained from vital registration.[0619] Two Latin American studies found similar discrepancies. In Sao Paolo, Brazil, an analysis of death certificates in 1986 revealed 118 maternal deaths in addition to 100 officially designated as such, making

the true rate more than double the official rate.[1992] In Greater Cordoba, Argentina, analysis of death certificates revealed 24 maternal deaths in addition to 17 officially declared as such in 1987.[2316]

It is clear that even in the most favourable circumstances such as those pertaining in developed countries and certainly in the far less favourable conditions of most of the developing world special efforts have to be made – and additional costs incurred – in order to get good data on maternal mortality.

Moreover, in most developed countries, a maternal death is a very rare event and is no longer a very good indicator of the risks to women's health which result from their reproductive functions. A more holistic view of reproductive health of women in these circumstances must include the risks women run in order *not* to get pregnant, i.e. the risks of death resulting from contraceptive use. This notion has given rise to the development of what is called the reproductive mortality rate which includes not only pregnancy-related deaths but also deaths from the side-effects of contraceptive methods. Whereas in 1955, 99 per cent of the reproductive deaths in the United States were pregnancy related, only slightly more than one-half (53 per cent) were in 1975. Virtually all of the remainder (45 per cent) were due to oral contraceptive use.[0629] By way of contrast, in Menoufia, Egypt in 1981-83 and in Bali, Indonesia 1980-82, 98% of reproductive mortality was pregnancy related.[0258]

Intermediate between countries with good vital registration and those where there is no or incomplete registration, there are many countries where the registration of deaths is fairly complete but registration of the cause of death is poor. Maternal mortality rates based on data derived from such systems can be extremely misleading. An indication of the degree of incompleteness of cause of death certification can be gleaned from the number of deaths classified as being due to "symptoms and ill-defined causes". In Thailand,[1445] for example, out of the 18,985 deaths of women aged 15 to 44 years registered in 1981, 863, or 5%, were registered as being from maternal causes; giving a maternal mortality rate of 81.2 per 100 000 births. However, an additional 6,061, or 32%, women died from "symptoms and ill-defined causes". Bearing in mind the problems of definition described above one can safely guess that at least an equivalent proportion (i.e. at least 5% of 6 061, or 300) also died from maternal causes, bringing the maternal mortality rate up to at least 109 per 100 000 births. If *all* the 6 061 deaths from ill-defined causes were maternal, the maternal mortality rate would be 651, which is clearly an overestimate but is indicative of the degree of confidence that the "official" maternal rate can inspire. Thailand is far from being unique in this respect – in some countries as many as 63% of women's deaths are without specified cause.[0226]

In areas where health care is largely provided by primary health care workers who do not have the necessary medical qualifications to certify deaths by the sophisticated categories of the ICD an alternative system of cause of death certification has to be used. WHO has developed a framework of classification[0896] based on lay reporting of symptoms on which health personnel can build and which can be used for classifying causes of death.

3.3 Community Studies

In situations where civil registration is incomplete or nonexistent – as it is for two thirds of the world's population – other sources of information and other methods have to be used. Different approaches have been tried, with varying success; the main ones are described below. Each method has its advantages and its drawbacks and not all approaches are feasible in all settings. It is possible to visualize a hierarchy of situations depending on the sort of records available and the degree of contact of the health system or other infrastructure and the population of childbearing women. These will range from countries such as Bangladesh, where some 95% of the births are attended by untrained TBA's or family members and no civil registration exists,[1087] through countries like Niger, with good PHC records and poor civil registration,[0697] Brazil with 75% coverage of civil registration[0107] and India, with a 1% sample registration system.[0339, 0340] Clearly no one method is the best in each of these diverse situations. The choice of method will depend not only on such circumstances but also on the purposes for which the data are to be used. Are they to be used for monitoring over time? Or for planning health services and infrastructure? Or for determining health care priorities? In each case the degree of precision has to be balanced against the cost in money and human resources.

3.3.1 Household surveys

Questions relating to maternal deaths can be incorporated into one-off or on-going (large-scale) household inquiries. It is possible for example to ask questions on pregnancy status and to make a repeat visit one year later to ascertain the pregnancy outcome.

Alternatively, retrospective questions can be asked about household members. A recent community survey in Addis Ababa was based on a sample of households to identify births, abortions and deaths over a period of two years. These were then followed up and details of care received, social and other characteristics of the women and households, as well as circumstances and causes of deaths were recorded. A sample of nearly 10 000 pregnancies yielded 45 deaths and an estimated maternal mortality rate of 480. Nevertheless at the 95% level of significance this gives a sampling error of about 30%, i.e. the population rate could lie anywhere between 370 and 660.[1120, 0980]

In a similar study carried out in Central Java, Indonesia, investigators had to visit 150 000 households, and record some 15 000 births in order to identify 50 maternal deaths.[2494]

These figures vividly illustrate the major drawback of using household surveys to measure maternal mortality, namely the enormous expense involved. Whilst they can provide interesting in-depth information on the circumstances surrounding each death, as was the case in Addis Ababa, household surveys are far too expensive to be used solely for the purpose of measuring maternal mortality.

It is however sometimes possible to add questions regarding maternal mortality on to large ongoing demographic or other household surveys. In such circumstances there are a number of recently developed techniques which make the most of the information that can be obtained.

3.3.2 Sisterhood and other indirect measures

A technique which has been receiving considerable attention in recent years is the so called "Sisterhood method". This consists of asking all adult women (sometimes also all adult men) interviewed in a household survey a number of simple questions about the survival of their sisters.[2355] Through a fairly complex, but well defined mathematical calculation it is possible to convert the information thus obtained into life-time chances of dying from maternal causes and hence into estimates of maternal mortality. The technique has proved successful in some countries, and, for reasons not yet fully understood, less so in others. Although somewhat smaller than in a straightforward household survey the sample size required is still very large.

Moreover, this method yields no information on the causes of the maternal deaths or of the circumstances surrounding them.

A similar approach is used in enquiries carried out among ever-married men about the survival of their spouses. One such study of 30 000 men in Egypt, drawn from a rural area and the city of Alexandria, revealed that husbands could be a good source of information for maternal deaths.[0269] This method however presents problems with the denominator.

Another new technique, which is a cross between a household survey and a reproductive age mortality survey (see below) was used in Kenya where women being interviewed in a child survival survey were asked whether they knew of any women who had died from maternal causes in the preceding year.[2230] Their answers were collated and the deaths identified were followed up in order to ascertain the circumstances surrounding each and ascribe the cause of death. The number of births, needed for the denominator, was obtained from the household survey. This technique called *networking* seems very promising for use in well defined geographic areas.

3.3.3 Reproductive age mortality surveys

Perhaps the most successful and economical way of measuring the extent and causes of maternal mortality is to identify and investigate the causes of all deaths of women of reproductive age; the so called Reproductive Age Mortality Surveys (RAMOS). This technique has now been used successfully in countries as different as Guinea [2757] and Honduras.[2776] In the latter, the maternal mortality rate was found to be four times that based on civil registration. The manner in which the deaths are identified prior to investigation differs according to the records and/or the types of knowledgeable informants available. A feature of all successful studies of this type is the use of multiple and varied sources of information on maternal deaths – civil registers, hospitals and health centres, community leaders, schoolchildren, religious authorities, undertakers, cemetary officials etc. (See, for example, the study in Jamaica.[1343]) An early study,[0131] used record matching of adult female death reports from a sample vital registration system in Matlab Thana, Bangladesh. The resulting estimate of 570 maternal deaths per 100 000 live births remained the definitive estimate for Bangladesh until more recent community studies [1254,1279] showed even this to be on the low side.

In areas with reasonable civil registration systems death certificates alone are a useful means of identifying deaths of reproductive age women. They were successfully used in Latin America already in the 1960s [0589] and have lately been widely used elsewhere.

An early RAMOS study in Menoufia, Egypt,[0226] first identified all deaths to women of reproductive age by this means. Interviews with the family of the deceased (most often with the husband) were conducted on average between 30 and 40 days after death to ascertain the symptoms. The interview schedules were then given to a panel of medical specialists for diagnosis. To estimate the maternal mortality rate in the district, the annual number of live births was derived by applying estimated age-specific fertility rates for Egypt as a whole to projections of the female population of Menoufia at these ages based on the latest available census results. The resulting estimate of maternal mortality was 190 per 100 000 live births, compared with the national rate of maternal mortality, based on civil registration, of 93.[0753] Looked at another way, the "official" rate was less than half of that found in Menoufia, a relatively privileged area of Egypt.

In Indonesia family planning workers were asked to list all deaths in their villages during the previous month. This method proved less successful – only about half the estimated number of deaths were traced, those taking place in remote areas being under-represented.[0258] In two Bangladesh studies, which both covered rural areas, traditional midwives were asked to report all births and deaths of women of reproductive age. These were followed up by supervisors who interviewed close relatives to ascertain the circumstances surrounding the death, including menstrual history preceding the death (to identify cases of early pregnancy and abortion).[1254,1279]

In India [1259] and Jamaica,[1343] multiple sources of information were used to identify deaths of women of reproductive age (hospitals, civil registers, schools, mortuaries etc.). Each death was then similarly investigated to determine cases. A notable feature of these two studies was that no single source of information uncovered all the deaths.

All these inquiries used lay reporters and interviewers and a medical review panel who, after examining the lay reports (the symptoms leading to the death), assigned the cause of death to ICD categories. A similar procedure, but using health professionals as interviewers and tracing the deaths back through the health care system was used some 20 years earlier to investigate the causes of adult mortality in 12 cities in the United Kingdom, North and South America.[0589] In every city it was found that maternal deaths had been underenumerated. Overall, some 30% of the final assignments to maternal causes had not originally been so classified. In eight cities the additions to maternal causes represented over 1/4 of the final assignments.

In a study in Bangladesh [0610] specially trained interviewers visited health facilities (MCH centres, FP clinics, hospitals etc.) throughout Bangladesh to obtain reports about pregnancy-related deaths. Of the nearly 2 000 reports only 40% were from hospitals. Family planning workers in rural clinics recalled more such deaths than did health workers in hospitals. Because family planning workers are most likely to know about reproductive health conditions they can be a very useful source of information. Even so, a comparison with the expected number of maternal deaths (using a previous estimate of the maternal mortality rate for Bangladesh [0131]) showed considerable under-reporting of maternal deaths.

Attractive as it is, the RAMOS approach only works if the area under study is well defined. A pilot study in Karachi, Pakistan [3123] found the technique impossible to apply in a large urban setting. In addition to the fact that the area covered by each source of information (or informant) was impossible to delineate, there were additional difficulties due to women who had left the city to give birth in their home villages and/or to those who had come into the district in order to give birth at the city hospital.

3.4 HEALTH SERVICE RECORDS

3.4.1 Hospital Data

In the absence of civil registration or other community data many researchers use hospital data to estimate the maternal mortality rate in a larger catchment area. There are, however, many limitations to this approach and estimates calculated on hospital data alone tend on the whole to be very high. In general, the smaller the proportion of births taking place inside the hospital the greater the discrepancy between the true – usually unknown – community rate and the hospital rate.

In Bogota, Colombia, in 1971-3, deliveries at the Instituto Materno Infantil accounted for 35% of all births in Bogota. The maternal mortality rate was 306 per 100 000 live births. [0632] During the same period the maternal mortality rate for the whole of Colombia (based on civil registration) was 190. [0827] Bearing in mind that Bogota probably has lower maternal mortality than the average for Colombia there still remains a differential of about 2 to 1 in the two rates.

The reason for such discrepancies between hospitals and community mortality rates is that either the numerator (the women who died), or the denominator (the women who gave birth in the hospital), or both, are not a representative sample of all maternal deaths and of all women giving birth respectively.

The usually upward bias found in rates coming from government (non fee-paying) hospitals is due to two factors:

- Firstly, a large proportion of the women who die in such hospitals are emergency admissions, women who had intended to give birth at home but who were transported to hospital when they developed a life-threatening condition. Often they arrive too late and their deaths swell the number of hospital deaths. Births to women delivering safely at home do not of course appear in the denominator. This phenomenon emerges very clearly when hospital data are divided into booked and unbooked patients. At the Black Lion Hospital in Addis Ababa, Ethiopia, for example, the overall maternal mortality rate in 1980-81 was 960, but for booked patients it was 210 compared with 1,050 for unbooked patients. [0550]

- Secondly, if a referral system is working efficiently most high-risk women – at least those who present themselves for prenatal care – are referred to the hospital for delivery. This means that among the women giving birth at the hospital there is a disproportionate number with obstetric complications, and hence of women who die there. The women who have been referred to the hospital for delivery will appear in the statistics as booked patients. It is not possible, therefore, to estimate the degree of bias introduced into the maternal mortality rate as a result.

Another source of bias inherent in hospital rates is that of socioeconomic selection. If a hospital is fee-paying or caters for patients with a certain type of insurance, e.g. private clinic, military hospital, it will attract economically advantaged women. Such hospitals may have a lower maternal mortality rate then that prevailing in the community.

All this is not to suggest that hospital-based studies are of little value. On the contrary, valuable information can be obtained from this source which can shed light on many avoidable factors and point to the need for specific interventions. A number of studies have used hospital deaths as a starting point in tracing back the path followed by the dead woman – her prenatal care, who attended the birth, problems encountered in transport, financial and social barriers to the use of services, as well as shortcomings in the health care system.

Care must, however, be taken in using hospital data for cause of death information. In general, emergency complications from which women die quickly, such as haemorrhage, will be underrepresented because many women will not reach the hospital in time. The study carried out in the Tangail district of Bangladesh [1279] showed that only 1 of the 58 deaths identified took place in hospital and this was from eclampsia whereas the majority of deaths taking place at home were from haemorrhage. Another source of possible bias is that deaths occurring early in pregnancy, e.g. from abortions or ectopic pregnancies, will not be included because they occur in a different part of the hospital. Furthermore, deaths occurring after the discharge of the woman from hospital, will not be recorded.

3.4.2 Combining hospital data with data from other sources

Much of the bias inherent in maternal mortality rates based on hospital data stems from the fact that the numerator and the denominator represent different population groups. Sometimes this can be corrected for.

In places where the catchment area of the hospital is well defined and transport and cultural factors are such that most women in serious difficulty in childbirth, or following an abortion, are transported to hospital even if moribund, it is possible to assume that almost all maternal deaths take place in hospital. The number of such deaths can then be a good approximation to the numerator of the community maternal mortality rate. The problem of estimation then becomes one of defining the denominator, i.e. adding the estimated number of domiciliary births to the known number of hospital births. Rates derived in this fashion tend to be underestimates (due to the unknown number of deaths outside the hospital) but are very useful as minimum estimates. In Madras City, for example, during 1974 to 1975, there were, in the four main teaching hospitals, some 393 maternal deaths and 87 438 deliveries giving a maternal mortality rate of 449. If, instead of hospital deliveries the total number of births in the city – 192,642 – is used as denominator the estimated maternal mortality rate for the city becomes 204.[0605] This compares with the official estimate of 370 for the whole of India.[0336]

3.4.3 Other health records

Numerous community studies testify to the fact that good records at the primary care level can provide all the information necessary for computing infant mortality rates for specific communities. Theoretically, maternal mortality rates can be calculated in the same way. The only difficulty is that of numbers. Even in countries with high maternal mortality rates a maternal death is a relatively rare event and to establish a maternal mortality rate of, for example, 300, correct to within 20% (95% confidence level), would require a sample size of 50 000 births!

The task is not impossible and several health development projects have produced reliable estimates of maternal mortality rates based on maternity records, but in most instances this has been as a by-product of other efforts. The keeping of records only aimed at measuring maternal mortality would throw an unacceptable burden on already busy health workers and is not therefore a viable proposition.

Complete record coverage of all births is not very common in countries without registration systems. Nevertheless, a maternal death is a sufficiently memorable event for it to be possible to gather (numerator only) information on the number of maternal deaths occurring in a given area.

3.5 INDIRECT INDICATORS AND OTHER MEASURES

There is considerable promise in the use of indirect methods to indicate high maternal mortality. Advances in demographic estimation techniques and improved health surveillance measures have yielded estimates of age-sex-specific mortality rates for many countries, or areas within countries where vital registration is poor or nonexistent. Higher female than male mortality in the reproductive ages can, in the absence of knowledge about other factors, be taken as indicative of high maternal mortality. This does not, of course, yield a precise quantitative estimate of the level of maternal mortality but nonetheless should be sufficient to broadly identify the order of magnitude of the problem.

The results of the record matching study in Bangladesh [0131] vividly demonstrate the impact of maternity-related deaths on overall female mortality in the childbearing ages. In the absence of maternity-related deaths, the age-specific death rates for the sexes would have been quite similar. However, when maternal deaths are included, overall death rates for females are roughly 550 per cent higher at ages 20-34 years and 150 per cent higher at ages 15-19 years.

While sex ratios of mortality (male death rate divided by the female death rate) markedly less than unity are almost surely indicative of high maternal mortality, sex ratios close to one may well conceal a similar situation. Thus in societies where the male is much more exposed to hazards at the workplace, accidental death rates for working-age men could be sufficiently high to counterbalance a high maternal mortality rate. Much the same effect could arise if male mortality from wars or other conflicts was known to be particularly high.

Imbalanced population sex ratios can also be indicative of excess female mortality and, by implication, of high maternal mortality. Perhaps the best example of this approach is a study [0204] of the census returns for India, Pakistan and what was then Ceylon. Contrary to the normal pattern, population sex ratios (number of males divided by the number of females) *increased* with age in these countries so that at ages 45 years and over, there were roughly 10 to 15 per cent more men than women. At the childbearing ages (15-44 years), sex ratios were generally in the range 1.05-1.10.

Considerable caution is necessary in using this approach, however. In general it requires supportive evidence based on sex-specific-mortality rates as well as information about sex differences in other confounding factors such as migration rates, underreporting of births and deaths, and differential enumeration in the census.

Indirect estimates of male and female survival during adulthood can also be obtained from other demographic techniques. A convenient overview of these methods, including their data requirements and examples of their application, has recently been published by the United Nations.[0981] Essentially, these techniques permit the estimation of adult mortality based on information about either the orphanhood or widowhood status of respondents. Rather than providing estimates of conventional age-specific mortality rates, these techniques provide conditional probabilities of survival. The *relative* survival of the sexes can then be used to estimate the level of maternal mortality.

In addition to statistical techniques such as those described above it is often possible to discover the frequency of maternal death using various social science techniques to elicit people's opinion on priority health problems.[0982] Such techniques will not yield any quantitative estimates but may provide useful pointers. The clue may even lie in local folklore. As when Tanzanian mothers, about to give birth, bid their older children farewell, telling them "I am going to the sea to fetch a new baby, but the journey is long and dangerous and I may not return."

3.6 REFERENCES

WHE 0107 Brazil, Ministerio de Saude, Secretaria Nacional de Acoes Basicas de Saude, Divisao Nacional de Epidemiologica. *Estadisticas de mortalidade, Brazil, 1980*. Brasilia, Centro de documentacao do Ministerio de Saude, 1983.

WHE 0131 Chen, L.C. et. al. Maternal Mortality in Rural Bangladesh. *Studies in Family Planning*, 1974; 5(11): 334-341.

WHE 0204 El Badry, M.A. Higher female than male mortality in some countries of South-East Asia: a digest. *American Statistical Association Journal*, 1969; 64(328): 1234-1244.

WHE 0226 Fortney, J.A. et al. *Causes of death to women of reproductive age in Egypt*. Michigan State University, Working Paper no. 49, 1984.

WHE 0258 Fortney, J.A. et. al. Reproductive mortality in two developing countries. *American Journal of Public Health*, 1986; 76(2): 134-136.

WHE 0269 El Sherbini, A.F. et al. *The feasibility of getting information about maternal mortality from the husband*. (Unpublished document), 1983.

WHE 0336 India, Ministry of Health and Family Welfare. *Family welfare programme in India: Yearbook 1979-1980*. New Delhi: Ministry of Health and Family Welfare. 1981.

WHE 0339 India, Ministry of Home Affairs, Office of the Registrar General. *Vital statistics of India, 1976*, (16th issue). New Delhi: Office of the Registrar General, 1981.

WHE 0340 India, Ministry of Home Affairs, Office of the Registrar General, Vital Statistics Division. *Survey of causes of death (rural) 1979: a report*. New Delhi: Office of the Registrar General (Series 3, No 12), 1982.

WHE 0550 Horvath, B. and Muletta, E. *Maternal mortality in Black Lion Hospital (1981, 1982)*. Addis Ababa, Department of Gynaecology and Obstetrics, Faculty of Medicine. Unpublished document.

WHE 0589 Puffer, R.R. and Wynne Griffith, G. *Patterns of urban mortality*. PAHO Scientific Publication No. 151. Pan American Health Organization, Washington, 1967.

WHE 0605 Bhasker Rao, K. and Malitta, P.E. A study of maternal mortality in Madras City. *Journal of Obstetrics and Gynaecology of India*, 1977; 27(6): 876-880.

WHE 0610 Rochat, R.W. et al. Maternal and abortion related deaths in Bangladesh, 1978-79. *International Journal of Gynaecology and Obstetrics*, 1981; 19: 155-164.

WHE 0619 Rubin, G. et al. The risk of childbearing re-evaluted. *American Journal of Public Health*, 1981; 71(7): 712-716.

WHE 0629 Sachs, B.P. et al. Reproductive mortality in the United States. *Journal of the American Medical Association*. 1982; 247(20): 2789-2792.

WHE 0632 Sanchez Torres, F. Maternal mortality at the Mother and Child Institute, Bogota (1971-1973). *Revista Colombiana Obstetrica y Ginecologica*, 1974; 25(6): 395-401.

WHE 0697 Thuriaux, M.C. and Lamotte, J.M. Maternal mortality in developing countries: a note on the choice of a denominator. *International Journal of Epidemiology.* 1984; 13(2): 246-247.

WHE 0753 United Nations. *Demographic yearbook.* New York, United Nations, various years.

WHE 0757 United States, Department of Health, Education and Welfare. *Methodology for intensive surveillance of pregnancy related deaths, Puerto Rico, 1978-79.* Atlanta, Center for Disease Control (undated document).

WHE 0827 World Health Organization. Pan American Health Organization. *Health conditions in the Americas, 1977-80.* (PAHO) scientific publication No.427). Washington, 1982

WHE 0846 Ziskin, L.Z. et al. Improved surveillance of maternal deaths. *International Journal of Gynaecology and Obstetrics*, 1979; 16: 282-286.

WHE 0881 World Health Organization. *International classification of diseases. Manual of international statistical classification of diseases, injuries and causes of death.* Ninth revision, WHO, Geneva 1977 and 10th revision in press.

WHE 0891 Smith, J.C. et al. An assessment of the incidence of maternal mortality in the United States. *American Journal of Public Health*, 1984; 74(8): 780-783.

WHE 0896 World Health Organization. *Lay reporting of health information.* WHO, Geneva, 1978.

WHE 0980 World Health Organization. *Adequacy of sample size.* WHO document HSM 73.1, 1973.

WHE 0981 United Nations, Population Division and US National Academy of Science. Manual X. *Indirect techniques for demographic estimation.* UN, New York, 1983.

WHE 0982 Coeytaux, F. *The role of the family in health: appropriate research methods.* WHO document No. FHE/84.2, 1982.

WHE 1087 Bangladesh, Ministry of Health and Popu-lation Control, MCH Task Force. *National strategy for a comprehensive MCH programme.* Dhaka, Ministry of Health and Population Control, 1985.

WHE 1120 Kwast, B.E. et al. Epidemiology of maternal mortality in Addis Ababa: a community-based study. *Ethiopian medical journal*, 1985; 23(7): 7-16.

WHE 1254 Khan, A.R. et al. Maternal mortality in rural Bangladesh. The Jamalpur District. *Studies in Family Planning*, 1986; 17(1): 7-12.

WHE 1259 Bhatia, J.C. *A study of maternal mortality in Anantapur district, Andhra Pradesh, India.* Bangalore, Indian Institute of Management, 1986.

WHE 1279 Alauddin, M. Maternal mortality in rural Bangladesh. The Tangail District. *Studies in Family Planning*, 1986; 17(1): 13-21.

WHE 1343 Walker, G.J. et al. Maternal mortality in Jamaica. *Lancet*, 1986; 1 (8479); 486-488.

WHE 1445 World Health Organization. Data reported by Member States and retained on WHO Data Bank.

WHE 1992 Laurenti, R. *Mortalidade de mulheres de 10 a 49 anos no municipio de Sao Paulo (com enfase a mortalidade materna) – alguns resultados de uma investigacao.* Paper presented at WHO/PAHO Workshop on Maternal Mortality, 12 – 15th April, 1988, Sao Paulo, Brazil.

WHE 2230 Boerma, J.T. and Mati, J.K.G. Identifying maternal mortality through networking: results from coastal Kenya. *Studies in Family Planning*, 1989; 20(6): 245-253.

WHE 2316 Molina Morey de Illia, M. et al. *Resumen de la metodologia y resultados de la investigacion sobre mortalidad materna en la provincia de Cordoba, Argentina.* Unpublished, 1989.

WHE 2355 Graham, W. et al. Estimating maternal mortality: the sisterhood method. *Studies in Family Planning*, 1989; 20(3): 125-135.

WHE 2494 Agoestina, T. and Soejoenoes, A. *Technical report on the study of maternal and perinatal mortality, Central Java Province, Republic of Indonesia,* 1989.

WHE 2757 Toure, B. et. al. *Mortalité maternelle en Guinée.* (Unpublished), 1990

WHE 2776 Castellanos, M. et al. *Mortalidad materna: Investigaçion sobre mortalidad de mujeres en edad reproductiva con enfasis en mortalidad materna.* Honduras, 1990.

WHE 3123 Aga Khan University, Karachi – *Personal communication*, 1988.

WHE 3147   Ruzicka, L.T. and Lopez, A.D. The use of cause-of death statistics for health situation assessment: national and international experiences. *World Health Statistics Quarterly 1990;* 43(4): 249-258.

4.
HOW TO READ
THE COUNTRY PROFILES

The country profiles, which make up the remainder of this book, bring together all available information pertaining to a given area or country in order to build up a picture of maternal health and mortality. Each country profile is as complete as it was possible to make it. There are inevitably gaps where information exists of which we were not aware. Anyone having such information is strongly encouraged to send it to the Maternal Health and Safe Motherhood programme, World Health Organization, Geneva, thus enabling us to improve our data base from which all the information used has been drawn.

The information on the WHO database comes from a wide variety of sources including government statistics, health service and hospital records, research results, journal articles, consultants' reports, doctoral and other theses, and from concerned individuals, agencies and organizations. The year the study was undertaken is given wherever possible. Where this was not available, the date of issue is given in brackets.

4.1 GEOGRAPHIC COVERAGE

There is a country profile for every developing country with a population of more than 200 000. Exceptions were made to this rule when particularly interesting information was available about a smaller country. For a complete listing of the countries please see the index at the front of the book. Information relating to the developed countries is given in the form of a table, chiefly in order to serve as a yardstick. Specific issues relating to all developed countries, such as patterns of causes of death or problems of underregistration are discussed in the introductory chapters.

4.2 HOW THE INFORMATION IS ORGANIZED

The layout of the profiles follows a uniform pattern, as shown below, so that a given section number always relates to the same subject.

1. BASIC INDICATORS
   1.1 Demographic
   1.2 Social and economic
2. HEALTH SERVICES
   2.1 Health expenditure
   2.2 Primary health care
   2.3 Coverage of maternity care
3. COMMUNITY STUDIES
4. HOSPITAL STUDIES
5. CIVIL REGISTRATION DATA/GOVERNMENT ESTIMATES
6. OTHER SOURCES/ESTIMATES
7. SELECTED ANNOTATED BIBLIOGRAPHY
8. FURTHER READING
9. DATA SOURCES

4.3 NOTES, DEFINITIONS AND EXPLANATIONS

BASIC INDICATORS

Demographic

Population rate of growth (%) – annual rate of change.

Life expectancy (years) – the number of years newborn children would live if subject to the mortality risks prevailing for the cross-section of population at the time of their birth.

Crude Birth Rate (CBR) – annual number of births per 1 000 population.

Total Fertility Rate (TFR) – the number of children that would be born per woman, if she were to live to the end of her child-bearing years and bear children at each age in accordance with prevailing age-specific fertility rates.

Crude Death Rate (CDR) – annual number of deaths per 1 000 population.

Infant Mortality Rate (IMR) – annual number of deaths of infants under one year of age per 1 000 live births or the probability of dying between birth and exactly one year of age.

1-4 years mortality rate – annual number of deaths of children aged between 1 and 4 years old per 1 000 children of that age group.

Population, life expectancy, fertility measures and the crude death rate are United Nations Population Division projections for 1980-85 or 1985-90. For most developing countries, with nonexistent or incomplete civil registration systems, these are more stable and realistic than other estimates. The choice of date was determined by the date of completion of the country profiles. Those completed before publication of the most recent version of the projections contain data for the earlier time period. This includes all countries in Africa.

Attention should be paid to sex differentials in life expectancy at birth. Females benefit from an innate biological advantage over males which renders them more resistant to infections during infancy and childhood. This, coupled with the fact that many men work in dangerous occupations and are more likely to die from external causes such as accidents or violence, means that women often outlive men. Where this is not the case, the explanation is usually to be found in the additional risks which women face during pregnancy and childbirth. The relative advantage in life expect-

ancy for women is usually in the region of 5%. Thus a difference of less than 5%, or a female life expectancy actually lower than the male figure, indicates discrimination against female children and/or a particularly high maternal mortality rate.

The same reasoning applies to differences between male and female infant and child mortality, where again a difference of less than 5% in favour of females indicates discrimination in feeding practices and/or health care utilisation on the basis of sex. Further information on this issue is provided in "Health implications of sex discrimination in childhood", document No. WHO/UNICEF/FHE 86.2. obtainable from WHO.

In some instances the infant and child death rates for girls and boys separately relate to an earlier year than do the overall rates, or are derived from a different source, giving rise to apparent inconsistencies.

Social and economic

Adult literacy rate (%)- percentage of persons aged 15 and over who can read and write.

Primary school enrolment rate (%)- the total number of children enrolled in primary level schooling whether or not they belong in the relevant age group for that level expressed as a percentage of the total number of children in the relevant age group for that level. This measure is also known as the gross enrolment rate.

Female mean age at first marriage (years) – the estimated mean age at first marriage.

GNP per capita (US $) – the gross national product expressed in current US dollars, per person.

Daily per capita calorie supply – as defined by the Food and Agriculture Organization.

Literacy rates and school enrolment are both good indicators of social development. Sex differentials in either of these indicators reflect the social status of women. A smaller differential in school enrolment than in literacy is indicative of an improvement of women's status. A primary school enrolment rate higher than 100% can arise when children older than the relevant age group are enrolled in primary school.

Female mean age at first marriage again reflects the social status of women. A particularly low age not only indicates low status, but also predicts a large number of very young mothers who are particularly vulnerable to the risks of pregnancy and childbirth. And, of course, the younger women are when they marry the larger their total fertility is likely to be. It should be noted that the existence of a legal minimum age at marriage does not alone guarantee its enforcement.

Gross National Product (GNP) per capita gives a measure of economic development and hence the type of health services a country can realistically hope to provide. Average GNP, however, tells nothing about how equitably income is distributed in the country and hence about economic disparities between rich and poor.

Daily per capita calorie supply as a percentage of requirements is based on Food and Agriculture Organization (FAO) estimates. When these are low they indicate substantial malnutrition. A higher indicator, however, does not imply a lack of malnutrition because, as is the case with GNP per capita, this indicator tells nothing about social disparities.

HEALTH SERVICES

Health expenditure

These data are usually those reported by countries as part of the WHO Health For All monitoring. The assumption is that they relate to central government health expenditure, although this is not often clearly stated. If this is the case, then in countries where health care is the responsibility of local or provincial governments, or even where most health care is funded through insurance companies, the government expenditure figure will underestimate the amount spent on health care.

Primary Health Care

PHC coverage, safe water and sanitation data are those reported by governments.

Contraceptive prevalence data usually relate to married women of reproductive age. The age groups vary slightly between countries. In some countries cohabiting women are included. Most of the data are from the Demographic and Health Surveys (DHS) or from the World Fertility Surveys (WFS).

Coverage of maternity care

Data on the percentage of pregnant women receiving prenatal and postnatal care, the percentage of births attended by trained attendants and the percentage taking place in institutions derive from a wide variety of sources. Where the information comes from a survey the sample size is also given. The definitions used are those of the originating source. In general "prenatal care" means at least one visit, regardless of when it took place or what care was given. The term "trained attendant" is taken to mean physicians, nurses, midwives or trained TBAs. In some countries it is

possible to obtain a more detailed breakdown, but because different categories have different meanings in different countries, no attempt was made here to give more detail. Interested readers are referred to the original source.

COMMUNITY STUDIES

Before using this and the two sections that follow, readers are strongly advised to carefully read Chapter 3, which describes in some detail the different ways of measuring maternal mortality and the strengths and weaknesses of each.

Sections 3 and 4 of the profiles give details of the findings of all available community and hospital studies and surveys. The two sections follow the same layout and most of the notes given below apply to both types of studies. Additional notes and caveats specific to hospital studies are given separately.

National surveys are reported on first, followed by local studies in date order. The date and place in which the study was undertaken is followed by a brief summary of the methodology used. Where it is known, sample size is also shown. This is important because it gives an indication of the reliability of the findings.

Maternal mortality rate

Following WHO practice, maternal mortality is generally expressed as the number of maternal deaths per 100 000 live births. Where the latter is not available total births, maternity cases or pregnancies may be used in the denominator. Where possible, the rate per 100 000 women of reproductive age is also given. When rates for sub-regions are given in national studies, these are also shown.

Causes of maternal deaths

The causes listed are those given by the authors of the study and no attempt has been made to redefine them. Causes are generally classified as direct, indirect and fortuitous but it has not always been possible to follow this classification where the authors of the study did not themselves do so.

It is not always clear whether abortion deaths are included. Usually only the final cause of death is given, and deaths due to abortion may be classified as being due to sepsis or haemorrhage, with no mention of the abortion which caused the complication. In many countries, but particularly where abortion is illegal, many doctors are reluctant to certify it as a cause of death. All data on deaths due to abortion should, therefore, be viewed with caution.

Whilst medically less reliable, cause of death information derived from lay reports, such as that used in RAMOS studies, is more likely to include abortion and other early pregnancy causes.

Avoidable factors

The avoidable factors given are those reported by the authors of each study. No attempt has been made to judge the validity of the conclusions made by the authors, nor has any attempt been made to evaluate or categorize the factors.

Analyses included in this section concern such factors as distance of the woman from the hospital, transport problems, delays in seeking help by those attending a home delivery, shortage of money to pay for treatment and inadequate referral from lower levels of the health care system.

High risk groups

Most frequently, this section presents an analysis of maternal deaths by age and parity, the most easily available factors. Information is only included if it was possible to relate maternal deaths either to births, to the obstetric population in general, or to a control group of women who survived. Numerator data alone have not been included.

Some studies examine other risk factors such as residence (urban/rural), marital status, type of housing (usually a proxy for socio-economic status), income, and educational level.

Other findings

This sections contains findings which did not fit readily into the previous sections, such as an analysis of time and/or place of death or selected demographic characteristics of the women who died.

HOSPITAL STUDIES

The layout of the section relating to hospital studies follows that already described for the community studies. It contains all information derived from the analysis of hospital records.

Data relating to groups of hospitals at the national or regional level are given first, followed by those relating to individual hospitals in the capital city and then by those from hospitals in other cities.

Most of the points made above also apply to hospital studies. Only additional points are made below.

Maternal mortality rate

In most developing countries where only a minority of all deliveries take place in an institutional setting, there are difficulties in generalizing from maternal mortality rates derived from hospital statistics. Maternal deaths which occur at home or en route to the hospital or health centre are not included in the numerator, and the denominator does not include all the births which took place outside the hospital. See Chapter 3 for a more detailed discussion of this issue.

Another serious limitation of hospital derived statistics is the fact that deaths occurring after the discharge of the woman from hospital are excluded.

Causes of maternal deaths

Care needs to be exercised in generalizing from the pattern of causes of maternal deaths occurring in hospital, particularly as they relate to emergency admissions. The time between the onset of an obstetric emergency and death is not the same for all life-threatening complications. For example women with a haemorrhage are less likely to reach hospital in time for effective treatment than those with an infection and the proportion of deaths from this cause will be underestimated.

It is rarely clear from the study reports whether deaths occurring in departments other than those of obstetrics are included. This issue is particularly important as complications occurring early in pregnancy, such as ectopic pregnancy or abortion, are likely to be treated in other wards.

Avoidable factors

Care should be taken in drawing conclusions from the differences in mortality rates for booked and unbooked patients (which are often given separately, as are rates for women who did and did not receive prenatal care). See Chapter 3 for a discussion of the biases involved.

Despite their constraints, some hospital studies provide important information on the reasons for maternal deaths. Case studies/confidential enquiries identify the avoidable factors surrounding each death, especially insofar as they relate to medical practice, emergency transport, referral procedures etc.

VITAL REGISTRATION DATA/GOVERNMENT ESTIMATES

This section contains data known to be derived from civil registration systems, as well as government data for which the source is not always known. Where civil registration is known to be incomplete, this fact is mentioned. The data reported in the UN Demographic Yearbook and the World Health Statistics are based on government reporting to the UN system and are included in this section.

The layout of the subsections is identical to that followed in the two preceding sections.

OTHER SOURCES/ ESTIMATES

This section contains maternal mortality rates derived from sources other than those already mentioned. These are many and varied, including estimates made by independent researchers, international organizations, field workers, consultants, professional groups etc.

SELECTED ANNOTATED BIBLIOGRAPHY

This section gives a short summary of additional materials relevant to maternal health and maternity care which, because they contain no numerical information, have not been included elsewhere in the profiles. Topics covered include traditional practices related to pregnancy and childbirth, training and use of traditional birth attendants, nutritional practices and sex discrimination, severe maternal morbidities such as obstetric fistulae, the issue of unwanted pregnancy and abortion, and differentials in the rates of operative deliveries.

FURTHER READING

This section includes references not considered suitable for inclusion in section 7 which are, nevertheless, of general interest.

DATA SOURCES

All the information contained in the profiles is drawn from the WHO women's health database and the data source is identified in the text and tables by a bracketed four digit number in superscript. The data sources listed at the end of each country profile are identified by means of these four digit numbers preceded by the letters WHE which distinguishes them from references in other WHO databases.

4.4 ABBREVIATIONS

b	births
d	deliveries
DHS	Demographic and health survey
E	Eastern
EPI	Expanded Programme of Immunization
FIGO	International Federation of Gynecology and Obstetrics
FP	Family Planning
GNP	Gross National Product
GP	General practitioner
HFA	Health For All
ICD	International Classification of Diseases
l.b.	live births
MCH	Maternal and Child Health
MMR	Maternal mortality rate/ratio
N	Northern
n.a.	Not available
No.	Number
PHC	Primary Health Care
RAMOS	Reproductive age mortality study
S	Southern
TBA	Traditional birth attendant
UVF	Urethro-vaginal fistula
VVF	Vesico-vaginal fistula
W	Western
w	women
WHE	Women's Health Database
WHO	World Health Organization

5.
GENERAL RESOURCE MATERIALS

Backett, E.M. et al. *The risk approach in health care, with special reference to maternal and child health, including family planning.* WHO Public Health Papers, number 76, 1984. ISBN 92 4 130076 0. (Accompanying slide set and presentation notes available, INT/83/P48).

Bergstrom, S. *The road to death.* Video in two 22 minute versions, one for medical personnel and the other for a more general audience. Uppsala, Sweden, 1990.

Center for Population and Family Health, Columbia University. *Prevention of maternal mortality program: multidisciplinary literature review.* New York.

Cook, J., Sankaran, B. and Wasunna, A.E.O. *Anaesthesia at the district hospital - a handbook for guidance of medical officers in small hospitals.* ISBN 92 4 154228 4. WHO, Geneva 1988

Cook, J., Sankaran, B. and Wasunna, A.E.O. *Surgery at the district hospital: obstetrics, gynaecology, orthopaedics and traumatology.* WHO, Geneva, 1991.

Dogget, M.A. *Women's views of antenatal care: a review of recent literature.* Institute of Population Studies, Exeter, UK, 1984.

Ferguson, J. *Reproductive health of adolescent girls.* World Health Statistics Quarterly, 1987; 40(3): 211-213.

Family Care International. *NGO participation in improving women's reproductive health in Africa.* New York, 1989.

Family Care International. *Women's perspectives on maternal mortality and morbidity.* New York, 1990.

International Planned Parenthood Federation. *Better health for women and children through family planning.* Report on an international conference held in Nairobi in October 1987. IPPF, London, 1987.

Jacobson, J.L. *The global politics of abortion.* Worldwatch Institute, Washington DC, 1990.

Jacobson, J.L. *Women's reproductive health: the silent emergency.* Worldwatch Institute, Washington DC, 1991.

Maine, D. *Safe motherhood programs: options and issues.* Columbia University, 1991.

Phillips, D.R. *Health and health care in the third world.* ISBN 0582 01418 2. The Longman Group. Harlow, UK.

Population Council. *Medical services to save mothers' lives: feasible approaches to reducing maternal mortality.* New York.

Population Reports. *Mothers' lives matter: maternal health in the community.* Population Information Program, John Hopkins University, Baltimore, USA. 1990.

Royston, E. and Armstrong S. (Eds). *Preventing maternal deaths.* ISBN 92 4 1561289. WHO, Geneva, 1989.

Smyke, P. *Women and health.* Zed Books. London, 1991.

Thaddeus, S. and Maine, D. *Too far to walk: maternal mortality in context.* Prevention of maternal mortality program, Center for Population and Family Health, New York, 1990.

United Nations Children Fund (UNICEF). *State of the World's Children.* Oxford University Press, Oxford, various years.

United Nations Children Fund. *The girl child - an investment for the future.* New York, 1990. E 90 XX USA 7 000595.

World Bank. *Preventing the tragedy of maternal deaths.* A report on the International Safe Motherhood Conference, Nairobi, February 1987.

World Bank. *The safe motherhood initiative: proposals for action.* Discussion Paper number 9. World Bank Publications, Washington DC and Paris, 1987.

World Health Organization. *Abortion - a tabulation of available data on the frequency and mortality of unsafe abortion.* WHO document number: WHO/MCH/90.14.

World Health Organization. *AIDS prevention: guidelines for MCH/FP programme managers - I. AIDS and family planning.* WHO, Geneva, 1990.

World Health Organization. *AIDS prevention: guidelines for MCH/FP programme managers - II. AIDS and maternal and child health (MCH).* WHO, Geneva, 1990.

World Health Organization. *Coverage of maternity care – a tabulation of available information.* Second edition. WHO document number: WHO/FHE/89.2.

World Health Organization. *Emergency obstetric care.* (in preparation).

World Health Organization. *Essential elements of obstetric care at first referral level.* ISBN 92 4 154424 4. Geneva, 1991.

World Health Organization. *Guidelines for introducing simple delivery kits at the community level.* WHO document number: MCH/87.4.

World Health Organization. *Guidelines on the prevention of severe anaemia in pregnancy.* (in preparation).

World Health Organization. *Health implications of sex discrimination in childhood.* WHO document number: WHO/UNICEF/FHE/86.2.

World Health Organization. *The hypertensive disorders of pregnancy.* Report of a WHO Study Group, Geneva 1985. Technical Report Series 758, 1987. ISBN 92 4 1207582.

World Health Organization. *Iron supplementation in pregnancy: Why aren't women complying?* A review of available information. WHO document number: WHO/MCH/90.5.

World Health Organization. *Maternal mortality: helping women off the road to death.* WHO Chronicle 1986; 40(5): 175-183.

World Health Organization. *Measuring reproductive morbidity.* Report of a technical working group, August 1989. WHO document number: WHO/MCH/90.4.

World Health Organization. *Safe motherhood - an information kit.* Presented at the International Conference held in Nairobi, Kenya, February 1987 and continuously updated.

World Health Organization. *Studying maternal mortality in developing countries: rates and causes.* WHO document number: WHO/FHE/87.7.

World Health Organization. *The Partograph: A managerial tool for the prevention of prolonged labour,* available in four parts: the principle and the strategy (WHO/MCH/88.3); a user's manual (WHO/MCH/88.4); facilitator's manual (WHO/MCH/89.2); guidelines for operations research (WHO/MCH/89.1), plus accompanying slide set. WHO, Geneva, 1989.

World Health Organization. *The prevention and management of a postpartum haemorrhage.* A report of a technical working group. WHO document number: WHO/MCH/90.7.

World Health Organization. *The prevention and treatment of obstetric fistulae.* Report of a Technical Working Group. WHO document number: WHO/FHE/89.5

World Health Organization. *The reproductive health of adolescents - a strategy for action.* Joint WHO/UNFPA/UNICEF statement. WHO, Geneva, 1989. ISBN 94 156125 4.

World Health Organization. *The risks to women of adolescent pregnancy and childbirth: a bibliography.* WHO document number: WHO/MCH/89.5.

World Health Organization. *The role of women's organizations in primary health care with special reference to maternal and child health including family planning.* WHO document number: WHO/FHE/WHD/88.1.

World Health Organization. *Women's health and safe motherhood; The role of the obstetrician and gynaecologist.* Report of a WHO/FIGO workshop prior to FIGO congress in Rio de Janeiro, Brazil. Report: WHO/MCH/89.3 and Statement of key speakers: WHO/MCH/89.4.

World Health Organization. *Women, health and development.* A report by the Director General. Offset publication number 90. 1985.

World Health Organization. *Women's health and the midwife: a global perspective.* Report of a WHO/UNICEF/International Confederation of Midwives (ICM) workshop prior to ICM Congress in The Hague, The Netherlands in August 1987. WHO MCH/87.5

World Health Organization/United Nations Population Fund/United Nations Children Fund. *The reproductive health of adolescents: a strategy for action.* ISBN 92 4 130076 0. (Accompanying slide set and presentation notes, reference INT/83/P48).

World Health Organization. *Why did Mrs X die?.* Video explaining the concept of "the road to maternal death". WHO, Geneva, 1989.

AFRICA

ALGERIA

	Year	Source

1. BASIC INDICATORS

1.1 Demographic

1.1.1 Population

		Year	Source
Size (millions)	23.8	1988	(1914)
Rate of growth (%)	3.1	1980-87	(1914)

1.1.2 Life expectancy

		Year	Source
Female	62	1980-85	(1915)
Male	59	1980-85	(1915)

1.1.3 Fertility

		Year	Source
Crude Birth Rate	40	1988	(1914)
Total Fertility Rate	6.0	1988	(1914)

1.1.4 Mortality

		Year	Source
Crude Death Rate	9	1988	(1914)
Infant Mortality Rate	73	1988	(1914)
Female	161	1969-71	(1917)
Male	162	1969-71	(1917)
1-4 years mortality rate			
Female	24	1969-71	(1917)
Male	22	1969-71	(1917)

1.2 Social and economic

1.2.1 Adult literacy rate (%)

		Year	Source
Female	37	1985	(1914)
Male	63	1985	(1914)

1.2.2 Primary school enrolment rate (%)

		Year	Source
Female	87	1986-88	(1914)
Male	105	1986-88	(1914)

1.2.3 Female mean age at first marriage

		Year	Source
(years)	21	1977	(1918)

1.2.4 GNP/capita

		Year	Source
(US $)	2 680	1987	(1914)

1.2.5 Daily per capita calorie supply

		Year	Source
(as % of requirements)	112	1984-86	(1914)

2. HEALTH SERVICES

2.1 Health expenditure

2.1.1 Expenditure on health
(as % of GNP)

2.1.2 Expenditure on PHC
(as % of total health expenditure)

2.2 Primary Health Care
(Percentage of population covered by):

2.2.1 Health services

		Year	Source
National	88	1985-87	(1914)
Urban	100	1985-87	(1914)
Rural	80	1985-87	(1914)

2.2.2 Safe water

		Year	Source
National	77	1980	(0834)
Urban	100	1980	(0834)
Rural	70	1980	(0834)

2.2.3 Adequate sanitary facilities

		Year	Source
National	75	1980	(0834)
Urban	95	1980	(0834)
Rural	70	1980	(0834)

2.2.4 Contraceptive prevalence rate

		Year	Source
(%)	7	1977	(1712)

2.3   Coverage of maternity care (%)

Area	Prenatal care	Trained attendant	Institutional deliveries	Postnatal care	Sample size	Year	Source
National			57			1980	(2114)
National	27	15				1984	(2008)
National:							
rural			7			1969-70	(0611)
urban			40			1969-70	(0611)
North-urban			73		1 334	1974-75	(0026)
North-rural			46		559	1974-75	(0026)
15 western Wilayate			62			1987	(2500)
Cheraga dt.			60			1979	(0821)
Hussein-Dey	14				506	1979	(2114)
Oran	60	93	85			1981	(0628)

3. COMMUNITY STUDIES

4. HOSPITAL STUDIES

4.1   All health institutions, by Wilayate, 1979 [(0025, 0027)]

4.1.1   Rate

Wilayate	Live births	Maternal deaths	MMR (per 100 000 live births)
All	297 256	403	136
Adrar	1 209	3	248
Chleff	11 266	221	195
Laghouat	5 868	5	85
Oum el Bouaghi	8 901	7	79
Batna	12 191	23	189
Bejaia	9 383	14	149
Biskra	9 954	15	151
Bechar	3 314	7	211
Blida	20 843	14	67
Bouira	10 970	18	164
Tamanrasset	331	2	604

Wilayate (Continued)	Live births	Maternal deaths	MMR (per 100 000 live births)
Tebessa	2 082	11	528
Tlemcen	8 421	9	107
Tiaret	4 901	8	163
Tizi Ouzou	27 039	33	122
Alger	28 187	269	92
Djelfa	1 457	11	755
Jijel	5 898	7	119
Setif	21 060	24	114
Saida	4 987	6	120
Skikda	8 627	6	70
Sidi Bel Abbes	6 114	9	147
Annaba	11 872	19	160
Guelma	8 082	4	49
Constantine	16 850	19	113
Medea	6 619	12	181
Mostaganem	9 740	23	236
M'sila	5 158	9	174
Mascara	9 249	8	86
Ouargla	4 445	5	112
Oran	12 238	24	196

4.2   Public maternity services, 1981 [(0025)]

4.2.1   Rate
MMR (per 100 000 live births)   129

4.3 Public hospitals in 15 western Wilayate, 1987 [(2500)]

4.3.1 Rate

Deliveries	116 809
Maternal deaths	88
MMR (per 100 000 deliveries)	75

4.4 Bab El Oued Teaching Hospital Algiers, 1977-84 [(1525)]

4.4.1 Rate

Deliveries	30 562
Maternal deaths	32
MMR (per 100 000 deliveries)	105

4.4.2 Causes of maternal deaths

	Number	%
Ruptured uterus	10	31
Haemorrhage	8	25
Sepsis	4	13
Abortion	3	9
Complications of surgery	3	9
Kidney failure	2	6
Other	2	6
TOTAL	32	100

4.5 All health institutions, Oran, 1971-88 [(0233, 1895, 2114)]

4.5.1 Rate

Year	Live births	Maternal deaths	MMR (per 100 000 live births)
1971	20 683	31	150
1972	19 779	28	142
1973	21 160	35	165
1974	22 237	37	166
1975	23 112	37	160
1976	23 539	34	146
1977	23 539	19	81
1978	23 928	25	104
1979	22 827	12	53
1980	23 429	16	68
1971-80	224 001	274	122

The decrease in maternal mortality rates after 1976 is attributed to the establishment of several new maternity hospitals in Oran. Moreover, fees for medical services were abolished in 1973-74, thus reducing the numbers of unassisted home deliveries.

4.5.2 Causes of maternal deaths (available for 206 cases)

Two-thirds of the maternal deaths were from direct obstetric causes of which haemorrhage was the most important, followed by sepsis and hypertensive disorders of pregnancy. Women aged between 30 and 45 years were found to be most at risk of haemorrhage, and those below 20 years old were more likely to suffer from hypertensive disorders of pregnancy.

Cardiorespiratory problems contributed to about half of the deaths from indirect obstetric causes. Cardiac problems arising from articular rheumatism are relatively frequent in the Maghreb. Anaemia is another important indirect obstetric cause of death: 50% of the women are known to be anaemic.

	Number	%
Haemorrhage	53	26
Sepsis	37	18
Hypertensive disorders of pregnancy	29	14
Embolisms	17	8
Other direct obstetric causes	4	2
DIRECT CAUSES	140	68
Cardiorespiratory problems	32	16
Anaemia	13	6
Cancer	11	5
Other indirect causes	10	5
INDIRECT CAUSES	66	32
TOTAL	206	100

4.5.3 Avoidable factors

4.5.4 High risk groups

According to estimates made on the basis of age-specific fertility rates available from a demographic survey conducted in 1970, women above 45 years of age had the highest maternal mortality rates, followed by those between 15 and 19 years old.

Age group	Live births	Maternal deaths	MMR (per 100 000 live births)
15-19	15 118	31	205
20-24	45 771	39	85
25-29	52 429	46	88
30-34	47 852	41	86
35-39	37 726	65	172
40-44	19 973	28	140
45+	5 132	22	429
Unknown	–	2	–

4.5 Other findings

Maternal mortality rates were higher in winter and spring at 138 and 126 per 100 000 live births respectively compared with 114 and 108 per 100 000 live births in summer and autumn.

Twenty-one of the 29 deaths from hypertensive disorders occurred during the winter. Sepsis was more common during the summer months. Of the 37 sepsis deaths 22 occurred during the summer.

4.6 Hussein-Dey Maternity Hospital, 1963-71 [(2114)]

4.6.1 Rate

	Live births	Maternal deaths	MMR (per 100 000 live births)
1963-71	45 000	145	322

4.6.2 Causes of maternal deaths

	Number	%
Haemorrhage	43	30
Ruptured uterus	22	15
Sepsis	18	12
Associated with caesarean section	16	11
Hypertensive disorders of pregnancy	12	8
DIRECT CAUSES	111	77
Cardiorespiratory conditions	15	10
Other indirect causes	17	12
INDIRECT CAUSES	32	22
Unknown	2	1
TOTAL	145	100

4.6.3 Avoidable factors

4.6.4 High risk groups

Age

Women aged 41 years and over had the highest maternal mortality rates.

	MMR* (per 100 000 live births)
15-20	275
21-25	258
26-30	320
31-35	500
36-40	600
41+	1 500

*   Estimated using age-specific fertility rates.

Parity

Mortality rates were higher among primiparous women and grand multiparas.

	MMR (per 100 000 live births)
primiparous	305
para 2-3	212
para 4-6	261
para 7+	435

5. CIVIL REGISTRATION DATA/GOVERNMENT ESTIMATES

6. OTHER SOURCES/ESTIMATES

6.1 National, 1973 [(0028)]

6.1.1 Rate

A paper presented at a WHO Regional meeting quotes a rate of 150-300 maternal deaths per 100 000 live births in 1973.

7. SELECTED ANNOTATED BIBLIOGRAPHY

8. FURTHER READING

Ait Ouyahia, B. et al. Les ruptures utérines, de 1963 à 1983. *Bulletin de l'Académie Nationale de Médecine* 1984; 168(7&8): 917-925. WHE 1877

Des Forts, J. *Evaluation de la mortalité maternelle dans la région d'El-Mohgoun (Oran)*. Projet de recherche agréé par l'INSP 1988. WHE 2104

Des Forts, J. Facteurs de risque de la mortalité maternelle en Algérie à partir des registres d'état civile et de registres d'admission à l'hôpital. *Revue d'épidemiologie et de santé publique* 1988; 36: 498-499. WHE 2111

Des Forts, J. *Maternal mortality: a difficult study.* Paper presented at the XXIst International Population Conference, New Delhi, India, 20-27 September 1989. WHE 2337

Faour, M. Fertility policy and family planning in the Arab countries. *Studies in Family Planning* 1988; 20(5): 254-263. WHE 2367

Merillet, D. *Aide à l'évaluation du programme d'espacement des naissances* (Unpublished WHO document ALG/MCH/001) 1980. WHE 0454

Nouasria, B. et al. Fulminant viral hepatitis in pregnancy in Algeria and France. *Annals of Tropical Medicine and Parasitology* 1986; 80(6): 623-629. WHE 1852

9. DATA SOURCES

WHE 0025   Algeria, Direction Nationale des Statistiques. *Annuaire statistique de l'Algérie, 1980.* 9ème édition 1981

WHE 0026   Algeria, Ministère de la Santé Publique. *Mortalité infantile et juvenile en rapport avec les tendances de la fécondité, 1974-75.* Alger, Ministère de la Santé Publique and World Health Organization 1980

WHE 0027   Algeria, Ministère de la Santé Publique, Direction des Services Sanitaires, Sous-direction des Statistiques. *Infrastructure sanitaire et activités des secteurs sanitaires, 1978.* Alger 1979

WHE 0028   Alihonou, E. *Pregnancy and delivery.* in WHO Regional Multidisciplinary Consultative Meeting on Human Reproduction, Yaounde, 4-7 December 1978

WHE 0233   Gana, B. and Louadi, T. *La mortalité maternelle en milieu hospitalier - le cas d'Oran,* Université d'Oran, Institut des Sciences Sociales, Département de Démographie 1982

WHE 0611   Rooth, G. and Engstrom, L. (eds.) *Perinatal care in developing countries* Uppsala Perinatal Research Laboratory, University of Uppsala 1977

WHE 0628   Saada, C. *Enquête d'information socio-démographique en liason avec la contraception en 1981 chez les femmes en âge de procréer à Oran* Université d'Oran, Département de Médecine Sociale (unpublished document)

WHE 0821   World Health Organization. European Regional Office. *Report of perinatal study group* Unpublished, undated document.

WHE 0834   World Health Organization *World Health Statistics annual - vital statistics and causes of death.* Geneva, various years

WHE 1525   Belkhodja, J. et al. Evolution de la mortalité maternelle dans le secteur sanitaire et universitaire de Bab El Oued de 1977 à 1984. *1er Congrès Maghrébin de Planification Familiale* Tunis, 18-20 October 1985.

WHE 1712   Mauldin, W.P. and Segal, S.J. *Prevalence of contraceptive use in developing countries. A chart book.* New York, Rockefeller Foundation 1986

WHE 1895   Des Forts, J. La mortalité maternelle: facteurs de risque en Oranie. *Mahgreb Informations Médicales* 1983; 18: 65-69

WHE 1914   United Nations Children's Fund (UNICEF). *The state of the world's children,* various years, Oxford, Oxford University Press

WHE 1915   United Nations. Department of International Economic and Social Affairs. *World population prospects: estimates and projections as assessed in 1984.* Population Studies No. 98. New York 1986

WHE 1917   United Nations. Department of International Economic and Social Affairs. *Age structure of mortality in developing countries. A database for cross-sectional and time-series research* New York 1986

WHE 1918   United Nations. Department of International Economic and Social Affairs. *First marriage: patterns and determinants.* New York 1988

WHE 2008   World Health Organization. African Regional Office. *Evaluation of the strategy for health for all by the year 2000.* Seventh report on the world health situation. Vol 2. Brazzaville 1987

WHE 2114   Des Forts, J. *Projet de recherche: Mortalité maternelle en Algérie.* Oran, Algérie, INESSM 1986

WHE 2500   Des Forts, J. *Mortalité maternelle hospitalière dans les 15 Wilayate de l'ouest Algérien.* (unpublished paper presented at "Journées medico-chirugicales du CHU de Telmcen"), 23-24 May 1990

NOTES

ANGOLA

	Year	Source

1. BASIC INDICATORS

1.1 Demographic

1.1.1 Population
Size (millions)	9.5	1988	(1914)
Rate of growth (%)	2.6	1980-87	(1914)

1.1.2 Life expectancy
Female	44	1980-85	(1915)
Male	40	1980-85	(1915)

1.1.3 Fertility
Crude Birth Rate	47	1988	(1914)
Total Fertility Rate	6.4	1988	(1914)

1.1.4 Mortality
Crude Death Rate	20	1988	(1914)
Infant Mortality Rate	172	1988	(1914)
Female			
Male			
1-4 years mortality rate			
Female			
Male			

1.2 Social and economic

1.2.1 Adult literacy rate (%)
Female	33	1985	(1914)
Male	49	1985	(1914)

1.2.2 Primary school enrolment rate (%)
Female	121	1982	(1914)
Male	146	1982	(1914)

1.2.3 Female mean age at first marriage
(years)	17.9	1960	(1918)

1.2.4 GNP/capita
(US $)	470	1980	(1914)

1.2.5 Daily per capita calorie supply
(as % of requirements)	82	1984-86	(1914)

2. HEALTH SERVICES

2.1 Health expenditure

2.1.1 Expenditure on health
(as % of GNP)

2.1.2 Expenditure on PHC
(as % of total health expenditure)

2.2 Primary Health Care
(Percentage of population covered by):

2.2.1 Health services
National	30	1985-87	(1914)
Urban			
Rural			

2.2.2 Safe water
National	28	1983	(0834)
Urban	90	1983	(0834)
Rural	12	1983	(0834)

2.2.3 Adequate sanitary facilities
National	18	1983	(0834)
Urban	29	1983	(0834)
Rural	15	1983	(0834)

2.2.4 Contraceptive prevalence rate
(%)	1	1977	(1712)

2.3   Coverage of maternity care (%)

Area	Prenatal care	Trained attendant	Institutional deliveries	Postnatal care	Sample size	Year	Source
National	27	34				1982	(2008)
National			16			1984	(2008)
National	27	15				1984	(0834)
Luanda urban	20					(1983)	(0037)

3. COMMUNITY STUDIES

4. HOSPITAL STUDIES

5. CIVIL REGISTRATION DATA/GOVERNMENT ESTIMATES

5.1   National, 1973 (0753)

5.1.1   Rate

According to the United Nations Demographic Year Book, the maternal mortality rate for Angola was 113 per 100 000 live births in 1973.

6. OTHER SOURCES/ ESTIMATES

7. SELECTED ANNOTATED BIBILOGRAPHY

8. FURTHER READING

9. DATA SOURCES

WHE 0037   World Health Organization and United Nations Children's Fund, *Basis for a food and nutrition program in the context of primary health care in Angola.* (unpublished document) 1983

WHE 0753   United Nations. *Demographic yearbook.* Various years, New York

WHE 0834   World Health Organization *World Health Statistics annual - vital statistics and causes of death.* Geneva, various years

WHE 1712   Mauldin W.P. and Segal, S.J., *Prevalence of contraceptive use in developing countries. A chart book.* Rockefeller Foundation, New York 1986

WHE 1914   United Nations Children's Fund (UNICEF). *The state of the world's children*, various years, Oxford, Oxford University Press

WHE 1915   United Nations. Department of International Economic and Social Affairs. *World population prospects: estimates and projections as assessed in 1984.* Population Studies No. 98. New York 1986

WHE 1918   United Nations. Department of International Economic and Social Affairs. *First marriage: patterns and determinants.* New York 1988

WHE 2008   World Health Organization. Regional Office for Africa *Evaluation of the strategy for health for all by the year 2000. Seventh report on the world health situation* Vol 2, African region, Brazzaville 1987

BENIN

		Year	Source

1. BASIC INDICATORS

1.1 Demographic

1.1.1 Population

Size (millions)	4.4	1988	(1914)
Rate of growth (%)	3.0	1980-87	(1914)

1.1.2 Life expectancy

Female	46	1980-85	(1915)
Male	42	1980-85	(1915)

1.1.3 Fertility

Crude Birth Rate	50	1988	(1914)
Total Fertility Rate	7.0	1988	(1914)

1.1.4 Mortality

Crude Death Rate	19	1988	(1914)
Infant Mortality Rate	109	1988	(1914)
Female			
Male			
1-4 years mortality rate			
Female			
Male			

1.2 Social and economic

1.2.1 Adult literacy rate (%)

Female	16	1985	(1914)
Male	37	1985	(1914)

1.2.2 Primary school enrolment rate (%)

Female	43	1986-88	(1914)
Male	84	1986-88	(1914)

1.2.3 Female mean age at first marriage

(years)	18.3	1982	(1918)

1.2.4 GNP/capita

(US $)	310	1987	(1914)

1.2.5 Daily per capita calorie supply

(as % of requirements)	95	1984-86	(1914)

2. HEALTH SERVICES

2.1 Health expenditure

2.1.1 Expenditure on health

(as % of GNP)	1	1983	(0800)

2.1.2 Expenditure on PHC
(as % of total health expenditure)

2.2 Primary Health Care
(Percentage of population covered by):

2.2.1 Health services

National	18	1985-87	(1914)
Urban			
Rural			

2.2.2 Safe water

National	14	1983	(0834)
Urban	45	1983	(0834)
Rural	9	1983	(0834)

2.2.3 Adequate sanitary facilities

National	10	1983	(0834)
Urban	45	1983	(0834)
Rural	4	1983	(0834)

2.2.4 Contraceptive prevalence rate

(%)	9	1980-87	(1914)

2.3   Coverage of maternity care (%)

Area	Prenatal care	Trained attendant	Institutional deliveries	Postnatal care	Sample size	Year	Source
National	27	34				1982	(0834)
National			19			1982	(0800)

3.   COMMUNITY STUDIES

4.   HOSPITAL STUDIES

4.1   67 maternity centres throughout the country, 1975-86 [0219, 0851, 2271, 2490]

4.1.1   Rate

MMR (per 100 000 live births)

1975	160
1977	181
1978	164
1979	186
1980	124
1981	158
1982	95
1983	168
1984	135
1985	141
1986	161

4.1.2   Causes of maternal deaths, 1977 and 1987

	1977		1987	
	Number	%	Number	%
Sepsis	22	23	66	30
Haemorrhage	28	29	41	18
Rupture of the uterus	27	28	26	12
Hypertensive disorders of pregnancy	3	3	23	10
Abortion	n.a.	n.a.	12	5
Post operative shock	4	4	0	–
Embolisms	2	2	0	–
Ectopic pregnancy	0	–	5	2
DIRECT CAUSES	86	91	173	77
Anaemia	n.a.	n.a.	37	17
Hepatitis	9	9	14	6
INDIRECT CAUSES	9	9	51	23
TOTAL	95	100	224	100

4.2   Maternity hospitals, 1986 and 1987 [2271]

4.2.1   Rate

MMR (per 100 000 live births)

1986	137	(212 hospitals)
1987	161	(217 hospitals)

4.2.2   Causes of maternal deaths 1987

	Number	%
Sepsis	66	27
Haemorrhage	41	17
Ruptured uterus	26	11
Obstructed labour	23	9
Abortion	12	5
Ectopic pregnancy	5	2
DIRECT CAUSES	173	71
Anaemia	37	15
Hepatitis	14	6
Other	20	8
INDIRECT CAUSES	71	29
TOTAL	244	100

4.3   Maternité de Cotonou, 1982 [0219]

4.3.1   Rate
MMR (per 100 000 live births)   160

4.3.2   Causes of maternal deaths.
Haemorrhage, sepsis, toxaemia, and parasitic infections resulting in anaemia are mentioned as the principal causes of maternal deaths. Haemorrhage alone accounted for 57% of all maternal deaths.

4.4   University Clinic of Gynaecology and Obstetrics, (CUGO) 1981-1987 [2490]

4.4.1   Rate

MMR (per 100 000 live births)

1981	1 030
1982	1 331
1983	1 358
1984	1 219
1985	1 062
1986	977
1987	809

5. CIVIL REGISTRATION DATA/GOVERNMENT ESTIMATES

6. OTHER SOURCES/ ESTIMATES

6.1 National 1973-75 [1899]

6.1.1 Rate

	MMR (per 100 000 live births)
1973	174
1974	153
1975	168

6.2 National 1975 [0028]

6.2.1 Rate

A paper presented at a WHO regional seminar quotes a maternal mortality rate of 170 per 100 000 live births.

6.3 National 1977 and 1981 [1732]

6.3.1 Rate

	MMR (per 100 000 live births)
1977	170
1981	160

7. SELECTED ANNOTATED BIBLIOGRAPHY

Sargent, C. Obstetrical choice among urban women in Benin. *Social Science and Medicine* 1985; 20(3): 287-292. WHE 0928

An analysis of the relationship between ethnicity, occupational status and reproductive behaviour of urban Bariba and non-Bariba women in Parakou, an urban centre of some 60,000 inhabitants, was undertaken during 1982-83. The comparison between Bariba and non-Bariba reproductive histories showed that only 26% of all Bariba delivered at home but that 94% of all home births were among Bariba women. Considerable pressures are exerted by the authorities to persuade women to have institutional deliveries. Women who deliver at home risk convocations and fines from government authorities and difficulties in obtaining birth certificates which are essential for receiving family allowances. Among Bariba women, however, cultural factors play a predominant role in the decision to deliver at home. To Bariba birth represents a rare opportunity for a women to demonstrate courage and bring honour to her family by her stoical demeanour during labour and delivery. The author concludes that home delivery may be seen as a strategy available to women for achieving power in the urban environment.

8. FURTHER READING

Alihonou, E. et al La prematurité en milieu hospitalier Beninois. *Afrique Médicale* 1980; 19(180): 315-325. WHE 0029

Frank, O. The demand for fertility control in sub-Saharan Africa. Working paper no. 117. *Studies in Family Planning* 1987; 18(4): 181-201. WHE 1371

Goudotte, E. Pathologie des organes genitaux en practique chirurgicale à Cotonou. *Médecine d'Afrique Noire* 1974; 21(12): 963-966. WHE 1072

Kodja, A. *Contribution à l'étude des avortements provoqués en République Populaire de Benin* (Doctoral dissertation) Université Nationale du Benin 1978. WHE 0394

9. DATA SOURCES

WHE 0028   Alihonou, E. *Pregnancy and delivery* in World Health Organization Regional Multidisciplinary Consultative Meeting on Human Reproduction, , 4-7 December 1978 (unpublished WHO document no. HRP/RMC/78.6)

WHE 0219   Feliho, F. and Houdegbe, A. *Information sur la République de Benin* (unpublished seminar background paper) 1978

WHE 0800   World Health Organization. *Country reports to regional offices of the progress in implementing Health for All by the Year 2000.* (Unpublished documents) 1983

WHE 0834   World Health Organization *World Health Statistics annual – vital statistics and causes of death.* Geneva, various years

WHE 0851   Benin, University of Benin. *Human reproduction resource strengthening at the University of Benin, Cotonou.* (unpublished paper)

WHE 1732   Alihonou, E. *Proposition de recherche dans le cadre du programme de recherche opérationelle sur la maternité sans risques.* 1987

WHE 1899   Faboumy, H. *Le stage en zone rurale dans le cadre de la formation pratique des élèves sage femmes en République Populaire de Benin.* Dissertation presented to the School of Midwifery, Dijon, France 1979-80

WHE 1914   United Nations Children's Fund (UNICEF). *The state of the world's children,* various years, Oxford, Oxford University Press

WHE 1915   United Nations. Department of International Economic and Social Affairs. *World population prospects: estimates and projections as assessed in 1984.* Population Studies No. 98. New York 1986

WHE 1918   United Nations. Department of International Economic and Social Affairs. *First marriage: patterns and determinants.* New York 1988

WHE 2271   Alihonou, E. and Takpara, I. Mortalité maternelle en République Populaire de Benin: causes et stratégies de lutte. In Bouyer, J. et al (eds.) *Réduire la mortalité maternelle dans les pays en developpement* 1988; 63-80: INSERM

WHE 2490   World Health Organization/Centre international de l'enfance, *Mortalité et morbidité maternelles* Seminar INFOSEC, Cotonou, 28 November - 4 December 1989.

BOTSWANA

	Year	Source

1. BASIC INDICATORS

1.1 Demographic

1.1.1 Population

Size (millions)	1.2	1988	(1914)
Rate of growth (%)	3.6	1980-87	(1914)

1.1.2 Life expectancy

Female	56	1980-85	(1915)
Male	53	1980-85	(1915)

1.1.3 Fertility

Crude Birth Rate	47	1988	(1914)
Total Fertility Rate	6.2	1988	(1914)

1.1.4 Mortality

Crude Death Rate	11	1988	(1914)
Infant Mortality Rate	66	1988	(1914)
Female			
Male			
1-4 years mortality rate			
Female			
Male			

1.2 Social and economic

1.2.1 Adult literacy rate (%)

Female	69	1985	(1914)
Male	73	1985	(1914)

1.2.2 Primary school enrolment rate (%)

Female	117	1986-88	(1914)
Male	111	1986-88	(1914)

1.2.3 Female mean age at first marriage

(years)	26.4	1981	(1918)

	Year	Source

1.2.4 GNP/capita

(US $)	1 050	1985	(1914)

1.2.5 Daily per capita calorie supply

(as % of requirements)	96	1988	(1914)

2. HEALTH SERVICES

2.1 Health expenditure

2.1.1 Expenditure on health

(as % of GNP)	3	1984	(0800)

2.1.2 Expenditure on PHC

(as % of total health expenditure)	48	1984	(0800)

2.2 Primary Health Care
(Percentage of population covered by):

2.2.1 Health services

National	89	1985-87	(1914)
Urban	100	1985-87	(1914)
Rural	85	1985-87	(1914)

2.2.2 Safe water

National	77	1984	(0834)
Urban	98	1984	(0834)
Rural	72	1984	(0834)

2.2.3 Adequate sanitary facilities

National	36	1983	(0834)
Urban	79	1984	(0834)
Rural	13	1984	(0834)

2.2.4 Contraceptive prevalence rate

(%)	33	1983-88	(2075)

2.3 Coverage of maternity care (%)

Area	Prenatal care	Trained attendant	Institutional deliveries	Postnatal care	Sample size	Year	Source
National	90	67	66	54	1 523w	1984	(1349)
National							
urban	96	88	87	63	289w	1984	(1349)
rural	89	61	61	52	1 234w	1984	(1349)
National	92	77		71	3 174	1984-88	(2075)
urban	97	94		68	819	1984-88	(2075)
rural	91	72		80	2 355	1984-88	(2075)
Thamaga	86		31		620w	(1981)	(0722)

3. COMMUNITY STUDIES

3.1 Kgalagadi District, 1987 [2477]

3.1.1 Rate
MMR (per 100 000 live births)   380

This study covered both institutional and home deliveries.

4. HOSPITAL STUDIES

4.1 All hospitals, 1982 [0252]

4.1.1 Rate
Live births   24 457
Maternal deaths   22
MMR (per 100 000 live births)   90

4.1.2 Causes of maternal deaths

	Number	%
Hyptertensive disorders of pregnancy	6	27
Haemorrhage	4	18
Obstructed labour	1	5
Complications of the puerperium	7	32
Other complications of pregnancy and childbirth	4	18
TOTAL	22	100

5. CIVIL REGISTRATION DATA/GOVERNMENT ESTIMATES

5.1. National, 1981 and 1985 [0280, 1090]

5.1.1 Rate
The maternal mortality rate for the country was estimated to be between 200 and 300 per 100 000 live births in 1981 and 1985.

6. OTHER SOURCES/ ESTIMATES

6.1 National, 1982-87 [2477]

6.1.1 Rate
Expected births   199 775
Notified maternal deaths*   82
MMR (per 100 000 births)   41

*   These figures are based on maternal notification forms and are almost entirely institutional. Only nine of the 82 deaths occurred at home and were reported to health facilities. It is not known how many deaths occurred at home but were not reported.

6.1.2   Causes of maternal deaths, 1982-86

	%
Sepsis	25
Hypertensive disorders of pregnancy	17
Haemorrhage	9
Abortion	7
Ectopic pregnancy	7
Prolonged labour	4
Ruptured uterus	3
Embolisms	3
Associated medical complications	10
Unknown	14
TOTAL	100

6.1.3   Avoidable factors

The author estimates that avoidable factors were present in 72% of the deaths.

7.   SELECTED ANNOTATED BIBLIOGRAPHY

8.   FURTHER READING

Boerma, J. T., *Maternal mortality in sub-Saharan Africa: levels, causes and interventions.* (unpublished document) 1987. WHE 1655

Watson, A.J. and Phillips, K. Postpartum haemorrhage is associated with poor housing, not multiparity in Botswana (letter) *The Lancet,* 20/27 December 1986 1462-1463. WHE 1491

9.   DATA SOURCES

WHE 0252   Botswana, Medical Statistics Unit, Ministry of Health *Medical statistics, 1982* Gabarone 1984

WHE 0280 Beattie, J.K. *Botswana country presentation.* Government/WHO/UNFPA Meeting, Brazzaville, 2-6 April 1984

WHE 0722   Ulin, P. and Ulin, R. The use and nonuse of preventive health services in a Southern African village. *International Journal of Health Education* 1981; 24: 45-53

WHE 0800   World Health Organization. *Country reports to regional offices of the progress in implementing Health for All by the Year 2000.* (Unpublished documents) 1983

WHE 0834   World Health Organization *World Health Statistics annual – vital statistics and causes of death.* Geneva, various years

WHE 1090   Botswana, Ministry of Health *Statistical information* (personal communication) 4 September 1985

WHE 1349   Manyeneng, W.G. et al. *Botswana family health survey 1984.* Gabarone, Family Health Division, Ministry of Health, 1985

WHE 1914   United Nations Children's Fund (UNICEF). *The state of the world's children*, various years, Oxford, Oxford University Press

WHE 1915   United Nations. Department of International Economic and Social Affairs. *World population prospects: estimates and projections as assessed in 1984.* Population Studies No. 98. New York 1986

WHE 1918   United Nations. Department of International Economic and Social Affairs. *First marriage: patterns and determinants.* New York 1988

WHE 2075   Demographic and health surveys, *Botswana: family health survey 1988.* Botswana Central Statistics Office/Family Health Division, Ministry of Health/Westinghouse

WHE 2477   Mwalali, P.N. Perinatal project consultant – UNDP, *Strategy for the programme on control of maternal and perinatal morbidity and mortality in Botswana.* (unpublished document), 1989

NOTES

BURKINA FASO

	Year	Source

1. BASIC INDICATORS

1.1 Demographic

1.1.1 Population

Size (millions)	8.5	1988	(1914)
Rate of growth (%)	2.5	1980-87	(1914)

1.1.2 Life expectancy

Female	47	1980-85	(1915)
Male	44	1980-85	(1915)

1.1.3 Fertility

Crude Birth Rate	47	1988	(1914)
Total Fertility Rate	6.5	1988	(1914)

1.1.4 Mortality

Crude Death Rate	18	1988	(1914)
Infant Mortality Rate	137	1988	(1914)
Female			
Male			
1-4 years mortality rate			
Female			
Male			

1.2 Social and economic

1.2.1 Adult literacy rate (%)

Female	6	1985	(1914)
Male	21	1985	(1914)

1.2.2 Primary school enrolment rate (%)

Female	24	1986-88	(1914)
Male	41	1986-88	(1914)

1.2.3 Female mean age at first marriage

(years)	17.4	1975	(1918)

		Year	Source

1.2.4 GNP/capita

(US $)	190	1987	(1914)

1.2.5 Daily per capita calorie supply

(as % of requirements)	86	1984-86	(1914)

2. HEALTH SERVICES

2.1 Health expenditure

2.1.1 Expenditure on health

(as % of GNP)	1	1981	(0800)

2.1.2 Expenditure on PHC

(as % of total expenditure)	5	1983	(0800)

2.2 Primary Health Care
(Percentage of population covered by):

2.2.1 Health services

National	49	1985-87	(1914)
Urban	51	1985-87	(1914)
Rural	48	1985-87	(1914)

2.2.2 Safe water

National	35	1984	(0834)
Urban	50	1984	(0834)
Rural	26	1984	(0834)

2.2.3 Adequate sanitary facilities

National	9	1984	(0834)
Urban	38	1984	(0834)
Rural	5	1984	(0834)

2.2.4 Contraceptive prevalence rate

(%)	1	1981-87	(1914)

2.3   Coverage of maternity care (%)

Area	Prenatal care	Trained attendant	Institutional deliveries	Postnatal care	Sample size	Year	Source
National	14	12				1980	(2008)
National	40					1984	(0834)
National		20				(1986)	(1910)
National	54	30				1986	(2095)

3. COMMUNITY STUDIES

4. HOSPITAL STUDIES

5. CIVIL REGISTRATION DATA/GOVERNMENT ESTIMATES

5.1   National, 1986 [2095]

5.1.1   Rate
Live births	90 353
Maternal deaths	732
MMR (per 100 000 live births)	810

5.1.2   Causes of maternal deaths
(for 384 cases where cause is known)

	Number	%
Haemorrhage	225	59
Obstructed labour	97	25
Sepsis	57	15
Hypertensive disorders of pregnancy	5	1
Total of known cases	384	100

5.1.3   Avoidable factors
Nationwide, very few of the 54 medical centres are capable of carrying out blood tests and blood transfusions; only two national hospitals and six regional centres are able to do so.

Maternity centres remain inaccessible due to transportation difficulties, especially during bad weather.

The costs of transfer accrue to the patient's family; delays in collecting adequate funds are frequently fatal.

There are severe shortages of suitable qualified medical personnel and such trained staff as are available tend to concentrate in particular areas.

5.1.4   High risk groups

5.1.5   Other findings

6. OTHER SOURCES/ ESTIMATES

6.1   National, 1986 [1910]

6.1.1   Rate
According to a joint report published in 1986 by the Government of Burkina Faso and UNICEF, the maternal mortality rate for the country was 350 per 100 000 live births for births assisted by trained persons and 650 per 100 000 live births for all births.

6.1.2   Causes of maternal deaths.
According to an enquiry conducted in 1960-61 the most common causes of maternal deaths were rupture of the uterus, postpartum haemorrhage, puerperal infections, eclampsia and tetanus, in that order of importance. Maternal deaths constituted 25% of all deaths to women in the age group 15-44 years and resulted in a higher mortality rate for women than for men in that age group.

7. SELECTED ANNOTATED BIBLIOGRAPHY

Sauerborn, R., Nougtara, A. et al. Assessment of MCH services in the District of Solenzo, Burkina Faso. I, II and III. *Journal of Tropical Pediatrics* 1989; 35: 1-17 WHE 2400, WHE 2401, WHE 2402

A representative household survey of a district of Burkina Faso was carried out in order to study the utilization of trained birth attendants versus professional health workers as providers of child, prenatal and maternity care. Overall utilization by target groups was around 31% for both prenatal and maternity care. The presence of a village health post did not increase utilization of MCH care and women who did utilize it preferred a combination of the professional midwife for prenatal care and the traditional "old woman" for delivery.

A large proportion of mothers had difficulties in using the service; in particular, it was felt that there was time wasting through inappropriate opening hours, that there were organizational problems and that there was poor communication with staff.

An analysis of the functioning of the "risk approach" found that there was a consistent lack of any action taken as a consequence of a recognized risk factor. This was due to a combination of implementation failure, inappropriateness of cutoff points for risk definition and conceptual problems such as the reluctance of both staff and patients to act on the basis of risk prediction.

8. FURTHER READING

Damas, R. et al, Fistules vesico-vaginales obstétricales africaines (à propos de 47 observations). *Médecine Tropicale* 1972; 32(4): 493-498. WHE 1060

Segbo, M.P. Catastrophes à Ouaga. *Sages femmes* January 1985; IX(9). WHE 0645

Van de Walle, F. and Ouaidou, N. Status and fertility among urban women in Burkina Faso. *International Family Planning Perspectives* 1985; 11(2): 60-64. WHE 1672

9. DATA SOURCES

WHE 0800 World Health Organization. *Country reports to regional offices of the progress in implementing Health for All by the Year 2000.* (Unpublished documents) 1983

WHE 0834 World Health Organization *World Health Statistics annual - vital statistics and causes of death.* Geneva, various years

WHE 1910 Burkina Faso Government and United Nations Children's Fund *Analyse de la situation des femmes et des enfants.* Ouagadougou 1986

WHE 1914 United Nations Children's Fund (UNICEF). *The state of the world's children*, various years, Oxford, Oxford University Press

WHE 1915 United Nations. Department of International Economic and Social Affairs. *World population prospects: estimates and projections as assessed in 1984.* Population Studies No. 98. New York 1986

WHE 1918 United Nations. Department of International Economic and Social Affairs. *First marriage: patterns and determinants.* New York 1988

WHE 2008 World Health Organization. Regional Office for Africa *Evaluation of the strategy for health for all by the year 2000. Seventh report on the world health situation* Vol 2, African region, Brazzaville 1987

WHE 2095 Sokal, D. et al *Mortalité maternelle à Burkina Faso.* (unpublished) 1987

NOTES

BURUNDI

		Year	Source

1. BASIC INDICATORS

1.1 Demographic

1.1.1 Population

		Year	Source
Size (millions)	5.1	1988	(1914)
Rate of growth (%)	2.8	1980-87	(1914)

1.1.2 Life expectancy

		Year	Source
Female	48	1982	(2008)
Male	45	1982	(2008)

1.1.3 Fertility

		Year	Source
Crude Birth Rate	46	1988	(1914)
Total Fertility Rate	6.3	1988	(1914)

1.1.4 Mortality

		Year	Source
Crude Death Rate	17	1988	(1914)
Infant Mortality Rate	111	1988	(1914)
Female	76	1977-86	(1795)
Male	99	1977-86	(1795)
1-4 years mortality rate	114	1977-86	(1795)
Female	114	1977-86	(1795)
Male	101	1977-86	(1795)

1.2 Social and economic

1.2.1 Adult literacy rate (%)

		Year	Source
Female	26	1986-88	(1914)
Male	43	1986-88	(1914)

1.2.2 Primary school enrolment rate (%)

		Year	Source
Female	50	1986-88	(1914)
Male	68	1986-88	(1914)

1.2.3 Female mean age at first marriage
(years)

1.2.4 GNP per capita

		Year	Source
(US $)	250	1987	(1914)

1.2.5 Daily per capita calorie supply

		Year	Source
(as % of requirements)	97	1984-86	(1914)

2. HEALTH SERVICES

2.1 Health expenditure

2.1.1 Expenditure on health
(as % of GNP)

2.1.2 Expenditure on PHC

(as % of total health		Year	Source
expenditure)	30	1984	(2008)

2.2 Primary Health Care
(Percentage of population covered by):

2.2.1 Health services

		Year	Source
National	45	1984	(0834)
Urban			
Rural			

2.2.2 Safe water

		Year	Source
National	23	1983	(0834)
Urban	33	1985	(0834)
Rural	22	1985	(0834)

2.2.3 Adequate sanitary facilities

		Year	Source
National	52	1983	(0834)
Urban	90	1983	(0834)
Rural	25	1983	(0834)

2.2.4 Contraceptive prevalence rate

		Year	Source
(%)	7	1982-87	(1795)

2.3   Coverage of maternity care (%)

Area	Prenatal care	Trained attendant	Institutional deliveries	Postnatal care	Sample size	Year	Source
National	14					1980	(0834)
National	30					1988	(2033)
National:	79	19			3841	1982-87	(1795)
urban	97	85			129	1982-87	(1795)
rural	79	17			3712	1982-87	(1795)
National			24			1984-85	(1905)
Ruyaga	57				362w	(1982)	(1905)

3. COMMUNITY STUDIES

4. HOSPITAL STUDIES

5. CIVIL REGISTRATION DATA/GOVERNMENT ESTIMATES

6. OTHER SOURCES/ ESTIMATES

7. SELECTED ANNOTATED BIBLIOGRAPHY

8. FURTHER READING

9. DATA SOURCES

WHE 0834   World Health Organization *World Health Statistics annual – vital statistics and causes of death.* Geneva, various years

WHE 1795   Demographic and Health Surveys, *Enquête démographique et de santé au Burundi 1987.* Ministère de l'interieur/Institute for Resource Development, Westinghouse 1988

WHE 1905   United Nations Children's Fund (UNICEF), *Etudes préliminaires à la situation de la femme et de l'enfant au Burundi.* UNICEF/CURDES, juin 1985

WHE 1914   United Nations Children's Fund (UNICEF), *The state of the world's children,* various years, Oxford, Oxford University Press

WHE 2008   World Health Organization. Regional Office for Africa *Evaluation of the strategy for health for all by the year 2000. Seventh report on the world health situation* Vol 2, African region, Brazzaville 1987

WHE 2033   World Health Organization. *Global strategy for health for all by the year 2000. Second report on monitoring progress.* WHO document EB83/2 Add. 1, 1988

CAMEROON

		Year	Source

1. BASIC INDICATORS

1.1 Demographic

1.1.1 Population
		Year	Source
Size (millions)	10.7	1988	(1914)
Rate of growth (%)	2.7	1980-87	(1914)

1.1.2 Life expectancy
		Year	Source
Female	53	1980-85	(1915)
Male	49	1980-85	(1915)

1.1.3 Fertility
		Year	Source
Crude Birth Rate	41	1988	(1914)
Total Fertility Rate	5.7	1988	(1914)

1.1.4 Mortality
		Year	Source
Crude Death Rate	15	1988	(1914)
Infant Mortality Rate	93	1988	(1914)
Female	165	1976	(1554)
Male	186	1976	(1554)
1-4 years mortality rate			
Female	21	1976	(1554)
Male	22	1976	(1554)

1.2 Social and economic

1.2.1 Adult literacy rate (%)
		Year	Source
Female	45	1985	(1914)
Male	68	1985	(1914)

1.2.2 Primary school enrolment rate (%)
		Year	Source
Female	100	1986-88	(1914)
Male	119	1986-88	(1914)

1.2.3 Female mean age at first marriage
		Year	Source
(years)	18.8	1978	(1918)

1.2.4 GNP/capita
		Year	Source
(US $)	970	1987	(1914)

1.2.5 Daily per capita calorie supply
		Year	Source
(as % of requirements)	88	1984-86	(1914)

2. HEALTH SERVICES

2.1 Health expenditure

2.1.1 Expenditure on health
		Year	Source
(as % of GNP)	5	1983	(0800)

2.1.2 Expenditure on PHC
		Year	Source
(as % of total health expenditure)	8	1983	(0800)

2.2 Primary Health Care
(Percentage of population covered by):

2.2.1 Health services
		Year	Source
National	41	1985-87	(1914)
Urban	44	1985-87	(1914)
Rural	39	1985-87	(1914)

2.2.2 Safe water
		Year	Source
National	36	1985	(0834)
Urban	46	1985	(0834)
Rural	30	1985	(0834)

2.2.3 Adequate sanitary facilities
		Year	Source
National	36	1985	(0834)
Urban			
Rural			

2.2.4 Contraceptive prevalence rate
		Year	Source
(%)	3	1978	(1712)

2.3   Coverage of maternity care (%)

Area	Prenatal care	Trained attendant	Institutional deliveries	Postnatal care	Sample size	Year	Source
National		57	42		4 400	1978	(0919)
National	96	10				1983	(2008)
National	85	25				1980s	(2490)

3.   COMMUNITY STUDIES

4.   HOSPITAL STUDIES

4.1   All health establishments, 1973 [0422]

4.1.1   Rate

Live births	74 202
Maternal deaths	117
MMR (per 100 000 live births)	158

4.2   Twenty five hospitals throughout the country, 1975 [0120]

4.2.1   Rate

Province	Live births	Maternal deaths	MMR (per 100 000 live births)
East	3 328	13	391
West	22 041	11	50
North	8 573	39	455
Centre-South	13 510	18	133
Coastal	12 036	18	150
North West	4 289	5	117
South West	2 249	5	222
TOTAL	66 026	109	165

4.3   Maternité centrale de Yaoundé, 1973-77 and 1980-85 [0479, 1679, 1680, 2018]

4.3.1   Rate

	Live births	Maternal deaths	MMR (per 100 000 deliveries)
1973-76	–	–	147*
1977	–	–	201
1980	9 650	15	155
1985	13 899	9	65

* Excluding abortions and ectopic pregnancies

The reduction in the maternal mortality rate between 1980 and 1985 is thought to be the result of the adoption of the "Risk Approach". This involved the introduction of a maternity clinic for high risk pregnancies, a clinic using contraceptive technologies to encourage birth spacing and the use of the partograph during labour.

4.3.2   Causes of maternal deaths, 1980-85

	Number	%
Haemorrhage	40	45
Sepsis	11	12
Hypertensive disorders of pregnancy	4	4
Pulmonary embolism	4	4
Ruptured uterus	2	2
Other medical complications	14	15
Anaemia	7	8
Unknown	9	10
TOTAL	91	100

A study of cases of uterine rupture admitted to the hospital between 1973-76 (0479) reported that rupture of the uterus was the fourth major cause of maternal death, with an incidence of one rupture per 528 deliveries, or 1.9 per 1000. Of the 70 cases admitted during the period, six died, four of them before receiving treatment.

4.3.3   Avoidable factors

The study of uterine rupture found that maternal deaths were mainly due to:

- inadequate prenatal and intrapartum care;
- poor communications and inadequate logistic support precluding early transfer of difficult cases to referral hospitals;
- inadequate obstetric experience of midwives in rural maternity centres;
- inadequate experience in management of uterine rupture on the part of specialists in urban hospitals.

Three of the six deaths from uterine rupture could have been prevented. Two women died on the operating table from cardiac arrest due to lack of oxygen in the hospital. Another death was probably related to surgical procedure (hysterectomy) by inexperienced staff, undertaken on a patient already exhausted by prolonged labour.

The 1980-85 study mentions lack of materials, lack of qualified personnel and overcrowding as factors contributing to maternal deaths.

4.4 University Teaching Hospital, Yaoundé, 1982-1986 [(2470)]

4.4.1 Rate

Deliveries	5 614
Maternal deaths	2
MMR (per 100 000 deliveries)	36

5. CIVIL REGISTRATION DATA/GOVERNMENT ESTIMATES

6. OTHER ESTIMATES/ SOURCES

6.1 National, 1974 [(0729)]

6.1.1 Rate

The UNFPA Report of Mission on Needs Assessment for Population Assistance quotes a maternal mortality rate of 210 per 100 000 live births in 1974 for all births in health institutions.

6.2 National, 1978 [(0422)]

6.2.1 Rate

A paper presented at a WHO regional meeting in 1978 quotes a maternal mortality rate of 303 per 100 000 live births.

6.3 National, 1980s [(2490)]
6.3.1 Rate

MMR (per 100 000 births)	430

6.4 Limba Province, 1980s [(2490)]
6.4.1 Rate

MMR (per 100 000 births)	570

7. SELECTED ANNOTATED BIBLIOGRAPHY

Klefstad-Sillonville, F., Le traitement des fistules vesico-vaginales africaines et leur prévention. *Médecine Tropicale* 1973; 31 (3): 311-321. WHE 1169

An analysis of 40 women (in Chad in 1964-66 and Cameroon in 1967-70) who were operated for vesico-vaginal fistulae, showed that 23 women were small and less than 20 years old. All came from villages far away from the hospitals. Thirty women were cured. The author stresses that prevention is the only long-term solution, and that education of village midwives is of major importance.

Nchinda, T.C., A household study of illness prevalence and health care preferences in a rural district of Cameroon. *International Journal of Epidemiology* 1977; 6(3): 235-241. WHE 2203

A health interview survey was carried out in rural Cameroon between November 1973 and March 1974 on a random selection of 1 886 families consisting of 9 362 individuals. The disease prevalence in the study area (a positive illness rate of 28% for a four-week recall period) is analyzed by age, sex and treatment preference. A significant finding was lower abdominal pain as a persistent complaint among women of reproductive age. This accounted for over 9% of the illness in women aged 15-44 years. The study emphasizes the importance of interview surveys despite the lack of diagnostic accuracy. It is the perception of illness by a respondent that will determine his or her use or non-use of any form of health care.

8. FURTHER READING

Boerma, J.T. *Maternal mortality in sub-Saharan Africa: levels, causes and interventions* 1987. WHE 1655

Frank, O. The demand for fertility control in sub-Saharan Africa. Working paper 117. *Studies in Family Planning* 1987; 18(4): 181-201. WHE 1373

Gubry, F. et al, *Les enquêtes sur la mortalité infantile et juvenile* 2 (1): Yaoundé 1987. WHE 1995

Nasah, B.T. et al, Gonorrhoea, trichomonas and candida among gravid and non-gravid women in Cameroon. *International Journal of Gynaecology and Obstetrics* 1980; 18(1): 48-52. WHE 1194

9. DATA SOURCES

WHE 0120 Cameroun, Service des Statistiques Sanitaires et Démographiques, *Rapport statistique d'activités des services de santé publique.* 1975

WHE 0422 Mafiamba, P.C. *Problems in human reproduction in Cameroon.* in World Health Organization Regional Multidisciplinary Consultative Meeting on Human Reproduction, Yaoundé, 4-7 December 1978

WHE 0479 Nasah, B.T. and Drouin, P., Review of 70 cases of ruptured uterus in Cameroon. *Tropical Doctor* 1978; 8: 127-131

WHE 0729 United Nations Fund for Population Activities UNFPA, *Report of a mission on needs assessment for population assistance – Cameroon.* UNFPA New York 1979

WHE 0800 World Health Organization. *Country reports to regional offices of the progress in implementing Health for All by the Year 2000.* (Unpublished documents) 1983

WHE 0834 World Health Organization *World Health Statistics annual – vital statistics and causes of death.* Geneva, various years

WHE 0919 Cameroon, United Republic of, *Enquête nationale sur la fécondité du Cameroun.* Ministère de l'economie et du plan, World Fertility Survey, Yaoundé 1978

WHE 1554 United Nations and World Health Organization, *Levels and trends of mortality since 1950.* New York 1982

WHE 1679 Nasah, B.T., Maternal mortality in Cameroon (editorial). *Annales universitaires des sciences de la santé* 1987; 4(1): 301-302

WHE 1680 Leke, R.J., Outcome of pregnancy and delivery at the Central Maternity Hospital Yaoundé. *Annales universitaires des sciences de la santé* 1987; 4(1): 322-330

WHE 1712 Mauldin, W.P. and Segal, S.J. *Prevalence of contraceptive use in developing countries. A chart book.* New York, Rockefeller Foundation 1986

WHE 1914 United Nations Children's Fund (UNICEF). *The state of the world's children,* various years, Oxford, Oxford University Press

WHE 1915 United Nations. Department of International Economic and Social Affairs. *World population prospects: estimates and projections as assessed in 1984.* Population Studies No. 98. New York 1986

WHE 1918 United Nations. Department of International Economic and Social Affairs. *First marriage: patterns and determinants.* New York 1988

WHE 2008 World Health Organization. Regional Office for Africa *Evaluation of the strategy for health for all by the year 2000. Seventh report on the world health situation* Vol 2, African region, Brazzaville 1987

WHE 2018 Leke, R.J. at al Introduction of high risk pregnancy care in rural Cameroon: Health service research approach. *Journal of Obstetrics and Gynaecology of East and Central Africa* 1988; 7(7): 7-10

WHE 2470 Doh, A.S. et al. The outcome of labor at the University Teaching Hospital (CHU), Yaoundé, Cameroon. *International Journal of Gynecology and Obstetrics* 1989; 30: 317-323

WHE 2490 World Health Organization Mortalité et morbidité maternelles. *Séminaire-Aterlier INFOSEC* Cotonou, 28 November - 4 December 1989

CAPE VERDE

		Year	Source

1. BASIC INDICATORS

1.1 Demographic

1.1.1 Population

		Year	Source
Size (millions)	0.3	1987	(1915)
Rate of growth (%)	1.9	1980-85	(1915)

1.1.2 Life expectancy

Female	61	1980-85	(1915)
Male	57	1980-85	(1915)

1.1.3 Fertility

Crude Birth Rate	31	1980-85	(1915)
Total Fertility Rate	4.8	1980-85	(1915)

1.1.4 Mortality

Crude Death Rate	11	1980-85	(1915)
Infant Mortality Rate	66	1984	(2008)
Female			
Male			
1-4 years mortality rate			
Female	7	1981	(0834)
Male	8	1981	(0834)

1.2 Social and economic

1.2.1 Adult literacy rate (%)

Female	39	1985	(1914)
Male	61	1985	(1914)

1.2.2 Primary school enrolment rate (%)

Female	105	1983-86	(1914)
Male	112	1983-86	(1914)

1.2.3 Female mean age at first marriage
(years)

1.2.4 GNP/capita

		Year	Source
(US $)	430	1985	(1914)

1.2.5 Daily per capita calorie supply
(as % of requirements)

2. HEALTH SERVICES

2.1 Health expenditure

2.1.1 Expenditure on health

(as % of GNP)	1	1981	(0800)

2.1.2 Expenditure on PHC
(as % of total health expenditure)

2.2 Primary Health Care
(Percentage of population covered by):

2.2.1 Health services
National
Urban
Rural

2.2.2 Safe water

National	31	1983	(0834)
Urban	99	1983	(0834)
Rural	21	1983	(0834)

2.2.3 Adequate sanitary facilities

National	10	1983	(0834)
Urban	36	1983	(0834)
Rural	9	1983	(0834)

2.2.4 Contraceptive prevalence rate
(%)

2.3 Coverage of maternity care (%)

Area	Prenatal care	Trained attendant	Institutional deliveries	Postnatal care	Sample size	Year	Source
National	96	10				1983	(0834)
Sal	85	50	27		197	1979	(0549)
Sao Vicente	92	53	51		307	1979	(0549)

3. COMMUNITY STUDIES

4. HOSPITAL STUDIES

5. CIVIL REGISTRATION DATA/GOVERNMENT ESTIMATES

5.1 National, 1975 [(0753)]

5.1.1 Rate

The United Nations Demographic Year Book gives a maternal mortality rate of 134 per 100 000 live births in 1975, and 107 per 100 000 live births in 1980. The rates are based on fewer than 30 maternal deaths.

6. OTHER SOURCES/ ESTIMATES

7. SELECTED ANNOTATED BIBLIOGRAPHY

8. FURTHER READING

9. DATA SOURCES

WHE 0549   Pina de, A. et al, *Health of women and young children at the Cape Verde Islands.* (unpublished document)

WHE 0753   United Nations, *Demographic Yearbook.* New York, various years

WHE 0800   World Health Organization. *Country reports to regional offices of the progress in implementing Health for All by the Year 2000.* (Unpublished documents) 1983

WHE 0834   World Health Organization *World Health Statistics annual – vital statistics and causes of death.* Geneva, various years

WHE 1914   United Nations Children's Fund (UNICEF). *The state of the world's children,* various years, Oxford, Oxford University Press

WHE 1915   United Nations. Department of International Economic and Social Affairs. *World population prospects: estimates and projections as assessed in 1984.* Population Studies No. 98. New York 1986

WHE 2008   World Health Organization. Regional Office for Africa *Evaluation of the strategy for health for all by the year 2000. Seventh report on the world health situation* Vol 2, African region, Brazzaville 1987

CENTRAL AFRICAN REPUBLIC

		Year	Source

1. BASIC INDICATORS

1.1 Demographic

1.1.1 Population

		Year	Source
Size (millions)	2.8	1988	(1914)
Rate of growth (%)	2.3	1980-87	(1914)

1.1.2 Life expectancy

Female	45	1980-85	(1915)
Male	41	1980-85	(1915)

1.1.3 Fertility

Crude Birth Rate	44	1988	(1914)
Total Fertility Rate	5.9	1988	(1914)

1.1.4 Mortality

Crude Death Rate	20	1988	(1914)
Infant Mortality Rate	131	1988	(1914)
Female			
Male			
1-4 years mortality rate			
Female			
Male			

1.2 Social and economic

1.2.1 Adult literacy rate (%)

Female	29	1985	(1914)
Male	53	1985	(1914)

1.2.2 Primary school enrolment rate (%)

Female	51	1986-88	(1914)
Male	82	1986-88	(1914)

1.2.3 Female mean age at first marriage
(years)

1.2.4 GNP/capita

(US $)	330	1987	(1914)

1.2.5 Daily per capita calorie supply

(as % of requirements)	86	1984-86	(1914)

2. HEALTH SERVICES

2.1 Health expenditure

2.1.1 Expenditure on health

(as % of GNP)	6	1986-88	(2033)

2.1.2 Expenditure on PHC
(as % of total health expenditure)

2.2 Primary Health Care
(Percentage of population covered by):

2.2.1 Health services

National	45	1985-87	(1914)
Urban			
Rural			

2.2.2 Safe water

National	16	1980	(0834)
Urban	24	1983	(0834)
Rural	5	1980	(0834)

2.2.3 Adequate sanitary facilities

National	19	1984	(0834)
Urban	36	1984	(0834)
Rural	9	1984	(0834)

2.2.4 Contraceptive prevalence rate
(%)

2.3   Coverage of maternity care (%)

Area	Prenatal care	Trained attendant	Institutional deliveries	Postnatal care	Sample size	Year	Source
National		71				1971	(0796)
National	69	66		68		1988	(2033)

3. COMMUNITY STUDIES

4. HOSPITAL STUDIES

5. CIVIL REGISTRATION DATA/GOVERNMENT ESTIMATES

6. OTHER SOURCES/ ESTIMATES

6.1   National, 1983 (0751)

6.1.1   Rate
The UNFPA report on the Mission on Needs Assessment for Population Assistance published in 1983 quotes a maternal mortality rate of over 600 per 100 000 live births.

7. SELECTED ANNOTATED BIBLIOGRAPHY

8. FURTHER READING

9. DATA SOURCES

WHE 0751   United Nations Fund for Population Activities UNFPA, République Centrafricaine, *Rapport de mission sur l'évaluation des besoins d'aide en matière de population.* UNFPA, New York 1983

WHE 0796   World Health Organization, *Global strategy for Health For All by the year 2000.* Thirty-sixth World Health Assembly. Provisional agenda item 21. WHO document no. A36/INF.DOC/1), Geneva 1983

WHE 0834   World Health Organization *World Health Statistics annual – vital statistics and causes of death.* Geneva, various years

WHE 1914   United Nations Children's Fund (UNICEF). *The state of the world's children,* various years, Oxford, Oxford University Press

WHE 1915   United Nations. Department of International Economic and Social Affairs. *World population prospects: estimates and projections as assessed in 1984.* Population Studies No. 98. New York 1986

WHE 2033   World Health Organization. *Global strategy for health for all by the year 2000. Second report on monitoring progress.* WHO document EB83/2 Add. 1, 1988

CHAD

		Year	Source

1. BASIC INDICATORS

1.1 Demographic

1.1.1 Population

		Year	Source
Size (millions)	5.4	1987	(1914)
Rate of growth (%)	2.3	1980-87	(1914)

1.1.2 Life expectancy

Female	45	1980-85	(1915)
Male	41	1980-85	(1915)

1.1.3 Fertility

Crude Birth Rate	44	1988	(1914)
Total Fertility Rate	5.9	1988	(1914)

1.1.4 Mortality

Crude Death Rate	19	1988	(1914)
Infant Mortality Rate	131	1988	(1914)
Female			
Male			
1-4 years mortality rate			
Female			
Male			

1.2 Social and economic

1.2.1 Adult literacy rate (%)

Female	11	1985	(1914)
Male	40	1985	(1914)

1.2.2 Primary school enrolment rate (%)

Female	29	1986-88	(1914)
Male	73	1986-88	(1914)

1.2.3 Female mean age at first marriage

(years)	16.5	1964	(1918)

1.2.4 GNP/capita

		Year	Source
(US $)	150	1987	(1914)

1.2.5 Daily per capita calorie supply

(as % of requirements)	69	1984-86	(1914)

2. HEALTH SERVICES

2.1 Health expenditure

2.1.1 Expenditure on health
(as % of GNP)

2.1.2 Expenditure on PHC
(as % of total health expenditure)

2.2 Primary Health Care
(Percentage of population covered by):

2.2.1 Health services

National	30	1985	(2033)
Urban			
Rural			

2.2.2 Safe water

National	31	1984	(0834)
Urban	27	1980	(0834)
Rural	30	1980	(0834)

2.2.3 Adequate sanitary facilities

National	15	1984	(0834)
Urban			
Rural			

2.2.4 Contraceptive prevalence rate

(%)	1	1980-87	(1914)

2.3 Coverage of maternity care (%)

Area	Prenatal care	Trained attendant	Institutional deliveries	Postnatal care	Sample size	Year	Source
National			60			1972	(1907)
National		45				1975	(0796)
National	69	24				1980-82	(2008)

3. COMMUNITY STUDIES

4. HOSPITAL STUDIES

4.1 N'Djamena Maternity Hospital, 1986 [2030]

4.1.1 Rate
Live births	5 760
Maternal deaths	48
MMR (per 100 000 live births)	833

4.1.2 Causes of maternal deaths

	Number	%
Hypertensive disorders of pregnancy	10	21
Ruptured uterus	7	15
Sepsis	7	15
Abortion	3	6
Obstetric shock	1	2
Other direct causes	4	8
DIRECT CAUSES	32	67
Hepatitis	9	19
Other infections	5	10
Other indirect causes	2	4
INDIRECT CAUSES	16	33
TOTAL	48	100

4.1.3 Avoidable factors
Nineteen of the deaths followed caesarean section. 13% of all caesarean sections resulted in the death of the patient. Of the seven cases of ruptured uterus, five had experienced rupture of the membranes between five and ten days prior to entry into hospital. Over half the women were classified as anaemic.

5. CIVIL REGISTRATION DATA/GOVERNMENT ESTIMATES

5.1 National, 1972 [1907]

5.1.1 Rate
Deliveries	26 122
Maternal deaths	224
MMR (per 100 000 deliveries)	858

6. OTHER SOURCES/ ESTIMATES

7. SELECTED ANNOTATED BIBLIOGRAPHY

Klefstad-Sillonville, F., Le traitement des fistules vesico-vaginales africaines et leur prévention. *Médecine Tropicale* 1973; 31(3): 311-321. WHE 1169

An analysis of 40 women (in Chad in 1964-66 and Cameroon in 1967-70) who were operated for vesico-vaginal fistulae, showed that 23 women were small and less than 20 years old. All came from villages far away from the hospitals. Thirty women were cured. The author stresses that prevention is the only long-term solution, and that education of village midwives is of major importance.

8. FURTHER READING

9. DATA SOURCES

WHE 0796   World Health Organization, *Global strategy for Health For All by the year 2000.* Thirty-sixth World Health Assembly. Provisional agenda item 21. WHO document no. A36/INF.DOC/1), Geneva 1983

WHE 0834   World Health Organization *World Health Statistics annual – vital statistics and causes of death.* Geneva, various years

WHE 1907   Chad, Ministry of Public Health and Social Affairs, Department of Public Health, *Statistiques sanitaires, Bulletin année 1972.* 1973

WHE 1914   United Nations Children's Fund (UNICEF). *The state of the world's children,* various years, Oxford, Oxford University Press

WHE 1915   United Nations. Department of International Economic and Social Affairs. *World population prospects: estimates and projections as assessed in 1984.* Population Studies No. 98. New York 1986

WHE 1918   United Nations. Department of International Economic and Social Affairs. *First marriage: patterns and determinants.* New York 1988

WHE 2008   World Health Organization. Regional Office for Africa *Evaluation of the strategy for health for all by the year 2000. Seventh report on the world health situation* Vol 2, African region, Brazzaville 1987

WHE 2030   Bernis, L. de, *Mortalité maternelle à N'Djamena (Tchad).* 1986

WHE 2033   World Health Organization. *Global strategy for health for all by the year 2000. Second report on monitoring progress.* WHO document EB83/2 Add. 1, 1988

NOTES

COMOROS

	Year	Source

1. BASIC INDICATORS

1.1 Demographic

1.1.1 Population

		Year	Source
Size (millions)	0.5	1988	(1914)
Rate of growth (%)	2.7	1988	(0753)

1.1.2 Life expectancy

		Year	Source
Female	52	1980-85	(0753)
Male	48	1980-85	(0753)

1.1.3 Fertility

		Year	Source
Crude Birth Rate	46	1980-85	(0753)
Total Fertility Rate	6.3	1980-85	(0753)

1.1.4 Mortality

		Year	Source
Crude Death Rate	16	1980-85	(0753)
Infant Mortality Rate	79	1988	(1914)
Female			
Male			
1-4 years mortality rate			
Female			
Male			

1.2 Social and economic

1.2.1 Adult literacy rate (%)

		Year	Source
Female	40	1985	(1914)
Male	56	1985	(1914)

1.2.2 Primary school enrolment rate (%)

		Year	Source
Female	70	1986-88	(1914)
Male	90	1986-88	(1914)

1.2.3 Female mean age at first marriage

		Year	Source
(years)	19.5	1980	(1918)

1.2.4 GNP/capita

		Year	Source
(US $)	370	1987	(1914)

1.2.5 Daily per capita calorie supply
(as % of requirements)

2. HEALTH SERVICES

2.1 Health expenditure

2.1.1 Expenditure on health
(as % of GNP)

2.1.2 Expenditure on PHC
(as % of total health expenditure)

2.2 Primary Health Care
(Percentage of population covered by):

2.2.1 Health services

		Year	Source
National	82	1983	(0834)
Urban			
Rural			

2.2.2 Safe water

		Year	Source
National	58	1982	(0834)
Urban	99	1980	(0834)
Rural	52	1980	(0834)

2.2.3 Adequate sanitary facilities

		Year	Source
National			
Urban	90	1986	(2033)
Rural	80	1986	(2033)

2.2.4 Contraceptive prevalence rate
(%)

2.3   Coverage of maternity care (%)

Area	Prenatal care	Trained attendant	Institutional deliveries	Postnatal care	Sample size	Year	Source
National	69	24				1988	(2033)

3. COMMUNITY STUDIES

4. HOSPITAL STUDIES

5. CIVIL REGISTRATION DATA/GOVERNMENT ESTIMATES

5.1   National, 1980 [2008]

MMR (per 100 000 births)   500

6. OTHER SOURCES/ ESTIMATES

7. SELECTED ANNOTATED BIBLIOGRAPHY

8. FURTHER READING

9. DATA SOURCES

WHE 0753   United Nations, *Demographic Yearbook.* New York, various years

WHE 0834   World Health Organization *World Health Statistics annual – vital statistics and causes of death.* Geneva, various years

WHE 1914   United Nations Children's Fund (UNICEF). *The state of the world's children,* various years, Oxford, Oxford University Press

WHE 1918   United Nations. Department of International Economic and Social Affairs. *First marriage: patterns and determinants.* New York 1988

WHE 2008   World Health Organization. Regional Office for Africa *Evaluation of the strategy for health for all by the year 2000. Seventh report on the world health situation* Vol 2, African region, Brazzaville 1987

WHE 2033   World Health Organization. *Global strategy for health for all by the year 2000. Second report on monitoring progress.* WHO document EB83/2 Add. 1, 1988

CONGO

		Year	Source

1. BASIC INDICATORS

1.1 Demographic

1.1.1 Population

		Year	Source
Size (millions)	1.9	1988	(1914)
Annual growth rate (%)	2.6	1988	(1914)

1.1.2 Life expectancy

		Year	Source
Female	56	1985-87	(2033)
Male	52	1985-87	(2033)

1.1.3 Fertility

		Year	Source
Crude Birth Rate	44	1988	(1914)
Total Fertility Rate	6.0	1988	(1914)

1.1.4 Mortality

		Year	Source
Crude Death Rate	17	1988	(1914)
Infant Mortality Rate	72	1988	(1914)
Female			
Male			
1-4 years mortality rate			
Female			
Male			

1.2 Social and economic

1.2.1 Adult literacy rate (%)

		Year	Source
Female	55	1985	(1914)
Male	71	1985	(1914)

1.2.2 Primary school enrolment rate (%)

Female
Male

1.2.3 Female mean age at first marriage
(years)

1.2.4 GNP per capita

		Year	Source
(US $)	870	1987	(1914)

1.2.5 Daily per capita calorie supply

		Year	Source
(as % of requirements)	117	1984-86	(1914)

2. HEALTH SERVICES

2.1 Health expenditure

2.1.1 Expenditure on health
(as % of GNP)

2.1.2 Expenditure on PHC
(as % of total health expenditure)

2.2 Primary Health Care
(Percentage of population covered by):

2.2.1 Health services
National
Urban
Rural

2.2.2 Safe water

		Year	Source
National	21	1985-87	(1914)
Urban	42	1983	(0834)
Rural	7	1983	(0834)

2.2.3 Adequate sanitary facilities

		Year	Source
National	40	1985	(0834)
Urban			
Rural			

2.2.4 Contraceptive prevalence rate
(%)

2.3   Coverage of maternity care (%)

Area	Prenatal care	Trained attendant	Institutional deliveries	Postnatal care	Sample size	Year	Source
National	35		47			1970	(0345)

3. COMMUNITY STUDIES

4. HOSPITAL STUDIES

4.1   Brazzaville and Pointe-Noire urban areas, 1978-82 [(2393)]

Retrospective studies were carried out between 1 January 1978 and 31 December 1981 in hospitals in Brazzaville and Pointe-Noire, and between 1 January and 30 June 1982 in Brazzaville.

4.1.1   Rate
Live births	161 679
Maternal deaths	120
MMR (per 100 000 live births)	74

4.1.2   Causes of maternal deaths

	Number	%
Abortion	48	40
Post-caesarean infection	37	31
Haemorrhage	15	13
Hypertensive disorders of pregnancy	10	8
Embolisms	2	2
Other	4	3
Unknown	4	3
TOTAL	120	100

4.2   Hospitals in three rural areas, 1981 [(2393)]

4.2.1   Rate
Live births	4 140
Maternal deaths	9
MMR (per 100 000 live births)	217

5. CIVIL REGISTRATION DATA/GOVERNMENT ESTIMATES

6. OTHER SOURCES/ ESTIMATES

6.1   National, 1971 [(0345)]

6.1.1   Rate
A report by the International Federation of Gynaecologists and Obstetricians and the International Confederation of Midwives estimated the maternal mortality rate to be 1 000 per 100 000 live births.

7. SELECTED ANNOTATED BIBLIOGRAPHY

8. FURTHER READING

Boerma, J.T. *Maternal mortality in sub-Saharan Africa: levels, causes and interventions* 1987. WHE 1655

Locko-Mafouta, C. et al, L'avortement clandestine à Brazzaville. *Médecine d'Afrique Noire* 1986; 33(3): 199-213. WHE 1903

9. DATA SOURCES

WHE 0345 International Federation of Gynaecologists and Obstetricians, International Confederation of Midwives, *Maternity care in the world.* London 1976

WHE 0834 World Health Organization *World Health Statistics annual – vital statistics and causes of death.* Geneva, various years

WHE 1914 United Nations Children's Fund (UNICEF). *The state of the world's children,* various years, Oxford, Oxford University Press

WHE 2033 World Health Organization. *Global strategy for health for all by the year 2000. Second report on monitoring progress.* WHO document EB83/2 Add. 1, 1988

WHE 2393 Locko-Mafouta, C. et al, La mortalité maternelle au Congo: étude préliminaire. *Médecine d'Afrique Noire* 1988; 35(7): 517-518

NOTES

CÔTE D'IVOIRE

		Year	Source

1. BASIC INDICATORS

1.1 Demographic

1.1.1 Population

		Year	Source
Size (millions)	11.6	1988	(1914)
Rate of growth (%)	4.2	1980-87	(1914)

1.1.2 Life expectancy

Female	52	1980-85	(1915)
Male	49	1980-85	(1915)

1.1.3 Fertility

Crude Birth Rate	51	1988	(1914)
Total Fertility Rate	7.4	1988	(1914)

1.1.4 Mortality

Crude Death Rate	14	1988	(1914)
Infant Mortality Rate	95	1988	(1914)
Female			
Male			
1-4 years mortality rate			
Female			
Male			

1.2 Social and economic

1.2.1 Adult literacy rate (%)

Female	31	1985	(1914)
Male	53	1985	(1914)

1.2.2 Primary school enrolment rate (%)

Female	65	1983-86	(1914)
Male	92	1983-86	(1914)

1.2.3 Female mean age at first marriage

(years)	18.9	1978	(1918)

1.2.4 GNP/capita

		Year	Source
(US $)	740	1985	(1914)

1.2.5 Daily per capita calorie supply

(as % of requirements)	110	1984-86	(1914)

2. HEALTH SERVICES

2.1 Health expenditure

2.1.1 Expenditure on health

(as % of GNP)	3	1986	(2033)

2.1.2 Expenditure on PHC

(as % of total health expenditure)	30	1986	(2033)

2.2 Primary Health Care
(Percentage of population covered by):

2.2.1 Health services

National			
Urban			
Rural			

2.2.2 Safe water

National	20	1980	(0834)
Urban	30	1980	(0834)
Rural	10	1980	(0834)

2.2.3 Adequate sanitary facilities

National	17	1980	(0834)
Urban	13	1980	(0834)
Rural	20	1980	(0834)

2.2.4 Contraceptive prevalence rate

(%)	3	1980-81	(1712)

2.3   Coverage of maternity care (%)

Area	Prenatal care	Trained attendant	Institutional deliveries	Postnatal care	Sample size	Year	Source
National		13	42			1984	(2084)
National		20				(1987)	(1530)
Rural areas			42			1980-81	(1900)
Abidjan			90			(1986)	(1502)
Abidjan	40					1988	(2084)
Interior	36					1988	(2084)

3.   COMMUNITY STUDIES

4.   HOSPITAL STUDIES

4.1   Centre Hospitalier Universitaire de Cocody, Abidjan, 1978-82 [1882, 1898, 1900, 2026, 2490]

4.1.1   Rate

	Births	Maternal deaths	MMR (per 100 000 births)
1978	2 340	11	470
1979	2 531	16	632
1980	2 635	15	569
1981	3 310	34	1 027
1982	3 083	105	3 406
1984	n.a.	n.a.	1 302

4.1.2   Causes of maternal deaths
70% of all maternal deaths were caused by sepsis, haemorrhage and uterine rupture; a further 9% were due to hypertensive disorders of pregnancy.

Cause	Number	%
Sepsis	56	31
Haemorrhage	39	22
Ruptured uterus	30	17
Hypertensive disorders of pregnancy	16	9
Complications of anaesthesia	8	4
Anaemia	7	4
Medical causes	11	6
Others	14	7
TOTAL	181	100

4.1.3   Avoidable factors

4.1.4   High risk groups
85% of the maternal deaths occurred among women who had been transferred to the CHU de Cocody from other hospitals.

4.1.5   Other findings
One study (1882, 2496) examined maternal deaths occurring among women who had been transferred to the CHU de Cocody from three other maternity hospitals – at Divo, Agboville, and Yopougon – between 1980 and 1985. The study found that obstructed labour was the most important reason for transfer, although obstetric trauma resulting from haemorrhage and sepsis were the principal causes of maternal death. The authors concluded that sepsis and haemorrhage were, in fact, secondary complications arising from obstructed labour.

Haemorrhage did not feature frequently as a cause for transfer, probably because death occurred very soon after the onset of the problem leaving no time for transfer.

The study quotes a doctoral thesis giving a maternal mortality rate for women who had been transferred to CHU de Cocody in 1986 of 2 700 per 100 000 deliveries. The mortality rates increased with the distance of transfer – varying from 2 000 per 100 000 live births for those transferred from within the urban zone, to 3 000 per 100 000 live births for those transferred from the suburban area, and 6 000 per 100 000 live births for those transferred from rural areas.

4.2 Centre Hospitalier Universitaire de Treichville, Abidjan, 1967-70 and 1989 (1901, 2490)

4.2.1 Rate

A doctoral thesis (1901) quotes a maternal mortality rate of 135 per 100 000 live births in 1967-70. A report of a seminar held in 1989 (2490) reports a figure of 1 800 per 100 000 live births.

4.2.2 Causes of maternal deaths

	1967-70		1988-89	
	Number*	%	Number	%
Haemorrhage	22	33	56	60
Ruptured uterus	18	27	n.a.	n.a.
Associated with caesarean section	17	26	n.a.	n.a.
Sepsis	13	19	32	34
Hypertensive disorders of pregnancy	4	3	5	5
Total	n.a.	n.a.	93	100

* Causes not mutually exclusive.

4.2.3 Avoidable factors, 1967-70

The large proportion of maternal deaths associated with caesarean section and with rupture of the uterus was mainly due to the poor pre-operative condition of the women, resulting from the long delay before intervention. The delays were caused by one or more of the following:

- distance to first health centre;
- wrong diagnosis and delay in transfer to a referral hospital;
- absence of ambulance facilities for transfer;
- lack of trained personnel in first level health facility.

4.3 Maternité de Divo, 1985 (1882, 2496)

4.3.1 Rate
Deliveries	4 097
Maternal deaths	23
MMR (per 100 000 deliveries)	560

4.3.2 Causes of maternal deaths

	Number
Haemorrhage	13
Sepsis	9
Phlebitis	1
Total	23

4.3.3 Avoidable factors

4.3.4 High risk groups

The large majority of the patients at the hospital come from the town of Divo itself. During a two-month period in 1985, only 27% of the patients were found to have come from the rural area. Extrapolating this figure to the entire year it would appear that only 1 093 of the 4 097 deliveries were from women in this group. However, 22 of the 23 deaths were among women from the rural area giving a maternal mortality rate of 2 013 per 100 000 live births compared with 33 per 100 000 for women from within the town.

4.3.5 Other findings

In 1982 the Divo hospital was upgraded to handle obstetric emergencies and provided with a specialist obstetrician. Subsequently, the number of emergency transfers to the CHU de Cocody, nearly 190 kilometres away, has fallen. Whereas 65 women were transferred in a critical condition in 1980, there were no transfers at all in 1985. The Divo hospital is developing into a referral centre for all obstetric complications in the surrounding area, thus replacing the CHU de Cocody.

5. CIVIL REGISTRATION DATA/GOVERNMENT ESTIMATES

6. OTHER SOURCES/ ESTIMATES

7. SELECTED ANNOTATED BIBLIOGRAPHY

Bohoussou, K.M. et al. Ruptures uterines au cours du travail. *Revue médicale de Côte d'Ivoire* 1979; 44: 2-9. WHE 1038

At the University Hospital in Cocody, Côte d'Ivoire, over the period 1974-76 there were 128 cases of uterine rupture during labour out of a total of 6 662 deliveries, a frequency of one per 520 deliveries. Only six cases occurred at the hospital itself, the remainder were patients admitted with uterine rupture. The majority of the patients were young multiparas of low socioeconomic status from poor urban or rural areas. Most of the ruptures followed prolonged labours attended by traditional birth attendants. Half the cases were caused by ob-

structed labour due to cephalo-pelvic disproportion, 21% were scar ruptures, 20% were due to fetal
dystocia and 5% resulted from the use of traditional
oxytocic drugs. There were 18 maternal deaths, a
case fatality rate of 14.8%, representing a maternal
mortality rate from uterine rupture alone of 270 per
100 000 deliveries. There were 19 cases of
vesicovaginal fistulae.

Tiacoh, G.M. et al. Bilan chirurgical de 6 années
d'activité dans le service de gynécologie-
obstétrique de l'hôpital de Treichville (C.H.U.
d'Abidjan) 1967-1972. *Revue Médicale de Côte
d'Ivoire* 1973; 31: 9-14. WHE 0956

From January 1967 to December 1972, 4 106
obstetric and gynaecological operations were
carried out in the Treichville Hospital in Abidjan,
Côte d'Ivoire, of which 105 were fistula repairs
(2.5%). Not all of these were successful. It is
suggested that decentralization of services, good
nursing care and health education can contribute
to better management and prevention.

Regnard, P.J. and Fraser, M. Traitement chirurgical des
fistules vesico-vaginales africaines en hôpital rural.
Médecine Tropicale 1978; 38(1): 87-90. WHE 2128

A case report of surgery carried out in the Protestant
Hospital in Dabou , Côte d'Ivoire, on 19 women
with vesicovaginal fistula is presented. Nine patients
were cured at the first operation, one at the third,
and there were nine failures.

Ribault, L., L'activité obstetricale d'un centre
hospitalier régional au Nord de la Côte d'Ivoire.
Revue français de Gynécologie et Obstétrique 1989;
84(5): 377-379. WHE 2358

A report on the obstetrical activity of a Regional
Hospital Centre at Korhogo, Côte d'Ivoire, is
presented. An average of 7 000 deliveries take
place annually and the patients come from an area
of up to 100 kilometres from the hospital. The
hospital thus serves as a referral centre for the
area. Of the 321 surgical interventions which took
place during 1985, 246 were caesarean sections
and 75 due to uterine rupture. The majority of
both caesarean sections and uterine ruptures
were due to dystocia. Many of the patients had
been labouring for several days before being
brought to the hospital and were in a very poor
condition. There were 18 maternal deaths, a death
to case ratio of 5.6%. There were 22 cases of
vesicovaginal fistula.

8. FURTHER READING

9. DATA SOURCES

WHE 0834   World Health Organization *World Health
Statistics annual – vital statistics and causes of
death.* Geneva, various years

WHE 1502   Family Health International, Pregnancy
surveillance in Africa. *Network* 1986; 7(3): 1-3

WHE 1530   International Bank for Reconstruction
and Development, *The Côte d'Ivoire in transition:
from structural adjustment to self-sustained growth.*
Vol.2, Washington, IBRD 1987

WHE 1712   Mauldin W.P. and Segal, S.J., *Prevalence
of contraceptive use in developing countries. A chart
book.* Rockefeller Foundation, New York 1986

WHE 1882   Berardi, J.C. et al, *Evaluation of the
benefit of setting up a decentralised obstetric-surgical
structure in order to reduce maternal mortality
and transfers in the Côte d'Ivoire.* (unpublished
document) 1987

WHE 1898   Bohoussou, K.M., et al, La mortalité
maternelle au cours de la parturition et le postpartum immédiat: étude hospitalière. *Afrique
Médicale* 1986; 25(239): 125-130

WHE 1900   Suchet, A., *Formation pratique des
élèves sages-femmes en Côte d'Ivoire.* Dissertation
presented to the School of Midwifery, Dijon, France
1980-81

WHE 1901   Diarra, S., *Données sur la protection de la
mere et de l'enfant en Côte d'Ivoire.* Paper presented
to the meeting on "L'enseignement des aspects
préventifs et sociaux de l'obstetrique." Paris, 28
February – 17 March 1978

WHE 1914   United Nations Children's Fund
(UNICEF). *The state of the world's children,* various
years, Oxford, Oxford University Press

WHE 1915   United Nations. Department of International Economic and Social Affairs. *World population prospects: estimates and projections as assessed in 1984.* Population Studies No. 98. New York 1986

WHE 1918   United Nations. Department of International Economic and Social Affairs. *First marriage: patterns and determinants.* New York 1988

WHE 2026   Papiernik, E., Principales causes de morts maternelles. Quotient de mortalité. Fréquence dans la population des accouchées. Une méta-analyse. in: Bouyer, J. et al, *Réduire la mortalité maternelle dans les pays en développement,* Centre International de 'Enfance/INSERM, Paris, 3-7 October 1988

WHE 2033   World Health Organization. *Global strategy for health for all by the year 2000. Second report on monitoring progress.* WHO document EB83/2 Add. 1, 1988

WHE 2084   Welffens-Ekra, G., *Pour une maternité sans risques: système de soins de santé élémentaire en Afrique au sud du Sahara.* Conference régionale sur la maternité sans risques (unpublished paper), 1989

WHE 2490   World Health Organization Mortalité et morbidité maternelles. *Séminaire-Aterlier INFOSEC* Cotonou, 28 November – 4 December 1989

WHE 2496   Berardi, J.C. et al. Decentralization of maternity care. *World Health Forum* 1989; 10: 322-326

NOTES

DJIBOUTI

		Year	Source

1. BASIC INDICATORS

1.1 Demographic

1.1.1 Population
Size (millions)   0.4   1986   (2033)
Rate of growth (%)

1.1.2 Life expectancy
Female   44   1984   (2033)
Male   56   1984   (2033)

1.1.3 Fertility
Crude Birth Rate
Total Fertility Rate

1.1.4 Mortality
Crude Death Rate
Infant Mortality Rate   121   1988   (1914)
Female
Male
1-4 years mortality rate
Female
Male

1.2 Social and economic

1.2.1 Adult literacy rate (%)
Female   9   1985   (1914)
Male   15   1985   (1914)

1.2.2 Primary school enrolment rate (%)
Female
Male

1.2.3 Female mean age at first marriage
(years)

1.2.4 GNP/capita
(US $)   276   1984   (2033)

1.2.5 Daily per capita calorie supply
(as % of requirements)

2. HEALTH SERVICES

2.1 Health expenditure

2.1.1 Expenditure on health
(as % of GNP)   13   1985   (2033)

2.1.2 Expenditure on PHC
(as % of total health
   expenditure)   10   1984   (2033)

2.2 Primary Health Care
(Percentage of population covered by):

2.2.1 Health services
National   37   1980   (0834)
Urban
Rural

2.2.2 Safe water
National   45   1985   (0834)
Urban   53   1985   (0834)
Rural   20   1985   (0834)

2.2.3 Adequate sanitary facilities
National   37   1985   (0834)
Urban   43   1985   (0834)
Rural   19   1985   (0834)

2.2.4 Contraceptive prevalence rate
(%)

2.3   Coverage of maternity care (%)

Area	Prenatal care	Trained attendant	Institutional deliveries	Postnatal care	Sample size	Year	Source
National:							
urban			40			1970	(0232)
rural			20			1970	(0232)
National	76	79				1987	(2033)

3. COMMUNITY STUDIES

3.1   Djibouti City and four rural districts, 1989 [(2565)]

A survey carried out for the Expanded Programme on Immunization was used as a vehicle to implement the "sisterhood method" of estimating the number of maternal deaths. Interviews were conducted with 7 463 women of reproductive age who reported 374 maternal deaths over the preceding 11.6 years.

3.1.1   Rate
MMR (per 100 000 live births)   740

4. HOSPITAL STUDIES

5. CIVIL REGISTRATION DATA/GOVERNMENT ESTIMATES

6. OTHER SOURCES/ ESTIMATES

6.1   National [(1950)]

6.1.1   Rate
According to an assignment report by a WHO consultant, the maternal mortality rate for Djibouti was 1 490 per 100 000 live births in 1965, 600 per 100 000 live births in 1974 and around 700 per 100 000 live births during the 1980s.

7. SELECTED ANNOTATED BIBLIOGRAPHY

8. FURTHER READING

9. DATA SOURCES

WHE 0232   Gamboa de Barnardi, R. *La santé maternelle et infantile dans la République de Djibouti.* (unpublished WHO document no. EM/MCH/138) 1979

WHE 0834   World Health Organization *World Health Statistics annual - vital statistics and causes of death.* Geneva, various years

WHE 1914   United Nations Children's Fund (UNICEF). *The state of the world's children.* Various years. Oxford. Oxford University Press.

WHE 1950   Ramakavelo, M.P. *Rapport de mission sur le développement des statistiques sanitaires et de la surveillance épidémiologique en République de Djibouti.* (unpublished Project No. DJI/HST/001) 1985

WHE 2033   World Health Organization. *Global strategy for health for all by the year 2000. Second report on monitoring progress.* WHO document EB83/2 Add. 1, 1988

WHE 2565   Graham, W. *Results of the application of the sisterhood method for estimating maternal mortality.* London School of Hygiene and Tropical Medicine (Unpublished) 1990

EGYPT

	Year	Source

1. BASIC INDICATORS

1.1. Demographic

1.1.1 Population

Size (millions)	51.5	1988	(1914)
Rate of growth (%)	2.7	1980-87	(1914)

1.1.2 Life expectancy

Female	60	1980-85	(1915)
Male	57	1980-85	(1915)

1.1.3 Fertility

Crude Birth Rate	36	1988	(1914)
Total Fertility Rate	4.8	1988	(1914)

1.1.4 Mortality

Crude Death Rate	10	1988	(1914)
Infant Mortality Rate	83	1988	(1914)
Female	77	1980	(2166)
Male	75	1980	(2166)
1-4 years mortality rate			
Female	18.9	1975-77	(1917)
Male	16.4	1975-77	(1917)

1.2 Social and economic

1.2.1 Adult literacy rate (%)

Female	30	1985	(1914)
Male	59	1985	(1914)

1.2.2 Primary school enrolment rate (%)

Female	79	1986-88	(1914)
Male	100	1986-88	(1914)

1.2.3 Female mean age at first marriage

(years)	21.4	1980	(1918)

	Year	Source

1.2.4 GNP/capita

(US $)	680	1987	(1914)

1.2.5 Daily per capita calorie supply

(as % of requirements)	132	1984-86	(1914)

2. HEALTH SERVICES

2.1 Health Expenditure

2.1.1 Expenditure on health
(as % of GNP)

2.1.2 Expenditure on PHC

(as % of total health expenditure)	90	1987	(2033)

2.2 Primary Health Care
(Percentage of population covered by):

2.2.1 Health services

National	99	1986	(2033)
Urban			
Rural			

2.2.2 Safe water

National	90	1981	(0834)
Urban	93	1981	(0834)
Rural	61	1981	(0834)

2.2.3 Adequate sanitary facilities

National	70	1981	(0834)
Urban	95	1981	(0834)
Rural	49	1981	(0834)

2.2.4 Contraceptive prevalence rate

(%)	38	1983-88	(2113)

2.3 Coverage of maternity care (%)

Area	Prenatal care	Trained attendant	Institutional deliveries	Postnatal care	Sample size	Year	Source
National:							
urban	48	4	22	32	4 754	1977-82	(0195)
rural	19	5	2	12	7 714	1977-82	(0195)
National		24				1978	(0834)
National	40					1982	(0834)
National		47	40		12 000	1986	(1688)
National:	52	34	22		8 643	1983-88	(2113)
urban	68	56	40		3 483	1983-88	(2113)
rural	42	19	11		5 160	1983-88	(2113)
Alexandria			14			1980	(0813)
Cairo		22	22			(1983)	(0324)
Upper Egypt			<20			1985	(1266)

3. COMMUNITY STUDIES

3.1 Alexandria, 1963-82 [0269, 2321, 2396]

3.1.1 Rate

A community study obtained data about the death of the wife by interviewing widowers. A total of 30 000 husbands were interviewed and reported 183 deaths which could be attributed to complications of pregnancy, childbirth and the puerperium. The maternal mortality rate was estimated as 163 per 100 000 live births.

3.2 Menoufia, 1981-83 [0226, 1006, 1260, 2072]

3.2.1 Rate

The Reproductive Age Mortality Survey (RAMOS) was carried out during 1981-83. Information on deaths was obtained from the vital registration system.

Live births	202 806
Maternal deaths	385
MMR (per 100 000 live births)	190
MMR (per 100 000 women aged 15-49)	45

3.2.2 Causes of maternal deaths

	Number	%
Haemorrhage	125	29
Sepsis	44	10
Hypertensive disorders of pregnancy	24	6
Associated with caesarean section	24	6
Abortion	21	5
Ectopic pregnancy	3	1
Other direct causes	24	6
DIRECT CAUSES	265	60
Circulatory diseases	65	15
Hepatitis	6	1
Other infections	8	2
Other indirect causes	23	5
Unknown	18	4
INDIRECT CAUSES	120	27
Trauma	27	6
Other	27	6
OTHER CAUSES	54	12
TOTAL	439	100

3.2.3 Avoidable factors

3.2.4 High risk groups

Age group	MMR (per 100 000 live births)
15-19	268
20-24	163
25-29	154
30-34	147
35-39	298
40-44	271
45-49	344
TOTAL	190

3.3 Governorates of Assiut, Suhag and Kena, 1984-85 [1266]

A study was carried out over the period July 1984 to June 1985 in El-Kossia, Suhag city and Nagaa Hammadi, in the governorates of Assiut, Suhag and Kena respectively. With the help of medical personnel, TBAs, social workers and others, data were collected about all maternal deaths occurring within and outside health facilities.

3.3.1 Rate

	El-Kossia (Assiut)	Suhag City (Suhag)	Nagaa Hammadi (Kena)	Total
Live births	8 976	4 887	10 528	24 391
Maternal deaths	16	23	34	73
MMR (per 100 000 live births)	178	471	323	299
MMR (per 100 000 women aged 15-49)	41	51	51	n.a.

3.3.2 Causes of maternal deaths

	Number	%
Haemorrhage	28	38
Hypertensive disorders of pregnancy	13	18
Associated with caesarean section	8	11
Sepsis	8	11
Ruptured uterus	6	8
Abortion	3	4
Ectopic pregnancy	1	1
Associated diseases	4	6
Unknown	2	3
TOTAL	73	100

3.4 Giza, 1985-86 [2396]

All maternal deaths occurring in five Giza health sectors during the 13-month period from August 1985 to August 1986 were identified by social/health workers, hospital staff, and local health unit clerks. Information on the maternal deaths was obtained from interviews with family members of the deceased using a series of detailed questions on the sequence of events, symptoms and complications due to pregnancy, septic abortions and childbirth.

3.4.1 Rate

Births	104 000
Maternal deaths*	156
MMR (per 100 000 births)	150
MMR (per 100 000 women aged 15-49)	30

* Includes ten non-obstetric deaths

3.4.2 Causes of maternal deaths

	Number	%
Haemorrhage	47	31
Sepsis	23	15
Other obstetric complications	9	6
Procedural, operative and anaesthetic	5	3
Other medical complications	39	25
Other, including non-obstetric causes	14	9
Unknown	19	12
TOTAL	156	100

3.4.3 Avoidable factors

Approximately 40% of the mothers who died received no prenatal care.

3.4.4 High risk groups

Women who died of maternal causes were more likely to be illiterate than women who died of non-maternal causes. Illiteracy among maternal deaths (72%) and non-maternal deaths (59%) were both higher than the general level of illiteracy for all women of reproductive age living in Giza in 1986.

About 25% of the women who died from maternal causes had a known illness prior to the last pregnancy. The most common illnesses were kidney problems, hypertension, diabetes, anaemia, mitral stenosis and asthma. 20% of the women who died from maternal causes had a previous history of surgery prior to the last pregnancy. Caesarean section and uterine operations (including induced abortion) were the most frequently mentioned interventions.

Almost one third of all maternal deaths were among women who were both over 35 years old and had four or more previous births.

4. HOSPITAL STUDIES

4.1 National sample of health facilities, 1977-83 [0571]

4.1.1 Rate

Live births	20 688
Maternal deaths	55
MMR (per 100 000 live births)	266

4.2 Ain Shams University hospital, Cairo, 1973-76, 1976-81, 1980-84 [2321]

4.2.1 Rate

	Deliveries	Maternal deaths	MMR (per 100 000 deliveries)
1973-76	15 326	69	450
1976-81	–	–	435
1980-84	–	–	279

4.2.2 Causes of maternal deaths, 1976-81 and 1980-84

	1976-81		1980-84	
	Number	%	Number	%
Hypertensive disorders of pregnancy	28	26	23	27
Haemorrhage	35	33	17	20
Sepsis	22	21	14	16
Uterine rupture	13	12	4	5
Other	8	8	27	32
TOTAL	106	100	85	100

4.3 Al-Hussein University Hospital and Al-Galaa Hospital, Cairo, 1975-76 [0839]

4.3.1 Rate

	Al-Hussein	Al-Galaa	Total
Deliveries	1 966	7 489	9 455
Maternal deaths	10	82	92
MMR (per 100 000 deliveries)	509	1 094	973

4.3.2 Causes of maternal deaths

	Number	%
Haemorrhage	33	36
Sepsis	16	17
Hypertensive disorders of pregnancy	13	14
Abortion	9	10
Ruptured uterus	7	8
Complications of anaesthesia	4	4
Hepatitis	2	2
Other	8	9
TOTAL	92	100

4.3.3 Avoidable factors

4.3.4 High risk groups

Parity	Deliveries	Maternal deaths	MMR (per 100 000 deliveries)
1	3 403	30	880
2-3	2 684	18	670
4-5	1 871	12	640
6+	1 497	32	2 130
TOTAL	9 455	92	970

4.4 General and district Hospitals, Assiut, Suhag and Kena Governorates, 1981-83 [1266, 1955]

4.4.1 Rate

	Assiut	Suhag	Kena	Total
Deliveries	6 687	8 092	5 022	19 801
Maternal deaths	105	198	83	386
MMR (per 100 000 deliveries)	1 570	2 446	1 653	1 949

4.4.2 Causes of maternal deaths

	Assiut	Suhag	Kena	Total No.	%
Haemorrhage	28	76	31	135	35
Ruptured uterus	9	41	7	57	15
Hypertensive disorders of pregnancy	10	31	13	54	14
Associated with caesarean section	21	15	8	44	11
Sepsis	7	13	13	33	9
Abortion	13	4	4	21	5
Ectopic pregnancy	1	2	3	6	2
Associated diseases	16	16	4	36	9
TOTAL	105	198	83	386	100

4.5 El-Minshawy Hospital, 1978-82 [2321]

4.5.1 Rate

MMR (per 100 000 live births)	371

4.5.2 Causes of maternal deaths

	Number	%
Haemorrhage	10	26
Sepsis	9	23
Hypertensive disorders of pregnancy	7	18
Uterine rupture	6	15
Other	8	21
TOTAL	39	100

4.6 Helwan Hospital, 1979-83 [2321]

4.6.1 Rate

MMR (per 100 000 live births)	505

4.6.2 Causes of maternal deaths

	Number	%
Haemorrhage	42	43
Sepsis	19	20
Hypertensive disorders of pregnancy	12	12
Uterine rupture	11	11
Other	14	14
TOTAL	98	100

4.7 Boulak El-Dakrour Hospital, Giza, 1980 and 1985-86 [2321, 2396]

4.7.1 Rate

	Births	Maternal deaths	MMR (per 100 000 deliveries)
1980	–	–	602
1985-86	6 676	17	255

4.8 Shobra Hospital, 1980-85 [2321]

4.8.1 Rate

MMR (per 100 000 live births)	483

4.8.2 Causes of maternal deaths

	Number	%
Haemorrhage	21	30
Sepsis	17	24
Hypertensive disorders of pregnancy	10	14
Rupture of the uterus	5	7
Other	17	24
TOTAL	70	100

4.9 Hospital and MCH centre in El-Kossia, Assiut Governorate, 1985 [1771]

4.9.1 Rate

Deliveries	2 591
Maternal deaths	8
MMR (per 100 000 deliveries)	309

4.10 Kasr el Aini Hospital, 1981-82 [2249]

4.10.1 Rate

Live births	10 115
Maternal deaths	34
MMR (per 100 000 live births)	336

5. CIVIL REGISTRATION DATA/GOVERNMENT ESTIMATES

5.1 National, 1980 [1430]

5.1.1 Rate

The source quotes a Ministry of Health report giving a maternal mortality rate of 80 per 100 000 live births in 1980 compared with 140 per 100 000 live births in 1952.

5.2 National, 1979 and 1987 [0834]

5.2.1 Rate

	MMR (per 100 000 live births)
1979	78
1987	60

5.3 National, 1970-1980 [0753]

5.3.1 Rate

	MMR (per 100 000 live births)
1970	107
1971	96
1972	98
1973	92
1975	73
1976	81
1977	85
1978	82
1980	93

6. OTHER SOURCES/ESTIMATES

6.1 National, 1981 [0708]

6.1.1 Rate

The overall maternal mortality rate in Egypt was estimated to be around 500 per 100 000 live births in 1981, with a hospital rate at around 800 per 100 000 live births.

7. SELECTED ANNOTATED BIBLIOGRAPHY

Fortney, J.A. et al. Causes of death to women of reproductive age in two developing countries. *Population Research and Policy Review* 1987; 6: 137-148. WHE 1267

Deaths among women of reproductive age (15-49 years) in Menoufia, Egypt and Bali, Indonesia were located and family members interviewed. Local physicians reviewed the completed interviews and determined the cause of death. Complications of childbirth were the cause of 23% of the deaths in Menoufia and Bali. In Egypt the first cause of death was circulatory system disease (28%) followed by complications of pregnancy and childbirth (23%) and trauma (14%, primarily burns). The death rate for complications of pregnancy was found to be three times higher than that reported in official statistics. Underreporting of maternal deaths is thought to be widespread in developing countries.

Gadalla, S. et al, How the number of living sons influences contraceptive use in Menoufia Governorate, Egypt. *Studies in Family Planning* 1985; 16(3): 164-169. WHE 1271

In 38 rural villages in Menoufia Governorate in Egypt, women's responses to a community-based contraceptive distribution programme were examined, taking into account both the number of living children and the number of living sons each woman reported having. Controlling for number of living children, women with more sons were more likely to be using contraception before the distribution programme began. Among women not using contraception before the programme, those with more sons were more likely to initiate and continue contraceptive use following the distribution. These findings imply that in addition to obstacles related to contraceptive availability, there are several cultural, social and economic factors that influence fertility behaviour and exert considerable pressure on married couples to have large families, including several sons. Unless the pressure exerted by these factors is changed or reduced, the impact of family planning programmes is likely to reach a plateau at a relatively low prevalence level.

Grubb G.S. et al, A comparison of two cause-of-death classification systems for deaths among women of reproductive age in Menoufia, Egypt. *International Journal of Epidemiology* 1988; 17(2): 385-391. WHE 2392

Data on 1979 deaths among reproductive age women were collected in the 1981-83 Reproductive Age Mortality Survey (RAMOS) in the governorate of Menoufia, Egypt and compared with data on these deaths as recorded by the Egyptian death registration system. Although the distribution of the causes of death were similar, there were substantial differences between classification systems for deaths due to particular causes. The percentage of deaths assigned to maternal causes was three times higher in RAMOS (19.2%) than on death certificates (6.1%). Reported mortality rates for pregnancy-related causes have been substantially underestimated in national death registration systems.

8. FURTHER READING

Assaad, M. and El Katsha, S. Villagers' use of and participation in formal and informal health services in an Egyptian delta village. *Contact* 1981; 65: 1-13. WHE 0003

Cook, R. *Damage to physical health from pharaonic circumcision (infibulation) of females.* Paper prepared for Seminar on Traditional Practices Affecting the Health of Women and Children in Africa, 1984, 6-10 February, Dakar, Senegal. WHE 1911

El Kady, A. et al. *Dayas' practices and maternal mortality in Giza, Egypt.* National Population Council, Egypt, July 1989. WHE2397

Family Health International. RAMOS study confirms contraception saves lives. *Network* 1985; 6(4): 4-5. WHE 1256

Faour, M. Fertility policy and family planning in the Arab countries. *Studies in Family Planning* 1988; 20(5): 254-263. WHE 2367

Gadalla, S. et al. Maternal mortality in Egypt. *Journal of Tropical Pediatrics* 1987; 33(4): 11-13. WHE 1857

Kamel, N.M. Determinants and patterns of female mortality associated with women's reproductive role. in: ANU/UN/WHO Meeting on *Sex Differentials in Mortality: Trends, Determinants and Consequences,* Canberra 1981 (unpublished document). WHE 0374

Nadim, N.E. *Rural health care in Egypt.* International Development Research Centre, Ottawa, Canada 1980. WHE 0477

Toppozada, H.K. Epidemiology of abortion in Alexandria. *Alexandria Medical Journal* 1980; 26(1,2): 1-167. WHE 1355

Van der Most van Spijk, M. *Who cares for her health? An anthropological study of women's health care in a village in Upper Egypt.* Women and Development Series: Egypt, Cairo/Leiden 1982. WHE 2211

9. DATA SOURCES

WHE 0195   Egypt, Ministry of Health, and National Center for Health Statistics. Survey of ever-married females. Medical care during last pregnancy and labour. *Health Profile of Egypt* 1982: 3 (5)

WHE 0226   Fortney, J.A. et al. *Causes of death to women of reproductive age in Egypt.* Michigan State University, Working Paper no. 49 1984

WHE 0269   El Sherbini, A.F. et al. *The feasibility of getting information about maternal mortality from the husband.* (unpublished document) 1983.

WHE 0324   Hassouna, W.A. *Study of urban health care: the case of the Cairo health sector assessment study.* in: Joint UNICEF/WHO Meeting on Primary Health Care in Urban Areas, Geneva 1983

WHE 0571   International Fertility Research Program. *Maternity record study: standard analysis input parameters, tables for pooled Egyptian data* (unpublished) 1983

WHE 0708   Tomkinson, J.S. *Establishment of a system of confidential enquiries into maternal deaths in Egypt.* (unpublished WHO document no. EM/MCH/163 1982

WHE 0753   United Nations. *Demographic Yearbook.* New York, various years

WHE 0813   World Health Organization. Eastern Mediterranean Regional Office. *Report of the EMR/SEAR meeting on the prevention of neonatal tetanus.* WHO document No. EM/IMZ/27, EM/BD/14, Lahore 1982

WHE 0834   World Health Organization.*World Health Statistics annual - vital statistics and causes of death.* Geneva, various years

WHE 0839   Younis, N. et al. *Analysis of maternal deaths in two Egyptian maternity hospitals.* (mimeographed undated document)

WHE 1006   Gadalla, S. *Reproductive age mortality survey.* (unpublished data) 1984

WHE 1260   Fortney, J.A. et al. *Maternal mortality in Indonesia and Egypt.* in: Interregional Meeting on the Prevention of Maternal Mortality, Geneva, 11-15 November 1985 (unpublished WHO document no. FHE/PMM/85.9.13)

WHE 1266   Abdullah, S.A. et al. *Maternal mortality in Upper Egypt.* in: Interregional Meeting on the Prevention of Maternal Mortality, Geneva, 11-15 November 1985 (unpublished WHO document no. FHE/PMM/85.9.18)

WHE 1430   United Nations Fund for Population Activities UNFPA. *Egypt: Report of the second mission on needs assessment. Report no. 78.* UNFPA, New York 1985

WHE 1688   World Health Organization, Expanded Programme on Immunization. Neonatal tetanus mortality surveys. *Weekly Epidemiological Record,* 30.10.1987: 332-335

WHE 1771   Abdullah, S.A.. *Study of unmet needs in maternal health and family planning: Upper Egypt.* (unpublished document) 1987

WHE 1914   United Nations Children's Fund (UNICEF). *The state of the world's children,* various years, Oxford, Oxford University Press

WHE 1915   United Nations. Department of International Economic and Social Affairs. *World population prospects: estimates and projections as assessed in 1984.* Population Studies No. 98 New York 1986

WHE 1917   United Nations. Department of International Economic and Social Affairs. *Age structure of mortality in developing countries. A database for cross-sectional and time-series research.* New York 1986

WHE 1918   United Nations. Department of International Economic and Social Affairs. *First marriage: patterns and determinants.* New York 1988

WHE 1955   Sharawi, A.A.. *Maternal mortality study.* Cairo, Ministry of Health 1987

WHE 2033   World Health Organization. *Global strategy for health for all by the year 2000. Second report on monitoring progress.* WHO document EB83/2 Add. 1 1988

WHE 2072   Saleh, S. et al. *Maternal mortality in Menoufia. A study of reproductive age mortality.* American University of Cairo, Cairo 1987

WHE 2113   Demographic and Health Surveys. *Egypt Demographic and health survey 1988.* Egypt National Population Council and Institute for Resource Development/Westinghouse 1989

WHE 2166   Nawar, L. et al, *Infant and child mortality in Egypt.* Central Agency for Public Mobilization and Statistics 1988

WHE 2249   Darwish, N. and Sarhan, D. Maternal mortality in cases of pregnancy toxaemia in Kasr el Aini Hospitals: a two-year study. in: Fayad, M.M. and Abdalla, M.I., (eds.) *Medical education in the field of primary maternal child health care:* Proceedings of an international conference, Cairo, 5-7 December 1983

WHE 2321   El-Mouelhy, M.T. *Maternal mortality in Egypt.* Cairo Family Planning Association (unpublished) 1987

WHE 2396   El Kady, A. et al. *Maternal mortality in Giza, Egypt.* Family Health International July 1989

EQUATORIAL GUINEA

		Year	Source

1. BASIC INDICATORS

1.1 Demographic

1.1.1 Population

		Year	Source
Size (millions)	0.5	1987	(0753)
Rate of growth (%)	2.4	1987	(0753)

1.1.2 Life expectancy

		Year	Source
Female	46	1980-85	(0753)
Male	42	1980-85	(0753)

1.1.3 Fertility

		Year	Source
Crude Birth Rate	43	1980-85	(0753)
Total Fertility Rate	5.7	1980-85	(0753)

1.1.4 Mortality

		Year	Source
Crude Death Rate	21	1980-85	(0753)
Infant Mortality Rate	126	1988	(1914)
Female			
Male			
1-4 years mortality rate			
Female			
Male			

1.2 Social and economic

1.2.1 Adult literacy rate (%)
Female
Male

1.2.2 Primary school enrolment rate (%)
Female
Male

1.2.3 Female mean age at first marriage
(years)

1.2.4 GNP/capita

		Year	Source
(US $)	180	1987	(1914)

1.2.5 Daily per capita calorie supply
(as % of requirements)

2. HEALTH SERVICES

2.1 Health expenditure

2.1.1 Expenditure on health
(as % of GNP)

2.1.2 Expenditure on PHC
(as % of total health expenditure)

2.2 Primary Health Care
(Percentage of population covered by):

2.2.1 Health services
National
Urban
Rural

2.2.2 Safe water

		Year	Source
National			
Urban	47	1983	(0834)
Rural			

2.2.3 Adequate sanitary facilities

		Year	Source
National			
Urban	28	1983	(0834)
Rural			

2.2.4 Contraceptive prevalence rate
(%)

2.3 **Coverage of maternity care (%)**

Area	Prenatal care	Trained attendant	Institutional deliveries	Postnatal care	Sample size	Year	Source
–	–	–	–	–	–	–	–

3. COMMUNITY STUDIES

4. HOSPITAL STUDIES

5. CIVIL REGISTRATION DATA/GOVERNMENT ESTIMATES

6. OTHER SOURCES/ ESTIMATES

6.1 **National, (1987)** [1655]

6.1.1 **Maternal mortality was estimated on the basis of model life tables.**
MMR (per 100 000 births)   430
MMR (per 100 000 women of reproductive age)   79

7. SELECTED ANNOTATED BIBLIOGRAPHY

8. FURTHER READING

9. DATA SOURCES

WHE 0753   United Nations. *Demographic Yearbook.* New York, various years

WHE 0834   World Health Organization. *World Health Statistics annual – vital statistics and causes of death.* Geneva, various years

WHE 1655   Boerma, J.T. *Maternal mortality in sub-Saharan Africa: levels, causes and interventions.* (Unpublished document) 1987

WHE 1914   United Nations Children's Fund (UNICEF). *The state of the world's children,* various years, Oxford, Oxford University Press

ETHIOPIA

		Year	Source

1. BASIC INDICATORS

1.1 Demographic

1.1.1 Population.

		Year	Source
Size (millions)	44.7	1988	(1914)
Rate of growth (%)	1.8	1980-87	(1914)

1.1.2 Life expectancy

Female	43	1980-85	(1915)
Male	39	1980-85	(1915)

1.1.3 Fertility

Crude Birth Rate	44	1988	(1914)
Total Fertility Rate	6.2	1988	(1914)

1.1.4 Mortality

Crude Death Rate	24	1988	(1914)
Infant Mortality Rate	153	1988	(1914)
Female			
Male			
1-4 years mortality rate			
Female			
Male			

1.2 Social and economic

1.2.1 Adult literacy rate (%)

Female	1	1970	(1914)
Male	8	1970	(1914)

1.2.2 Primary school enrolment rate (%)

Female	28	1986-88	(0834)
Male	46	1986-88	(0834)

1.2.3 Female mean age at first marriage

(years)	17.7	1981	(1918)

1.2.4 GNP/capita

		Year	Source
(US $)	130	1987	(1914)

1.2.5 Daily per capita calorie supply

(as % of requirements)	71	1984-86	(1914)

2. HEALTH SERVICES

2.1 Health expenditure

2.1.1 Expenditure on health

(as % of GNP)	1.8	1981	(0800)

2.1.2 Expenditure on PHC

(as % of total health expenditure)	27.2	1984	(0800)

2.2 Primary Health Care
(Percentage of population covered by):

2.2.1 Health services

National	46	1985-87	(1914)
Urban			
Rural			

2.2.2 Safe water

National	16	1985-87	(1914)
Urban	69	1985-87	(1914)
Rural	9	1985-87	(1914)

2.2.3 Adequate sanitary facilities

National			
Urban			
Rural	5	1984	(0834)

2.2.4 Contraceptive prevalence rate

(%)	2	1982	(1712)

2.3   Coverage of maternity care (%)

Area	Prenatal care	Trained attendant	Institutional deliveries	Postnatal care	Sample size	Year	Source
National	14	58				1984	(0834)
National	20	10		15		1988	(2033)
National: rural* urban	50 50-81	11 21-58				(1988) (1988)	(2008) (2008)
Addis Ababa 12 areas	70	65 3	56		8724w 5394	1981-3 1981-3	(1979) (1318)

* Areas where EPI/MCH programmes are being undertaken

3.   COMMUNITY STUDIES

3.1   Addis Ababa, 1981-83 (0596, 1446, 1967, 1979)

A household survey was conducted to obtain data on pregnancy outcomes for all women aged 13-49 in 32 215 households. There were 9 954 pregnancies resulting in 9 154 live births. The survey covered a two-year period, from 11 September 1981 to 10 September 1983. A total of 45 women died from complications of pregnancy, delivery and the puerperium.

3.1.1   Rate

	1981-82	1982-83	1981-83
MMR (per 100 000 live births)	353	566	457

3.1.2.   Causes of maternal deaths, 1981-83

Abortion was the single most important cause of direct obstetric deaths. Unskilled interference was reported by relatives in twelve of the thirteen cases. Infectious hepatitis was the most important indirect obstetric cause of death. The two deaths from poisoning (one in the first trimester and the other in the last trimester), were attributable to unwanted pregnancies.

	Number	%
Abortion	13	29
Haemorrhage	3	7
Hypertensive disorders of pregnancy	3	7
Ruptured uterus	2	4
Sepsis	1	2
DIRECT CAUSES	24	53
Hepatitis	7	17
Complications of anaesthesia	2	4
Poisoning	2	4
"Zar"*	2	4
Anaemia	1	2
Others	4	9
Unknown	5	11
TOTAL	45	100

*   Involves erratic behaviour, convulsions, and extreme apathy.

3.1.3   Avoidable factors

Mortality rates were highest among women who had no prenatal care and among those who delivered at home without the assistance of a TBA.

Prenatal care

	MMR (per 100 000 live births)	
	Including abortion deaths	Excluding abortion deaths
No prenatal care	1100	620
Prenatal care	240	240

Delivery by TBAs

	MMR (per 100 000 live births)
Delivered at home with TBA	132
Delivered at home without TBA	411
Delivered at MCH clinic	68

3.1.4 High risk groups

Mortality rates were highest for young, primiparous women, for those in the lowest income groups, those who were widowed, divorced or separated and for those whose pregnancy was unwanted.

Age group

	MMR (per 100 000 live births)	
	Including abortion deaths	Excluding abortion deaths
15-19	1 270	630
20-24	700	500
25-29	360	250
30-34	280	190
35+	420	420

Parity

	MMR (per 100 000 live births)	
	Including abortion deaths	Excluding abortion deaths
0	1 321*	377*
1	810	590
2-3	320	250
4	540	390
5+	300	300

* Calculated per 100 000 nulliparous women.

Income group

	MMR (per 100 000 live births)	
	Including abortion deaths	Excluding abortion deaths
< US$ 25 monthly	1 530	940
> US$ 25 monthly	320	240

Marital status

	MMR (per 100 000 live births)	
	Including abortion deaths	Excluding abortion deaths
Married	320	280
Single	1 300	820
Divorced/separated	2 020	580
Widowed	2 170	1 090

Unwanted pregnancy

	MMR (per 100 000 live births)	
	Including abortion deaths	Excluding abortion deaths
Unwanted pregnancy	560	330
Wanted pregnancy	320	280

3.1.5 Other findings

Use of maternity services

- 32% of the pregnant women received no prenatal care. 35% of the women received prenatal care in Maternal and Child Health Clinics where services are free, 30% in hospitals and 3% in private clinics.

- Younger women were more likely to seek prenatal care and to deliver in health institutions. Use of prenatal care both in hospitals and in MCH clinics decreased with rising parity. Non attendance among the high risk para 5-8 and 8+ was 35% and 44% respectively.

- Attendance at prenatal clinics was closely related to the level of the women's education. Half of the illiterate women received no prenatal care compared with only 7% of women who had more than 12 years of education.

- 45% of the women delivered at home, 39% in hospitals and 15% in clinics. Uneducated women were more likely to deliver at home.

- The use of prenatal care and delivery at health institutions increased with higher incomes.

Wanted and unwanted pregnancies

- Half of all pregnancies were unwanted. 59% of women with unwanted pregnancies received no prenatal care compared with only 26% of women with wanted pregnancies. The majority of women with unwanted pregnancies delivered at home or in MCH clinics where the services are free.

Abortion

- Of the total pregnancies, 92% ended in live births, 2% in stillbirths and 6% in abortions.

- For 71% of pregnancies resulting in abortions no prenatal care was received.

4. HOSPITAL STUDIES

4.1. Black Lion Hospital and Yekatit 12 Hospital, Addis Ababa, 1981-83 [0596, 2577]

This was a confidential enquiry carried out in the two hospitals over the two-year period, September 1981 - September 1983. There were 70 direct obstetric deaths and 30 deaths due to associated causes. The cause of death in another six deaths could not be determined.

4.1.1   Rate

	Black Lion Hospital *	Yekatit 12 Hospital
Live births	7 018	3 763
Maternal deaths	89	17
MMR (per 100 000 live births)	1 268	452

    * Tikur Anbessa

4.1.2   Causes of maternal deaths

	Black Lion Hospital		Yekatit 12 Hospital	
	Number	%	Number	%
Abortion	21	24	5	29
Ruptured uterus	11	12	0	0
Sepsis	10	11	3	18
Haemorrhage	7	8	1	6
Obstructed labour	5	6	0	0
Hypertensive disorders of pregnancy	4	5	0	0
Ectopic pregnancy/ Anaesthesia/Unknown	6	7	1	6
DIRECT CAUSES	64	72	10	58
Hepatitis	17	19	3	18
Other indirect causes	8	8	4	23
INDIRECT CAUSES	23	26	7	4
TOTAL	89	100	17	100

4.1.3   Avoidable factors* (available for 92 cases from both hospitals).

	Prenatal	Labour/ delivery	Post-abortion/ delivery
Patient and home circumstances	55**	14	12
Medical staff factors	10	17	37
Nursing staff factors	5	3	12
Shortage of blood	4	4	18
Inadequate facilities	21	18	14

*   In most cases more than one avoidable factor was involved.
** Includes 25 patients who procured illegal abortions.

4.1.4   High risk groups

At the Black Lion Hospital mortality rates were lowest for women aged 20-24 years and at parity 2-4. The mortality rate was significantly higher in primiparous women and grand multiparae older than 30.

	MMR (per 100 000 live births)		
Age in years	Parity 1	Parity 2-4	Parity 5+
15-19	880	0	0
20-24	860	620	0
25-29	850	1060	900
30-34	4 680	830	1 270
35+	21 420*	760	1 620

*   Based on two deaths.

4.2   Black Lion Hospital, Addis Ababa, 1980-1985 [2247, 2580]

4.2.1   Rate

	Live births	Maternal deaths	MMR (per 100 000 live births)
1980	3 729	30	805
1981	4 049	47	1 161
1982	3 538	33	933
1983	3 400	43	1 265
1984	3 973	25	629
1985	3 715	38	1 023
1980-1985	22 404	216	964

4.2.2   Causes of maternal deaths

	Number	%
Abortion	48	22
Sepsis	36	17
Ruptured uterus	29	13
Haemorrhage	20	9
Hypertensive disorders of pregnancy	12	6
Ectopic pregnancy	4	2
DIRECT CAUSES	149	69
Hepatitis	29	13
Malaria	4	2
Other indirect causes	30	14
INDIRECT CAUSES	63	29
Unknown	4	2
TOTAL	216	100

4.2.3   Avoidable factors

Of the 216 deaths, 91% occurred in unbooked patients.

4.3   Gandhi, Paulos and Zewditu Hospitals, Addis Ababa, 1981-83 [0596]

4.3.1   Rate

	Gandhi Hospital	Paulos Hospital	Zewditu Hospital	TOTAL
Live births	7 578	5 623	4 601	17 802
Maternal deaths	38	18	20	76
MMR (per 100 000 live births)	501	320	435	427

4.3.2   Causes of maternal deaths

	No.	%
Abortion	19	25
Sepsis	13	17
Hypertensive disorders of pregnancy	13	17
Haemorrhage	12	16
Obstructed labour	2	3
Other direct causes	2	3
DIRECT CAUSES	61	80
Hepatitis	4	5
Other indirect causes	3	4
INDIRECT CAUSES	7	9
TOTAL	76	100

4.4 Five city hospitals, Addis Ababa, 1981-83 [(1803)]

A study of maternal mortality associated with viral hepatitis was conducted by a Maternal Mortality Review Committee under the auspices of the medical faculty of Addis Ababa University.

4.4.1 Rate

Live births	28 538
Maternal deaths	198
MMR (per 100 000 live births)	694

4.4.2 Causes of maternal deaths

26 deaths were classified as being associated with viral hepatitis, giving a hospital maternal mortality rate for viral hepatitis alone of 91 per 100 000 live births. Viral hepatitis ranked third among the causes of maternal mortality behind septic abortion and puerperal sepsis.

4.4.3 Avoidable factors

Although 30% of women who died from maternal causes received prenatal care in Addis Ababa, only 13% of the women who died from viral hepatitis received prenatal care. Preventive strategies should include education for women, application of good hygiene, provision of safe water and improvements in basic sanitation in order to prevent disease transmission.

5. CIVIL REGISTRATION DATA/GOVERNMENT ESTIMATES

5.1. National, 1972 [(0436,0731,1120 2008)]

5.1.1 Rate

A number of sources quote a rate of 2000 per 100 000 live births as being the official maternal mortality rate for 1972, an estimate based on institutional figures.

6. OTHER SOURCES/ ESTIMATES

7. SELECTED ANNOTATED BIBLIOGRAPHY

Abbo, A.H. and Mukhtar, M. *New trends in the operative management of urinary fistulae.* Sudan Medical Journal 1975: 13(4): 126-132 WHE2147.

An analysis of 70 cases of urinary fistulae treated from April to December 1974 is presented. Thirty of the cases were operated in Addis Ababa, Ethiopia and 40 in Khartoum Civil Hospital, Sudan. Sixty-two (88%) of the fistulae were caused by prolonged labour, and eight (12%) by hysterectomy. Four of the post hysterectomy cases were obstetrical in origin because they followed ruptured uteri for which a hysterectomy was done.

Eighty-five percent of the women were between ages 12 and 30 and were primiparae. Forty-nine percent of the women had undergone previous unsuccessful attempts at fistula repair. Most patients were extremely poor and malnourished and many were suffering from malaria, dysentery, helminthic diseases and anaemia. Associated conditions included bladder calculus in four cases.

Surgical techniques are described. Of the eight cases with urethro-vaginal fistulae, all were successfully repaired, with complete restoration of function in five cases and partial restoration of function in three cases. Of the 60 cases of vesico-vaginal fistulae, 57 (95%) were successfully repaired, with 83% restoration of continence and seven cases with stress incontinence. In three cases the repair failed.

Bal, J.S. *The vesico-vaginal and allied fistulae - a report on 40 cases.* Medical Journal of Zambia 1975: 9(3): 69-71. WHE1033

The results of treatment in a series of 40 women with vesico-vaginal and allied fistulae carried out at the Public Health College Hospital, Gondar, Ethiopia, from 1969-71 are reported. Located in the highlands of Ethiopia, Gondar has no facilities for vehicular transport into the villages. If labour becomes obstructed at home, it sometimes takes up to three or four days before the relatives can bring the woman to the hospital.

The average age of the 37 patients with obstetric fistulae was 22 years with a range of 15-40. The average height was 147cm. Thirty women (81%) were primiparae, six were para 2-6 and one was para 10.

Surgical methods are described. Repair was mostly carried out through the vaginal route. Thirty-six (90%) of the fistulae were successfully cured. There were seven cases (20%) where the fistula was closed but the women suffered stress incontinence. This was considered to be related to the amount of fibrosis and tissue destruction at the site of the fistula. In the four unsuccessful cases urinary diversion was done.

Gurovsky, S. *Rupture of the gravid uterus* Ethiopian Medical Journal 1971: 9: 193-196. WHE1076

A series of 60 cases of ruptured uterus in 13,090 deliveries at the Gandhi Memorial Hospital in Addis Ababa is given, an incidence of 1:216 deliveries. There were 39 spontaneous ruptures, 13 traumatic ruptures and eight ruptured scars. Of the patients with spontaneous ruptures, 13 were aged 15 years or under, twelve were aged from 21 to 30 and only four were older than 30. Three patients were primiparous, 31 were para 2 or 3 and 26 were para four or more. There were ten maternal deaths giving a case fatality rate for the series of 16.7%. The large number of spontaneous and traumatic ruptures is a reflection of the absence of prenatal care and the inadequate maternity services available to most of the patients.

Habte-Gabr, E. et al. *Analysis of admissions to Gondar Hospital in North-western Ethiopia, 1971-1972.* Ethiopian Medical Journal 1976: 14: 49-59. WHE1153

An analysis of 3,611 patient records over one year showed that gynaecological admissions represented 3% (120) of all admissions to this hospital, and of these, the highest percentage (30%) were for fistulae, followed by dysfunctional uterine bleeding (19%), pelvic inflammatory diseases (18%), and uterovaginal prolapse (19%). Fistulae accounted for 1% of all admissions.

Haile, A. *Fistula – a sociomedical problem.* Ethiopian Medical Journal 1983: 21(2): 71-78. WHE1155

An inquiry using clinical records and a questionnaire was made into the condition of 18 obstetric fistula patients who came for treatment at the Gondar Hospital, Ethiopia, between December 1979 and February 1981.

All patients were Amharas, illiterate and poor. All the women were dependent economically on their husbands, and their marriages had been arranged by parents at ages as young as five, with a mean marriage age of 11.5 years. Age distribution showed that 50% of the women were aged between 15 and 20 years. Only six women had been

delivered in hospital or a clinic, and this was only after prolonged obstructed labour. All but one of the deliveries leading to the formation of fistulae had resulted in the baby's death. Only half of the patients had received some advice about pregnancy and birth from traditional birth attendants. The others had had no information. The problem of lack of transport to health services and distances to be travelled, is stressed.

Most of the women felt extreme shame at their condition. Two-thirds of them had stopped attending church and other social services, and more than half of them were divorced - ten of them had been abandoned by their husbands when they acquired fistulae. Ten women were too severely incapacitated to carry out their normal duties as housewives. Six were reduced to begging.

Recommendations for preventive measures are given and include the training of traditional birth attendants and midwives, literacy campaigns and health education with a strong bias towards maternal and child health care, and raising by law the minimum age of marriage.

Kelly, J. *Vesico-vaginal fistulae.* British Journal of Urology 1979: 51: 208-210 WHE2141.

A report on repair of 161 obstetric fistulae in women aged between 16 and 68 is presented. One hundred and twenty-eight of the women were in Africa (mostly Ethiopia) and 33 in Britain. Twenty-six of the cases (79%) in Britain were caused through obstetric or gynaecological surgery, while 121 cases (95%) in Africa were caused by pressure necrosis from obstructed labour. Surgical techniques are described. In Africa 100 women (81%) were cured at the first attempt, with 15 (12%) having stress incontinence, and 13 (8%) not cured. Those with stress incontinence all had fistulae involving the urethra and bladder base. With perineal exercises over several months, the incontinence disappeared in 7 women.

Thirty-three of the patients became pregnant within one year of the repair, 18 of whom were delivered by caesarean section and 12 vaginally, all with satisfactory outcomes and no breakdown of the fistulae repair. The three remaining African women, delayed by poor roads, had unattended deliveries which resulted in stillbirths and breakdown of the fistulae repair.

Perine, P.L. et al. *Pelvic inflammatory disease and puerperal sepsis in Ethiopia, 1. Etiology.* American Journal of Obstetrics and Gynecology 1980; 138(7): 969-973: WHE1201

A survey of hospital records of 1,329 women admitted to the gynaecology wards of St. Paul's Hospital, Addis Ababa, from 1983-85, revealed that 297 (30%) had pelvic inflammatory disease and another 132 (10%) had puerperal sepsis. Twelve of these 529 patients died of their infections and the remainder were hospitalized for an average of 12.4 days. A similar pattern of illness was seen in the outpatient clinics. Lack of obstetric services and hence delivery at home frequently resulted in women presenting on an emergency basis with a diagnosis of obstructed labour, intrauterine infection, ruptured uterus or fistula formation, causing gross pelvic sepsis and peritonitis.

Neissera gonorrhoeae is probably the prime cause of genital sepsis in Ethiopia. Moreover, N. gonorrhoeae was also frequently isolated from asymptomatic parturient women and from those with puerperal sepsis. The former went untreated since they were discharged the day after delivery, before the results of the culture were known. The majority of the patients with puerperal sepsis had a polymicrobial endometritis, which was initiated by retained placental tissue or blood clots. Most of these women were delivered at home, attended only by traditional midwives, and could not be given oxytocic drugs to prevent postpartum haemorrhage or retention of blood clots and placental tissue.

Tsega, E. *Viral hepatitis during pregnancy in Ethiopia.* East African Medical Journal 1976; 53(5): 270-277. WHE1451

Both retrospective and prospective studies were undertaken to evaluate the effects of viral hepatitis during pregnancy at St. Paul's Hospital in Addis Ababa between July 1972 and August 1973. In the retrospective group there were 37 pregnant and 28 non-pregnant cases and in the prospective group 47 pregnant and 36 non-pregnant, making a total of 84 pregnant patients and 64 non-pregnant. The incidence of fulminant hepatitis was significantly higher in the pregnant group (30 with 19 deaths) than in the non-pregnant group (12 with seven deaths).

Hepatitis had adverse effects on the outcome of pregnancy and the survival of the foetus. Fulminant hepatitis with maternal and foetal mortality was more common in the third trimester. Undernutrition is probably an important factor in adversely influencing the course of hepatitis in pregnancy.

8. FURTHER READING

Boerma, T. *The magnitude of the maternal mortality problem in Sub-Saharan Africa.* Social Science and Medicine 1987; 24(6): 551-558. WHE1532

Chang, W.P. *Population studies in Ethiopia: knowledge, attitudes and practice surveys in population and health.* Journal of Ethiopian Studies 1974; XII(1): Addis Ababa, Ethiopia. WHE0127

Cook, R. *Damage to physical health from pharaonic circumcision (infibulation) of females.* Paper pre-pared for Seminar on Traditional Practices Affecting the Health of Women and Children in Africa 1984, 6-10 February, Dakar, Senegal WHE1911

Duncan, M.E. et al. *Pelvic inflammatory disease and puerperal sepsis in Ethiopia, II. Treatment.* American Journal of Obstetrics and Gynecology 1980; 138(7.2): 1059-1063. WHE1624

Hamlin, R.H.J. and Nicholson, E.C. Experiences in the treatment of 600 vaginal fistulas and in the management of 80 labours which have followed the repair of these injuries. *Ethiopian Medical Journal* 1966; 4: 189-192. WHE 2576

Kelly, J. Vesicovaginal fistula (letter). *Lancet,* 1989; 8654: 109. WHE 2581

Kloos, H. et al. *Illness and health behaviour in Addis Ababa and rural Central Ethiopia.* Social Science and Medicine 1987; 25(9): 1003-1019 WHE1777

Kwast, B. E. *Unsafe motherhood - a monumental challenge. A study of maternal mortality in Addis Ababa* Leiderdorp, Netherlands 1988. WHE 2583

McGinley, M.M. (ed.) *Poverty and pregnancy – a deadly combination.* Medical Mission Sisters News 1988: XVIII9(3): Philadelphia, USA. WHE2246

Naeye, R.L. et al. *Epidemiological features of perinatal death due to obstructed labour in Addis Ababa.* British Journal of Obstetrics and Gynaecology 1977; 84: 747-750. WHE1830

Okubagzhi, G.S. *Fulfilling the potential of traditional birth attendants.* World Health Forum 1988; 9: 426-431. WHE2056

Tadesse, E. et al. Determinants of perinatal deaths: a five-year retrospective survey at Tikur Anbessa Teaching Hospital. *Journal of Obstetrics and Gynaecology of Eastern and Central Africa,* 1989; 8: 15-17. WHE 2578

Tafari, N. et al. *Health services research towards health for all by the year 2000 in Ethiopia.* (Unpublished document) 1980 WHE0687

Vorperian, K.A. *Rupture of the uterus: a clinical study of 97 cases.* Department of Obstetrics and Gynaecology, Addis Ababa University. WHE0961

9. DATA SOURCES

WHE 0436 Mariam, W.K. *Data on reproductive health in Ethiopia.* in: WHO Regional Multidisciplinary Meeting on Human Reproduction, Yaounde 4-7 December 1978. (Unpublished WHO document No. HRP/REM/78.11).

WHE 0596 Kwast, B. et al. *Maternal mortality in Addis Ababa, Ethiopia,* Swedish Save the Children Federation 1984

WHE 0731 United Nations Fund for Population Activities. *Report of mission on needs assessment for population assistance – Ethiopia.* New York 1980

WHE 0800 World Health Organization. *Country reports to regional offices of the progress in implementing Health for All by the Year 2000.* (Unpublished documents) 1983

WHE 0834 World Health Organization *World Health Statistics annual – vital statistics and causes of death.* Geneva, various years

WHE 1120 Kwast, B. et al. *Epidemiology of maternal mortality in Addis Ababa: a community based study.* Ethiopian Medical Journal 1985; 23(7): 7-26

WHE 1318 Ethiopia. *Health survey.* Unpublished tabulations, 1983

WHE 1446 Kwast, B. et al. *Maternal mortality in Addis Ababa, Ethiopia.* Studies in Family Planning 1986; 17(6): 288-301

WHE 1712 Mauldin, W.P. and Segal, S.J. *Prevalence of contraceptive use in developing countries. A chart book.* New York, Rockefeller Foundation 1986

WHE 1803 Kwast, B. and Stevens, J.A. *Viral hepatitis as a major cause of maternal mortality in Addis Ababa, Ethiopia.* International Journal of Gynaecology and Obstetrics 1987; 25: 99-106

WHE 1914 United Nations Children's Fund (UNICEF). *The state of the world's children,* various years, Oxford, Oxford University Press

WHE 1915 United Nations. Department of International Economic and Social Affairs. *World population prospects: estimates and projections as assessed in 1984.* Population Studies No. 98. New York 1986

WHE 1918 United Nations. Department of International Economic and Social Affairs. *First marriage: patterns and determinants.* New York 1988

WHE 1967 Kwast, B. and Liff, J.M. *Factors associated with maternal mortality in Addis Ababa, Ethiopia.* International Journal of Epidemiology 1988; 17(1): 115-121

WHE 1979 Kwast, B. *Maternity services and TBAs in Addis Ababa: biosocial factors related to birth place and outcome of pregnancy.* Health Policy and Planning 1988; 3(2): 109-118

WHE 2008 World Health Organization. Regional Office for Africa *Evaluation of the strategy for health for all by the year 2000. Seventh report on the world health situation* Vol 2, African region, Brazzaville 1987

WHE 2033 World Health Organization. *Global strategy for health for all by the year 2000. Second report on monitoring progress.* WHO document EB83/2 Add. 1 1988

WHE 2247 Yoseph, S. and Kifle, G. *A six-year review of maternal mortality in a teaching hospital in Addis Ababa.* Ethiopian Medical Journal 1988; 26: 115-120

WHE 2577 Kwast, B. et al. Confidential enquiries into maternal deaths in Addis Ababa, Ethiopia 1981-1983. *Journal of Obstetrics and Gynaecology of East and Central Africa* 8, 1989; 75-82

WHE 2580 Frost, O. Maternal and perinatal deaths in an Addis Ababa hospital, 1980. *Ethiopian Medical Journal,* 1984; 22: 143-146

GABON

	Year	Source

1. BASIC INDICATORS

1.1 Demographic

1.1.1 Population

Size (millions)	1.1	1888	(1914)
Rate of growth (%)	3.8	1988	(1914)

1.1.2 Life expectancy

Female	51	1980-85	(1915)
Male	47	1980-85	(1915)

1.1.3 Fertility

Crude Birth Rate	39	1988	(1914)
Total Fertility Rate	5.0	1988	(1914)

1.1.4 Mortality

Crude Death Rate	16	1988	(1914)
Infant Mortality Rate	102	1988	(1914)
Female			
Male			
1-4 years mortality rate			
Female			
Male			

1.2 Social and economic

1.2.1 Adult literacy rate (%)

Female	53	1985	(1914)
Male	70	1985	(1914)

1.2.2 Primary school enrolment rate (%)

Female	
Male	

1.2.3 Female mean age at first marriage

(years)	17.7	1960	(1918)

1.2.4 GNP/capita

(US $)	2 700	1987	(1914)

1.2.5 Daily per capita calorie supply

(as % of requirements)	107	1984-86	(1914)

2. HEALTH SERVICES

2.1 Health expenditure

2.1.1 Expenditure on health

(as % of GNP)	3	1987	(2033)

2.1.2 Expenditure on PHC

(as % of total health expenditure)	34	1987	(2033)

2.2 Primary Health Care
(Percentage of population covered by):

2.2.1 Health services

National	80	1983	(0834)
Urban			
Rural			

2.2.2 Safe water

National	50	1983	(0834)
Urban	75	1980	(0834)
Rural	34	1980	(0834)

2.2.3 Adequate sanitary facilities

National	50	1983	(0834)
Urban			
Rural			

2.2.4 Contraceptive prevalence rate
(%)

2.3 Coverage of maternity care (%)

Area	Prenatal care	Trained attendant	Institutional deliveries	Postnatal care	Sample size	Year	Source
National	73					1983	(0834)
National	90	80				1983	(2008)

3. COMMUNITY STUDIES

4. HOSPITAL STUDIES

4.1 Centre Hospitalier de Libreville, 1984-87 [1904, 2420]

4.1.1 Rate

	1984-86	1987
Live births	23 187	8 271
Maternal deaths	34	14
MMR (per 100 000 live births)	147	169

4.1.2 Causes of maternal deaths, 1984-87

	Number	%
Haemorrhage	9	19
Abortions	8	17
Ectopic pregnancy	7	15
Sepsis	6	13
Ruptured uterus	4	8
Hypertensive disorders of pregnancy	5	10
Embolism	1	2
Complication of caesarean section	1	2
DIRECT CAUSES	41	85
Cardiopathies	3	6
Hepatitis	2	4
Other infections	1	2
INDIRECT CAUSES	6	13
Unknown	1	2
TOTAL	48	100

There were 12 postoperative deaths, of which seven followed intervention for ectopic pregnancy and five were subsequent to caesarean section. There were 509 admissions for ectopic pregnancy in all, a death-to-case ratio of 13.6 per 1000, and there were a total of 682 caesarean sections, a death-to-case ratio of 7.3 per 1000.

4.1.3 Avoidable factors.
Lack of trained personnel

Six of the nine provinces of Gabon were without the services of a specialist obstetrician. In addition, neither the health centres nor the provincial hospitals had a 24 hour service.

Delays in transfer

The absence of proper roads made transfer of emergency cases very difficult. Even within the hospital, there were inordinate delays in transfer of the patient to the operative block.

Absence of a blood bank

Patients suffering haemorrhage were often kept waiting for operative intervention until a donor with a matching blood group was found.

Inadequate equipment in the hospital

There was severe overcrowding, with a bed occupancy rate of 130%. Supplies of drugs were inadequate, and treatment was sometimes delayed until the patient's family bought drugs from a pharmacy.

4.1.4 High risk groups
Multiparity [2352]

A study of the risks to mothers of multiple pregnancies was carried out at the Centre Hospitalier de Libreville between 1985 and 1988. The perinatal mortality of twins is four times higher than in single pregnancies, maternal pathology consists in frequent hypertensive complications and severe anaemia. Maternal morbidity and mortality are higher than in single deliveries. Death is mainly due to haemorrhage. Haemorrhage occurred in 7.6% of multiple pregnancies compared with 4.6% of all pregnancies. The maternal mortality rate for multiple pregnancies was 244 per 100 000 pregnancies compared with 100 per 100 000 for singleton pregnancies. There is no blood bank available; transfusion is dependent on relatives and there are no blood screening tests.

5. CIVIL REGISTRATION DATA/GOVERNMENT ESTIMATES

5.1 Six provinces, 1983 [1904, 2389]

5.1.1 Rate

Province	MMR (per 100 000 live births)
Estuaire (Libreville)	220
Haut Ogooue (Franceville)	160
Nyanga (Tchibanga)	220
Ogooue Ivindo (Makokou)	990
Ogooue Maritime (Port-Gentil)	400
Woleu-Ntem (Oyem)	530
Gabon	190

6. OTHER SOURCES/ESTIMATES

7. SELECTED ANNOTATED BIBLIOGRAPHY

Picaud, A. et al, Les ruptures utérines: à propos de 31 cas observés au Centre Hospitalier de Libreville (Gabon). *Revue français de Gynécologie et Obstétrique* 1989; 84(5): 411-416. WHE 2394

Over the period 1985-87 there were 31 cases of ruptured uterus for 24 046 deliveries, a frequency of 129 per 100 000 deliveries. 30 of the ruptures occurred during labour; eleven cases resulted from neglected dystocia and a further twelve were ruptures of caesarian scars. There were two maternal deaths, a death-to-case ratio of 6.5%. Only eight patients were treated by simple suturing of the uterus. In all the other cases treatment consisted of total or partial hysterectomy. In Africa, where hysterectomy and the ensuing disappearance of reproductive function entails a loss of status and even social ostracism the consequences of uterine rupture are particularly grave.

8. FURTHER READING

9. DATA SOURCES

WHE 0834   World Health Organization.*World Health Statistics annual – vital statistics and causes of death.* Geneva, various years

WHE 1904   Nlome-Nze, R. et al. *La mortalité maternelle au Centre Hospitalier de Libreville (Gabon).* (unpublished document) 1986

WHE 1914   United Nations Children's Fund (UNICEF). *The state of the world's children,* various years, Oxford, Oxford University Press

WHE 1915   United Nations. Department of International Economic and Social Affairs. *World population prospects: estimates and projections as assessed in 1984.* Population Studies No. 98. New York 1986

WHE 1918   United Nations. Department of International Economic and Social Affairs. *First marriage: patterns and determinants.* New York 1988

WHE 2008   World Health Organization. Regional Office for Africa. *Evaluation of the strategy for health for all by the year 2000. Seventh report on the world health situation* Vol 2, African region, Brazzaville 1987

WHE 2033   World Health Organization. *Global strategy for health for all by the year 2000. Second report on monitoring progress.* WHO document EB83/2 Add. 1, 1988

WHE 2352   Picaud, A. et al. Risques périnatal et maternel des grossesses multiples. *Revue français de Gynécologie et Obstétrique* 1989; 84(5): 381-391

WHE 2389   Belgharbi, L. *Rapport sur la situation socio-sanitaire des femmes et des enfants en République Gabonaise.* Ministère de la Santé Publique et de la Population 1986

WHE 2420   Picaud, A. et al. La mortalité maternelle au Centre Hospitalier de Libreville (1984-87). *Journal de Gynécologie et d'Obstétrique et Biologie Réproductive* 1989; 18: 445-450

NOTES

NOTES

GAMBIA

		Year	Source

1. BASIC INDICATORS

1.1 Demographic

1.1.1 Population

		Year	Source
Size (millions)	0.7	1987	(1915)
Rate of growth (%)	1.9	1980-85	(1915)

1.1.2 Life expectancy

		Year	Source
Female	37	1980-85	(1915)
Male	34	1980-85	(1915)

1.1.3 Fertility

		Year	Source
Crude Birth Rate	48	1980-85	(1915)
Total Fertility Rate	6.4	1980-85	(1915)

1.1.4 Mortality

		Year	Source
Crude Death Rate	29	1980-85	(1915)
Infant Mortality Rate	162	1987	(2033)
Female			
Male			
1-4 years mortality rate			
Female			
Male			

1.2 Social and economic

1.2.1 Adult literacy rate (%)

		Year	Source
Female	15	1985	(1914)
Male	36	1985	(1914)

1.2.2 Primary school enrolment rate (%)

		Year	Source
Female	47	1986-88	(1914)
Male	76	1986-88	(1914)

1.2.3 Female mean age at first marriage
(years)

1.2.4 GNP/capita

		Year	Source
(US $)	250	1983	2008

1.2.5 Daily per capita calorie supply
(as % of requirements)

2. HEALTH SERVICES

2.1 Health expenditure

2.1.1 Expenditure on health
(as % of GNP)

2.1.2 Expenditure on PHC

(as % of total health expenditure)	7	1983	(2008)

2.2 Primary Health Care
(Percentage of population covered by):

2.2.1 Health services

		Year	Source
National	90	1985	(0834)
Urban			
Rural			

2.2.2 Safe water

		Year	Source
National	45	1983	(0834)
Urban	100	1983	(0834)
Rural	33	1983	(0834)

2.2.3 Adequate sanitary facilities

		Year	Source
National	77	1983	(0834)
Urban			
Rural			

2.2.4 Contraceptive prevalence rate

(%)	1	1977	(1712)

2.3   Coverage of maternity care (%)

Area	Prenatal care	Trained attendant	Institutional deliveries	Postnatal care	Sample size	Year	Source
National	90	80				1983	(0834)
National	90	85				1984	(2008)
National: rural			15		314	1985	(1971)
Farafenni	34	5	5			1982-83	(2333)
Farafenni	40	48	6			1984-87	(2333)

3.   COMMUNITY STUDIES

3.1   Kaneba and Manduar villages, West Kiang district, 1951-83 [0289, 1131]

An intensive longitudinal study of two adjacent Gambian villages, Kaneba and Manduar, gives data on a range of demographic issues including maternal mortality, for the period 1951-1983.

3.1.1   Rate

1951-1975	Kaneba	Manduar
Live births	1 138	423
Maternal deaths	12	4
MMR (per 100 000 live births)	1 054	946

There were no maternal deaths in either of the villages between 1975 and 1983. This decline in maternal mortality was a direct outcome of the opening of an outpatient clinic in the area with 24-hour availability of a physician or qualified midwife. On the basis of estimates of maternal mortality elsewhere in rural Gambia, around 16 deaths could have been expected. Some idea of potential mortality can be gained from the fact that in 1983 alone, 19 women were referred to hospital, nine prenatally and ten perinatally, for various complications including severe antepartum or postpartum haemorrhage, preeclampsia and obstructed labour.

3.2   41 villages and hamlets, Farafenni area, North Bank Division, 1982-87 [1772, 2333]

The study was carried out during a five-year period, 1982-87, in 41 villages and hamlets on the north bank of the River Gambia around the town of Farafenni. The population of the study area at the mid point of the survey was 13 780 of which 2 738 were women aged 15-44 years. During the period of the investigation the town nearly doubled in size and although transport remained difficult there were considerable improvements.

Prior to the introduction of a primary health care programme a survey on the outcome of pregnancy was carried out during 1982-83. New pregnancies were identified by a member of each study village selected as reporter. This information was relayed to a group of field workers who were each responsible for about five villages. The outcome of pregnancy was determined by field staff who visited each village regularly. All reports of a maternal death were investigated by a physician.

In 1983 the Government's PHC programme was introduced into the Farafenni district. 15 of the 16 eligible villages have joined the project. Selected traditional birth attendants received a ten-week training course and were supplied with an obstetric pack at the end of the course.

Also in 1983 a new health centre manned by a team of 2-4 doctors was opened in Farafenni town. However, this health centre does not have any facilities for major surgery or for blood transfusions and patients who require either of these have to cross the river by an uncertain ferry to reach the specialist hospital at Banjul, a journey of nearly 200km.

Maternal deaths occurring after the introduction of the new health centre and the TBA training courses were investigated using the same techniques as before. It is thought that very few pregnancies were missed. (It is worth noting, however, that in view of the relatively small numbers involved the confidence limits are very wide).

	Pre-intervention 1982-83	Post-intervention 1984-87
Deliveries	672	1 963
Maternal deaths	15	20
MMR (per 100 000 deliveries)	2 232	1 019

The decline in the maternal mortality rate was observed in both villages which were the object of the PHC programme and in those which were not, but the decline was more marked in the former. However, the differences are not statistically significant.

	1982-83	1984-87
PHC-villages		
Deliveries	405	1 236
Maternal deaths	11	13
MMR (per 100 000 deliveries)	2 716	1 052
Non-PHC-villages		
Deliveries	267	727
Maternal deaths	4	7
MMR (per 100 000 deliveries)	1 498	963

3.2.2 Causes of maternal deaths (PHC villages only)

	1982-83	1984-87
Haemorrhage	5	5
Sepsis	2	0
Hypertensive disorders of pregnancy	0	3
Jaundice	0	1
Other	2	2
Unknown	2	2
TOTAL	11	13

3.2.3 Avoidable factors, 1982-83 (All villages)

In eleven of the fifteen cases, death occurred either before or within four hours of delivery and was associated with haemorrhage or sudden collapse. There were no resuscitation facilities at the nearest dispensary, and the government hospital at Banjul, the nearest place where blood transfusion and obstetric services were available, is several hours journey away, including a ferry crossing of the river Gambia.

Eleven of the fifteen women who died had been seen at least once at a prenatal clinic but none had been referred for health centre delivery. The author concludes that since maternal deaths in the area are mainly due to catastrophic episodes at the time of delivery, ways of preventing these should include:

- upgrading health centres to provide blood transfusion facilities and the services of an obstetrician;

- encouraging 'at risk' mothers to deliver in health centres, and making available a place for mothers to stay near a health centre prior to delivery.

3.2.4 High risk groups, 1982-83

The mean age of the mothers who died was very similar to that of the 657 pregnant women who survived. Death occurred more frequently among primigravidae (2 out of 7; 286 per 1000) and among women who had five or more pregnancies (8 out of 176; 45 per 1000) than among women who had had one to four pregnancies (5 out of 420; 12 per 1000).

3.3 Six villages around Farafenni, 1987 [2355]

The study describes a field trial of a new indirect technique, the "sisterhood method", for deriving population-based estimates of maternal mortality, using the proportions of adult sisters dying during pregnancy, childbirth or the puerperium reported by adults during a survey.

3.3.1 Rate

Maternal deaths	91
MMR (per 100 000 live births)	1 005

3.4 Eastern, Central and Western Regions 1985 [1652]

3.4.1 Rate

A community study carried out in 1985 based on interviews with 6 000 married men with 9 195 wives.

Region	Western	Central	Eastern	Total
Live births	897	690	1 315	2 902
Maternal deaths	9	8	13	30
MMR (per 100 000 live births)	1 003	1 159	989	1 034

4. HOSPITAL STUDIES

5. CIVIL REGISTRATION DATA/GOVERNMENT ESTIMATES

6. OTHER SOURCES/ ESTIMATES

6.1 National, 1984 [1338]

6.1.1 Rate

According to a WHO report, the maternal mortality rate for 1984 was estimated to be 1 500 per 100 000 live births.

7. SELECTED ANNOTATED BIBLIOGRAPHY

8. FURTHER READING

Brabin, B.J., An analysis of malaria in pregnancy in Africa. *Bulletin of the World Health Organization* 1983; 61(6): 1005-1016. WHE 0104

Graham, W. and Brass, W., Estimating maternal mortality in developing countries. Letter. *Lancet* 20 February 1988. WHE 1958

Heini, A. et al, Total daily energy expenditure and heart rate during pregnancy in free-living Gambian women. *Nestlé Foundation Annual Report* 1988. WHE 2197

Lawrence, M. et al, The composition of weight gained during pregnancy and its relationship to birthweight. *Nestlé Foundation Annual Report* 1988. WHE 2221

Prentice, A.M. et al, Dietary supplementation of lactating Gambian women. II. Effect on maternal health, nutritional status and biochemistry. *Human Nutrition* Clinical Nutrition 1983; 37(1): 65-74. WHE 1206

9. DATA SOURCES

WHE 0289   Billewicz, W.Z. and McGregor, I.A., The demography of two west African (Gambian) villages, 1951-1975. *Journal of Biosocial Science* 1981; 13(2): 219-240

WHE 0834   World Health Organization *World Health Statistics annual - vital statistics and causes of death.* Geneva, various years

WHE 1131   Lamb, W.H. et al, Changes in maternal and child mortality rates in three isolated villages over ten years. *Lancet* October 20 1984

WHE 1338   World Health Organization, Africa Regional Office, *Where are we in PHC? Countries take a close look at themselves through PHC reviews.* Part 2. Swaziland 7-15 October 1985

WHE 1652   Yaya Sanyang, *Maternal mortality survey: preliminary results.* (memorandum to the Director of Medical Services) 1985

WHE 1712   Mauldin W.P. and Segal, S.J., *Prevalence of contraceptive use in developing countries. A chart book.* Rockefeller Foundation, New York 1986

WHE 1772   Greenwood A. et al, A prospective study of pregnancy in a rural area of The Gambia, West Africa. *Bulletin of the World Health Organization* 1987; 65(5): 635-644

WHE 1914   United Nations Children's Fund (UNICEF). *The state of the world's children,* various years, Oxford, Oxford University Press

WHE 1915   United Nations. Department of International Economic and Social Affairs. *World population prospects: estimates and projections as assessed in 1984.* Population Studies No. 98. New York 1986

WHE 1971   Gambia, Ministry of Health and Social Welfare, *National primary health care review, 1985.* Gambia 1986

WHE 2008   World Health Organization. Regional Office for Africa *Evaluation of the strategy for health for all by the year 2000. Seventh report on the world health situation* Vol 2, African region, Brazzaville 1987

WHE 2033   World Health Organization. *Global strategy for health for all by the year 2000. Second report on monitoring progress.* WHO document EB83/2 Add. 1, 1988

WHE 2333   Greenwood, A.M. et al, Evaluation of a primary health care programme in The Gambia. I The impact of trained traditional birth attendants on the outcome of pregnancy. *Journal of Tropical Medicine and Hygiene.* 1990; 93: 58-66

WHE 2355   Graham, W. et al. Estimating maternal mortality: the sisterhood method. *Studies in Family Planning* 1989; 20(3): 125-135

GHANA

		Year	Source

1. BASIC INDICATORS

1.1 Demographic

1.1.1 Population

Size (millions)	14.1	1988	(1914)
Rate of growth (%)	3.4	1980-87	(1914)

1.1.2 Life expectancy

Female	54	1980-85	(1915)
Male	50	1980-85	(1915)

1.1.3 Fertility

Crude Birth Rate	44	1988	(1914)
Total Fertility Rate	6.4	1988	(1914)

1.1.4 Mortality

Crude Death Rate	13	1988	(1914)
Infant Mortality Rate	89	1988	(1914)
Female	74	1978-87	(2009)
Male	89	1978-87	(2009)
1-4 years mortality rate			
Female	79	1978-87	(2009)
Male	78	1978-87	(2009)

1.2 Social and economic

1.2.1 Adult literacy rate (%)

Female	43	1985	(1914)
Male	64	1985	(1914)

1.2.2 Primary school enrolment rate (%)

Female	63	1986-88	(1914)
Male	78	1986-88	(1914)

1.2.3 Female mean age at first marriage

(years)	19.4	1971	(1918)

1.2.4 GNP/capita

(US $)	390	1987	(1914)

1.2.5 Daily per capita calorie supply

(as % of requirements)	76	1984-86	(1914)

2. HEALTH SERVICES

2.1 Health expenditure

2.1.1 Expenditure on health

(as % of GNP)	1	1987	(2033)

2.1.2 Expenditure on PHC

(as % of total health expenditure)	25	1987	(2033)

2.2 Primary Health Care
(Percentage of population covered by):

2.2.1 Health services

National	60	1985-87	(1914)
Urban	90	1985-87	(1914)
Rural	45	1985-87	(1914)

2.2.2 Safe water

National	56	1985-87	(1914)
Urban	93	1985-87	(1914)
Rural	39	1985-87	(1914)

2.2.3 Adequate sanitary facilities

National	26	1983	(0834)
Urban	47	1983	(0834)
Rural	17	1983	(0834)

2.2.4 Contraceptive prevalence rate

(%)	13	1983-88	(2009)

2.3   Coverage of maternity care (%)

Area	Prenatal care	Trained attendant	Institutional deliveries	Postnatal care	Sample size	Year	Source
National	88	73				1984	(0834)
National	82	40			4 096	1983-88	(2009)
National:							
urban	94	70			1 114	1983-88	(2009)
rural	78	31			2 982	1983-88	(2009)
Western	89	40			360	1983-88	(2009)
Central	78	31			466	1983-88	(2009)
Eastern	88	39			591	1983-88	(2009)
Greater Accra	91	72			400	1983-88	(2009)
Volta	81	33			532	1983-88	(2009)
Upper West, East & Northern	54	13			544	1983-88	(2009)

3.   COMMUNITY STUDIES

3.1   Danfa district, 1972 [1280]

3.1.1   Rate

An attempt to estimate maternal mortality was undertaken by the Danfa comprehensive rural health and family planning project. A rate of 400 per 100 000 live births was found for 1972, but with wide confidence intervals.

4.   HOSPITAL STUDIES

4.1   All health units and private maternity homes, 1983 [1010]

4.1.1   Rate

Region	Live births	Maternal deaths	MMR (per 100 000 live births)
Greater Accra	15 068	21	139
Eastern Region	11 760	32	272
Western Region	1 003	1	100
Ashanti	2 970	33	1 111

4.1.1   Rate *(Continued)*

Region	Live births	Maternal deaths	MMR (per 100 000 live births)
Central Region	3 949	47	1 190
Brong Ahafo	6 737	27	400
Northern Region	173	0	—
Upper Region	2 767	14	506
Volta Region	2 069	17	822
TOTAL	46 496	192	413

4.2   Maternity Hospital, Accra, 1963-67 [0033]

4.2.1   Rate

Deliveries	35 193
Maternal deaths	378
MMR (per 100 000 deliveries)	1 074

4.2.2   Causes of maternal deaths

Haemorrhage, obstructed labour and uterine rupture together accounted for a third of all maternal deaths. Cephalo-pelvic disproportion was widely prevalent and was the most common indication for caesarean section. In 28 of the 33 deaths from ruptured uterus, the rupture was the result of untreated obstructed labour, and in only five cases was there rupture of a previous scar. Ectopic pregnancy was far more common in this series than is usually the case, and was due to widespread chronic salpingitis in the area. Infective hepatitis was the most common infectious disease causing maternal deaths.

	Number	%
Haemorrhage	63	17
Hypertensive disorders of pregnancy	35	9
Abortion	33	9
Uterine rupture	33	9
Ectopic pregnancy	27	7
Obstructed labour	26	7
Sepsis	24	6
Complications of anesthesia	8	2
DIRECT CAUSES	249	66
Hepatitis	28	7
Sickle cell disease	23	6
Anaemia	7	2
Other infections	26	7
Other indirect causes	45	12
INDIRECT CAUSES	129	34
TOTAL	378	100

4.2.3 Avoidable factors

Although a blood bank was available, supply was inadequate. Patients requiring transfusion had to depend on blood donations from relatives. Supply was, therefore, very unreliable and blood was not always available when most urgently needed.

4.3 Korle-Bu University Teaching Hospital, Accra, 1981-82 (0398, 1112)

4.3.1 Rate

Live births	4 990
Maternal deaths	11
MMR (per 100 000 live births)	220

4.3.2 Causes of maternal deaths for 69 cases, 1962-64 (0398)

	Number	%
Hypertensive disorders of pregnancy	11	16
Sepsis	10	15
Haemorrhage	7	10
Uterine rupture	5	7
Postoperative shock	5	7
Embolisms	4	6
Ectopic pregnancy	3	4
DIRECT CAUSES	45	65
Hepatitis	8	12
Sickle cell disease	3	4
Other indirect causes	13	19
INDIRECT CAUSES	24	35
TOTAL	69	100

5. CIVIL REGISTRATION DATA/GOVERNMENT ESTIMATES

5.1 National, 1984 (1338)

5.1.1 Rate

At the 1984 census the maternal mortality rate was estimated at between 500 and 1 500 per 100 000 live births.

6. OTHER ESTIMATES

6.1 National, 1974 (0028)

6.1.1 Rate

A rate of 390 per 100 000 live births in 1974 is quoted in a review paper presented at a WHO regional seminar.

6.2 Accra, 1974 (0503)

6.2.1 Rate

The source quotes a maternal mortality rate of 800 per 100 000 live births for 1974.

6.3 National (0036)

6.3.1 Rate

An article published in 1977 mentions a maternal mortality rate of 500 to 1000 per 100 000 live births for Ghana.

7. SELECTED ANNOTATED BIBLIOGRAPHY

Ashworth, F.L. Urinary vaginal fistulae: a series of 152 patients treated in a small hospital in Ghana. *West African Medical Journal* 1973; 22(2): 39-43. WHE 1030

A study was carried out over a period of seven years of 152 cases of urinary vaginal fistulae at the Baptist Medical Centre at Nalerigu, a rural area of Northern Ghana, about 340 miles from the nearest specialist gynaecological unit. All but one case were obstetric in origin. It was not possible to establish the age of the women, but in terms of parity, the highest percentage (28%) were parity 1, with 16% at parity 2, and steadily declining numbers with increased parity. Multiple fistulae were present in 35 patients. Associated conditions included excoriation of the vulva, and there were three cases of vesical calculus.

There was a 74% operative success rate, with 12% of stress incontinence, and 8% of cases where urinary diversion into the rectum was the only solution. The author discusses the operative procedures, stressing the difficulties of such an operation. He also points out that subsequent pregnancy is not indicated, but given that nearly half the women had no living children in a society which regards childlessness as a great affliction, societal pressures make this difficult.

8. FURTHER READING

Ampofo, D.A., The dynamics of induced abortion and its social implications in Ghana. *Ghana Medical Journal* 1970; 9(4): 295-302. WHE 0035

Belcher, D.W. et al, A household morbidity survey in rural Africa. *International Journal of Epidemiology* 1976; 5(2): 113-120. WHE 2200

Boerma, J.T. *Maternal mortality in sub-Saharan Africa: levels, causes and interventions* 1987. WHE 1655

Frank, O. The demand for fertility control in sub-Saharan Africa. Working paper no. 117. *Studies in Family Planning 1987;* 18(4): 181-201. WHE 1371

Lamptey, P. et al, Abortion experience among obstetric patients at Korle-Bu Hospital, Accra, Ghana. *Journal of Biosocial Science* 1985; 17(2): 195-203. WHE 0347

9. DATA SOURCES

WHE 0028   Alihonou, E. *Pregnancy and delivery* in World Health Organization Regional Multidisciplinary Consultative Meeting on Human Reproduction, , 4-7 December 1978 (unpublished WHO document no. HRP/RMC/78.6)

WHE 0033   Ampofo, D.A., Causes of maternal deaths and comments, Maternity Hospital, Accra 1963-67. *West African Medical Journal* 1969; 18(3): 75-81

WHE 0036   Ampofo, D.A. et al, The training of traditional birth attendants in Ghana: experience of the Danfa rural health project. *Tropical and Geographical Medicine* 1977; 29(2): 197-203

WHE 0398   Kovi, J. and Laing, W.N., Pathology of maternal deaths in Accra. *Ghana Medical Journal* 1965; 4(4): 146-149

WHE 0503   Ojo, O.A. and Savage, V.Y., A ten-year review of maternal mortality rates in the University Hospital, Ibadan, Nigeria. *American Journal of Obstetrics and Gynecology* 1974; 118(4): 517-522

WHE 0834   World Health Organization *World Health Statistics annual – vital statistics and causes of death.* Geneva, various years

WHE 1010   Ghana, *Annual report: midwives' monthly returns – all regions.* 1983

WHE 1112   Janowitz, B. et al, *Reproductive health in Africa: issues and options.* Family Health International, North Carolina 1984

WHE 1280   Danfa. *Comprehensive rural health and family planning project, Ghana.* University of Ghana Medical School, Department of Community Health, Accra 1979

WHE 1338   World Health Organization. African Regional Office, *Where are we in PHC? Countries take a close look at themselves through PHC reviews.* Part II. 7-15 October 1985

WHE 1712   Mauldin W.P. and Segal, S.J., *Prevalence of contraceptive use in developing countries. A chart book.* Rockefeller Foundation, New York 1986

WHE 1914   United Nations Children's Fund (UNICEF). *The state of the world's children,* various years, Oxford, Oxford University Press

WHE 1915   United Nations. Department of International Economic and Social Affairs. *World population prospects: estimates and projections as assessed in 1984.* Population Studies No. 98. New York 1986

WHE 1918   United Nations. Department of International Economic and Social Affairs. *First marriage: patterns and determinants.* New York 1988

WHE 2009   Demographic and Health Surveys, *Ghana demographic and health survey 1988.* Ghana Statistical Service and Westinghouse 1988

WHE 2033   World Health Organization. *Global strategy for health for all by the year 2000. Second report on monitoring progress.* WHO document EB83/2 Add. 1, 1988

GUINEA

		Year	Source

1. BASIC INDICATORS

1.1 Demographic

1.1.1 Population

Size (millions)	6.5	1988	(1914)
Rate of growth (%)	2.4	1980-87	(1914)

1.1.2 Life expectancy

Female	42	1980-85	(1915)
Male	39	1980-85	(1915)

1.1.3 Fertility

Crude Birth Rate	47	1988	(1914)
Total Fertility Rate	6.2	1988	(1914)

1.1.4 Mortality

Crude Death Rate	22	1988	(1914)
Infant Mortality Rate	146	1988	(1914)
Female			
Male			
1-4 years mortality rate			
Female			
Male			

1.2 Social and economic

1.2.1 Adult literacy rate (%)

Female	17	1985	(1914)
Male	40	1985	(1914)

1.2.2 Primary school enrolment rate (%)

Female	18	1986-88	(1914)
Male	41	1986-88	(1914)

1.2.3 Female mean age at first marriage
(years)

1.2.4 GNP/capita

(US $)	320	1987	(2033)

1.2.5 Daily per capita calorie supply

(as % of requirements)	77	1987	(1914)

2. HEALTH SERVICES

2.1 Health expenditure

2.1.1 Expenditure on health

(as % of GNP)	2	1987	(2033)

2.1.2 Expenditure on PHC
(as % of total health expenditure)

2.2 Primary Health Care
(Percentage of population covered by):

2.2.1 Health services

National	32	1985-87	(2033)
Urban			
Rural			

2.2.2 Safe water

National	19	1985-87	(1914)
Urban	62	1987	(2033)
Rural	12	1987	(2033)

2.2.3 Adequate sanitary facilities

National	12	1980	(0834)
Urban	54	1980	(0834)
Rural	1	1980	(0834)

2.2.4 Contraceptive prevalence rate

(%)	1	1977	(1712)

2.3   Coverage of maternity care (%)

Area	Prenatal care	Trained attendant	Institutional deliveries	Postnatal care	Sample size	Year	Source
National			20			(1987)	(1975)
National	36	25				1988	(2033)
Conakry			90			1988	(2757)
Kankan			60-75			1989	(2415)
Labé			10-20			1989	(2415)

3.   COMMUNITY STUDIES

3.1   Conakry, 1989-90 [2757]

A community study was carried out in the urban centre of Conakry (total population 1 million) between July 1989 and June 1990. The area comprises two referral maternity centres attached to the two university hospitals and capable of performing all types of intervention. There are also six maternity homes within the urban agglomeration which cannot, however, undertake any of the major surgical procedures such as caesarean section, forceps delivery, oxytocic treatment etc. In addition there are several private delivery centres run by doctors, midwives or traditional birth attendants.

Data on births were collected from all the maternity centres, both public and private. It was estimated that only 10% of all deliveries took place at home with the assistance of a traditional birth attendant or midwife. A standard reporting form was set up in all the maternity centres and medical and para-medical personnel were trained to identify and report maternal deaths. Additional information on maternal deaths was gathered through the local religious leaders and burial grounds. Detail on the circumstances surrounding each death were obtained from the family. Deaths of women not normally resident in the city were excluded from the analysis.

3.1.1   Rate
Live births	29 860
Maternal deaths	167
MMR (per 100 000 live births)	559

4.   HOSPITAL STUDIES

4.1   Centre Hospitalier Universitaire Donka, Conakry, 1980-82 and 1986 [1908, 1951]

4.1.1   Rate

	MMR (per 100 000 live births)
1980	780
1981	1 030
1982	630
1986	1 247

4.2   Maternité d'Ignace Deen, Conakry 1980-86 [1951, 2395]

4.2.1   Rate

	Births	Maternal deaths	MMR (per 100 000 births)
1980	2 970	27	909
1981	3 028	31	1 024
1982	3 371	30	890
1983	3 222	28	869
1984	3 487	33	946
1985	4 802	32	666
1986	4 592	31	675
1980-86	25 472	212	833

4.2.2 Causes of maternal deaths

	Number	%
Haemorrhage	92	43
Sepsis	42	20
Hypertensive disorders of pregnancy	32	15
Rupture of the uterus	15	7
DIRECT CAUSES	181	85
Cardiopathies	10	5
Pneumonia	7	3
Diabetes	4	2
Hemopathies	4	2
INDIRECT CAUSES	25	12
Other causes	6	3
TOTAL	212	100

4.2.3 Avoidable factors

Over 40% of the deaths occurred within 24 hours of admission and 72% within 72 hours of admission. The vast majority of the patients were in a grave condition or moribund on arrival indicating the need for more rapid referral and for adequate treatment at local level.

4.2.4 High risk groups
Age-group (for 187 deaths)

	Births	Maternal deaths	MMR (per 100 000 births)
<15	226	17	7 522
16-20	3 721	55	1 478
21-25	6 173	30	486
26-30	9 972	34	341
36+	2 030	51	2 512

Parity

	Births	Maternal deaths	MMR (per 100 000 births)
Primiparous	4 613	46	997
Para 2-4	9 718	35	360
Para 5-7	7 419	53	714
Para 7+	3 722	78	2 096

4.2.5 Other findings

4.3 Conakry, 1989 [(2490)]

A study was carried out at the Donka and Ignace Deen hospitals during January and February 1989.

4.3.1 Rate

Live births	3 110
Maternal deaths	28
MMR (per 100 000 live births)	900

5. CIVIL REGISTRATION DATA/GOVERNMENT ESTIMATES

6. OTHER SOURCES/ ESTIMATES

6.1 Kissidougou and Gueckedou, 1986 [(1908)]

6.1.1 Rate

	MMR (per 100 000 live births)
Kissidougou	1 120
Gueckedou	700

6.2 Kankan and Labé, 1989 [(2415)]

6.2.1 Rate

	MMR (per 100 000 live births)
Kankan	500-700
Labé	2 000

7. SELECTED ANNOTATED BIBLIOGRAPHY

Balde, M.D. and Bastert, G. Decrease in uterine rupture in Conakry, Guinea by improvements in transfer management. *International Journal of Gynecology and Obstetrics* 1990; 31: 21-24. WHE 2398

The teaching hospitals of Donka and Ignace Deen receive patients from peripheral maternity units without operative capacities. In most cases patients are transferred by private means of transportation because ambulance and medical personnel are unavailable. In January 1988 a collaborative programme was established between the teaching hospitals and the seven peripheral units. The aim of the programme was to reduce the number of obstetric complications, especially uterine rupture. The incidence of uterine rupture decreased markedly during the study period compared with the two years prior to the study, from 0.20% in 1986 and 0.18% in 1987 to 0.12% during the intervention period 1988. The maternal mortality rate from uterine rupture fell from 56 per 100 000 deliveries in 1986 to 25 per 100 000 deliveries in 1988. The percentage of all maternal deaths due to uterine rupture declined from 28% to 21% over the same period. The authors conclude that the incidence of uterine rupture may be lowered by integration, consultation and feedback between the two levels of medical care. The intensive collaboration leads to better prenatal care as well as earlier transfer of high risk pregnancies and deliveries. From internal evidence it is possible to calculate that the overall maternal mortality fell from 210 per 100 000 deliveries in 1986 to 119 per 100 000 during the study period in 1988.

8. FURTHER READING

9. DATA SOURCES

WHE 0834   World Health Organization. *World Health Statistics annual - vital statistics and causes of death.* Geneva, various years

WHE 1712   Mauldin W.P. and Segal, S.J. *Prevalence of contraceptive use in developing countries. A chart book.* Rockefeller Foundation, New York 1986

WHE 1908   Konde, M.K. *Santé de l'enfant en Guineé. Etat actuel et perspectives.* Memoire pour le certificat d'études spéciales de santé publique, Université de Nancy, Faculté de Médecine, 1986

WHE 1914   United Nations Children's Fund (UNICEF). *The state of the world's children,* various years, Oxford, Oxford University Press

WHE 1915   United Nations. Department of International Economic and Social Affairs. *World population prospects: estimates and projections as assessed in 1984.* Population Studies No. 98. New York 1986

WHE 1951   Toure, B. *Etude descriptive de la mortalité maternelle des les maternités de Conakry. Projet d'étude.* Ministère de la Santé Publique et de la Population, 1988

WHE 1975   Guinea. Ministry of Health and Social Affairs, *Evaluation and analysis of maternal mortality in Guinea. Project proposal.* (unpublished documents) 1987

WHE 2033   World Health Organization. *Global strategy for health for all by the year 2000. Second report on monitoring progress.* WHO document EB83/2 Add. 1, 1988

WHE 2395   Diallo, M.S. et al. La mortalité maternelle: à propos de 212 observations en sept ans (1980-1985) à la Maternité Ignace-Deen de Conakry (Guinée). *Revue français de Gynécologie et Obstétrique* 1989; 84(5): 419-422

WHE 2415   Thonneau, P. Rapport de mission en Guinée du 11.12.1989 au 19.12.1989 (unpublished)

WHE 2490   World Health Organization and Centre Internationale de l'Enfance. Mortalité et morbidité maternelles. *Séminaire-Aterlier INFOSEC* Cotonou, 28 November – 4 December 1989

WHE 2757   Touré, B. et al. *Mortalité maternelle en Guineé.* (unpublished), 1990.

GUINEA-BISSAU

		Year	Source

1. BASIC INDICATORS

1.1 Demographic

1.1.1 Population

		Year	Source
Size (millions)	0.9	1987	(1915)
Rate of growth (%)	1.9	1980-85	(1915)

1.1.2 Life expectancy

Female	45	1980-85	(1915)
Male	41	1980-85	(1915)

1.1.3 Fertility

Crude Birth Rate	41	1980-85	(1915)
Total Fertility Rate	5.4	1980-85	(1915)

1.1.4 Mortality

Crude Death Rate	22	1980-85	(1915)
Infant Mortality Rate	180	1987	(2033)
Female			
Male			
1-4 years mortality rate			
Female			
Male			

1.2 Social and economic

1.2.1 Adult literacy rate (%)

Female	17	1985	(1914)
Male	46	1985	(1914)

1.2.2 Primary school enrolment rate (%)

Female	39	1986-88	(1914)
Male	73	1986-88	(1914)

1.2.3 Female mean age at first marriage
(years)

1.2.4 GNP/capita

(US $)	200	1986	(2033)

1.2.5 Daily per capita calorie supply
(as % of requirements)

2. HEALTH SERVICES

2.1 Health expenditure

2.1.1 Expenditure on health

(as % of GNP)	2	1986	(2033)

2.1.2 Expenditure on PHC

(as % of total health expenditure)	40	1986	(2033)

2.2 Primary Health Care
(Percentage of population covered by):

2.2.1 Health services

National	64	1984	(0834)
Urban			
Rural			

2.2.2 Safe water

National	31	1984	(0834)
Urban	21	1983	(0834)
Rural	37	1983	(0834)

2.2.3 Adequate sanitary facilities

National	25	1984	(0834)
Urban	21	1980	(0834)
Rural	13	1980	(0834)

2.2.4 Contraceptive prevalence rate

(%)	1	1976	(1712)

2.3 Coverage of maternity care (%)

Area	Prenatal care	Trained attendant	Institutional deliveries	Postnatal care	Sample size	Year	Source
National		31				1972	(0790)
National	29					1988	(2033)

3. COMMUNITY STUDIES

3.1 Bafata, 1988-89 [2756]

A pilot study was carried out in an attempt to identify all maternal deaths in the region. It is thought that both the number of births and the number of maternal deaths were underestimated.

3.1.1 Rate
Live births	2 077
Maternal deaths	31
MMR (per 100 000 live births)	1 490

3.1.2 Causes of maternal deaths

	Number
Sepsis	11
Haemorrhage	7
Abortion	1
Malaria	3
Other	5
Unknown	4

3.1.3 Avoidable factors
Lack of prenatal care and living more than 10 kilometres from the place of delivery were the most important risk factors together with illiteracy.

4. HOSPITAL STUDIES

4.1 All hospitals, 1979-83 [1537]

4.1.1 Rate

	Live births	Maternal deaths	MMR (per 100 000 live births)
1979	4 640	36	776
1980	5 396	53	982
1981	5 922	39	659
1982	5 371	39	726
1983	6 042	41	679
1979-83	27 371	208	760

4.2 Simao Mendes Maternity Hospital, Bissau, 1977, 1979-83 and 1986-87 [0096, 1537, 1639]

4.2.1 Rate

	Live births	Maternal deaths	MMR (per 100 000 live births)
1977	3 239	9	278
1979-83	18 325	98	535
1986-1987*	2 000**	24	1 200

*   November to April
**   Deliveries

It is thought that the 1977 figure is an underestimate due to incomplete registers and the exclusion of maternal deaths occurring outside the maternity wards, in, for example, intensive care units. The author estimates that the rate cannot be lower than 400 per 100 000 live births.

In the 1986-87 study the most frequent causes of death were haemorrhage and infection, followed by toxaemia and septic abortion. More than half the deliveries in the hospital were of women transferred from regional hospitals. 50% of all deliveries were to adolescents below 18 years of age.

4.3 Cachungo Regional Maternity Hospital, 1979-83 and 1986 [1537, 1639]

4.3.1 Rate

	Live births	Maternal deaths	MMR (per 100 000 live births)
1979-83	1 545	6	388
1986	318*	1	315

*   deliveries

4.4 Farim Maternity Hospital, 1979-86 [1537, 1639]

4.4.1 Rate

	Live births	Maternal deaths	MMR (per 100 000 live births)
1979-83	680	7	1 029
1984-86	589*	24	4 074

* deliveries

4.5 Bafata Maternity Hospital, 1979-83, 1986 [1639]

4.5.1 Rate

	Deliveries	Maternal deaths	MMR (per 100 000 live births)
1979-83	1 729	38	2 198
1986	608	12	1 974

4.5.2 Causes of maternal deaths 1986

	Number
Haemorrhage	5
Ruptured uterus	3
Sepsis	2
Hypertensive disorders of pregnancy	2
Total	12

4.5.3 Avoidable factors

The hospital did not have an ambulance and the transportation of women with complications from villages or from health centres was difficult. The result was that a high proportion of transferred women died. Nine of the twelve women who died in 1986 had been transferred.

4.5.4 High risk groups

4.5.5 Other findings

Discussions with the hospital staff revealed that induced abortion was an important cause of maternal death, although the incidence and frequency was not known.

4.6 Four regional hospitals, 1979-83 [1537]

4.6.1 Rate

Hospital	Live births	Maternal deaths	MMR (per 100 000 live births)
Bolama	1 255	9	717
Bubaque	413	2	484
Catio	754	6	796
Gabu	1 359	31	2 281

5. CIVIL REGISTRATION DATA/GOVERNMENT ESTIMATES

6. OTHER SOURCES/ ESTIMATES

6.1 National, 1980, 1982, 1986 [1639]

6.1.1 Rate

On the basis of figures for all institutional births and of maternal deaths between 1980 and 1986, maternal mortality rates for the country were estimated to be 900, 600 and 700 per 100 000 live births in 1980, 1982 and 1986 respectively.

7. SELECTED ANNOTATED BUBLIOGRAPHY

8. FURTHER READING

9. DATA SOURCES

WHE 0096   Boal, M. *Observations on problems in human reproduction.* in: World Health Organization Regional Multidisciplinary Consultative Meeting on Human Reproduction, Yaoundé 4-7 December 1978 (unpublished WHO document No. HRP/RMC/78.10)

WHE 0790   World Health Organization. *Fifth report of the world health situation 1969-72.* Official records of the World Health Organization No. 225, Geneva 1975

WHE 0834   World Health Organization *World Health Statistics annual - vital statistics and causes of death.* Geneva, various years

WHE 1537   Woodall, J. *Data on maternal deaths in all hospitals.* 1986

WHE 1639   Berardi, J.C. *Rapport de mission effectuée en Guinée Bissau du 19 au 26 avril 1987.* WHO 1987

WHE 1712   Mauldin W.P. and Segal, S.J. *Prevalence of contraceptive use in developing countries. A chart book.* Rockefeller Foundation, New York 1986

WHE 1914   United Nations Children's Fund (UNICEF). *The state of the world's children,* various years, Oxford, Oxford University Press

WHE 1915   United Nations. Department of International Economic and Social Affairs. *World population prospects: estimates and projections as assessed in 1984.* Population Studies No. 98. New York 1986

WHE 2033   World Health Organization. *Global strategy for health for all by the year 2000. Second report on monitoring progress.* WHO document EB83/2 Add. 1, 1988

WHE 2756   Costa, C.M.M. et al. *La mortalité maternelle dans la région de Bafata,* (unpublished). Ministère de la santé publique, Bissau, 1989

KENYA

		Year	Source

1. BASIC INDICATORS

1.1 Demographic

1.1.1 Population
Size (millions)	23.1	1988	(1914)
Rate of growth (%)	4.1	1980-87	(1914)

1.1.2 Life expectancy
Female	55	1980-85	(1915)
Male	51	1980-85	(1915)

1.1.3 Fertility
Crude Birth Rate	54	1988	(1914)
Total Fertility Rate	8.1	1988	(1914)

1.1.4 Mortality
Crude Death Rate	12	1988	(1914)
Infant Mortality Rate	71	1988	(1914)
Female	54	1979-89	(2283)
Male	63	1979-89	(2283)
1-4 years mortality rate			
Female	33	1979-89	(2283)
Male	35	1979-89	(2283)

1.2 Social and economic

1.2.1 Adult literacy rate (%)
Female	49	1985	(1914)
Male	70	1985	(1914)

1.2.2 Primary school enrolment rate (%)
Female	93	1986-88	(1914)
Male	98	1986-88	(1914)

1.2.3 Female mean age at first marriage
(years)	20.4	1979	(1918)

		Year	Source

1.2.4 GNP/capita
(US $)	330	1987	(1914)

1.2.5 Daily per capita calorie supply
(as % of requirements)	92	1984-86	(1914)

2. HEALTH SERVICES

2.1 Health expenditure

2.1.1 Expenditure on health
(as % of GNP)	2	1982-83	(0800)

2.1.2 Expenditure on PHC
(as % of total health expenditure)

2.2 Primary Health Care
(Percentage of population covered by):

2.2.1 Health services
National
Urban
Rural

2.2.2 Safe water
National	27	1983	(0834)
Urban	61	1983	(0834)
Rural	21	1983	(0834)

2.2.3 Adequate sanitary facilities
National	44	1983	(0834)
Urban	75	1983	(0834)
Rural	39	1983	(0834)

2.2.4 Contraceptive prevalence rate
(%)	27	1984-89	(2283)

2.3   Coverage of maternity care (%)

Area	Prenatal care	Trained attendant	Institutional deliveries	Postnatal care	Sample size	Year	Source
National	40	28				1984	(2008)
National: rural	80		36		1 065w	1984	(0899)
National: urban rural	77 82 77	50 78 46			7 046 1 006 6 040	1984-89 1984-89 1984-89	(2283) (2283) (2283)
Central	69	73			976	1984-89	(2283)
Coast	69	41			417	1984-89	(2283)
Eastern	80	40			1 218	1984-89	(2283)
Nairobi	83	83			428	1984-89	(2283)
Nyanza	84	53			1 310	1984-89	(2283)
Rift Valley	80	45			1 536	1984-89	(2283)
Western	71	35			1 162	1984-89	(2283)
Chogoria	96	73	69	11	1 800	1985	(1983)
Machakos	40	25			1 586	(1982)	(0475)
Nairobi	96	59	56			(1983)	(0442)
10 districts	92	59	56			1985	(1338)
3 divisions			36			1984-85	(1360)

3.   COMMUNITY STUDIES

3.1   Machakos project area, rural Kenya, 1975-76 [0772, 0773]

3.1.1   Rate

The study covering the Machakos project area (population 25 000; location 60kms. east of Nairobi) made use of a surveillance system comprising fortnightly home visits to all 3 700 households by twelve field workers. The majority of the women, irrespective of where they chose to deliver, attended prenatal clinics at the nearest hospital at least once during the pregnancy. The maternal mortality rate was 46 per 100 000 live births but this figure is based on only one death.

3.1.2   Causes of maternal deaths

3.1.3   Avoidable factors

3.1.4   High risk groups

3.1.5   Other findings

During their pregnancy 84% of the women had attended a prenatal clinic at least once. When asked during pregnancy 56% of the women stated that they intended to deliver in hospital but only 26% ultimately did so. Hospital delivery seemed to depend mostly on opportunity and habit. There was little interference during labour or deliveries attended by traditional birth attendants and few harmful practices were discovered.

The authors propose a more efficient way of screening high and low risk women. An improved transport system would give women the opportunity to reach hospital once labour has started. The provision of maternity waiting homes near hospitals would further encourage hospital delivery.

3.2 Kambusu, Kingoti, Katheka, Katitu, Ulaani rural areas, 1975-79 [2073]

3.2.1 Rate

The outcome of pregnancy of all women included in the study population was investigated by field workers in collaboration with traditional birth attendants.

Live births	4 768
Maternal deaths	4
MMR (per 100 000 live births)	84

3.2.2 Causes of maternal deaths

3.2.3 Avoidable factors

3.3.4 High risk groups

3.3.4 Other findings

A total of 4 716 women participated in the study of which 84% attended a prenatal clinic at least once; 13% never attended. The majority of the women went to the clinic at Kangundo Hospital which is between six and twenty-six kilometers from the study locations. Around 27% of the women delivered in hospital. The lowest percentage of hospital deliveries occurred during the rainy seasons. Regular public transport to Kangundo was available only to people living in the western part of the study area comprising the sublocations Kingoti and Kambusu. Women from the eastern area who wanted to go to a prenatal clinic or who required hospital delivery either had to walk or to wait for a passing lorry. Attendance was closely related to the distance the women had to travel.

Previous caesarean section and short stature were recognized as risk factors by the women themselves and by their relatives and TBAs. So too, though to a lesser degree was primiparity. However, for the majority of women, whether or not to deliver in hospital was largely a question of opportunity. Distance and public transport were the most important obstacles.

3.3 Kwale District, Coastal Province, 1987 [2230, 2275]

3.3.1 Rate

This is a rural area with a relatively undeveloped infrastructure except in the coastal strip where tourism is a major source of income. Total population in 1987 was nearly 400 000. Fertility was estimated at 7.6 in 1984. Fewer than one in ten of ever married women used modern contraceptive methods.

During the second half of 1987, in conjunction with an ongoing survey, an enquiry was carried out comprising interviews with 3 835 women of reproductive age (15-44 years). Every interviewee was asked whether she knew of any deaths of women during pregnancy or the postpartum period. A "network" of deaths was reported and after eliminating multiple reporting, deaths occurring outside the survey location, those which occurred more than five years previously and deaths which were not thought to be related to pregnancy or associated conditions, a final total of 32 maternal deaths was identified over the period 1984-87.

Live births	4 870
Maternal deaths	32
MMR (per 100 000 live births)	657

3.3.2 Causes of maternal deaths

(includes an additional three deaths of women who did not strictly conform to the residence qualifications imposed by the study.)

	Number	%
Haemorrhage	12	34
Sepsis	4	11
Rupture of the uterus	3	9
Hypertensive disorders of pregnancy	1	3
Renal failure due to toxic herbs	1	3
DIRECT CAUSES	21	60
Anaemia	4	11
Malaria	1	3
Cardiac disease	1	3
INDIRECT CAUSES	6	17
Unknown	8	23
TOTAL	35	100

3.3.3 Avoidable factors

3.3.4 High risk groups

A comparison of the frequencies of a number of risk factors between maternal deaths and surviving mothers in the survey found that nulliparous women appeared to have higher mortality risks. For first pregnancies the maternal mortality rate was as high as 1 100 per 100 000 live births. Women delivering at very young or old ages or women with higher parity did not have higher maternal mortality rates. No significant differences in attendance at prenatal clinics between maternal deaths and survivors were found.

3.3.5 Other findings

Fate of the child

Of the seventeen live births to the mothers who died, five died during the first week, two at ages 2-4 weeks and five in the post neonatal period. Thus only five (29%) survived infancy.

Anaemia

Anaemia was prevalent and caused many problems for the pregnant women. Major causes were malaria, hookworm infection and nutritional deficiencies which may have been aggravated by certain food taboos. There was widespread knowledge of the problem and TBAs and traditional healers had a variety of methods of dealing with it, only some of which were of value.

The role of the TBA and the traditional healer

With only 10% of deliveries taking place at hospital the traditional sector will continue to play a key role. However, a study of the biomedical aspects of the work of TBAs found that they had a low average number of deliveries and that there was an important division of labour between TBAs and traditional healers. In this context training programmes for TBAs can be of only limited value. The authors considered that it could be useful to concentrate on a number of leading TBAs and to teach them simple methods of arresting haemorrhage and, perhaps, manual removal of placenta. With respect to traditional healers, training of the most important among them should focus on the value of prenatal care especially in the prevention of anaemia.

4. HOSPITAL STUDIES

4.1. All health institutions, Nairobi, 1981 (June - August) [1622]

4.1.1 Rate

Deliveries	5 293
Maternal deaths	3
MMR (per 100 000 deliveries)	56

4.1.2 Causes of maternal deaths

4.1.3 Avoidable factors

4.1.4 High risk groups

4.1.5 Other findings

Complications during pregnancy

The leading complication during the prenatal period was hypertensive disorders of pregnancy. However, the incidence of eclampsia was only 0.6%. Other pregnancy complications included malaria (2.4%), threatened abortion (2.0%), antepartum haemorrhage (1.9%), and anaemia (1.6%).

Complications during labour

15% of the labours had complications. The main complications were fetal distress (5.2%) and prolonged labour (5.1%). Others included malpresentation (2.1%), and obstructed labour (1%). The incidence of intrapartum haemorrhage and of ruptured uterus was 0.5% and 0.1% respectively. Fourteen women developed eclampsia during labour.

Complications during the postpartum period

The major problem in the first 24 hours after delivery was infection of the genital tract. Four mothers developed eclampsia during the period.

4.2 Kenyatta National Hospital, Nairobi, 1972-78 [0015, 0016, 0017, 0427, 0494, 1288]

4.2.1 Rate

	1972-77	1978
Deliveries	20 510	–
Maternal deaths	99	–
MMR (per 100 000 deliveries)	196	350

4.2.2 Causes of maternal deaths

The leading cause of maternal mortality was infection. Of the 99 deaths during 1972-77, postabortal sepsis claimed 22 lives and puerperal sepsis, 21 lives. Nine of the 21 deaths from puerperal sepsis had delivered by caesarean section.

There were 15 cases of haemorrhage, of which one was postabortal and 14 were postpartum. There were no deaths from antepartum haemorrhage.

	1972-77	
	Number	%
Abortion	23	23
Sepsis	21	21
Haemorrhage	14	14
Rupture of the uterus	6	6
Ectopic pregnancy	5	5
Perforated uterus	3	3
Hypertensive disorders of pregnancy	3	3
Complications of anaesthesia	5	5
Anaemia	3	3
Other infections	3	3
Others	13	14
Total	99	100

4.2.3 Avoidable factors

Late referral

Several women who died arrived at the hospital in a poor condition, after futile management had been attempted for many days. This was especially true of women who had had illegal abortions. Women who died from puerperal sepsis were all referrals or had delivered at home.

Some cases of postpartum haemorrhage could have been saved by early referral: there were instances where the woman had gone from home to a peripheral hospital which did not have facilities for blood transfusion, and arrived nearly moribund at the Kenyatta National Hospital (KNH).

Inadequate facilities in KNH

Facilities in KNH were far from adequate to meet the inflow of obstetric patients. There was overcrowding, and patients often had to share beds and mattresses, leaving them vulnerable to cross-infection within the hospital. There was not enough clean linen, and even basic equipment such as gloves and antiseptic solution fell short of requirements.

Poor patient management

Patient management was poor. Lack of proper investigations with regard to aetiological causes of infections led to inappropriate choice of drugs and non-response of the microorganism to therapy. Decisions about operative interventions were sometimes taken too late, and then, the operations were entrusted to junior doctors.

Two women with ruptured ectopic pregnancies lost virtually their entire blood volume because cross-matching of blood for transfusion was inordinately delayed.

4.2.4 High risk groups

A study of obstetric emergency referrals from district and provincial hospitals to Kenyatta National Hospital in 1977 (0017) shows that they contributed to 59% of total maternal deaths although they accounted for only 3% of all deliveries. More than a third of the women referred had been in labour for between two and five days.

4.2.5 Other findings

- 30 of the 92 women referred from district and provincial hospitals in 1977 were suffering from obstructed labour. In all 47 women had to have an emergency caesarean section. Many of them were dehydrated, exhausted and infected. There were six cases of ruptured uterus, all of which had undergone previous caesarean sections and had been in prolonged labour. One patient died on arrival.

- There were various reasons for transfer from peripheral hospitals to KNH. In 43 cases, either the anaesthetist or the medical officer in charge was not available; in 19 cases the hospital had no facilities for operative delivery; in 21 cases blood was not available, and in nine cases the hospitals did not have water or electricity.

- 38 of the 92 women referred to KNH in 1977 had never attended any prenatal clinic, and had reached the district or provincial hospital after being in labour for a long time. However, in the remaining 54 cases, the problem lay with the local hospital – high risk patients had been admitted even though the hospital had no facilities to tackle the problem, or had diagnosed the problem late, delaying referral.

- 23% of all maternal deaths between 1972 and 1977 were due to abortion. A study of abortions in KNH in 1978 (0015) found that abortion constituted 60% of all emergency gynaecological admissions. The number of patients admitted following abortion increased by 65% between 1973 and 1978, and septic abortions increased by 100%. Patients in the septic group were mainly single adolescent girls and in most cases this was their first pregnancy.

- According to another study of abortions in KNH between 1974 and 1983 (1288), the abortion mortality rate was 290 per 100 000 admissions for the 10-year period (abortion deaths as a proportion of all maternal deaths is not stated). The death rate showed a tendency to decline after 1979. An analysis of 95 (of the 109) deaths from abortion showed that 65% had certainly undergone interference. 97% of those who died following induced abortion died of sepsis, and only 3% from haemorrhage.

- 11% of all primigravida admitted to KNH in 1978 were under 20 years old and 3% were under 16 years (0494). Pre-term delivery and premature rupture of the membranes was higher in this group, but there was no evidence of increase in preeclampsia. There were no maternal deaths in the under 20 years age group, while the maternal mortality rate for the total obstetric population was 350 per 100 000 births.

4.3 Kwale District Hospitals, Coastal Province, 1984-87 [2230]

4.3.1 Rate
MMR (per 100 000 live births)   400-500

4.4 Rural hospitals, Coastal Province, 1987 [2230]

4.4.1 Rate
MMR (per 100 000 live births)   300

4.5   Pumwani Maternity Hospital, 1975-84 [2461, 2462]

4.5.1   Rate

Births	223 111
Maternal deaths	150
MMR (per 100 000 births)	67

4.5.2   Causes of maternal deaths

	Number	%
Hypertensive disorders of pregnancy	31	21
Sepsis	29	19
Ruptured uterus	21	14
Haemorrhage	20	13
Cardiac disease	10	7
Complications of anaesthesia	9	6
Embolisms	8	5
Other	11	7
Unknown	11	7
TOTAL	150	100

Caesarean section [2461]

A study of caesarean section during 1983 found that there were 24 625 deliveries, of which 1 059 were by caesarean section, an incidence of 4.3%. There were four maternal deaths, a mortality rate of 3.78 per 1 000. Cephalopelvic disproportion, two previous caesarean sections, prolonged labour, fetal distress and cord prolapse were the most common indications for caesarean section. 21% of the caesarean sections were performed electively and 79% were emergencies. Of the 364 cases with two previous scars, cephalopelvic disproportion and one previous scar or placenta praevia, only 179 were electives whereas all should have been selected as such. In nine cases the uterus had ruptured before the patient could be operated. All four maternal deaths occurred in emergency patients. Because of overcrowding and inadequate surgical facilities at the hospital elective operations had to be postponed until the mother went into labour and became an emergency; emergencies were often further delayed until the situation became critical.

4.5.3   Avoidable factors

Among the women who died prenatal attendance was low. 48% attended for the first time after 28 weeks of gestation, 70% paid inadequate visits and in 69% no investigations were carried out during the prenatal period.

A few patients died because blood was not available in time. Of the mothers who died, 34% developed complications during the prenatal period. However, the remaining 66% of women who died had no prenatal problems and developed complications during labour or the puerperium.

4.5.4   High risk groups

Women over 35 years old, primigravidas and women of parity 5+ were overrepresented among the women who died compared with the overall delivery population.

	Maternal deaths		Total deliveries
	Number	%	%
Age			
< 15	0	0	0
15-20	33	22	23
21-25	34	23	35
26-30	23	15	13
31-35	9	6	4
35+	14	9	4
Unknown	37	25	22
Parity			
Primiparous	48	32	28
Parity 1-3	45	30	47
Parity 4	15	10	11
Parity 5+	39	26	14
Unknown	3	2	–
TOTAL	150	100	100

5.   CIVIL REGISTRATION DATA/GOVERNMENT ESTIMATES

5.1   National, 1977 [0386]

5.1.1   Rate

The maternal mortality rate was 168 per 100 000 pregnancies.

5.2   National, 1970 [0753]

5.2.1   Rate

According to the UN Demographic Year Book, the maternal mortality rate for Kenya was 204 per 100 000 live births in 1970.

6.   OTHER SOURCES/ ESTIMATES

7. SELECTED ANNOTATED BIBLIOGRAPHY

Bird, G.C. Obstetric vesico-vaginal and allied fistulae. *Journal of Obstetrics and Gynaecology of the British Commonwealth* 1967; 74: 749-752. WHE 2296.

A study of 69 cases of obstetric fistulae treated at the Rift Valley Provincial General Hospital in Nakuru, Kenya from 1958-1965 is presented. Types of fistulae are described and surgical methods briefly presented. Sixty-two (89%) of the fistulae were regarded as operable, and of these 49 (79%) were cured, while nine (15%) had their fistula closed but remained incontinent. Urinary diversion was performed in nine cases.

Gunaratne, M. and Mati, J.K.G. Acquired fistulae of the female lower genital tract: a comprehensive five-year review. *Journal of Obstetrics and Gynaecology of Eastern and Central Africa* 1982; 1: 11-15. WHE 1075

An examination of 254 cases of fistulae referred to Kenyatta National Hospital, Nairobi, Kenya, during a five-year period (1974-1978), is presented. 93% of the cases were urinary fistulae, and 7% recto-vaginal. Of the urinary fistulae, 207 (88%) were labour related. Nearly 8% of fistulae were associated with carcinoma of the cervix. There was a high incidence of juxta-cervical fistulae, associated with abdominal delivery and uterine rupture.

The age distribution showed a peak incidence for women aged 20-24 years, with primigravidae accounting for 42%. However 31% were of parity of five or above. The interval between fistula formation and the women seeking treatment varied from three months to 15 years. Approximately half the patients were seen within the first six months. The cure rate was analyzed by type of fistula and varied from 58% to 100%. Complications included haemorrhage, bladder calculus, ureteric occlusion and death.

Kaseje, Dan C.O. and Spencer, H.C.,, et al, Malaria chemoprophylaxis to pregnant women provided by community health workers in Saradidi, Kenya. I. and II. *Annals of Tropical Medicine and Parasitology* 1987; 81(1): 77-89. WHE 1926

Chloroquine prophylaxis for malaria was available free of charge to pregnant women in Saradidi, Kenya. The drug was supplied by village health helpers. However, only 29% of 357 pregnant women seen at prenatal clinics from 1983 to 1984 were on chemoprophylaxis despite the fact that malaria was generally perceived as an important cause of stillbirths and abortion. The major reason was lack of awareness that the service was available but other reasons included fear of toxic reactions. The authors conclude that delivery of antimalarial chemoprophylaxis may be better provided by prenatal clinics and that the additional responsibility may be too much for community health workers.

Rogo, K.O. Mortality in acute gynecology: a developing country perspective. *International Journal of Gynecology and Obstetrics* 1989; 30: 343-347. WHE 2467

Reports of maternal deaths in developing countries frequently describe only deaths occurring in maternity units and exclude pregnancy-related deaths in gynecology units which are, by definition, maternal. A study at the Acute Gynecology Ward, Kenyatta National Hospital, Nairobi, over a 20-month period in 1986-87, found 109 deaths. The records of 89 cases were examined. Of these, 37 deaths (41.6%) were due to pregnancy-related causes. Septic abortion accounted for more than two-thirds of the total.

Solomon, M.M. and Rogo, K.O. A needs assessment study of traditional birth attendants in rural Kenya. *International Journal of Gynecology and Obstetrics* 1989; 30: 329-334. WHE 2469

A study of TBAs serving one area in Kenya was conducted for the purpose of designing an appropriate intervention programme. 36 TBAs were interviewed. Together, they had attended a total of 116 deliveries within one month. The local hospital was conducting an average of 37 deliveries monthly. Although most TBAs were good at abdominal palpation, they did not conduct routine prenatal checks and rarely referred deserving cases to hospital They appeared to have a poor grasp of time making it difficult for them to refer patients with prolonged labour in good time. Haemorrhage and retained placenta were recognised as major indications for referral but there were usually long delays in referral giving the hospital little chance of saving mother or baby Sterility and asepsis were not observed during labour and there was generally poor handling of the cord.

Thornton, J.G. Should vesicovaginal fistula be treated only by specialists? *Tropical Doctor* 1986; April: 78-79. WHE 2040.

This paper reports the results of a small series of thirteen cases of vesicovaginal fistula from Chogoria in rural Kenya, operated on over a period of 12 years (1972-83). Only two women were operated on by a specialist gynaecologist, and all but one were repaired per vaginum. Twelve of the thirteen fistulae were successfully closed at the first attempt. In the remaining case a pinhole residual fistula was successfully repaired three months after the primary operation. It is concluded that good results can be obtained by relatively inexperienced doctors in a small hospital, provided that massive fistulae, those complicated by severe scarring, and failed repairs from previous operations, are referred to more specialized hospitals.

8. FURTHER READING

Cook, R. *Damage to physical health from pharaonic circumcision (infibulation) of females.* Paper prepared for Seminar on Traditional Practices Affecting the Health of Women and Children in Africa 1984, 6-10 February, Dakar, Senegal. WHE 1911

Cox, P.S.V. and Webster, D. Genital prolapse amongst the Pokot. *East African Medical Journal* 1975; 52(12): 694-699. WHE 1058

Hezekiah, J. and Wafula, F., Major health problems of women in a Kenyan village. *Health Care for Women International* 1989; 10: 15-25. WHE 2360

Malone, M.I. The quality of care in an antenatal clinic in Kenya. *East African Medical Journal* 1980; 57(2): 86-96. WHE 0430

Mbugua, I. Abortion in Kenya. *Viva Magazine* 1982; 8(4). WHE 1103

Mtimavalye, L.A.R. Reproductive health care among women in Africa: current trends and the future. *Journal of Obstetrics and Gynaecology of Eastern and Central Africa* 1982; 1(2): 48-53. WHE 0468

Raikes, A. *Pregnancy and birth in Kisii, utilization behaviour and culture.* (unpublished document) Centre for Development Research and Institute of Social Medicine, Copenhagen. WHE 1674

Raikes, A. Women's health in East Africa. *Social Science and Medicine* 1989; 5: 447-459. WHE 2220

Schulpen, T.W.J. and Swinkels, W.J.A.M., Machakos Project Studies. Agents affecting the health of mother and child in a rural area of Kenya. XIX. The utilization of health services in a rural area of Kenya. *Tropical and Geographical Medicine* 1980; 32: 340-349. WHE 2205

9. DATA SOURCES

WHE 0015   Aggarwal, V.P. and Mati, J.K.G. Review of abortions at Kenyatta National Hospital, Nairobi. *East African Medical Journal* 1980; 57(2): 138-143

WHE 0016   Aggarwal, V.P. and Mati, J.K.G. Epidemiology of induced abortion in Nairobi, Kenya. *Journal of Obstetrics and Gynaecology of Eastern and Central Africa* 1982; 1(2): 54-57

WHE 0017   Aggarwal, V.P. Obstetric emergency referrals to Kenyatta National Hospital. *East African Medical Journal* 1980; 57(2): 144-149

WHE 0386   Kenya, Registrar General. *Annual report of the Registrar General 1977.* Nairobi, Registrar General's Department, 1981

WHE 0427   Makokha, A.E. Maternal mortality – Kenyatta National Hospital, 1972-1977 *East African Medical Journal* 1980; 57(7): 451-460

WHE 0442   Mati, J.K.L. at al. The Nairobi Birth Survey II. Antenatal care in Nairobi. *Journal of Obstetrics and Gynaecology of Eastern and Central Africa* 1983; 2: 1-11

WHE 0475   Mwalali, P.N. The effectiveness of the training of the traditional birth attendants in a rural area - Machakos, Kenya. *Journal of Obstetrics and Gynaecology of Eastern and Central Africa* 1982; 1(1): 32-36

WHE 0494   Ngoka, W.M. and Mati, J.K.G. Obstetric aspects of adolescent pregnancy. *East African Medical Journal* 1980; 57(2): 124-130

WHE 0753   United Nations. *Demographic Yearbook.* New York, various years

WHE 0772   Voorhoeve, A.M. et al. Machakos project studies. Agents affecting the health of mother and child in a rural area of Kenya. XVI The outcome of pregnancy. *Tropical and Geographic Medicine* 1979; 31: 607-627

WHE 0773   Voorhoeve, A.M. et al. Machakos project studies. Agents affecting the health of mother and child in a rural area of Kenya. XXI Antenatal and delivery care. *Tropical and Geographic Medicine* 1982; 34(1): 91-101

WHE 0800   World Health Organization. *Country reports to regional offices of the progress in implementing Health for All by the Year 2000.* (Unpublished documents) 1983

WHE 0834   World Health Organization. *World Health Statistics annual – vital statistics and causes of death.* Geneva, various years

WHE 0899   Sempebwa, E.N. and Okello, M. *Status of women, infant and young child feeding.* (Draft report) Breastfeeding information group, Nairobi 1983

WHE 1250   Mandjale, A.E. *Mortalité infantile et juvenile en Afrique.* Louvain, CIACO 1985

WHE 1288   Wanjala, S. et al. Mortality due to abortion at Kenyatta National Hospital, 1974-83. *Ciba Foundation Symposium* 1985; 115:41-53

WHE 1338   World Health Organization. African Regional Office, *Where are we in PHC? Countries take a close look at themselves through PHC reviews.* Part II. 7-15 October 1985

WHE 1360   World Health Organization. Expanded Programme on Immunization, Neonatal tetanus mortality surveys. Kenya. *Weekly Epidemiological Record* 1986; 61(16): 117-118

WHE 1622   Mati, J.K.G. et al. The Nairobi birth survey I. The study design, the population and outline results. *Journal of Obstetrics and Gynaecology of Eastern and Central Africa* 1982; 1: 132-139

WHE 1712   Mauldin W.P. and Segal, S.J. *Prevalence of contraceptive use in developing countries. A chart book.* Rockefeller Foundation, New York 1986

WHE 1914   United Nations Children's Fund (UNICEF). *The state of the world's children,* various years, Oxford, Oxford University Press

WHE 1915   United Nations. Department of International Economic and Social Affairs. *World population prospects: estimates and projections as assessed in 1984.* Population Studies No. 98. New York 1986

WHE 1918   United Nations. Department of International Economic and Social Affairs. *First marriage: patterns and determinants.* New York 1988

WHE 1983   Chogoria Hospital and Community Health Department. *1985 Chogoria community health survey. Report of the principal findings.* Chogoria, 1987

WHE 2008   World Health Organization. Regional Office for Africa *Evaluation of the strategy for health for all by the year 2000. Seventh report on the world health situation* Vol 2, African region, Brazzaville 1987

WHE 2073   Voorhoeve, A.M. et al. Modern and traditional antenatal and delivery care. In: *Maternal and child health in rural Kenya. An epidemiological study.* London, Croome Helm, 1980

WHE 2230   Boerma, J.T. and Mati, J.K.G. Identifying maternal mortality through networking: results from coastal Kenya. *Studies in Family Planning* 1989; 20(6): 245-253

WHE 2275   Boerma, T. *Maternal mortality in Kwale.* (unpublished document) 1989

WHE 2283   Demographic and Health Surveys. *Demographic and health survey Kenya.* National Council for Population and Development and Ministry of Home Affairs and National Heritage, Institute for Resource Development/Macro Systems Inc. 1989

WHE 2461   Bansal,Y.P. Caesarean section: indications and maternal mortality at Pumwani Maternity Hospital, Nairobi, (1983). *East African Medical Journal* 1987; 64(11): 741-744

WHE 2462   Ngoka, W.M. and Bansal, Y.P. Maternal mortality – Pumwani Maternity Hospital – 1975-1984. *East African Medical Journal* 1987; 64(4): 277-283

NOTES

LESOTHO

		Year	Source

1. BASIC INDICATORS

1.1 Demographic

1.1.1 Population

		Year	Source
Size (millions)	1.7	1988	(1914)
Rate of growth (%)	2.8	1980-87	(1914)

1.1.2 Life expectancy

Female	52	1980-85	(1915)
Male	46	1980-85	(1915)

1.1.3 Fertility

Crude Birth Rate	41	1988	(1914)
Total Fertility Rate	5.8	1988	(1914)

1.1.4 Mortality

Crude Death Rate	12	1988	(1914)
Infant Mortality Rate	99	1988	(1914)
Female			
Male			
1-4 years mortality rate			
Female			
Male			

1.2 Social and economic

1.2.1 Adult literacy rate (%)

Female	84	1985	(1914)
Male	62	1985	(1914)

1.2.2 Primary school enrolment rate (%)

Female	127	1983-86	(1914)
Male	102	1983-86	(1914)

1.2.3 Female mean age at first marriage

(years)	20.5	1977	(1918)

1.2.4 GNP/capita

(US $)	370	1987	(1914)

1.2.5 Daily per capita calorie supply

(as % of requirements)	101	1984-86	(1914)

2. HEALTH SERVICES

2.1 Health expenditure

2.1.1 Expenditure on health

(as % of GNP)	1.4	1984	(0800)

2.1.2 Expenditure on PHC

(as % of total health expenditure)	43.0	1983	(0800)

2.2 Primary Health Care
(Percentage of population covered by):

2.2.1 Health services

National	50	1984	(0834)
Urban			
Rural			

2.2.2 Safe water

National			
Urban	37	1980	(0834)
Rural	14	1984	(0834)

2.2.3 Adequate sanitary facilities

National	12	1980	(0834)
Urban	22	1980	(0834)
Rural	11	1980	(0834)

2.2.4 Contraceptive prevalence rate

(%)	5	1977	(1712)

2.3 Coverage of maternity care (%)

Area	Prenatal care	Trained attendant	Institutional deliveries	Postnatal care	Sample size	Year	Source
National	22		32			1984	(1338)
National	40	28				1984	(0834)
National	50	40				1988	(2033)

3. COMMUNITY STUDIES

4. HOSPITAL STUDIES

5. CIVIL REGISTRATION DATA/GOVERNMENT ESTIMATES

6. OTHER SOURCES/ ESTIMATES

6.1 National, 1973 (0345)

6.1.1 Rate
A report of the International Federation of Gynaecology and Obstetrics quotes a maternal mortality rate of 1 600 per 100 000 live births in 1973.

7. SELECTED ANNOTATED BIBLIOGRAPHY

8. FURTHER READING

Andriessen, P.P. et al. The village health worker project in Lesotho: an evaluation. *Tropical Doctor* 20; 111-113: 1990

Boerma, J. T., *Maternal mortality in sub-Saharan Africa: levels, causes and interventions.* (unpublished document) 1987. WHE 1655

Frank, O. The demand for fertility control in sub-Saharan Africa. Working paper no. 117. *Studies in Family Planning* 1987; 18(4): 181-201. WHE 1371

Wicinski, R. *Development of health services in Lesotho: maternal and child health/child spacing* (unpublished WHO document No. AFR/MCH/74) 1977. WHE 0779

9. DATA SOURCES

WHE 0345   International Federation of Gynaecologists and Obstetricians and International Confederation of Midwives. *Maternity care in the world.* (2nd edition) London, FIGO/ICM 1976

WHE 0800   World Health Organization. *Country reports to regional offices of the progress in implementing Health for All by the Year 2000.* (Unpublished documents) 1983

WHE 0834   World Health Organization. *World Health Statistics annual – vital statistics and causes of death.* Geneva, various years

WHE 1338   World Health Organization. Africa Regional Office. *Where are we in PHC? Countries take a close look at themselves through PHC reviews* Part 2, October 7-15 1985

WHE 1712   Mauldin W.P. and Segal, S.J. *Prevalence of contraceptive use in developing countries. A chart book.* Rockefeller Foundation, New York 1986

WHE 1914   United Nations Children's Fund (UNICEF). *The state of the world's children,* various years, Oxford, Oxford University Press

WHE 1915   United Nations. Department of International Economic and Social Affairs. *World population prospects: estimates and projections as assessed in 1984.* Population Studies No. 98. New York 1986

WHE 1918   United Nations. Department of International Economic and Social Affairs. *First marriage: patterns and determinants.* New York 1988

WHE 2033   World Health Organization. *Global strategy for health for all by the year 2000. Second report on monitoring progress.* WHO document EB83/2 Add. 1, 1988

NOTES

LIBERIA

		Year	Source

1. BASIC INDICATORS

1.1 Demographic

1.1.1 Population

Size (millions)	2.4	1988	(1914)
Rate of growth (%)	3.2	1980-87	(1914)

1.1.2 Life expectancy

Female	51	1980-85	(1915)
Male	47	1980-85	(1915)

1.1.3 Fertility

Crude Birth Rate	45	1988	(1914)
Total Fertility Rate	6.5	1988	(1914)

1.1.4 Mortality

Crude Death Rate	13	1988	(1914)
Infant Mortality Rate	86	1988	(1914)
Female	128	1981-86	(1633)
Male	160	1981-86	(1633)
1-4 years mortality rate			
Female	90	1981-86	(1633)
Male	88	1981-86	(1633)

1.2 Social and economic

1.2.1 Adult literacy rate (%)

Female	23	1985	(1914)
Male	47	1985	(1914)

1.2.2 Primary school enrolment rate (%)

Female	50	1986-88	(1914)
Male	82	1986-88	(1914)

1.2.3 Female mean age at first marriage

(years)	19.3	1974	(1918)

1.2.4 GNP/capita

(US $)	450	1987	(1914)

1.2.5 Daily per capita calorie supply

(as % of requirements)	102	1984-86	(1914)

2. HEALTH SERVICES

2.1 Health expenditure

2.1.1 Expenditure on health

(as % of GNP)	3	1983	(0800)

2.1.2 Expenditure on PHC

(as % of total health expenditure)	23	1983	(0800)

2.2 Primary Health Care
(Percentage of population covered by):

2.2.1 Health services

National	35	1983	(0834)
Urban			
Rural			

2.2.2 Safe water

National	37	1983	(0834)
Urban	50	1983	(0834)
Rural	24	1983	(0834)

2.2.3 Adequate sanitary facilities

National	21	1983	(0834)
Urban	24	1983	(0834)
Rural	20	1983	(0834)

2.2.4 Contraceptive prevalence rate

(%)	8	1981-86	(1633)

2.3 Coverage of maternity care (%)

Area	Prenatal care	Trained attendant	Institutional deliveries	Postnatal care	Sample size	Year	Source
National	88	89				1983	(0834)
National	88	87				1984	(2008)
National:	83	58			3 178w	1981-86	(1633)
urban	92	77			1 179w	1981-86	(1633)
rural	78	47			1 999w	1981-86	(1633)

3. COMMUNITY STUDIES

4. HOSPITAL STUDIES

4.1 All hospitals, 1974 [0211]

4.1.1 Rate

Live births	13 858
Maternal deaths	24
MMR (per 100 000 live births)	173

5. CIVIL REGISTRATION DATA/GOVERNMENT ESTIMATES

6. OTHER SOURCES/ ESTIMATES

7. SELECTED ANNOTATED BIBLIOGRAPHY

8. FURTHER READING

9. DATA SOURCES

WHE 0211   Etzel, R.A. Liberian obstetrics: the birth and development of midwifery. Part II. *Journal of Nurse-Midwifery* 1977; 22(1): 18-30

WHE 0800   World Health Organization. *Country reports to regional offices of the progress in implementing Health for All by the Year 2000.* (Unpublished documents) 1983

WHE 0834   World Health Organization *World Health Statistics annual – vital statistics and causes of death.* Geneva, various years

WHE 1633   Demographic and Health Surveys, *Liberian demographic and health survey 1986,* Ministry of Planning and Economic Affairs/Institute for Resource Development, Westinghouse, 1987

WHE 1914   United Nations Children's Fund (UNICEF). *The state of the world's children,* various years, Oxford, Oxford University Press

WHE 1915   United Nations. Department of International Economic and Social Affairs. *World population prospects: estimates and projections as assessed in 1984.* Population Studies No. 98. New York 1986

WHE 1917   United Nations. Department of International Economic and Social Affairs. *Age structure of mortality in developing countries. A database for cross-sectional and time-series research.* New York 1986

WHE 1918   United Nations. Department of International Economic and Social Affairs. *First marriage: patterns and determinants.* New York 1988

WHE 2008   World Health Organization. Regional Office for Africa *Evaluation of the strategy for health for all by the year 2000. Seventh report on the world health situation* Vol 2, African region, Brazzaville 1987

LIBYAN ARAB JAMAHIRIYA

	Year	Source
1. BASIC INDICATORS		

1.1 Demographic

1.1.1 Population

		Year	Source
Size (millions)	4.2	1988	(1914)
Rate of growth (%)	4.1	1980-87	(1914)

1.1.2 Life expectancy

Female	60	1980-85	(1915)
Male	57	1980-85	(1915)

1.1.3 Fertility

Crude Birth Rate	44	1988	(1914)
Total Fertility Rate	6.8	1988	(1914)

1.1.4 Mortality

Crude Death Rate	9	1988	(1914)
Infant Mortality Rate	80	1988	(1914)
Female	73	1973	(0753)
Male	77	1973	(0753)
1-4 years mortality rate			
Female	10	1973	(0753)
Male	9	1973	(0753)

1.2 Social and economic

1.2.1 Adult literacy rate (%)

Female	50	1985	(1914)
Male	81	1985	(1914)

1.2.2 Primary school enrolment rate (%)

Female	
Male	

1.2.3 Female mean age at first marriage

(years)	18.7	1973	(1918)

		Year	Source
1.2.4 GNP/capita			
(US $)	5 460	1987	(1914)
1.2.5 Daily per capita calorie supply			
(as % of requirements)	153	1984-86	(1914)

2. HEALTH SERVICES

2.1 Health expenditure

2.1.1 Expenditure on health

(as % of GNP)	3	1983	(1888)

2.1.2 Expenditure on PHC
(as % of total health expenditure)

2.2 Primary Health Care
(Percentage of population covered by):

2.2.1 Health services

National	100	1983	(0834)
Urban			
Rural			

2.2.2 Safe water

National	90	1983	(0834)
Urban	100	1983	(0834)
Rural	77	1983	(0834)

2.2.3 Adequate sanitary facilities

National	70	1983	(0834)
Urban	100	1985	(2033)
Rural	53	1985	(2033)

2.2.4 Contraceptive prevalence rate
(%)

2.3 Coverage of maternity care (%)

Area	Prenatal care	Trained attendant	Institutional deliveries	Postnatal care	Sample size	Year	Source
National			49			1972	(0790)
National	76					1976	(0834)
National			64			1977	(0415)
National			70			(1982)	(0149)
National			68			(1983)	(0800)
National	76					1984	(0834)

3. COMMUNITY STUDIES

4. HOSPITAL STUDIES

4.1 Al-Jamahiriya Hospital, Benghazi, 1981-84 [1677]

4.1.1 Rate
Deliveries	61 161
Maternal deaths	13
MMR (per 100 000 deliveries)	21

4.1.2 Causes of maternal deaths
Eight of the 13 deaths followed emergency obstetric hysterectomy procedures carried out because of massive postpartum haemorrhage or rupture of the uterus.

5. CIVIL REGISTRATION DATA/GOVERNMENT ESTIMATES

6. OTHER SOURCES/ ESTIMATES

6.1 National, 1978 [0149]

6.1.1 Rate
An Assignment Report by a WHO consultant quotes a maternal mortality rate of 80 per 100 000 live births in 1978.

7. SELECTED ANNOTATED BIBLIOGRAPHY

8. FURTHER READING

9. DATA SOURCES

WHE 0149   Chowdhury, T.A. *Assignment report in connection with the establishment of a system of confidential enquiries into maternal deaths and other aspects of maternal health care – Libyan Arab Jamahiriya.* (unpublished WHO document no. EM/MCH/164) 1982

WHE 0415   Libya, Secretariat of Planning Census and Statistics Department. *Vital statistics of the Socialist People's Libyan Arab Jamahiriya* 1977 Vol. 5, Tripoli, 1979

WHE 0753   United Nations. *Demographic Yearbook.* New York, various years

WHE 0790   World Health Organization. *Fifth report of the world health situation 1969-72.* Official records of the World Health Organization No. 225, Geneva, 1975

WHE 0800   World Health Organization. *Country reports to regional offices of the progress in implementing Health for All by the Year 2000.* (Unpublished documents) 1983

WHE 0834   World Health Organization. *World Health Statistics annual – vital statistics and causes of death.* Geneva, various years

WHE 1677   Legnain, M. et al. Epidemiological analysis of cases of postpartum hysterectomy at Benghazi, 1981-84. *Eastern Mediterranean Region Health Services Journal* 1987; 3: 37-41

WHE 1888   World Health Organization. Eastern Mediterranean Regional Office, *Evaluation of the strategy for Health for All by the year 2000. Seventh report of the world health situation.* Alexandria, EMRO 1987

WHE 1914   United Nations Children's Fund (UNICEF). *The state of the world's children,* various years, Oxford, Oxford University Press

WHE 1915   United Nations. Department of International Economic and Social Affairs. *World population prospects: estimates and projections as assessed in 1984.* Population Studies No. 98. New York 1986

WHE 1918   United Nations. Department of International Economic and Social Affairs. *First marriage: patterns and determinants.* New York 1988

WHE 2033   World Health Organization. *Global strategy for health for all by the year 2000. Second report on monitoring progress.* WHO document EB83/2 Add. 1, 1988

NOTES

MADAGASCAR

		Year	Source

1. BASIC INDICATORS

1.1 Demographic

1.1.1 Population
		Year	Source
Size (millions)	11.2	1988	(1914)
Rate of growth (%)	3.1	1980-87	(1914)

1.1.2 Life expectancy
		Year	Source
Female	50	1980-85	(1915)
Male	49	1980-85	(1915)

1.1.3 Fertility
		Year	Source
Crude Birth Rate	46	1988	(1914)
Total Fertility Rate	6.6	1988	(1914)

1.1.4 Mortality
		Year	Source
Crude Death Rate	14	1988	(1914)
Infant Mortality Rate	119	1988	(1914)
Female			
Male			
1-4 years mortality rate			
Female			
Male			

1.2 Social and economic

1.2.1 Adult literacy rate (%)
		Year	Source
Female	62	1985	(1914)
Male	74	1985	(1914)

1.2.2 Primary school enrolment rate (%)
		Year	Source
Female	92	1986-88	(1914)
Male	97	1986-88	(1914)

1.2.3 Female mean age at first marriage
		Year	Source
(years)	20.3	1975	(1918)

1.2.4 GNP/capita
		Year	Source
(US $)	210	1987	(1914)

1.2.5 Daily per capita calorie supply
		Year	Source
(as % of requirements)	106	1984-86	(1914)

2. HEALTH SERVICES

2.1 Health expenditure

2.1.1 Expenditure on health
		Year	Source
(as % of GNP)	3.5	1986	(2033)

2.1.2 Expenditure on PHC
		Year	Source
(as % of total health expenditure)	23.6	1985	(1914)

2.2 Primary Health Care
(Percentage of population covered by):

2.2.1 Health services
		Year	Source
National	65	1984	(0834)
Urban			
Rural			

2.2.2 Safe water
		Year	Source
National	21	1983	(0834)
Urban	81	1985	(2033)
Rural	17	1985	(2033)

2.2.3 Adequate sanitary facilities
		Year	Source
National			
Urban	12	1985	(2033)
Rural			

2.2.4 Contraceptive prevalence rate
(%)

2.3   Coverage of maternity care (%)

Area	Prenatal care	Trained attendant	Institutional deliveries	Postnatal care	Sample	Year	Source
National	33		52	6		1979	(0421)
National		62				1984	(0834)

3. COMMUNITY STUDIES

3.1   Firaisana of Belamoty, 1988 [2509]

A household enquiry was carried out in the "befamio" (persons linked through lineage who recognise the authority of a chief) in the ten "Fokontany" (villages) comprising the Firaisana of Belamoty. The cooperation of the Head of the local Health Centre and of the village "killy" (old women) was obtained. The enquiry was carried out during the months of April and May (the latter part of the rainy season) during which time the women remain in the villages and the labour of the men is less onerous than at other times. The total population was estimated at 11 300 at the time of the survey. Information was collected on all births and deaths during the previous 24 months and on all deaths of women of reproductive age. Female interviewers were used throughout. There was a total of 38 deaths of women of reproductive age during the period of which 17 were assessed by the author to be maternal deaths.

3.1.1   Rate

Live births	473
Maternal deaths	17
MMR (per 100 000 live births)	3 594

3.1.2   Causes of maternal deaths

	Number
Haemorrhage	4
Sepsis	4
Obstructed labour	1
Ectopic pregnancy or abortion	1
DIRECT CAUSES	10
Malaria	3
Tuberculosis	3
Dysentery	1
INDIRECT CAUSES	7
TOTAL	17

3.1.3   Avoidable factors

Of the women who died only three had been assisted by a health worker (midwife or nurse), three had received no assistance and 11 had been assisted by a traditional birth attendant.

3.1.4   High risk groups
Age

	% of mothers	% of maternal deaths
<15 years	2	–
15-24	40	59
25-34	35	29
35-44	17	12
44 years+	2	–
Unknown	4	–

Parity

	% of mothers	% of maternal deaths
Primigravida	22	35
Gravida 2-4	35	12
Multigravida	43	24
Unknown	–	29

4. HOSPITAL STUDIES

4.1   General Hospital, Befelatanana, 1977-78 and 1980-83 [2509]

4.1.1   Rate

	1977-78	1980-83
Live births	n.a.	55 309
Maternal deaths	n.a.	398
MMR (per 100 000 live births)	565	720

4.2   Maternité de l'Hôpital Principal de Toamasina, 1977-85 [2509]

4.2.1   Rate

Live births	34 958
Maternal deaths	173
MMR (per 100 000 live births)	495

4.3 Maternité de l'Hôpital Joseph Pavoahangy Andrianavalona, Antananarivo, 1986-88 [2569]

4.3.1 Rate

Maternal deaths	5
MMR (per 100 000 live births)	257

4.3.2 Causes of maternal deaths

	Number
Haemorrhage	1
Hypertensive disorders of pregnancy	1
Complications of caesarean section	1
Anaesthetic accident	1
Pulmonary embolism	1

4.3.3 Avoidable factors

The case of pulmonary embolism was considered unavoidable but the remaining four deaths could have been prevented given more adequate care. Four of the women had received little or no prenatal care.

5. CIVIL REGISTRATION DATA/GOVERNMENT ESTIMATES

5.1 National, 1979 [0421]

5.1.1 Rate

According to figures reported by the Department of Public Health and the Ministry of Health, the maternal mortality rate in 1979 was 300 per 100 000 live births.

5.2 National, 1984 and 1986 [2509]

5.2.1 Rate

	1984	1986*
Live births	202 855	81 308
Maternal deaths	818	271
MMR (per 100 000 live births)	403	333

* First six months only

6. OTHER SOURCES/ ESTIMATES

6.1 National, 1974-75 [0791]

6.1.1 Rate

According to the World Health Organization's Sixth Report on the World Health Situation, the maternal mortality rate for Madagascar was 127 per 100 000 live births in 1974-75.

6.2 Faritany of Tuléar, 1987 [2509]

	MMR (per 100 000 live births)
Medical circumscription of Betioky-Sud	1 030
Medical circumscription of Tolanaro	400

6.3 National and town of Antananarivo, 1986-88 [2569]

6.3.1 Rate

	MMR (per 100 000 live births)
National	570
Antananarivo	474

7. SELECTED ANNOTATED BIBLIOGRAPHY

8. FURTHER READING

Boerma, J.T. *Maternal mortality in sub-Saharan Africa: levels, causes and interventions* 1987. WHE 1655

9. DATA SOURCES

WHE 0421   Madagascar, Ministère de la Santé, Direction des Services Sanitaire et Médicaux. Rapport annuel 1979. *Services des Statistiques Sanitaire et Démographique* 1979

WHE 0791   World Health Organization. *Sixth report on the world health situation 1973-77. Part II: review by country and area.* Geneva 1980

WHE 0834   World Health Organization. *World Health Statistics annual – vital statistics and causes of death.* Geneva, various years

WHE 1914   United Nations Children's Fund (UNICEF). *The state of the world's children,* various years, Oxford, Oxford University Press

WHE 1915   United Nations. Department of International Economic and Social Affairs. *World population prospects: estimates and projections as assessed in 1984.* Population Studies No. 98. New York 1986

WHE 1918   United Nations. Department of International Economic and Social Affairs. *First marriage: patterns and determinants.* New York 1988

WHE 2033   World Health Organization. *Global strategy for health for all by the year 2000. Second report on monitoring progress.* WHO document EB83/2 Add. 1, 1988

WHE 2509   Solange, M. *Mortalité maternelle dans le Firaisana de Belamoty - Toliara.* Thesis, Université d'Antananarivo, 1989

WHE 2569   Ramialison, L. *Etudes sur la mortalité maternelle à la Maternité de l'Hôpital Joseph Ravoahangy Andrianavalona.* Université d'Antananarivo/Hôpital Joseph Ravoahangy Andrianavalona. (unpublished document) 1989

MALAWI

	Year	Source

1. BASIC INDICATORS

1.1 Demographic

1.1.1 Population

		Year	Source
Size (millions)	7.9	1988	(1914)
Rate of growth (%)	3.2	1988	(1914)

1.1.2 Life expectancy

		Year	Source
Female	46	1980-85	(1915)
Male	44	1980-85	(1915)

1.1.3 Fertility

		Year	Source
Crude Birth Rate	53	1988	(1914)
Total Fertility Rate	7.0	1988	(1914)

1.1.4 Mortality

		Year	Source
Crude Death Rate	20	1988	(1914)
Infant Mortality Rate	149	1988	(1914)
Female	129	1977	(0753)
Male	151	1977	(0753)
1-4 years mortality rate			
Female	87	1977	(0753)
Male	98	1977	(0753)

1.2 Social and economic

1.2.1 Adult literacy rate (%)

		Year	Source
Female	31	1985	(1914)
Male	52	1985	(1914)

1.2.2 Primary school enrolment rate (%)

		Year	Source
Female	59	1986-88	(1914)
Male	73	1986-88	(1914)

1.2.3 Female mean age at first marriage

		Year	Source
(years)	17.8	1977	(1918)

1.2.4 GNP/capita

		Year	Source
(US $)	160	1987	(1914)

1.2.5 Daily per capita calorie supply

		Year	Source
(as % of requirements)	102	1984-86	(1914)

2. HEALTH SERVICES

2.1 Health expenditure

2.1.1 Expenditure on health

		Year	Source
(as % of GNP)	3	1983-84	(0800)

2.1.2 Expenditure on PHC

		Year	Source
(as % of total health expenditure)	46	1983-84	(0800)

2.2 Primary Health Care
(Percentage of population covered by):

2.2.1 Health services

		Year	Source
National	54	1984	(0834)
Urban			
Rural			

2.2.2 Safe water

		Year	Source
National	65	1984	(0834)
Urban	82	1984	(0834)
Rural	54	1984	(0834)

2.2.3 Adequate sanitary facilities

		Year	Source
National	55	1984	(0834)
Urban			
Rural			

2.2.4 Contraceptive prevalence rate

		Year	Source
(%)	1	1977	(1712)

2.3   Coverage of maternity care (%)

Area	Prenatal care	Trained attendant	Institutional deliveries	Postnatal care	Sample size	Year	Source
National	74	59				1984	(2008)
National	37	45				1988	(2033)
National:	78	52	52	28		1979-84	(1828)
urban	94	84	84	42		1979-84	(1828)
rural	75	48	48	26		1979-84	(1828)
24 districts	79	52	81			1984	(1338)

3.   COMMUNITY STUDIES

3.1   Central Region, 1977 [0114]

3.1.1   Rate

A study of the Central Region of Malawi (population about 2 million) found 118 maternal deaths for 114 103 "expected" live births, of which 112 occurred in hospital and six at home. The maternal mortality rate was 103 per 100 000 live births. Information on all maternal deaths known to have occurred within or outside all health institutions was obtained from doctors and midwives. The author suspects gross underreporting of deaths occurring at home.

3.1.2   Causes of maternal deaths *(available for 116 cases)*

Haemorrhage was the main cause of death, followed by rupture of the uterus. None of the latter were ruptures of a previous caesarean scar. In eight cases, the rupture had occurred at home after the women had been in labour for between 36 and 96 hours.

Cause	Number	%
Haemorrhage	28	24
Rupture of the uterus	19	16
Obstructed labour	13	11
Sepsis	10	9
Abortion	4	3
Ectopic pregnancy	3	3
Hypertensive disorders of pregnancy	3	3
Puerperal tetanus	3	3
Embolisms	2	2
Other direct obstetric causes	6	5
DIRECT CAUSES	91	78
Anaemia	7	6
Accidental poisoning by herbal medicines	7	6
Hepatitis	1	1
Other infections	5	4
Other indirect obstetric causes	5	4
INDIRECT CAUSES	25	22
TOTAL	116	100

3.1.3   Avoidable factors * *(available for 109 cases)*

	Number	%
Patient and home environment		
Delay at home	38	34
Use of herbal medicines	15	14
Refused admission	1	1
Medical services		
Shortage of blood	43	39
Medical staff factors	30	28
Nursing staff factors	26	24
Ambulance service inadequate	17	15
Lack of telephone	12	11
Poor equipment or facilities	5	5

*   categories not mutually exclusive.

While delay at home was an important avoidable factor, the number of cases in which the medical services were responsible in one way or another was significant. Medical and nursing staff factors were present in 56 cases. This included instances of patient mismanagement such as failure to diagnose the problem, failure to initiate appropriate treatment and failure to refer sufficiently early to a higher level of care.

3.1.4   High risk groups

3.1.5   Other findings

The study also gives the place of death for 109 of the 118 maternal deaths.

Place of death	Number
Home	6
Rural maternity unit	9
During transfer to district hospital	2
Mission hospital	23
District hospital	39
Central hospital	30
TOTAL	109

3.2 Southern Region, Thyolo District, 1985-89 [2484]

The Thyolo District is a densely populated area with a total population of 431 539 (1987 statistics). It is divided into eleven Traditional Areas, each of which is further subdivided into a number of Enumeration Areas, with a population of some 500-700 people. The study used the "sisterhood method" to estimate the number of maternal deaths occurring during the previous five years. This method has been described elsewhere (2355) and consists essentially of interviewing adults in a defined population to detect the number of sisters dying from pregnancy-related causes.

In this survey 4 000 adult respondents were selected from the Enumeration Areas which were selected at random and scattered proportionately throughout the Traditional Areas. In order to avoid duplication of information care was taken to avoid interviewing adults born to the same mother.

3.2.1 Rate
Maternal deaths	149
MMR (per 100 000 live births)	420

The study estimated that the lifetime risk of a woman dying through pregnancy related causes was 1 in 32.

3.2.2 Causes of maternal deaths (for 98 deaths only)
	%
Haemorrhage	25
Obstructed labour/ruptured uterus	20
Abortion	18
Sepsis	13
Complications of caesarean section	8
Hypertensive disorders of pregnancy	4
Injuries, accidents and other causes	10

4. HOSPITAL STUDIES

4.1 All health institutions, Central Region, 1977 [0114]

4.1.1 Rate
Live births	42 533
Maternal deaths	112
MMR (per 100 000 live births)	263

4.2 Six district hospitals, 1983 [0929]

4.2.1 Rate
District	Deliveries	Maternal deaths	MMR (per 100 000 deliveries)
Chikwawa	848	4	471
Chirazulu	4 850	1	21
Chitipa	2 133	7	328
Mchinji	1 409	5	354
Salima	1 704	14	822
Thyolo	1 693	2	118
Total	12 637	34	269

4.3 Twelve hospitals, 1989 [2472]

4.3.1 Rate
Births	35 160
Maternal deaths	214
MMR (per 100 000 births)	609

4.3.2 Causes of maternal deaths
	Number	%
Abortion	39	18
Sepsis	25	12
Haemorrhage	22	16
Ruptured uterus	18	8
Obstructed labour	11	5
Hypertensive disorders of pregnancy	6	3
Ectopic pregnancy	3	1
Hydatiform mole	2	1
Anaesthesia	1	1
DIRECT CAUSES	127	59
Anaemia	17	8
Meningitis	7	3
AIDS	5	2
Cardiac failure	4	2
Malaria	2	1
Intoxication with traditional medicines	1	1
Other infections	14	7
Other indirect causes	16	7
INDIRECT CAUSES	66	31
Unknown	21	10
TOTAL	214	100

4.3.3 Avoidable factors
	Number	%
Deficient hospital care	61	29
Patient's delay	42	19
Pregnancy contraindicated	11	5
Deficient care at health centre	6	3
Transfer problem between health units	4	2
Uncertain	47	22
No avoidable factors discerned	43	20
TOTAL	214	100

4.4 Kamuzu Central Hospital, Lilongwe, 1985 [1563]

4.4.1 Rate

Live births	8 075
Maternal deaths	69
MMR (per 100 000 live births)	854

4.4.2 Causes of maternal deaths* *(available for 60 cases)*

	Number	%
Anaemia	23	38
Sepsis	16	27
Rupture of the uterus	14	23
Associated with caesarean section	10	17
Abortion	8	13
Hypertensive disorders of pregnancy	5	8
Renal failure	5	8
Ectopic pregnancy	3	5
Hepatic failure	2	4
Others/Unknown	1	2

*   categories not mutually exclusive.

4.4.3 Avoidable factors*

	Number	%
Patient delay	29	48
Medical personnel responsible	14	23
Lack of blood	10	17
Donors unavailable	10	17
Peripheral unit delay	7	12
Anaesthetic death	3	5
Lack of transport	2	3
Appropriate drug unavailable	2	3
District medical officer absent	2	3
District laboratory officer absent	1	2

*   categories not mutually exclusive.

Transport problems were much more acute in the past but have been largely resolved by a more disciplined approach to the use of vehicles and by assuring residence for night-call staff within the hospital. Another problem was that medical staff were sometimes required simultaneously at the Central Hospital and the Old Wind Maternity Hospital, three kilometres away. This alone had contributed to death in some cases. Non-availability of adequate supplies of blood for transfusion remains a major problem.

The author asserts that much more could be learned about the relative importance of avoidable factors if more adequate hospital records were maintained. This would permit retrospective analysis of the data.

4.5 Ekwendeni Hospital, Ekwendeni, 1976-88 [1638, 1953, 2474]

4.5.1 Rate

	Deliveries	Maternal deaths	MMR (per 100 000 deliveries)
1976-85	8 711	30	344
1986-88	3 155	1	32

The hospital has a prenatal waiting shelter, which has greatly reduced the maternal mortality rate. Obstetrical emergencies are fast becoming a thing of the past. Other factors seen as contributing to the reduction of maternal mortality include:

- increased numbers of elective lower segment caesarean sections;

- blood transfusion service, and routine supply of iron to women attending clinics for prenatal care;

- aggressive use of antibiotics in puerperal sepsis and suspected illegal abortions;

- increasing supervision of prenatal patients to discourage intake of toxic herbal medicines;

- improved health education of "at risk" patients with the result that the majority made use of the maternity waiting home and subsequently delivered in hospital;

- the use of new and better facilities from 1986;

- supervision by well-trained and motivated staff and the routine in-service training of staff and refresher courses to maintain motivation;

- availability of ambulances for "flying squad" duties;

- early culdocentesis in cases of suspected ectopic pregnancy;

- introduction of family planning services with the aim of reducing the numbers of grand multiparas delivering.

Problems remain in four major areas:

- the nutritional status of women (during 1988, as a result of a series of poor harvests, there was a big increase in the proportion of women suffering from severe anaemia (less than 8 gm/dl);

- the availability of blood especially in emergencies (there is a marked reluctance on the part of many in the community to give blood to non-relatives);

- the failure of staff to adequately complete and analyse prenatal histories;

- HIV infection and AIDS

4.6 Mulanje Mission Hospital, 1989 [(2518)]

4.6.1 Rate
Deliveries	5 109
Maternal deaths	21
MMR (per 100 000 deliveries)	411

4.6.2 Causes of maternal deaths
Haemorrhage	5
Ruptured uterus	4
Sepsis	3
Meningitis	4
Pneumonia	3
Tetanus	1
Other	1
Total	21

4.6.3 Avoidable factors
Eleven of the patients died within 24 hours of admission indicating that they reached the hospital in a desperate condition. Long transport delays were an important contributory factor. In some cases there was insufficient blood available for transfusion.

4.6.4 High risk groups

4.6.5 Other findings
The hospital receives around 12 new fistula cases every year, of which half are treated on the spot, two or three cases are referred elsewhere and nothing is known about the fate of the remainder. The typical fistula patient is a young primipara without living children, abandoned by her husband, and is from a poor family.

5. CIVIL REGISTRATION DATA/GOVERNMENT ESTIMATES

6. OTHER SOURCES/ ESTIMATES

6.1 National and by region, 1980-87 [(2474)]

6.1.1 Rate
National	MMR (per 100 000 births)
1980-84	250
1985	180
1987	167
By region, 1987	
Northern	270
Central	180
Southern	100

7. SELECTED ANNOTATED BIBLIOGRAPHY

Bullough, C. et al Early suckling and postpartum haemorrhage: controlled trial in deliveries by traditional birth attendants *The Lancet* 1989, 8662. WHE 2347

A randomised, controlled trial was carried out to determine whether suckling immediately after birth reduces the frequency of postpartum haemorrhage, the mean blood loss, and the frequency of retained placenta. The trial subjects were attended by traditional birth attendants and randomisation was by TBA and not by mother. 23 TBAs in the early suckling group and 26 in the control group recorded blood loss in 2 104 and 1 123 deliveries of liveborn singletons respectively. The frequency of postpartum haemorrhage (loss greater than 500ml) was 7.9% in the suckling group and 8.4% in the control group and the mean blood loss was 258ml and 256ml respectively. Neither result is statistically significant. Analysis of the results by individual TBA showed no significant differences between the groups. The frequency of postpartum haemorrhage in women of higher parity and in those with multiple pregnancies and stillbirths was high, as expected, which seems to validate the results.

8. FURTHER READING

Armon, P.J. Rupture of the uterus in Malawi and Tanzania *East African Medical Journal* 1977 54(9): 462-471. WHE 0042

Boerma, T. The magnitude of the maternal mortality problem in sub-Saharan Africa. *Social Science and Medicine* 1987; 24(6): 551-558. WHE 1532

Boerma, T. *Maternal mortality in sub-Saharan Africa: levels, causes and interventions* 1987. WHE 1655

Chiphangwi, J.D. Obstetric problems in a developing country – experience in Malawi *Medical Quarterly* 1983; 13: 5-6. WHE 0145

Leigh, B. The urban poor and obstetric outcome *Journal of Tropical Pediatrics* 1983; 29(5): 265-267. WHE 0412

Mbvundula, M.W. Maternal and child health services in Malawi *Medical Quarterly* 1982; 10: 25-26. WHE 0445

Mtimavalye, L.A.R. Reproductive health care among women in Africa: current trends and the future. *Journal of Obstetrics and Gynaecology of Eastern and Central Africa* 1982; 1(2): 48-53. WHE 0468

9. DATA SOURCES

WHE 0114 Bullough, C. Analysis of maternal deaths in the Central Region of Malawi. *East African Medical Journal* 1981; 58(1): 25-36

WHE 0753 United Nations. *Demographic Yearbook.* New York, various years

WHE 0800 World Health Organization. *Country reports to regional offices of the progress in implementing Health for All by the Year 2000.* (Unpublished documents) 1983

WHE 0834 World Health Organization. *World Health Statistics annual – vital statistics and causes of death.* Geneva, various years

WHE 0929 World Health Organization/UNICEF/ Governmant of Malawi. *Joint programme review MCH, EPI, PHC,* August 1984, WHO document no. MCH/85.6, 1985

WHE 1338 World Health Organization, Regional Office for Africa. *Where are we in PHC? Countries take a close look at themselves through PHC reviews* Part II October 1985

WHE 1563 Keller, M.E. Maternal mortality at Kamazu Central Hospital for 1985. *Medical Quarterly (Malawi)* 1987; 4(1): 13-16

WHE 1638 Knowles, J.K. *The antenatal waiting shelter as an important factor in reducing maternal mortality.* 1986 (unpublished document)

WHE 1712 Mauldin W.P. and Segal, S.J. *Prevalence of contraceptive use in developing countries. A chart book.* Rockefeller Foundation, New York 1986

WHE 1828 Malawi, National Statistical Office. *Family formation survey.* Ministry of Health 1987

WHE 1914 United Nations Children's Fund (UNICEF). *The state of the world's children,* various years, Oxford, Oxford University Press

WHE 1915 United Nations. Department of International Economic and Social Affairs. *World population prospects: estimates and projections as assessed in 1984.* Population Studies No. 98. New York 1986

WHE 1918 United Nations. Department of International Economic and Social Affairs. *First marriage: patterns and determinants.* New York 1988

WHE 1953 Knowles, J.K. A shelter that saves mothers' lives *World Health Forum,* 1988; 9: 387-388

WHE 2008 World Health Organization. Regional Office for Africa *Evaluation of the strategy for health for all by the year 2000. Seventh report on the world health situation* Vol 2, African region, Brazzaville 1987

WHE 2033 World Health Organization. *Global strategy for health for all by the year 2000. Second report on monitoring progress.* WHO document EB83/2 Add. 1, 1988

WHE 2472 Driessen, F. *Maternal deaths in 12 Malawi hospitals in 1989.* (unpublished document) 1990

WHE 2474 Knowles, J.K. *The multifactorial approach in reducing maternal mortality* (personal communication) 1989

WHE 2484 Chiphangwi, J.D. et al. *Maternal mortality in Southern Malawi – Thyolo District* (unpublished draft document), 1989

WHE 2518 Kempf, M. *Mulanje Mission Hospital Annual Report 1989* and personal communication, 1990

MALI

		Year	Source

1. BASIC INDICATORS

1.1 Demographic

1.1.1 Population

		Year	Source
Size (millions)	8.8	1988	(1914)
Rate of growth (%)	2.9	1980-87	(1914)

1.1.2 Life expectancy

		Year	Source
Female	44	1980-85	(1915)
Male	40	1980-85	(1915)

1.1.3 Fertility

		Year	Source
Crude Birth Rate	50	1988	(1914)
Total Fertility Rate	6.7	1988	(1914)

1.1.4 Mortality

		Year	Source
Crude Death Rate	21	1988	(1914)
Infant Mortality Rate	168	1988	(1914)
Female	125	1977-86	(1978)
Male	138	1977-86	(1978)
1-4 years mortality rate			
Female	174	1977-86	(1978)
Male	166	1977-86	(1978)

1.2 Social and economic

1.2.1 Adult literacy rate (%)

		Year	Source
Female	11	1985	(1914)
Male	23	1985	(1914)

1.2.2 Primary school enrolment rate (%)

		Year	Source
Female	17	1986-88	(1914)
Male	29	1986-88	(1914)

1.2.3 Female mean age at first marriage

		Year	Source
(years)	18.1	1976	(1918)

1.2.4 GNP/capita

		Year	Source
(US $)	210	1987	(1914)

1.2.5 Daily per capita calorie supply

		Year	Source
(as % of requirements)	86	1984-86	(1914)

2. HEALTH SERVICES

2.1 Health expenditure

2.1.1 Expenditure on health

		Year	Source
(as % of GNP)	1	1983	(0800)

2.1.2 Expenditure on PHC

		Year	Source
(as % of total health expenditure)	25	1984	(0800)

2.2 Primary Health Care
(Percentage of population covered by):

2.2.1 Health services

		Year	Source
National	20	1980	(0834)
Urban			
Rural			

2.2.2 Safe water

		Year	Source
National	17	1985-87	(1914)
Urban	46	1985-87	(1914)
Rural	10	1985-87	(1914)

2.2.3 Adequate sanitary facilities

		Year	Source
National	21	1983	(0834)
Urban	90	1984	(0834)
Rural	5	1984	(0834)

2.2.4 Contraceptive prevalence rate

		Year	Source
(%)	3	1982-87	(1978)

2.3   Coverage of maternity care (%)

Area	Prenatal care	Trained attendant	Institutional deliveries	Postnatal care	Sample size	Year	Source
National		14				1984	(1744)
National		16				1988	(2033)
National	27	27			3 374	1982-87	(1978)
urban	69	74			810	1982-87	(1978)
rural	14	12			2 563	1982-87	(1978)

3. COMMUNITY STUDIES

4. HOSPITAL STUDIES

4.1   All hospitals, Bamako, 1981-82 [0296]

4.1.1   Rate

A study of abortion in Mali quotes an estimated 24 000 obstetric and gynaecological admissions and 50 maternal deaths during 1981-82, giving a maternal mortality rate of 208 per 100 000 admissions. Five of the 50 were abortion deaths, two from induced and three from spontaneous abortions. Although women with abortion complications represented only 0.5% of obstetric admissions, they accounted for at least 4% of maternal deaths.

4.2   Hamdallaye Maternity Hospital, Bamako, 1979-81 [1112]

4.2.1   Rate

Live births*	8 750
Maternal deaths	1
MMR (per 100 000 live births)	11

*   Includes some deliveries outside the hospital.

5. CIVIL REGISTRATION DATA/GOVERNMENT ESTIMATES

5.1   National, 1987 [1744]

5.1.1   Rate

A Ministry of Health report published in 1987 estimated the maternal mortality rate to be between 1 750 and 2 900 per 100 000 live births.

6. OTHER SOURCES/ ESTIMATES

7. SELECTED ANNOTATED BIBLIOGRAPHY

Chabot, H.T.J. and Rutten, A.M. Use of antenatal cards for literate health personnel and illiterate traditional birth attendants: an overview. *Tropical Doctor* January 1990. WHE 2444

Few antenatal/prenatal cards have been developed for use by illiterate traditional birth attendants. A version of an antenatal/prenatal card for illiterates which has been developed in Mali is presented. The authors emphasize that the particular value of the card is that it can be used at the various levels of the health care pyramid, including specifically, the village level, where traditional birth attendants are likely to continue to take care of pregnant women in rural areas for the foreseeable future.

Defontaine. P., A propos de cinquante ruptures utérines observées à l'hôpital du Point "G", Bamako, Mali. *Médecine Tropicale* 1976; 36(3): 217-222. WHE 1872

Between January 1971 and June 1974 there were 73 cases of uterine rupture at the hospital. An analysis of the 50 cases for which adequate records were available shows that the most important risk factors were grand multiparity, previous caesarean section and dystocia. The survival of the patient depends crucially on the rapidity of surgical intervention. Of the 50 uterine ruptures, 40 occurred prior to admission and there were 15 deaths. Of the ten ruptures which took place after hospitalization, there were two deaths. Overall, 34% of the patients died. There is an urgent need to upgrade the skills of local midwives, to encourage prenatal consultations, to improve the level of services available at rural maternity centres and to facilitate the transfer of patients if and when the need arises.

8. FURTHER READING

Frank, O. The demand for fertility control in sub-Saharan Africa. Working paper no. 117. *Studies in Family Planning* 1987; 18(4): 181-201. WHE 1371

9. DATA SOURCES

WHE 0296 Binkin, N.J. et al. Women hospitalized for abortion complications in Mali. *International Family Planning Perspectives* 1984; 10(1): 8-12

WHE 0800 World Health Organization. *Country reports to regional offices of the progress in implementing Health for All by the Year 2000.* (Unpublished documents) 1983

WHE 0834 World Health Organization. *World Health Statistics annual – vital statistics and causes of death.* Geneva, various years

WHE 1112 Janowitz, B. et al. *Reproductive health in Africa: issues and options.* Family Health International, North Carolina 1984

WHE 1744 Ministère de la Santé Publique et des Affaires Sociales, Division de la Santé Familiale. *Recherche/actions sur la maternité sans risque* 1987

WHE 1914 United Nations Children's Fund (UNICEF). *The state of the world's children,* various years, Oxford, Oxford University Press

WHE 1915 United Nations. Department of International Economic and Social Affairs. *World population prospects: estimates and projections as assessed in 1984.* Population Studies No. 98. New York 1986

WHE 1918 United Nations. Department of International Economic and Social Affairs. *First marriage: patterns and determinants.* New York 1988

WHE 1978 Traoré, B. et al. *Enquête Démographique et de Santé au Mali 1987.* Centre d'Etudes et de Recherches sur la Population pour le Développement, Institut du Sahel, Bamako, and Institute for Resource Development/Westinghouse 1988 (preliminary report)

WHE 2033 World Health Organization. *Global strategy for health for all by the year 2000. Second report on monitoring progress.* WHO document EB83/2 Add. 1, 1988

NOTES

MAURITANIA

	Year	Source

1. BASIC INDICATORS

1.1 Demographic

1.1.1 Population
Size (millions)	1.9	1988	(1914)
Rate of growth (%)	2.6	1980-87	(1914)

1.1.2 Life expectancy
Female	48	1988	(1914)
Male	44	1988	(1914)

1.1.3 Fertility
Crude Birth Rate	46	1988	(1914)
Total Fertility Rate	6.5	1988	(1914)

1.1.4 Mortality
Crude Death Rate	19	1988	(1914)
Infant Mortality Rate	126	1988	(1914)
Female			
Male			
1-4 years mortality rate			
Female			
Male			

1.2 Social and economic

1.2.1 Adult literacy rate (%)
Female
Male

1.2.2 Primary school enrolment rate (%)
Female	42	1986-88	(1914)
Male	61	1986-88	(1914)

1.2.3 Female mean age at first marriage
(years)

1.2.4 GNP/capita
(US $)	440	1987	(1914)

1.2.5 Daily per capita calorie supply
(as % of requirements)	92	1984-86	(1914)

2. HEALTH SERVICES

2.1 Health expenditure

2.1.1 Expenditure on health
(as % of GNP)	8	1986	(2033)

2.1.2 Expenditure on PHC
(as % of total health expenditure)	60	1986	(2033)

2.2 Primary health care
(Percentage of population covered by):

2.2.1 Health services
National	30	1983	(0834)
Urban			
Rural			

2.2.2 Safe water
National	37	1984	(0834)
Urban	80	1984	(0834)
Rural	16	1984	(0834)

2.2.3 Adequate sanitary facilities
National			
Urban	7	1983	(0834)
Rural			

2.2.4 Contraceptive prevalence rate
(%)	1	1980-87	(1914)

2.3   Coverage of maternity care (%)

Area	Prenatal care	Trained attendant	Institutional deliveries	Postnatal care	Sample size	Year	Source
National	58	23				1983	(2008)
National	26	20				1985	(2033)

3.   COMMUNITY STUDIES

4.   HOSPITAL STUDIES

5.   CIVIL REGISTRATION DATA/GOVERNMENT ESTIMATES

6.   OTHER SOURCES/ ESTIMATES

7.   SELECTED ANNOTATED BIBLIOGRAPHY

8.   FURTHER READING

9.   DATA SOURCES

WHE0834   World Health Organization. *World Health Statistics annual – vital statistics and causes of death.* Geneva, various years

WHE1914   United Nations Children's Fund (UNICEF). *The state of the world's children,* various years, Oxford, Oxford University Press

WHE2008   World Health Organization. Regional Office for Africa *Evaluation of the strategy for health for all by the year 2000. Seventh report on the world health situation* Vol 2, African region, Brazzaville 1987

WHE2033   World Health Organization. *Global strategy for health for all by the year 2000. Second report on monitoring progress.* WHO document EB83/2 Add. 1, 1988

MAURITIUS

	Year	Source

1. BASIC INDICATORS

1.1 Demographic

1.1.1 Population

Size (millions)	1.1	1988	(1914)
Rate of growth (%)	1.5	1980-87	(1914)

1.1.2 Life expectancy

Female	69	1980-85	(1915)
Male	64	1980-85	(1915)

1.1.3 Fertility

Crude Birth Rate	18	1988	(1914)
Total Fertility Rate	1.9	1988	(1914)

1.1.4 Mortality

Crude Death Rate	5	1988	(1914)
Infant Mortality Rate	22	1988	(1914)
Female	56	1971-73	(1917)
Male	69	1971-73	(1917)
1-4 years mortality rate			
Female	7	1971-73	(1917)
Male	6	1971-73	(1917)

1.2 Social and economic

1.2.1 Adult literacy rate (%)

Female	77	1985	(1914)
Male	89	1985	(1914)

1.2.2 Primary school enrolment rate (%)

Female	107	1986-88	(1914)
Male	105	1986-88	(1914)

1.2.3 Female mean age at first marriage

(years)	21.7	1983	(1918)

1.2.4 GNP/capita

(US $)	1 490	1987	(1914)

1.2.5 Daily per capita calorie supply

(as % of requirements)	121	1985	(1914)

2. HEALTH SERVICES

2.1 Health expenditure

2.1.1 Expenditure on health

(as % of GNP)	2	1986	(2033)

2.1.2 Expenditure on PHC

(as % total health expenditure)	10	1986	(2033)

2.2 Primary Health Care
(Percentage of population covered by):

2.2.1 Health services

National	100	1983	(0834)
Urban			
Rural			

2.2.2 Safe water

National	99	1984	(0834)
Urban	100	1984	(0834)
Rural	98	1984	(0834)

2.2.3 Adequate sanitary facilities

National	97	1984	(0834)
Urban	100	1984	(0834)
Rural	95	1984	(0834)

2.2.4 Contraceptive prevalence rate

(%)	56	1984	(1712)

2.3   Coverage of maternity care (%)

Area	Prenatal care	Trained attendant	Institutional deliveries	Postnatal care	Sample size	Year	Source
National	90	84	81			1983	(2008)
National	90	84				1983	(0834)
National		85	77		1 741	1985	(1969)
National:							
urban		96	91		700	1985	(1969)
rural		77	68		1 041	1985	(1969)
Rodrigues	100	85	70			1985	(1342)

3. COMMUNITY STUDIES

4. HOSPITAL STUDIES

5. CIVIL REGISTRATION DATA/GOVERNMENT ESTIMATES

5.1   National and by district, 1970-1980 (0443)

5.1.1   Rate

	Live births	Maternal deaths	MMR (per 100 000 deliveries)
1970-74	104 865	157	150
1975-79	115 778	136	117
1980	24 983	27	108

District	MMR (per 100 000 births) 1980
Port Louis	200
Pamplemousses	80
Riv. du rempart	40
Flacq	–
Grandport	170
Savanne	320
Plaines Wilhems	70
Moka	190
Black river	–

5.2   National, 1972-87 (0834)

5.2.1   Rate

	Live births	Maternal deaths	MMR (per 100 000 births)
1972			177
1973			153
1974			135
1975			112
1976			113
1977			167
1978			99
1979			100
1980			108
1982	21 247	21	99
1983	19 948	11	55
1984	19 222	18	94
1985	18 520	19	103
1986	18 225	23	126
1987	19 190	19	99

5.2.2   Causes of maternal deaths

Abortion, clandestinely induced in a majority of the cases, accounted for half the maternal deaths.

	1982-86	
	Number	%
Abortion	46	50
Haemorrhage	18	20
Hypertensive disorders of pregnancy	11	12
Complications of the puerperium	7	8
Other direct obstetric causes	8	8
Indirect causes	2	2
Total	92	100

5.3 National, 1982 [(0753)]

5.3.1 Rate

MMR (per 100 000 live births)	99

6. OTHER SOURCES/ ESTIMATES

6.1 National, 1984 [(1341)]

6.1.1 Rate

Live births	19 202
Maternal deaths	10
MMR (per 100 000 live births)	52

6.2 National, 1977-81 [(1141)]

6.2.1 Rate

Live births	120 689
Maternal deaths due to abortion	71
Abortion deaths per 100 000 live births	59

7. SELECTED ANNOTATED BIBLIOGRAPHY

8. FURTHER READING

9. DATA SOURCES

WHE 0443   Mauritius, Ministry of Health. *Vital health statistics of the Island of Mauritius* 1980, Post Louis.

WHE 0753   United Nations. *Demographic Yearbook.* New York, various years

WHE 0834   World Health Organization. *World Health Statistics annual – vital statistics and causes of death.* Geneva, various years

WHE 1141   International Bank for Reconstruction and Development, Mauritius. *Population sector review* No. 4486-MAS, Washington, 1983

WHE 1341   Radhakeesoon, B. *Impact of government family planning and child health services in Mauritius* (Unpublished MPH thesis) 1985

WHE 1342   World Health Organization. EPI as a component of MCH, *Weekly Epidemiological Record* 1986; 61: 77-79

WHE 1712   Mauldin W.P. and Segal, S.J. *Prevalence of contraceptive use in developing countries. A chart book.* Rockefeller Foundation, New York 1986

WHE 1914   United Nations Children's Fund (UNICEF). *The state of the world's children,* various years, Oxford, Oxford University Press

WHE 1915   United Nations. Department of International Economic and Social Affairs. *World population prospects: estimates and projections as assessed in 1984.* Population Studies No. 98. New York 1986

WHE 1917   United Nations. Department of International Economic and Social Affairs. *Age structure of mortality in developing countries. A database for cross-sectional and time-series research.* New York 1986

WHE 1918   United Nations. Department of International Economic and Social Affairs. *First marriage: patterns and determinants.* New York 1988

WHE 1969   Mauritius, Ministry of Health, Evaluation Unit. *Mauritius contraceptive prevalence survey* 1985, Georgia, Center for Disease Control

WHE 2008   World Health Organization. Regional Office for Africa *Evaluation of the strategy for health for all by the year 2000. Seventh report on the world health situation* Vol 2, African region, Brazzaville 1987

WHE 2033   World Health Organization. *Global strategy for health for all by the year 2000. Second Report.* Geneva 1988

NOTES

MOROCCO

		Year	Source

1. BASIC INDICATORS

1.1 Demographic

1.1.1 Population

		Year	Source
Size (millions)	23.9	1988	(1914)
Rate of growth (%)	2.6	1980-87	(1914)

1.1.2 Life expectancy

Female	60	1980-85	(1915)
Male	57	1980-85	(1915)

1.1.3 Fertility

Crude Birth Rate	35	1988	(1914)
Total Fertility Rate	4.8	1988	(1914)

1.1.4 Mortality

Crude Death Rate	10	1988	(1914)
Infant Mortality Rate	80	1988	(1914)
Female	71	1982-86	(2717)
Male	76	1982-86	(2717)
1-4 years mortality rate			
Female	31	1982-86	(2717)
Male	31	1982-86	(2717)

1.2 Social and economic

1.2.1 Adult literacy rate (%)

Female	22	1985	(1914)
Male	45	1985	(1914)

1.2.2 Primary school enrolment rate (%)

Female	56	1986-88	(1914)
Male	85	1986-88	(1914)

1.2.3 Female mean age at first marriage

(years)	22.3	1982	(1918)

1.2.4 GNP/capita

(US $)	610	1987	(1914)

1.2.5 Daily per capita calorie supply

(as % of requirements)	118	1984-86	(1914)

2. HEALTH SERVICES

2.1 Health expenditure

2.1.1 Expenditure on health

(as % of GNP)	4	1987	(2033)

2.1.2 Expenditure on PHC

(as % of total health expenditure)	57	1987	(2033)

2.2 Primary Health Care
(Percentage of population covered by):

2.2.1 Health services

National	93	1987	(2033)
Urban			
Rural			

2.2.2 Safe water

National	57	1984	(0834)
Urban	73	1987	(2033)
Rural	17	1987	(2033)

2.2.3 Adequate sanitary facilities

National	46	1984	(0834)
Urban	63	1986	(2033)
Rural	13	1986	(2033)

2.2.4 Contraceptive prevalence rate

(%)	36	1987	(0753)

2.3 Coverage of maternity care (%)

Area	Prenatal care	Trained attendant	Institutional deliveries	Postnatal care	Sample size	Year	Source
National		20	17			1979-80	(1210)
Rabat-Salé				41		1976	(1902)

3. COMMUNITY STUDIES

4. HOSPITAL STUDIES

4.1 Centre Hospitalier Universitaire Averroes de Casablanca, 1978-80 [0103]

4.1.1 Rate

Deliveries	28 706
Maternal deaths	94
MMR (per 100 000 live births)	327

4.1.2 Causes of maternal deaths

	Number	%
Haemorrhage	29	31
Ruptured uterus	15	16
Sepsis	12	13
Embolisms	9	10
Hypertensive disorders of pregnancy	7	7
Obstetric shock	4	4
Complications of anaesthesia	2	2
DIRECT CAUSES	78	83
Hepatitis	4	4
Other infections	3	3
Others	9	10
INDIRECT CAUSES	16	17
TOTAL	94	100

Sepsis was more frequently a cause of death in women of parity 1 and 2 than in women of higher parities (7 out of the 12 sepsis deaths), while haemorrhage and rupture of the uterus were the most frequent causes of death in grand multiparous women (parity 6-14). Of 32 maternal deaths among grand multiparae, 11 were from haemorrhage and a further 12 from rupture of the uterus.

4.1.3 Avoidable factors

19 cases were judged to be avoidable given intensive care and more adequate medication.

4.1.4 High risk groups.

Parity	Deliveries	Maternal deaths	MMR (per 100 000 births)
1-2	16 232	32	197
3-5	6 514	30	461
6+	5 960	32	537

4.2 Centre Hospitalier Universitaire de Rabat-Salé, 1976-77 [1902]

4.2.1 Rate

MMR (per 100 000 live births)	200

4.3 Oujda Maternity Hospital, 1975-81 [2114]

4.3.1 Rate

Year	Deliveries	Maternal deaths	MMR (per 100 000 births)
1975	2 653	15	565
1976	2 976	12	403
1977	3 026	13	429
1978	3 190	19	595
1979	3 409	15	440
1980	3 305	20	605
1981	2 232	28	1 254
1975-81	20 791	122	586

4.3.2 Causes of maternal deaths

	Number	%
Haemorrhage	32	27
Sepsis	21	18
Ruptured uterus	18	15
Hypertensive disorders of pregnancy	8	7
Obstetric shock	4	3
Embolisms	3	3
Other direct causes	5	4
DIRECT CAUSES	91	76
Cardiorespiratory conditions	11	9
Other indirect causes	11	9
INDIRECT CAUSES	22	18
Unknown	7	6
TOTAL	120	100

5. CIVIL REGISTRATION DATA/GOVERNMENT ESTIMATES

6. OTHER SOURCES/ ESTIMATES

6.1 National, 1974 [(1902)]

6.1.1 Rate

The maternal mortality rate was estimated at between 200 and 300 per 100 000 live births in 1974.

7. SELECTED ANNOTATED BIBLIOGRAPHY

8. FURTHER READING

Abdelhaq, J. and Boukhrissi, *Case study for the improvement of family planning in Morocco* Ministry of Public Health, 1981. WHE 0005

Faour, M. Fertility policy and family planning in the Arab countries *Studies in Family Planning* 1989; 20(5): 254-263. WHE 2367

Mernissi, F. Obstacles to family planning practice in urban Morocco *Studies in Family Planning* 1975; 6(12): 418-425. WHE 0455

9. DATA SOURCES

WHE 0103   Boutaleb, Y. at al. Mortalité maternelle et mortalité perinatale. *Journal de Gynaecologie Obstétrique et Biologie de la Réproduction* 1982; 2(1): 99-102

WHE 0753   United Nations. *Demographic Yearbook.* New York, various years

WHE 0834   World Health Organization. *World Health Statistics annual – vital statistics and causes of death.* Geneva, various years

WHE 1210   Morocco, Ministry of Health. World Fertility Survey *Enquête nationale sur la fécondité et la planification nationale 1979-80* Rapport national Vol 3, 1984

WHE 1902   Temmar, F.M. Paper presented to meeting on *L'enseignement des aspects préventifs et sociaux de l'obstétrique* Paris, 28 February – 17 March 1978

WHE 1914   United Nations Children's Fund (UNICEF). *The state of the world's children,* various years, Oxford, Oxford University Press

WHE 1915   United Nations. Department of International Economic and Social Affairs. *World population prospects: estimates and projections as assessed in 1984.* Population Studies No. 98. New York 1986

WHE 1918   United Nations. Department of International Economic and Social Affairs. *First marriage: patterns and determinants.* New York 1988

WHE 2033   World Health Organization. *Global strategy for health for all by the year 2000. Second report on monitoring progress.* WHO document EB83/2 Add. 1, 1988

WHE 2114   Des Forts, J. *Projet de recherche mortalité maternelle en Algérie* INESSM, 1986

WHE 2717   Demographic and Health Surveys. *Enquête nationale sur la planification familiale, la fécondité et la santé de la population au Maroc (ENPS) 1987,* Ministère de la Santé Publique/ Resource Development/Westinghouse, 1989

NOTES

MOZAMBIQUE

		Year	Source

1. BASIC INDICATORS

1.1 Demographic

1.1.1 Population

Size (millions)	14.8	1988	(1914)
Rate of growth (%)	2.6	1980-87	(1914)

1.1.2 Life expectancy

Female	46	1980-85	(1915)
Male	44	1980-85	(1915)

1.1.3 Fertility

Crude Birth Rate	45	1988	(1914)
Total Fertility Rate	6.4	1988	(1914)

1.1.4 Mortality

Crude Death Rate	18	1988	(1914)
Infant Mortality Rate	172	1988	(1914)
Female			
Male			
1-4 years mortality rate			
Female			
Male			

1.2 Social and economic

1.2.1 Adult literacy rate (%)

Female	22	1985	(1914)
Male	55	1985	(1914)

1.2.2 Primary school enrolment rate (%)

Female	59	1986-88	(1914)
Male	76	1986-88	(1914)

1.2.3 Female mean age at first marriage

(years)	17.6	1980	(1918)

		Year	Source

1.2.4 GNP/capita

(US $)	170	1987	(1914)

1.2.5 Daily per capita calorie supply

(as % of requirements)	69	1984-86	(1914)

2. HEALTH SERVICES

2.1 Health expenditure

2.1.1 Expenditure on health

(as % of GNP)	1	1987	(2033)

2.1.2 Expenditure on PHC

(as % of total health expenditure)	38	1987	(2033)

2.2 Primary Health Care
(Percentage of population covered by):

2.2.1 Health services

National	30	1987	(2033)
Urban			
Rural			

2.2.2 Safe water

National	9	1980	(0834)
Urban	82	1980	(0834)
Rural	2	1980	(0834)

2.2.3 Adequate sanitary facilities

National	10	1980	(0834)
Urban			
Rural			

2.2.4 Contraceptive prevalence rate

(%)	4	1981-85	(2033)

2.3   Coverage of maternity care (%)

Area	Prenatal care	Trained attendant	Institutional deliveries	Postnatal care	Sample size	Year	Source
National	46	28				1983	(0834)
Maputo	94					1981	(1493)

3. COMMUNITY STUDIES

4. HOSPITAL STUDIES

4.1   Maputo Central Hospital, Maputo, 1984 [0848, 1282]

4.1.1   Rate

Live births	10 769
Maternal deaths	40
MMR (per 100 000 live births)	371

4.1.2   Causes of maternal deaths

	Number	%
Hypertensive disorders of pregnancy	9	23
Sepsis	5	13
Haemorrhage	5	13
Abortion	3	7
Complications of anaesthesia	2	5
DIRECT CAUSES	24	60
Anaemia	2	5
Malaria	2	5
Other infections	5	13
INDIRECT CAUSES	9	38
Others	7	18
TOTAL	40	100

4.1.3   Avoidable factors

4.1.4   High risk groups

4.1.5   Other findings
   More than 80% of women who died had attended a prenatal clinic either in a peripheral hospital or a health centre. Nonetheless deaths occurred from preventable problems such as anaemia and eclampsia, leading to the conclusion that special attention needs to be paid to the quality of prenatal care.

5. CIVIL REGISTRATION DATA/GOVERNMENT ESTIMATES

5.1   National, 1981 [1148]

5.1.1   Rate
   A study of maternal morbidity in Mozambique quotes a Ministry of Health source giving a maternal mortality rate of 300 per 100 000 live births in 1981.

6. OTHER SOURCES/ ESTIMATES

7. SELECTED ANNOTATED BIBLIOGRAPHY

Jelley, D. and Madeley, R.J. Antenatal care in Maputo, Mozambique *Journal of Epidemiology and Community Health* 1983; 37: 111-116. WHE 1860

   In 1980 a prenatal control form was introduced into all Maputo's antenatal clinics to monitor pregnancies and to help direct specialist care to mothers at greatest risk. In this study three health centres were selected from contrasting areas of the city. Almost 1000 completed antenatal forms were analysed to determine the incidence of risk and to evaluate the implementation of this strategy. It was found that a considerable number of women at risk were identified, referred and successfully monitored throughout their pregnancies. Of those women at risk who were identified by the health centres, fewer than half were actually referred for specialist care. Those women at greatest risk were not the highest users of the services and many of them underused the services compared with women at lower risk.

8. FURTHER READING

9. DATA SOURCES

WHE 0834   World Health Organization. *World Health Statistics annual – vital statistics and causes of death.* Geneva, various years

WHE 0848   Songane, F. Analise dos casos de mortes maternas ocorridas nos primeiros 7 meses de 1984, Maputo, Hopital Central *Boletin Informativo do Servico de Ginecologia Obstetricia* February 1985

WHE 1148   Liljestrand, J. *Maternal mortality in Mozambique* University of Uppsala, 1985

WHE 1282   Songade, F. *Maternal mortality at Maputo Central Hospital* in: FIGO congress, Berlin September 1985

WHE 1493   Jelley, D. and Madeley, R.J. Preventive health care for mothers and children. A study in Mozambique. *Journal of Tropical Medicine and Hygiene* 1983; 86: 229-236

WHE 1914   United Nations Children's Fund (UNICEF). *The state of the world's children,* various years, Oxford, Oxford University Press

WHE 1915   United Nations. Department of International Economic and Social Affairs. *World population prospects: estimates and projections as assessed in 1984.* Population Studies No. 98. New York 1986

WHE 1918   United Nations. Department of International Economic and Social Affairs. *First marriage: patterns and determinants.* New York 1988

WHE 2033   World Health Organization. *Global strategy for health for all by the year 2000. Second report on monitoring progress.* WHO document EB83/2 Add. 1, 1988

NOTES

NAMIBIA

	Year	Source

1. BASIC INDICATORS

1.1 Demographic

1.1.1 Population

Size (millions)	1.8	1988	(1914)
Rate of growth (%)	3.1	1988	(1914)

1.1.2 Life expectancy

Female	50	1980-85	(0753)
Male	47	1980-85	(0753)

1.1.3 Fertility

Crude Birth Rate	44	1988	(1914)
Total Fertility Rate	6.1	1988	(1914)

1.1.4 Mortality

Crude Death Rate	10	1988	(1914)
Infant Mortality Rate	105	1988	(1914)
Female			
Male			
1-4 years mortality rate			
Female			
Male			

1.2 Social and economic

1.2.1 Adult literacy rate (%)
Female
Male

1.2.2 Primary school enrolment rate (%)
Female
Male

1.2.3 Female mean age at first marriage
(years)

	Year	Source

1.2.4 GNP/capita
(US $)

1.2.5 Daily per capita calorie supply

(as % of requirements)	82	1984-86	(1914)

2. HEALTH SERVICES

2.1 Health expenditure

2.1.1 Expenditure on health
(as % of GNP)

2.1.2 Expenditure on PHC
(as % of total health expenditure)

2.2. Primary Health Care
(Percentage of population covered by):

2.2.1 Health services
National
Urban
Rural

2.2.2 Safe water
National
Urban
Rural

2.2.3 Adequate sanitary facilities
National
Urban
Rural

2.2.4 Contraceptive prevalence rate
(%)

2.3   Coverage of maternity care (%)

Area	Prenatal care	Trained attendant	Institutional deliveries	Postnatal care	Sample size	Year	Source
	–	–	–	–	–	–	–

3. COMMUNITY STUDIES

4. HOSPITAL STUDIES

5. CIVIL REGISTRATION DATA/GOVERNMENT ESTIMATES

6. OTHER SOURCES/ ESTIMATES

7. SELECTED ANNOTATED BIBLIOGRAPHY

8. FURTHER READING

9. DATA SOURCES

WHE 0753   United Nations. *Demographic Yearbook.* New York, various years

WHE 1914   United Nations Children's Fund (UNICEF). *The state of the world's children,* various years, Oxford, Oxford University Press

NIGER

		Year	Source

1. BASIC INDICATORS

1.1 Demographic

1.1.1 Population
		Year	Source
Size (millions)	6.7	1988	(1914)
Rate of growth (%)	2.9	1980-87	(1914)

1.1.2 Life expectancy
		Year	Source
Female	44	1980-85	(1915)
Male	41	1980-85	(1915)

1.1.3 Fertility
		Year	Source
Crude Birth Rate	51	1988	(1914)
Total Fertility Rate	7.1	1988	(1914)

1.1.4 Mortality
		Year	Source
Crude Death Rate	21	1988	(1914)
Infant Mortality Rate	134	1988	(1914)
Female			
Male			
1-4 years mortality rate			
Female			
Male			

1.2 Social and economic

1.2.1 Adult literacy rate (%)
		Year	Source
Female	9	1985	(1914)
Male	19	1985	(1914)

1.2.2 Primary school enrolment rate (%)
		Year	Source
Female	20	1986-88	(1914)
Male	37	1986-88	(1914)

1.2.3 Female mean age at first marriage
(years)

1.2.4 GNP/capita
		Year	Source
(US $)	260	1987	(1914)

1.2.5 Daily per capita calorie supply
		Year	Source
(as % of requirements)	100	1984-86	(1914)

2. HEALTH SERVICES

2.1 Health expenditure

2.1.1 Expenditure on health
		Year	Source
(as % of GNP)	6	1982	(0800)

2.1.2 Expenditure on PHC
		Year	Source
(as % of total health expenditure)	53	1984	(0800)

2.2 Primary Health Care
(Percentage of population covered by):

2.2.1 Health services
		Year	Source
National	48	1984	(0834)
Urban			
Rural			

2.2.2 Safe water
		Year	Source
National	37	1983	(0834)
Urban	48	1983	(0834)
Rural	34	1983	(0834)

2.2.3 Adequate sanitary facilities
		Year	Source
National	9	1983	(0834)
Urban	36	1983	(0834)
Rural	3	1983	(0834)

2.2.4 Contraceptive prevalence rate
		Year	Source
(%)	1	1977	(1712)

2.3 Coverage of maternity care (%)

Area	Prenatal care	Trained attendant	Institutional deliveries	Postnatal care	Sample size	Year	Source
National		25				1980	(0697)
National	27					1982	(0586)
National	47	47				1983	(0834)
Agadez	54					1982	(0586)
Diffa	21					1982	(0586)
Dosso	24					1982	(0586)
Maradi	22					1982	(0586)
Niamey	46					1982	(0586)
Niamey	93		84			1988	(2088)
Tahoua	19					1982	(0586)
Zinder	15					1982	(0586)
Zinder	18		9			1987	(2088)

3. COMMUNITY STUDIES

4. HOSPITAL STUDIES

4.1 All institutions, 1982 [0586]

4.1.1 Rate

Area	Deliveries	Maternal deaths	MMR (per 100 000 births)
Agadez	2 630	8	304
Diffa	2 873	14	487
Dosso	17 451	83	476
Maradi	18 772	80	426
Niamey	30 372	82	263
Tahoua	25 116	107	426
Zinder	17 982	110	612
Total	115 196	484	420

4.2 Maternité Centrale, Niamey, 1973-88 [2112, 2164]

4.2.1 Rate

	Live births	Maternal deaths	MMR (per 100 000 deliveries)
1973-78	39 291*	122	311
1979-84	56 573*	202	357
1985-88	30 694	140	456

* Deliveries

During 1985-88 nearly 64% of the 140 maternal deaths were in women coming from outside the city although they constituted only 11% of deliveries. If deaths of women originating outside Niamey are excluded, maternal mortality rates are considerably lowered.

	MMR (per 100 000 live births)	
Year	Women from all areas	Women from within Niamey
1985	242	84
1987	394	172

4.2.2 Causes of death, 1973-83 and 1983-88

	1973-83		1983-88	
	Number	%	Number	%
Haemorrhage	59	30	36	27
Sepsis	55	28	28	21
Uterine rupture	53	27	37	28
Hypertensive disorders of pregnancy	31	16	31	23
TOTAL	198	100	132	100

An analysis of maternal deaths by cause and parity over the period 1973-83 shows that hypertensive disorders of pregnancy were the major cause of death among primiparae while haemorrhage was the leading cause of death among grand multiparae.

	Number of deaths at parity:			
	1	2-5	6+	TOTAL
Haemorrhage	1	12	46	59
Sepsis	18	22	15	55
Uterine rupture	2	8	43	53
Hypertensive disorders of pregnancy	28	3	0	31
TOTAL	49	45	104	198

4.2.3 Avoidable factors

4.2.4 High risk groups, 1985-88

Age group	Live births	Maternal deaths	MMR (per 100 000 births)
10-14	49	0	–
15-19	5 631	19	337
20-24	9 188	37	402
25-29	7 835	20	255
30-34	5 181	23	444
35-39	2 317	30	1 290
40-44	475	3	631
45-49	68	8	1 176

4.2.5 Other findings
Under-reporting

An examination of records at the National Hospital in Niamey indicates that during 1986 there were at least 24 deaths which could be classified as maternal although they occurred in a general rather than a maternity hospital. There were 32 maternal deaths in the three maternity hospitals in Niamey during 1986. There is, therefore, considerable undercounting of maternal deaths if data from the maternity hospitals alone are taken into consideration.

Fistulae

During a period of eight years, 1977-1984, there were 428 cases of urogenital and rectovaginal fistula at the National Hospital in Niamey of which 412 (96%) were obstetrical in origin. 58% of the patients were primiparous, two thirds were less than 25 years of age and 37% were younger than 19 years old.

5. CIVIL REGISTRATION DATA/GOVERNMENT ESTIMATES

6. OTHER SOURCES/ ESTIMATES

6.1 National, 1980 [0697]

6.1.1 Rate

An attempt was made to estimate maternal mortality rates for different areas of the country using "expected" births instead of "recorded" deliveries in the denominator since births were thought to be greatly underreported. The number of births expected was calculated on the basis of the 1977 Census which was considered to give a fair representation of the population distribution by age and sex. The birth rate of Niger was estimated to be of the order of 50 per 1000.

Area	Births expected	Births recorded *	Maternal deaths	MMR (per 100 000 births) expected	recorded
Agadez	7 450	2 540	10	134	394
Diffa	8 850	2 910	12	136	412
Dosso	37 250	9 650	47	126	487
Maradi	51 350	11 980	60	117	501
Niamey	64 600	25 370	90	139	355
Tahoua	52 950	10 210	90	170	881
Zinder	54 350	9 400	65	120	691
Total	276 800	72 070	374	135	519

* Rounded to nearest ten births.

It should be noted that although the authors felt that maternal deaths were sufficiently serious events to warrant reporting to the health authorities whenever they occurred, this view is not shared by all those working in the field and a case can be made that many maternal deaths occurring at home were not registered. (see section 8, Further Reading)

6.2 National and Zinder rural area, 1988 [2088]

6.2.1 Rate

	National	Zinder
MMR (per 100 000 live births)	700	860

7. SELECTED ANNOTATED BIBLIOGRAPHY

Docquier, J. and Sako. A. Fistules recto-vaginales d'origine obstetricale. *Médecine d'Afrique Noire* 1983; 30(5): 213-215. WHE 1063

This is the report of a four-year study (January 1977 - December 1980) carried out in Niamey Hospital in Niger, of 283 patients with vesico-vaginal fistulae, of which 277 were entirely obstetrical in origin. Of these, 28 recto-vesico-vaginal fistulae (RVVF) were found, and are presented in detail here. One woman died shortly after arrival in hospital and two others died later, not due to interventions.

Of the 25 women left, 20 (80%) were aged 15-19, and 18 (72%) were primiparae. Fourteen of the women were measured and of these, seven measured between 1.35m and 1.50m. It is concluded that these three characteristics – age, parity and height – are linked most closely with the occurrence of fistulae.

Surgical techniques are also described. There was an 88% cure rate, with the majority being operated via the vaginal route. One patient died.

8. FURTHER READING

Gray, R.H. Maternal mortality in developing countries (letter) *International Journal of Epidemiology* 1985; 14(2): 337. WHE 1093

Juncker, T. Maternal mortality in developing countries. (letter) *International Journal of Epidemiology* 1985; 14: 338. WHE 1227

Thuriaux, M.C. and Lamotte, J-M, Maternal mortality in developing countries (letter) *International Journal of Epidemiology* 1985; 14: 485-486. WHE 0975

9. DATA SOURCES

WHE 0586   Niger, Republic of, Ministère de la Santé Publique et des Affaires Sociales. *Rapport d'activités 1982.* Niamey, 1983

WHE 0697   Thuriaux, M.C. and Lamotte, J-M. Maternal mortality in developing countries: a note on the choice of denominator. *International Journal of Epidemiology* 1984; 13(2): 246-247.

WHE 0800   World Health Organization. *Country reports to regional offices of the progress in implementing Health for All by the Year 2000.* (Unpublished documents) 1983

WHE 0834   World Health Organization. *World Health Statistics annual – vital statistics and causes of death.* Geneva, various years

WHE 1712   Mauldin W.P. and Segal, S.J. *Prevalence of contraceptive use in developing countries. A chart book.* Rockefeller Foundation, New York 1986

WHE 1914   United Nations Children's Fund (UNICEF). *The state of the world's children,* various years, Oxford, Oxford University Press

WHE 1915   United Nations. Department of International Economic and Social Affairs. *World population prospects: estimates and projections as assessed in 1984.* Population Studies No. 98. New York 1986

WHE 2088   Guimba, A.D. *Santé maternelle au Niger.* Conférence régionale sur la maternité sans risques pour l'Afrique francophone, 1989

WHE 2112   Huguet, D. et al. Maternal mortality in a Sahelian capital (letter) *Lancet* 11 March 1989; 557.

WHE 2164   Huguet, D. and Prual, A. *La santé maternelle à Niamey – analyse de la situation.* Ministère de la Santé Publique et des Affaires Sociales, 1988

NIGERIA

		Year	Source

1. BASIC INDICATORS

1.1 Demographic

1.1.1 Population

		Year	Source
Size (millions)	105.5	1988	(1914)
Rate of growth (%)	3.4	1980-87	(1914)

1.1.2 Life expectancy

		Year	Source
Female	50	1980-85	(1915)
Male	47	1980-85	(1915)

1.1.3 Fertility

		Year	Source
Crude Birth Rate	50	1988	(1914)
Total Fertility Rate	7.0	1988	(1914)

1.1.4 Mortality

		Year	Source
Crude Death Rate	15	1988	(1914)
Infant Mortality Rate	104	1988	(1914)
Female			
Male			
1-4 years mortality rate			
Female			
Male			

1.2 Social and economic

1.2.1 Adult literacy rate (%)

		Year	Source
Female	31	1985	(1914)
Male	54	1985	(1914)

1.2.2 Primary school enrolment rate* (%)

		Year	Source
Female	85	1986-88	(1914)
Male	97	1986-88	(1914)

* Net

1.2.3 Female mean age at first marriage

		Year	Source
(years)	18.7	1981-82	(1918)

1.2.4 GNP/capita

		Year	Source
(US $)	370	1987	(1914)

1.2.5 Daily per capita calorie supply

		Year	Source
(as % of requirements)	90	1988	(1914)

2. HEALTH SERVICES

2.1 Health expenditure

2.1.1 Expenditure on health
(as % of GNP)

2.1.2 Expenditure on PHC

(as % of total health expenditure)	3	1986	(2033)

2.2 Primary Health Care
(Percentage of population covered by):

2.2.1 Health services

National
Urban
Rural

2.2.2 Safe water

National	36	1983	(0834)
Urban	60	1983	(0834)
Rural	30	1983	(0834)

2.2.3 Adequate sanitary facilities

National			
Urban	30	1983	(0834)
Rural			

2.2.4 Contraceptive prevalence rate

(%)	5	1981-82	(1712)

2.3   Coverage of maternity care (%)

Area	Prenatal care	Trained attendant	Institutional deliveries	Postnatal care	Sample size	Year	Source
National		40				1980	(1227)
Bendel State		57			3 958d	(1984)	(0267)
Ebendo rural		3	3		322w	1974	(0467)
Kainji Lake	8		3	9	4 508	(1989)	(2276)
Lagos urban	80		79		2 352w	1980	(0426)
Ogun State	76					1984	(1338)
Ondo State	80	56			4 213	1981-86	(2491)
Ondo State riverine areas	17	9				1981-86	(2491)
Oyo State	25		11			1978	(0495)
Plateau State	24	3				1977	(0793)
Udi rural	68	38		56	498	1986-88	(2457)
Western State	10					1976	(0908)
Zaria rural	70		40		22 774w	1983	(0313)

3.   COMMUNITY STUDIES

3.1   Imesi-ile village, South West Nigeria, 1961-69 [0321]

The data for this study was drawn from a Birth and Death Register maintained in the village dispensary run by the Wesley Guild Hospital in the town of Ilesha from 1957. The dispensary has a small room set aside for delivery. A dispensary car transported emergency cases to the Wesley Guild Hospital 40 kilometers (about an hour's ride) away.

3.1.1   Rate

Live births	2 324
Maternal deaths	4
MMR (per 100 000 live births)	171

The author affirms that, in the absence of the services described above, the rate would have been not lower than 600 per 100 000 live births, and probably as high as 1200 per 100 000 live births. At least 20 maternal deaths had been averted during the nine year period covered by the study.

3.1.2   Causes of maternal deaths

	Number
Postpartum haemorrhage	1
Hepatitis	1
Typhoid fever	1
Tuberculosis and typhoid fever	1
Total	4

3.1.3   Avoidable factors

3.1.4   High risk groups

3.1.5   Other findings

Sixteen percent of the 2 146 pregnancies studied were associated with a potentially dangerous condition such as haemorrhage (6%), multiple pregnancy (4%) and cephalo-pelvic disproportion (2%). Six percent of all deliveries were transferred to the Wesley Guild Hospital due to serious complications.

4. HOSPITAL STUDIES

4.1 Twenty-three hospitals, Western State, 1972-73 [(0506)]

4.1.1 Rate

	1972	1973
Births	24 332	25 415
Maternal deaths	93	119
MMR (per 100 000 births)	380	470

4.1.2 Causes of maternal deaths

	1972 Number	1972 %	1973 Number	1973 %
Obstructed labour	29	31	37	31
Haemorrhage	30	32	3	29
Hypertensive disorders of pregnancy	9	10	13	11
Sepsis	5	5	5	6
Abortion	2	2	4	3
DIRECT CAUSES	7	81	93	78
Anaemia	9	10	11	9
Haemoglobinopathies	1	1	3	3
Others	8	9	11	9
INDIRECT CAUSES	18	19	25	21
TOTAL	93	100	119	100

4.2 Ten hospitals in Anambra State, 1981-85 [(2237)]

4.2.1 Rate

The aim of the study was to investigate maternal deaths in forty institutions, including 17 maternity homes and 23 hospitals in Anambra State. However, major problems were encountered with regard to record keeping and collaboration with some of the institutions. The authors were, therefore, obliged to limit the research to ten hospitals which had retained some basic data.

Live births	48 046
Maternal deaths	239
MMR (per 100 000 live births)	497

4.2.2 Causes of maternal deaths

	Number	%
Uterine rupture	66	28
Haemorrhage	55	23
Obstructed labour	31	13
Sepsis	29	12
Hypertensive disorders of pregnancy	19	8
Abortion*	5	3
DIRECT CAUSES	205	86
Anaemia	7	3
Jaundice	7	3
INDIRECT CAUSES	14	6
Unknown	20	8
TOTAL	239	100

* The authors suspect under-reporting of abortion deaths in view of the grave social stigma attached.

4.2.3 Avoidable factors

Of the 232 deaths for which booking status was known, 203 (88%) occurred among unbooked patients.

4.2.4 High risk groups

Nearly 30% of the deaths occurred among women of parity 5 or higher and a further 17% among nulliparous women.

4.3 General Hospital, Benin, 1970-71 [(0164)]

4.3.1 Rate

Deliveries	7 080
Maternal deaths	33
MMR (per 100 000 deliveries)	466

4.3.2 Causes of maternal deaths (available for 30 cases)

	Number	%
Abortion	4	14
Haemorrhage	3	10
Hypertensive disorders of pregnancy	3	10
Ectopic pregnancy	1	3
Obstructed labour	1	3
Uterine rupture	1	3
DIRECT CAUSES	13	43
Tetanus	3	10
Hepatitis	2	7
Anaemia	1	3
Malaria	1	3
Other infections	6	20
Others	4	14
TOTAL	30	100

Severe anaemia (haemoglobin less than 30%) was not very common. Less than 3% of the women admitted for delivery had a mean haemoglobin level lower than 45%.

4.4. University of Benin Teaching Hospital, 1973-88 [(0511, 0514, 1112, 2152, 2419)]

4.4.1 Rate

	1973-85	1986-88
Deliveries	29 324	5 256
Maternal deaths	165	22
MMR (per 100 000 deliveries)	563	419

4.4.2 Causes of maternal deaths
Abortion [(0511, 2152)]

A study carried out over the six-year period 1974-79 found that induced abortion accounted for 27% of the total maternal deaths and that induced abortion among adolescents accounted for 17% of all maternal deaths.

Over the period 1973-85 abortion accounted for 37 (22%) of the 165 maternal deaths and illegally induced abortion for 34 of these deaths. The main cause of abortion related death was sepsis. The majority of the fatal cases were induced in the second trimester of pregnancy.

Causes of abortion-related deaths, 1973-85*

Sepsis	25
Haemorrhage	7
Perforated uterus	6
Tetanus	6
Cardiac problems	2
Other	6

* Categories not mutually exclusive

Obstructed labour [0514]

A study carried out from 1973 to 1977 found 6 369 deliveries and 136 cases of obstructed labour, an incidence of 2.1%. During the same period 520 caesarean sections were performed, 102 of which were carried out because of obstructed labour. Analysis of case notes was possible for 126 cases in all. Most of the women arrived at the hospital moribund having been in labour for several days. Some were originally booked for prenatal care but failed to attend to avoid possible caesarean delivery. A small group was referred from maternity homes where facilities were inadequate. The majority of the cases of obstructed labour (103 cases) were due to feto-pelvic disproportion. There was one maternal death and two cases of vesicovaginal fistulae.

4.4.3   Avoidable factors

4.4.4   High risk groups, 1973-85

Maternal mortality rates were highest among young women aged under 15 years and in women aged 39 years and over. The very high rate among under 15 patients was entirely accounted for by abortion deaths. The majority of all abortion deaths occurred among adolescents, induced abortion accounting for 70% of all maternal deaths in the 15-19 year-old age group and for all the deaths among girls aged 15 years or less.

Age	Deliveries	Maternal deaths	MMR (per 100 000 deliveries)	Abortion deaths	Abortion as % of total deaths
<15	47	3	6 383	3	100
15-19	3 230	26	805	18	69
20-24	8 391	36	429	3	8
25-29	9 829	36	366	5	14
30-34	5 730	16	279	–	–
35-39	1 774	15	846	1	7
39+	318	9	2 830	1	11
Total*	29 324	165	563	37	22

* Including 11 deliveries to women of unknown age.

4.5   Catholic Maternity Hospital, Benin City, 1985-86 [2404]

4.5.1   Rate

Live births	5 688
Maternal deaths	19*
MMR (per 100 000 live births)	334

* Including two deaths from abortion.

4.5.2   Causes of maternal deaths

4.5.3   Avoidable factors

Although 85% of all deliveries were to women who were booked for prenatal care and who had attended the prenatal clinics before delivery, they accounted for only 30% of maternal deaths.

	Booked	Unbooked
Live births	4 835	853
Maternal deaths	5	12
MMR (per 100 000 live births)	103	1 407

4.5.4   High risk groups

	Live births	Maternal deaths	MMR (per 100 000 live births)
Age group			
15-19	553	3	543
20-24	2 022	4	198
25-29	2 018	5	248
30-34	712	5	702
Parity			
Primiparous	1 084	6	554
Multiparous	4 225	5	118
Para 7 and higher	400	6	1 500
Educational level			
Nil	889	4	450
Primary	1 853	7	378
Secondary	2 228	5	224
Tertiary	550	1	182
Social class			
I and II	379	0	–
III	1 106	3	271
IV	1 668	6	360
V	1 725	7	406
unclassified	310	1	323

Social class was obtained through a scoring index combining a woman's level of education with the occupation of her husband, which allocates each woman to a social class I to V, social class V being at the bottom of the social stratification.

Ethnic group

There were no statistically significant differences in maternal mortality rates between the various ethnic groups.

4.5.5 Other findings

There were no significant differences in mortality by distance from the hospital.

4.6 Calabar Maternity Unit and Aba Maternity Unit, South Eastern State, [(0775)]

4.6.1 Rate

	Calabar 1964-65	Aba 1970-71
Deliveries	2 168	4 307
Maternal deaths	41	75
MMR (per 100 000 deliveries)	1 891	1 741

4.6.2 Causes of maternal deaths

	Calabar 1964-65		Aba 1970-71	
	Number	%	Number	%
Haemorrhage	13	33	16	21
Hypertensive disorders of pregnancy	8	20	10	13
Ruptured uterus	5	13	11	15
Prolonged labour	5	13	7	9
Sepsis	3	8	3	4
DIRECT CAUSES	34	83	47	63
Hepatitis	–	–	18	24
Anaemia	1	3	1	1
Tetanus	–	–	3	4
Others	6	10	6	8
TOTAL	41	100	75	100

4.6.3 Avoidable factors

Maternal mortality rates were higher among unbooked patients.

	Calabar 1964-65		Aba 1970-71	
	Booked	Unbooked	Booked	Unbooked
Deliveries	1 897	271	3 738	569
Maternal deaths	6	35	20	55
MMR (per 100 000 deliveries)	316	12 915	535	9 666

4.6.4 High risk groups

Primigravidae were at greater risk of death than multigravidae, with maternal mortality rates of 2 010 and 1 680 per 100 000 live births respectively. The higher primigravid mortality is attributable to higher incidence of eclampsia. Of 38 primigravid deaths, eclampsia alone caused 16 deaths and 16 of the 18 eclampsia deaths were in primigravidae.

4.7 University of Nigeria Teaching Hospital, Enugu, 1971-72 [(2419)]

4.7.1 Rate

MMR (per 100 000 deliveries)	1 350

4.7.2 Causes of maternal deaths [(0449)]

Between 1974 and 1979 there were 73 cases of jaundice, an incidence of 345 per 100 000 births. There were eight maternal deaths resulting from jaundice, a fatality rate of 11%. Viral hepatitis was found to be the commonest cause of jaundice, accounting for 69% of the total.

4.8 Wesley Guild Hospital, Ilesha, 1958-70 [(0320)]

4.8.1 Rate

Deliveries	14 485
Maternal deaths*	133
MMR (per 100 000 deliveries)	918

* Deaths from abortion, ectopic pregnancy and anaemia not included.

4.8.2 Causes of maternal deaths

	Number	%
Haemorrhage	34	26
Uterine rupture	29	22
Hypertensive disorders of pregnancy	21	16
Sepsis	10	7
Obstructed labour	9	7
Ectopic pregnancy	2	1
DIRECT CAUSES	105	79
Anaemia	12	9
Hepatitis	10	7
Tetanus	5	4
Others	1	1
INDIRECT CAUSES	28	21
TOTAL	133	100

4.8.3 Avoidable factors

Maternal mortality rates were higher among unbooked patients.

	Booked	Unbooked
Deliveries	10 163	4 322
Maternal deaths	29	104
MMR (per 100 000 deliveries)	285	2 406

4.9 Ife State Hospital and Wesley Guild Hospital, Ilesha, 1979-80 [(1897)]

4.9.1 Rate

Live births	6 308
Maternal deaths	66
MMR (per 100 000 live births)	1 046

4.9.2.   Causes of maternal deaths

4.9.3   Avoidable factors

47 (71%) of the deaths occurred among unbooked patients.

4.10   Baptist Medical Centre, Ile-Ife, 1966-75 [0049]

4.10.1   Rate

Births	13 182
Maternal deaths	90
MMR (per 100 000 births)	683

4.10.2   Causes of maternal deaths

	Number	%
Haemorrhage	30	33
Complications of caesarean section	16	18
Ruptured uterus	12	13
Hypertensive disorders of pregnancy	10	11
Anaemia	7	8
Sepsis	5	6
Embolisms	5	6
Complications of anaesthesia	4	4
Others	1	1
Total	90	100

4.11   University of Ilorin Teaching Hospital, Ilorin, Kwara State, 1972-83, 1984-87 and 1988 [1728, 2238, 2245, 2411, 2413, 2419]

4.11.1   Rate

	1972-83	1984-87	1988
Births	138 577	27 714	6 203
Maternal deaths	624	138	16
MMR (per 100 000 births)	450	498	258

	Deliveries*	Maternal* deaths	MMR* (per 100 000 deliveries)
1972	5 752	36	626
1973	6 756	45	666
1974	7 718	39	505
1975	9 058	52	574
1976	11 228	58	517
1977	12 530	59	471
1978	13 146	77	586
1979	14 844	70	472
1980	15 779	61	387
1981	15 908	41	258
1982	17 394	41	237
1983	11 373	31	273
1984	9 536	36	378
1985	5 909	26	440
1986	6 333	32	505
1987	5 936	44	741
1988	6 203	16	258

*   There are slight differences in the data taken from the two sources 1728 and 2411.

4.11.2   Causes of maternal deaths 1972-83 (for 624 deaths)

	Number	%
Haemorrhage	151	24
Ruptured uterus	87	14
Obstructed labour	74	12
Hypertensive disorders of pregnancy	70	11
Sepsis	52	8
Hemoglobinopathies	7	1
Anaesthetic death	4	1
Embolisms	4	1
DIRECT CAUSES	449	72
Anaemia	47	8
Meningitis	35	6
Pulmonary infections	31	5
Hepatitis	21	4
Native drug intoxication	18	3
Tetanus	7	1
Uremia	7	1
INDIRECT CAUSES	166	27
Unknown	9	1
TOTAL	624	100

Eclampsia [2411, 2478]

A study of maternal deaths during 1972-87 (2411) found that there were 169 200 deliveries and 748 maternal deaths in all, a maternal mortality rate for the 16-year period of 442 per 100 000 births. There were 651 cases of eclampsia, an incidence of 3.8/1000 births, and 94 maternal deaths, a case fatality rate of 14.4%. Eclampsia accounted for 12.6% of the total maternal deaths, a maternal mortality rate for eclampsia alone of 56 per 100 000 births. Maternal deaths were high in the very young primigravida and in elderly women of higher parity.

Age	Parity	Total eclampsia deaths	Survivors eclampsia cases	Total eclampsia cases
15-19	0	29	73	102
	1+	14	69	83
20-24	0	1	35	36
	1+	25	126	151
25-34	0-3	3	35	38
	4+	8	101	109
35 and older	0-3	1	27	28
	4+	13	91	104
Total		94	557	651

During the period 1968-87, the incidence of eclampsia was 4.2/1000 deliveries (2478). There was a seasonal distribution of eclampsia cases with greater frequency during the wet season. There were 3.5 cases of eclampsia during the wet season for every case occurring during the dry season. Long-term maternal morbidities included secondary amenorrhea, infertility, epilepsy and blindness from retinal haemorrhage. Maternal mortality was highest in elderly multiparous women although the majority of eclampsia cases occurred among young primigravidae.

Abortion [2413]

A study of abortion mortality over the 15-year period 1972-86 found that there were 53 maternal deaths associated with illegally induced abortion. In the same period there were 12 736 cases of abortion (induced and spontaneous) and 173 521 live births. The rate of abortion per 1000 live births was 73.4 and the abortion mortality rate was 416 per 100 000 total abortions. Septicemia accounted for 66% of the abortion deaths and haemorrhage for a further 21%. Seventeen of the maternal deaths occurred among women younger than 20 years old and 28 were nulliparous.

Caesarean section [2238]

A study of maternal deaths following caesarean section was carried out during the 5-year period 1982-86. During the study period there were 48 974 deliveries of which 1 992 were by caesarean section, a rate of 4.1%. The total number of maternal deaths was 125 with 36 deaths following caesarean section. The mortality rate for caesarean section was 18.1 per 1000 compared with 1.9 per 1000 for vaginal deliveries. Maternal sepsis was responsible for 81.5% of the caesarean deaths. Obstructed labour was the single most important indication for caesarean section and was the most significant predisposing factor for maternal sepsis. Avoidable factors included late admission in 20 cases and unbooked status in 14 cases. In all patients there was a failure to use prophylactic antibiotics. Some patients were not on any antibiotics until the third postoperative day because the relatives were not able to buy the drugs immediately when they were not in stock in the hospital pharmacy. There were difficulties in contacting medical staff during emergencies and no telephone services to doctors were available.

Haemorrhage [2245]

During a 16-year period (1972-87) there were 169 200 deliveries with 7 088 cases of haemorrhage. Of the 4 293 women who had no prenatal care 134 died, a fatality rate of 31.2 per 1000 cases of haemorrhage. Only 29 of the 2 795 booked patients died, a fatality rate of 10.4 per 1000. The overall maternal mortality rate for haemorrhage was 229 per 100 000 births. Maternal mortality was found to be greatly influenced by environmental factors, especially those related to transportation difficulties. The majority of the women who died had travelled a minimum of ten kilometers to reach the hospital and arrived in a very poor condition. There was a general shortage of blood and blood components at the hospital. The author asserts that there is a need to train primary health care workers in simple and effective techniques in order to reduce the risks of death from haemorrhage.

4.11.3 Avoidable factors

The author suggests that the majority of the maternal deaths could be avoided if expectant women attended prenatal clinics, accepted medical advice, declined unorthodox interference and reported to hospital early in labour. The large number of deaths from postpartum haemorrhage was attributed to unorthodox ways of conducting the third stage of labour, whereby a violent fundal pressure combined with uncontrolled cord traction was employed by midwives. Also ergometrine was administered when available after delivery of the placenta. Lack of adequate quantity of blood for transfusion coupled with the poor response from husbands or relations of the patients to donate blood when so requested compounded the problems posed by haemorrhage.

Over 80% of the deaths occurred among unbooked patients.

4.12 Ahmadu Bello University Teaching Hospital, Kaduna, 1964-72, 1976-77 and 1987-88 [0057, 0117, 2419]

4.12.1 Rate

	1964-72	1976-77	1987-88
Births	42 976	22 237	4 366
Maternal deaths	163*	141*	25
MMR (per 100 000 births)	379	634	573

* Excluding abortions and ectopic pregnancies.

4.12.2 Causes of maternal deaths

Rupture of the uterus and haemorrhage were the major causes of maternal deaths during 1964-72 and continued to be important causes of death during the years 1976-77. Hepatitis was a significant indirect cause of maternal deaths.

	1964-72		1976-77	
	Number	%	Number	%
Haemorrhage	39	15	14	10
Ruptured uterus	27	17	13	9
Hypertensive disorders of pregnancy	27	17	11	8
Sepsis	15	9	13	9
Obstructed labour	10	6	–	–
Complications of anaesthesia	4	3	–	–
DIRECT CAUSES	122	75	51	36
Hepatitis	11	7	10	7
Cardiac disease	9	6	–	–
Anaemia	7	4	–	–
INDIRECT CAUSES	27	17	10	8
Others/Unknown	14	16	80	56
TOTAL	163	100	141	100

4.13 Maternity Hospital, Katsina, 1974-81 and 1988 [1519, 2419]

4.13.1 Rate*

	1974-81	1988
Live births	10 492	3 370
Maternal deaths	63	151
MMR (per 100 000 live births)	600	4 481

* Only the women belonging to the Hausa ethnic group were considered for this study.

4.13.2 Causes of maternal deaths, 1974-81

	Number	%
Haemorrhage	26	41
Uterine rupture	20	31
Obstructed labour	13	20
Hypertensive disorders of pregnancy	2	4
DIRECT CAUSES	61	97
Anaemia	1	2
Cardiac diseases	1	2
INDIRECT CAUSES	2	3
TOTAL	63	100

4.14 Five hospitals, Ibadan City, 1982 [1658]

4.14.1 Rate

Deliveries	35 650
Maternal deaths	110
MMR (per 100 000 deliveries)	310

4.14.2 Causes of maternal deaths (available for 96 cases)

Infective hepatitis accounted for an unusually large number of maternal deaths in this series.

	Number	%
Haemorrhage	28	29
Hypertensive disorders of pregnancy	13	14
Ruptured uterus	8	8
Sepsis	6	6
Complications of anaesthesia	4	4
DIRECT CAUSES	59	61
Hepatitis	19	20
Others	13	14
INDIRECT CAUSES	32	33
Unexplained	5	5
TOTAL	96	100

4.14.3 Avoidable factors

Maternal mortality rates were higher in unbooked women.

	Booked	Unbooked
Deliveries	31 481	4 169
Maternal deaths*	37	59
MMR (per 100 000 deliveries)	120	1 420

* Booking status was not known for 14 deaths.

4.14.4 High risk groups

An analysis of maternal deaths by age and parity shows that women below 20 years of age and women of parity five and more had higher maternal mortality rates.

Age group	MMR (per 100 000 deliveries)
15-19	526
20-24	144
25-29	211
30-34	310
35-39	159
40+	337
Parity	
0	191
1	225
2	183
3	237
4	276
5+	508

4.15 University College Hospital, Ibadan, Oyo State, 1957-60, 1962-71, 1983-84 and 1988 [0503, 1393, 2371, 2419]

4.15.1 Rate

	1957-60	1962-71	1983-84*	1988
Deliveries	5 134	22 280	851	1 189
Maternal deaths	114	183	3	7
MMR (per 100 000 deliveries)	2 220	821	352	589

* March to November

4.15.2 Causes of maternal deaths, 1957-60 and 1962-71

Haemolytic anaemia in pregnancy is common in Ibadan, and in severe cases may result in death from congestive heart failure. This cause was responsible for 12% and 19% of the maternal deaths in the two periods under consideration. Acute hepatic failure was the second most frequent cause of death in the second period. The fatal course of infective hepatitis in this series is thought to be related to the poor nutritional status of the women.

	1957-60		1962-71	
	No.	%	No.	%
Haemorrhage	10	9	29	16
Sepsis	10	9	13	7
Abortion	1	1	12	7
Uterine rupture	8	7	7	4
Hypertensive disorders of pregnancy	6	5	7	4
Complications of anaesthesia	8	7	7	4
Ectopic pregnancy	1	1	6	3
Fatal sequelae of blood transfusion	5	4	–	–
Obstructed labour	4	4	–	–
DIRECT CAUSES	53	47	81	44
Anaemia	14	12	34	19
Hepatitis	5	4	28	15
Haemoglobinopathies	11	10	8	4
Other infections	6	5	6	3
INDIRECT CAUSES	36	32	76	42
Others	25	18	26	14
TOTAL	114	100	183	100

Haemolytic anaemia, 1975-84, [2471]

A study of the outcome of 78 pregnancies in 47 patients with homozygous sickle cell anaemia managed at the hospital from 1975-84 found two maternal deaths, a mortality rate of 25.6/1000.

4.15.3 Avoidable factors

4.15.4 High risk groups

4.15.5 Other findings

A comparison of the age and parity distribution of the women who died during 1962-71 with 10 577 randomly selected women who delivered in the hospital during the same period showed no significant differences. There was high incidence of anaemia in primigravidae whose immunity to malaria is reduced during pregnancy, and consequently, a high death rate among young primigravidae in this study.

4.16 Lagos University Teaching Hospital, Lagos, 1966-74 [0023, 0194, 0504]

4.16.1 Rate

	1966-72	1970-74
Deliveries	10 338	11 041
Maternal deaths	53	38*
MMR (per 100 000 deliveries)	513	344

* Excluding abortions

4.16.2 Causes of maternal deaths

During 1966-72, 18 of the 53 maternal deaths were due to abortion which accounted for 34% of all maternal deaths at the hospital. During 1970-74 abortion deaths were excluded. Haemorrhage and hypertensive disorders of pregnancy were the most frequent causes of maternal deaths during the period.

	1970-74	
	Number	%
Hypertensive disorders of pregnancy	17	45
Haemorrhage	10	26
Obstructed labour	6	16
Complications of anaesthesia	3	7
Hepatitis	1	3
Intestinal obstruction	1	3
TOTAL	38	100

4.16.3 Avoidable factors

4.16.4 High risk groups

A study of the obstetric performance of primigravidae aged under 16 years during the period 1967-73 (0194), showed an increased incidence of preeclampsia compared with a control group of primigravidae aged over 22 years. However, this was effectively controlled by good prenatal care.

4.16.5 Other findings

4.17 Lagos Island Maternity Hospital, Lagos, 1966-72 [0014, 0023]

4.17.1 Rate

Deliveries	131 673
Maternal deaths	1 089
MMR (per 100 000 deliveries)	827

4.17.2 Causes of maternal deaths

63 of the 1 089 maternal deaths during 1966-72 were due to abortion (6% of all maternal deaths).

4.18 Jos University Teaching Hospital, Plateau region, 1978-80 [2488]

4.18.1 Rate

Births	26 518
Maternal deaths	109
MMR (per 100 000 births)	411

4.18.2 Causes of maternal deaths

	Number	%
Haemorrhage	30	28
Sepsis	16	15
Hepatic failure	15	14
Ruptured uterus	13	12
Anaemia	11	10
Hypertensive disorders of pregnancy	6	6
Complications of anaesthesia	2	2
Embolisms	2	2
Cardiac disease	2	2
Haemoglobinopathy	1	1
Other	11	10
TOTAL	109	100

4.18.3 Avoidable factors

The authors assert that most of the deaths were preventable. The setting up of a blood bank and making blood readily available when required could help to correct anaemia and shock or replace blood lost through haemorrhage. Improvements in transport and communications systems could enable patients to summon help when needed and permit them to arrive at hospital early.

4.19 Sokoto University Teaching Hospital, 1985 and 1988 [2310, 2419]

4.19.1 Rate

	1985	1988
Deliveries	4 291	3 368
Maternal deaths	104	202
MMR (per 100 000 deliveries)	1 965	5 998

4.19.2 Causes of maternal deaths

4.19.3 Avoidable factors

4.19.4 High risk groups
Age

	Deliveries	Maternal deaths	MMR (per 100 000 deliveries)
16	377	26	6 897
17-19	528	31	5 871
20-29	2 558	32	1 251
30-39	783	13	1 660
40 and over	45	2	4 444

4.20 St. Mary's Hospital, Urua Akpan, 1979-85 [2244]

4.20.1 Rate

	Number of maternal deaths	MMR (per 100 000 live births)	Number of unbooked patients	Number of booked patients
1979	26	1 000	18	8
1980	16	600	12	4
1982	22	600	17	5
1983	23	700	14	9
1984	5	200	5	0
1985	12	400	9	3

4.20.2 Causes of maternal deaths

4.20.3 Avoidable factors

4.20.4 High risk groups

4.20.5 Other findings

In 1982 a Primary Health Care outreach programme was started for the areas surrounding the hospital. A survey found that up to 50% of women were delivered at home and attended by TBAs. Each year some 250 unbooked patients were transferred to the hospital with serious complications of labour. In order to reach the women delivering in the villages a TBA training programme was started in 1983, in consultation with Village Chiefs and Clan Heads. Each training course lasted three months and TBAs were given basic instruction in hygiene, prenatal care, labour and its complications and the care of mother and child. The most important objective was to gain the cooperation and confidence of the TBAs and to encourage referral of women at risk of complications as well as the transfer of patients to hospital in good time. Since 1983 TBAs have referred 320 patients and the maternal mortality rates have fallen as have the numbers of unbooked births.

4.21 Ahmadu Bello University Hospital, Zaria, Kaduna State, 1976-79 and 1988
(0197, 0314, 1244, 1356, 2419)

4.21.1 Rate

	1976-79	1988
Deliveries	22 725	2 647
Maternal deaths	238	75
MMR (per 100 000 deliveries)	1 047	2 833

4.21.2 Causes of maternal deaths for 219 unbooked women, 1976-79

	Main cause Number	Contributing cause * Number	%
Anaemia	14	98	46
Haemorrhage	6	70	33
Disproportion	0	56	26
Prolonged labour	1	55	26
Hypertensive disorders of pregnancy	18	47	22
Sepsis	26	28	13
Rupture of the uterus	1	28	13
Ectopic pregnancy	1	0	–
Non-induced abortion	0*	2	1
Sickle cell disease	0	1	1
Other infections	14	26	12
Traditional surgical practices	1	9	4
Other	4	7	3

*   Categories not mutually exclusive.

Eclampsia [0197]

Between 1978 and 1979, 100 eclamptic patients were admitted of whom nine died. All were under 20 years old and eight were younger than 16. Six patients were primiparous. Maternal deaths were twice as likely in the youngest patients as in those over 20 years of age. Abdominal delivery was associated with a lower mortality rate than vaginal delivery.

4.21.3 Avoidable factors
Maternal mortality rates were higher among unbooked women.

1976-79	Booked	Unbooked
Deliveries	15 020	7 654
Maternal deaths	19	219
MMR (per 100 000 deliveries)	126	2 861

4.21.4 High risk groups
Analysis of maternal deaths by age, parity and booking status for all singleton births indicated that maternal mortality was highest for the very young and for older women of parity five and above. Prenatal care was associated with a reduction in maternal mortality in all age and parity groups.

Age group and prenatal care

	MMR (per 100 000 deliveries)		
	No prenatal care	With prenatal care	Total
<15	5 610	1 050	3 780
15	7 130	210	3 970
16	3 200	0	1 430
17-19	2 080	90	760
20-24	1 960	100	580
25-29	2 490	130	740
29+	3 680	160	1 510

Age group, parity and prenatal care

	MMR (per 100 000 deliveries)					
	Primigravidae			Parity 5+		
	No prenatal care	With prenatal care	Total	No prenatal care	With prenatal care	Total
<15	5 670	1 080	3 850	–	–	–
15	7 360	240	4 190	–	–	–
16	3 290	0	1 460	–	–	–
17-19	2 100	0	800	0	0	0
20-24	1 180	110	480	2 200	0	970
25-29	1 750	0	610	2 710	150	1 160
29+	1 920	0	1 010	4 530	150	2 010

Education

There were significant difference in mortality rates between mothers with some formal education and those with none, probably as a result of several related intervening factors including prenatal care. Only 2% of the mothers with education were unbooked, compared with 38% of the mothers without any formal education.

	Formal education	No formal education	Total*
Deliveries	2 437	20 089	22 725
Maternal deaths	6	232	238
MMR (per 100 000 deliveries)	246	1 155	1 047

* Includes mothers whose educational status was unknown.

Ethnic group and religion

Among women who did not receive prenatal care, maternal mortality was still significantly related to both ethnic group and religion. The two variables were however, closely related to each other.

Ethnic group

	Hausa-Fulani	Other Nigerians	Others/ Unknown	Total
Deliveries	11 192	11 327	206	22 725
Maternal deaths	220	18	0	238
MMR (per 100 000 deliveries)	1 966	159	0	1 047

Religion

	Christian	Islam	Others/	Total
Deliveries	7 781	14 098	846	22 725
Maternal deaths	12	225	1	238
MMR (per 100 000 deliveries)	154	1 596	118	1 047

4.21.5 Other findings

Obstetric fistulae

A section of this study of births at Ahmadu Bello Hospital, Zaria, analyses modes of delivery. Among 20 028 singleton hospital births, neglected obstructed labour was the dominant problem in complicated deliveries, and resulted in uterine rupture in 203 women and vesicovaginal fistula in 79 cases. This excluded the hundreds of women and teenage girls with fistula seen for the first time after the puerperium. Most of the 79 women were short, unbooked, illiterate, of Islamic faith, young Hausa-Fulanis, resident outside Zaria. Twelve of the women died.

Ninety-seven women in the survey population had already undergone fistula repair. They suffered greater disadvantages than women having undergone other kinds of surgery (for example, caesarean section). They had the lowest rates for literacy and for child survival from previous births, and the worst fetal results in their current pregnancies. More than 20% had not attended for prenatal care, and reported at hospital in an already advanced stage of labour. The results included stillbirth, recurrence of fistulae, uterine rupture, embryotomy, maternal and perinatal deaths. It is proposed that appropriate social and health reforms need to be implemented.

Nutritional supplementation

Sixty-nine primigravidae, 59 of them aged between 13 and 16 years, were placed on various combinations of antimalarial drugs, folic acid and iron throughout the second half of the pregnancy and the puerperium. Between their first attendance at the prenatal clinic and 1-60 days after delivery, more than half of the women had increased in height by 2-16cm. Haematinic supplementation and growth of both the fetus and mother were found to be linked. When compared with girls who did not receive nutritional supplements, a significantly greater proportion of girls who were supplemented grew by at least 2cm during pregnancy. This acceleration of growth was associated with a statistically significant reduction in the proportion of those who had to have abdominal deliveries.

4.22 Hospitals in several States, 1988 [2419]

4.22.1 Rate

	Live births	Maternal deaths	MMR (per 100 000 live births)
General Hospital, Okigwe, Imo State	252	1	397
General Hospital, Owerri, Imo State	1 882	6	319
University of Calabar Teaching Hospital	1 633	30	1 837
Government Hospitals, Cross River State	5 665	11	194
Adeyoyo Maternity Hospital	6 996	12	172
General Hospital Okene, Kwara State	893	11	1 232
Specialist Hospital Akure, Ondo State	3 245	18	555
General Hospital Ikole Ekiti, Ondo State	414	2	483
Garki Health Centre, Abuja	1 611	3	186
General Hospital, Makurdi, Benue State	4 234	3	71
General Hospital, Minna, Niger State	3 552	32	901
Murtula Mohammed Hospital, Kano	13 737	386	2 810

5. CIVIL REGISTRATION DATA/GOVERNMENT ESTIMATES

5.1 Kaduna, Ogun, Ondo and Oyo states, 1981-83 [1217]

5.1.1 Rate

According to the Medical Statistics division (Ministry of Health) estimates, the maternal mortality rate for Kaduna, Ogun, Ondo and Oyo States for 1981-83 was 1 500 per 100 000 live births.

6. OTHER SOURCES/ ESTIMATES

6.1 Ogun State, 1984 [1338]

6.1.1 Rate

A WHO report quotes an estimated maternal mortality rate of 800 per 100 000 live births for Ogun State in 1984.

6.2 National, 1988 [2480]

6.2.1 Rate

MMR (per 100 000 live births)	800

7. SELECTED ANNOTATED BIBLIOGRAPHY

Adedoyin, M.A. and Adetoro, O.O. Pregnancy and its outcome among teenage mothers in Ilorin, Nigeria. *East African Medical Journal* 1989; 66(7): 448-452. WHE 2308

The records of pregnant women seen at the University of Ilorin Teaching Hospital between January and June 1986 were reviewed. 496 adolescents (15-19 years old) and 500 adult mothers (24-30 years), the latter acting as controls, were studied with respect to maternal and fetal outcome. Anaemia of pregnancy was commoner among the adolescents (60%) than the controls (15%). Toxaemia of pregnancy was also more common among the adolescents than the controls (5% and 2.4% respectively). However, hypertension was more common among the controls (13%) than the adolescents (2.6%).

Ademowore, A.S. et al, Anaemia in pregnancy – a ten-year review. *Journal of Obstetrics and Gynecology of Eastern and Central Africa* 1988; 7: 59-63. WHE 2239

A review of 6 167 obstetric admissions at Ife University Teaching Hospitals Complex over a ten-year period, 1978-87, was undertaken. All case notes of patients with packed red cell volume of 30% and below were studied with respect to booking status, age, parity, social class, causes of anaemia and the outcome of the pregnancy. It was found that anaemia was present in 7.9% of antenatal admissions all occurring in the second and third trimesters. Nutritional anaemia was the commonest, followed by blood loss anaemia, haemolytic anaemia and lastly by anaemia of undetermined causes. Complications occurred in half the patients and their frequency and severity was related to the severity of the anaemia. There were five maternal deaths out of a total of 294 deliveries, a maternal mortality rate for anaemic patients of 1 700 per 100 000 deliveries compared with an overall hospital maternal mortality rate of 900 per 100 000 deliveries.

Anaemia was more common among unbooked patients (53% compared with 47% among booked patients) and 78% of the severely anaemic patients were from the unbooked group. Of the patients who were successfully treated for anaemia on admission, 40% delivered outside the hospital. The authors note that the worsening of the economic situation from the early 1980s has resulted in fewer hospital deliveries and a rising rate of anaemia among obstetric admissions.

Adetoro, O.O. Personal communication. Ilorin. 1989. WHE 2297

Data from a total of 29 cases of obstetric fistula seen at the University of Ilorin Hospital, Ilorin, Nigeria, between January 1987 and June 1989 showed that 6 women (21%) were aged between 16 and 20, and 19 (65%) were aged 30 and under. However, seven (24%) were aged over 35, and 22 (76%) were at parity 2-4. Although 97% gave birth at a hospital, clinic or health centre, more than 50% had to be delivered by emergency caesarean section. Twenty women (69%) had had no formal education, while 52% of the husbands had had no education. None of the other women and husbands had had education beyond primary level. Of the 27 women operated upon, 15 had their fistulae cured, giving a success rate of 56%.

Aimakhu, V.E. Reproductive functions after the repair of obstetric vesicovaginal fistulae. *Fertility and Sterility* 1974; 25(7): 586-591. WHE 2136

This is a retrospective study of 246 women with obstetric traumatic vesicovaginal fistulae repaired at the University College Hospital, Ibadan, Nigeria, between 1957 and 1966. 125 (51%) of the women had sustained the fistulae during their first delivery; 179 patients (73%) were between 15 and 30 years of age at the time of the obstetric trauma.

Case notes of all patients were examined for the presence of coital difficulties, secondary amenorrhea and the outcome of any pregnancy after the repair of the fistulae. There were 41 cases of acquired gynatresia (vaginal stenosis). In eight of these women, coitus had led to reopening of the previously repaired fistulae. Before the repair of their fistulae, 108 patients (44%) had secondary amenorrhea varying from four months to eight years, and 33 of them were known to have resumed menstruation within two years after repair. A discussion of the possible causes of this amenorrhea is presented, with no clear conclusions.

Forty-eight women had 65 pregnancies after the repair of their fistulae, five of which ended in abortion before the 16th week. There were eight vaginal deliveries, 49 caesarean sections, two women lost to follow-up, and one woman who died at home in obstructed labour, undelivered. Of the eight women who delivered vaginally, 6 had no recurrence of fistula; there were three stillbirths and one neonatal death, but no maternal deaths. Of the 49 women delivered by caesarean section, one died due to pulmonary embolism, and two of the 49 babies died. There was no reopening of the fistula in any of these patients. It is concluded that vaginal delivery for a patient with a previously repaired vesicovaginal fistula is more hazardous to mother and infant than caesarean section.

Bentley, R.J. Abdominal repair of high rectovaginal fistula. *Journal of Obstetrics and Gynaecology of the British Commonwealth* 1973; 80: 364-367. WHE 2139

Five case reports from the Ahmadu Bello University, Zaria, Nigeria, show that the main indication for abdominal repair of a high rectovaginal fistula is severe stenosis of the vagina preventing access to the fistula even with a generous episiotomy or a Schuchardt incision. The author describes an abdominal operation which was successfully used in the five cases, in which the rectum is mobilized to the pelvic floor, separated from the vagina, repaired and a pedicle graft of greater omentum interposed between the rectum and vagina.

Cockshott, W.P. Pubic changes associated with obstetric vesicovaginal fistulae. *Clinical Radiology* 1973; 24: 241-247. WHE 2146

The radiological features of the pubic changes in 312 women with vesicovaginal fistulae following obstructed labour were reviewed at the University College Hospital, Ibadan, Nigeria (in 1972). Patients ranged in age from 16 to the early forties, and fistula followed the first pregnancy in 60%. One hundred (32%) patients showed abnormal pubic findings: bone resorption (17), separation of the pubes (5), marginal fractures and spurs (10), narrowing of the symphysis (40), bony obliteration of the symphysis (23), and distal inflammatory changes (3). Some of the changes represented more severe manifestations of processes that may follow normal delivery. Patients with obliteration of the symphysis had severe bladder neck fistulae. Factors in the pathogenesis are discussed.

Elkins, T. et al. Uterine rupture in Nigeria. *The Journal of Reproductive Medicine* 1985; 30(3): 195-199. WHE 1871

During the period 1978-83, 65 cases of uterine rupture were recorded at the Eku Baptist Hospital, Benin. During that time there were approximately 6 000 births, an incidence of 11 per thousand. Adequate records were available in 45 cases. The predisposing factors included cephalopelvic disproportion (62%), grand multiparity (33%), previous caesarean section (24%), placental pathology (15%) and abnormal presentation (20%). 84% of the patients had had no prenatal care and eight of the nine maternal deaths occurred among them, a mortality rate of 20%.

Evoh, N.J. and Akinla, O. Reproductive performance after the repair of obstetric vesicovaginal fistulae. *Annals of Clinical Research* 1978; 10: 303-306. WHE 2263

Between 1966 and 1976, 148 out of 162 patients with obstetrically acquired vesicovaginal fistulae were successfully repaired in Lagos University Teaching Hospital, Nigeria. The women were aged between 17 and 35 at the time the fistulae occurred. Eighty-five cases (52%) were primiparae, and 48 (30%) were grand multiparae. Before the repair of the fistulae 66 patients (41%) suffered from secondary amenorrhea, another seven from disturbed menstrual cycles, and 28 (17%) from gynatresia. It is suggested that amenorrhea may have been due to a combination of factors: severe malnutrition, anaemia, endometritis, psychological upsets and occasionally endocrine malfunction due to focal anterior pituitary necrosis.

After repair of the the fistulae, menstruation returned in 58 of the 66 women. Twelve patients had dyspareunia and three others had apareunia. Reopening of the fistula after early resumption of coitus occurred in five patients. Thirty-one women had 38 pregnancies within 24 months of the repair, most of which (81.5%) were delivered by caesarean section. Five women had vaginal deliveries, and there was one abortion at 12 weeks. Thirty infants delivered by caesarean section and three infants delivered vaginally survived. There were no maternal deaths, but four infants died neonatally. The crude perinatal mortality rate was 10.7%, but the corrected perinatal mortality rate (i.e. excluding antepartum deaths, congenital malformations incompatible with life, haemolytic disease of the newborn not due to delivery) was nil. Four women had a recurrence of the fistula after delivery, three of which followed emergency caesarean section. Two patients developed stress incontinence after caesarean section. It is proposed that elective caesarean section should be the preferred method of delivery after successful fistula repair, and that continuous health education of the patients and their husbands should be undertaken.

Harrison, K.A. *Obstetric fistulae*. Paper prepared for a Technical Working Group. Geneva: WHO, 1989. 38p. Unpublished. WHE 2121

A brief historical sketch indicates that poverty and famine are key underlying factors in the incidence of vesicovaginal fistula. A description of the epidemiology of obstetric fistula is given, based on the Zaria maternity survey, Nigeria. The risk of acquiring fistula was highest among the early teenage primigravidae aged 16 and under; young multigravidae and the oldest most parous group constituted the other high risk group. When

compared to taller women, short women were more likely to have pelvic contraction, the presence of which exposes them to the risk of cephalo-pelvic disproportion, to an increased risk of caesarean section and embryotomy delivery, and to an increased risk of acquiring obstetric fistula from neglected obstructed labour. Associated complications were uterine rupture and postpartum haemorrhage.

Other factors described as contributing to vesicovaginal fistula are: early marriage and early start to childbearing, lack of access to health facilities and/or lack of desire to use facilities, the traditional practice of gishiri cutting, low socioeconomic status, and lack of education. Protection against malaria and iron and folic acid deficiencies during pregnancy in young women through the administration of malarial chemoprophylaxis and iron and folic acid supplements showed that growth can be promoted and the incidence of obstetric fistula lowered. Increased hospital deliveries in Zaria from 1972-77 also helped eliminate fistula among women from Zaria itself.

The author concludes that measures to increase pelvic size and to prevent prolonged or obstructed labour are the key issues for prevention of obstetric fistula. Literacy and mass formal education are vital and must work in conjunction with better provision of appropriate health services.

Iloabachie, G.C. Two-stage repair of giant vesicovaginal fistula. *International Journal of Gynaecology and Obstetrics* 1989; 28: 27-31. WHE 2260

A review of 840 bladder fistulae over ten years (1973-1982) at the University of Nigeria Teaching Hospital, Enugu, Nigeria, revealed that 64 (7.6%) were giant vesicovaginal fistulae. Association with vaginal stenosis and rectovaginal fistulae occurred in 23% and 5% of cases respectively, and 50 patients (78%) had amenorrhea Operative treatment is presented. The results of direct one-stage repair were poor at 35% for the first attempt, while the two-stage repair achieved 80% success at the first attempt. The advantages of a staged operation are discussed.

Lagundoye, S.B. et al. Pelvic bone changes in vesicovaginal fistula. *West African Medical Journal* 1975; 23(4): 141-145. WHE 1171

The preliminary films taken in the course of intravenous urography in 216 women with vesicovaginal fistula due to obstructed labour were assessed for pelvic bone changes at the University College Hospital in Ibadan, Nigeria (before 1975). One hundred and sixteen (53%) showed no abnormality. Of the remaining 100, the changes were in the pubic symphysis in 82 and consisted of ten with diastasis, four with narrowing and eleven with bony ankylosis. Osteitis pubis was observed in twenty and steophytic spurs in the same number. The role of the trauma from obstructed labour and infection of pelvic and perineal tissues in the pathogenesis of the osseous changes are discussed.

Lawson, J. Tropical obstetrics and gynaecology. 3. Vesico-vaginal fistula - a tropical disease. *Transactions of the Royal Society of Tropical Medicine and Hygiene,* 1989: 83: 454-456. WHE 2148

The predominantly obstetric origin of vesico-vaginal fistulae in the tropics is contrasted with the mainly surgical aetiology of those in Europe by analysis of 543 cases treated in Nigeria and the United Kingdom. Of 369 obstetric fistulae in Ibadan, 343 (93%) resulted from obstructed labour. The basic reason for the common occurrence of obstetric fistulae in tropical countries is that cephalo-pelvic disproportion is common in environments unfavourable to childhood and adolescence, where malnutrition and untreated infections stunt the growth of future mothers and result in a high prevalence of contracted pelvis. An additional factor in many cultures is starting childbearing too early, the first pregnancy occurring soon after the menarche before growth of the pelvis is complete. In the absence of any obstetric care, obstructed labour in the multipara usually ends in fatal rupture of the uterus. In the primipara, the fetus dies and the surviving women are left with vesico-vaginal fistulae.

The general management of patients with obstetric fistulae is described, followed by the principles of their surgical treatment and postoperative nursing care. The importance of success at the first attempt at repair is stressed, and the small place for managing failures by urinary diversion is mentioned. It is concluded that obstetric fistulae should be preventable in the tropics, having now been effectively eliminated from industrialized countries.

Lister, U.G. Vesico-vaginal fistulae. *Postgraduate Doctor* 1984; October: 321-323. WHE 1620

Based on experience in northern Nigeria, the author outlines the problems of vesicovaginal fistulae. The two major causes are obstructed labour causing pressure necrosis and the traditional gishiri cut, or a combination of the two. The commonest reason for doing a gishiri cut is difficulty with delivery. It is a tradition that the first baby is born at home. The average age of patients with vesicovaginal fistula in Zaria is 16 years old. The social implications are outlined: if a girl delivers a stillborn child and becomes incontinent, she is generally returned to her parents' compound and divorced by her husband, yet it is often the husband who refuses to allow his wife to go to hospital. If vaginal scarring is such that sexual intercourse is impossible, the woman is unmarriageable and becomes a social outcast. If she does become pregnant again, she is at risk of premature labour associated with renal damage from infection. It is proposed that health education and good obstetric care should be able to eradicate obstetric fistulae.

Mabogunje, O.A. Burn injuries during the puerperium in Zaria, Nigeria. *International Journal of Gynecology and Obstetrics* 1989; 30: 133-137. WHE 2418

From 1971 to 1987, 35 parturient women were admitted to the Ahmadu Bello University Hospital for care of burns and scalds. 31 had practised ritual hot baths or "Wankan-jego" which caused severe scalds. They were all illiterate rural housewives of the Hausa-Fulani tribe. Five of the women developed peripartum cardiac failure and two died. Three of the newborns also died partly as a result of the mothers' illness. The author concludes that formal education and general economic development would help in eliminating this preventable source of maternal and infant mortality and morbidity.

Murphy, M. Social consequences of vesico-vaginal fistula in Northern Nigeria. *Journal of Biosocial Sciences* 1981; 13: 139-150. WHE 0473

In order to explore the social situation of women suffering from obstetric fistulae in Zaria, Nigeria, interviews were conducted with four sets of patients: 100 fistula patients attending a gynaecological clinic for the first time between October 1976 and June 1978; 52 long-term patients who had been incontinent for 2 years or more; 22 cured patients who had subsequent confinements in Zaria hospital; and 45 patients attending the cardiac clinic for postpartum cardiac failure, who provided controls. A second control group was provided from records of 207 patients with postpartum cardiac failure treated between 1969 and 1972. Further information was gathered from informal discussions with 40 patients in a rehabilitation programme.

Results showed that fistula patients were much younger than the controls: 69% of the new patients and over 50% of the long-term patients were aged 19 and under, as against 13% and 22% in the control groups. However, there was a close similarity in all groups in age at marriage (the vast majority being married by age 15), and age at first birth (over 60% by age 17). Fistula patients came mostly from poor subsistence farming backgrounds, and only 15% of the husbands of new fistula patients and 8% of long-term patients had received any form of modern education, compared with 31% of the control group. Although polygamous marriage is widespread in the area, 66% of fistula patients were the only wife, a factor also indicative of low socioeconomic status.

Seventy-seven percent of the long-term fistula patients had been living apart from their husbands for two years or more, while none of the control group was divorced or living apart. Childlessness was an important factor in marital breakdown. Of all 174 fistula patients, 50 had living children before developing fistula. Of these 50, 14% were divorced as a result of the disorder, compared with 36% of the 124 patients with no living children. Fistula patients enjoyed less support and interest from their husbands than other patient groups and the amount of practical support given by family members diminished with prolongation of the illness. Patients felt they were a social disgrace to the family and expected to be treated as outcasts. They were frequently segregated – not allowed to eat with the family, cook or pray.

Nnatu, S. Profile of obstetric fistula in a sub-Saharan centre. *Journal Obstetrics and Gynaecology of Eastern and Central Africa* 1986; 5: 13-15. WHE 1559

A study of 71 Nigerian women with vesicovaginal fistulae repaired at the Lagos University Teaching Hospital, from 1978-1982 is presented. Sixty-seven (94%) of the cases were due to prolonged obstructed labour (70% from pressure necrosis and 17% from uterine rupture) and 6% from caesarean section. The highest percentage (37% - 26 women) were aged 25-29, with 19% under 25 and 33% over 30. Sixty percent were parity 4 and over with only 15% (11 women) primiparae. Thirty-eight percent of the women were below 150cm in height and 86% below160 cm. Associated conditions included vulval and perineal excoriation (97%), secondary amenorrhea (52%), pre-operative vaginal stenosis (27%), anaemia, vesical calculus and nerve palsy. Fifty-three (74.6%) fistulae were successfully repaired, the majority by the vaginal approach. Blocked catheter, urinary tract and wound infection were the postoperative problems probably responsible for failure of the other 18 cases.

The author observes that patients were relatively older and more parous than those in studies from northern Nigeria. Fifteen percent, as opposed to 52% in the north (cf. Tahzib, WHE 0686) were having their first confinement. The fact that 32% of women in this series were overweight is suggested as a contributing factor: a tendency to have big babies whose weights increase with successive pregnancies, causing cephalopelvic disproportion, irrespective of parity.

Ojengbede, O.A. et al. Pregnancy performance of Nigerian women aged 16 years and below, as seen in Ibadan, Nigeria. *African Journal of Medicine and Medical Science* 1987; 16: 89-95. WHE 1923

A review of 84 women aged 16 years and below who gave birth at the University College Hospital, Ibadan, during the period 1978-82, found that the majority of the patients were unemployed women from a low socioeconomic class. 46 of the women were unbooked. Pregnancy and delivery were complicated by a higher than usual incidence of pregnancy-induced hypertension and by feto-pelvic disproportion. There were no maternal deaths but considerably more postpartum morbidity among these very young patients than among older women.

Ojo, V.A. and Okwerekwu, F.O. A critical analysis of the rates and indications for caesarean section in a developing country. *Asia-Oceania Journal of Obstetrics and Gynaecology* 1988; 14(2): 185-193. WHE 2349

A retrospective analysis of cases of caesarean section performed over the two-year period January 1985 to December 1986 at the University of Ilorin Teaching Hospital, Nigeria, was carried out. There were 12 138 deliveries of which 845 were by caesarean section, giving an incidence of 6.7%. Sufficient information was available for analysis in a total of 785 cases. The majority of the cases were for primary section the incidence being 6.1% and that of repeat section 0.8%. The most common indications for caesarean section were dystocia (38%), malpresentation and malposition (17%), previous caesarean section (12%), fetal distress (11%) and antepartum haemorrhage (9%). Maternal complications occurred in 84 patients. Wound sepsis was the single most important morbidity (74%). There were seven maternal deaths, a caesarean maternal mortality rate of 892 per 100 000. Most of the deaths were a consequence of septicaemia The author states that all the maternal deaths were preventable.

Okojie, S.E. Induced illegal abortion in Benin City, Nigeria. *International Journal of Gynaecology and Obstetrics* 1976; 14: 517-521. WHE 0505

Abortions constitute about 25% of gynaecological admissions at the University of Benin Teaching Hospital. Between July 1974 and February 1975, 59 patients admitted with confirmed illegally induced abortions were studied. The majority of the patients were single, young schoolgirls. There was one death.

Orhue, A.A.E. et al. The contribution of previous induced abortion to tubal ectopic pregnancy. *West African Journal of Medicine* 1989; 8(4): 257-263. WHE 2460

The incidence of ectopic pregnancy varies all over the world and conceivably each community may have a predominant etiologic factor underlying cases of ectopic pregnancy. This report presents data from a study involving cases of ectopic tubal pregnancy and matched controls collected prospectively with a view to determining the predominant clinical etiologic factors. During the study period there were 39 ectopic pregnancies and a total of 1 852 deliveries, an incidence of 2.1%. Compared with the controls, a history of induced abortion was significantly more frequent among the subjects and was also more likely to have been the outcome of the penultimate pregnancy.

Non-physicians provided 51.6% and 3.3% of induced abortions in the study group and controls respectively. Complications occurred in 51.6% of the study population and 6.5% of the controls. The authors conclude that induced abortions created the predisposition to tubal implantation in the study population and that a reduction in the incidence of induced abortion in the community can reduce the incidence of ectopic tubal gestation and tubal infertility.

Osefo, N.J. Cesarean and postpartum hysterectomy in Enugu, 1973-86. *International Journal of Gynecology and Obstetrics* 1989; 30: 93-97. WHE 2412

Over a thirteen-year period at the University of Nigeria Teaching Hospital, Enugu, there were 56 823 deliveries of which 6 664 (11.7%) were by caesarean section. Obstetric hysterectomies were performed on 163 patients, an incidence of 1 in 349 deliveries and 1 in 41 caesarean sections. Of the patients requiring hysterectomy, 116 (71%) had received no antenatal care during the pregnancy. This included 23 patients who had undergone caesarean section during previous deliveries. The majority of the patients were grandmultiparas. Fewer than 5% of the women were practising contraception.

The main indication for hysterectomy was ruptured uterus resulting from obstructed labour (119 patients or 73%). Rupture of a previous uterine scar occurred in 23 cases and in 20 cases the hysterectomy was necessitated by intractable haemorrhage.

Many of the patients had to travel long distances to reach the hospital and presented between four and fourteen hours after the uterine rupture. In some cases patients living near the hospital presented late because midwives or traditional birth atten-

dants failed to recognize the condition. Seventeen patients developed vesicovaginal fistulae. There were ten maternal deaths, a case fatality rate of 6.1%. Of the ten, six arrived at the hospital in a moribund condition more than twelve hours after the uterine rupture. Complications included pyrexia (69%) and anaemia (66%). There were 142 fetal deaths (87%).

Otubu, J.A. et al. Pregnancy and delivery after successful repair of vesicovaginal fistula. *International Journal of Gynaecology and Obstetrics* 1982; 20: 163-166. WHE 2138

A retrospective study of 110 women who gave birth after successful repair of fistula at the Ahmadu Bello University Teaching Hospital in Zaria, Nigeria, from 1977-1979, was carried out to assess pregnancy complications, mode of delivery and fetal outcome. Four controls were selected for each case and matched for age, parity, socioeconomic status and ethnicity.

Forty-six percent of the women were below age 20, the youngest being 12 years, and 89% were below age 25. Ninety-one percent of patients were of second parity and had sustained their fistula with the first delivery. The most frequently encountered antenatal complication was urinary tract infection (15%), followed by anaemia (12%), and toxaemia (4.5%), all of which were more common than in the control group, with the incidence of urinary tract infection being statistically significant.

101 women were delivered by caesarean section (22 emergency cases) and nine vaginally. The perinatal mortality rate for vaginal deliveries was 66%, and 36% for emergency caesarean section but only 6% for elective caesarean section. There were 92 live births, eight still births and eleven deaths within seven days of delivery. The overall perinatal mortality was 17.2%, with one maternal death from an emergency caesarean section. The authors suggest that, although caesarean section is the preferred method of delivery after successful fistula repair, the general dislike of caesarean section by most women in the Hausa-Fulani population is mostly responsible for late arrival to hospital.

Ozumba, B.C. Destructive operation in obstetric practice in Nigeria. *International Surgeon* 1989; 74: 64-66. WHE 2382

An analysis of the use of destructive operation in obstetric practice at the University of Nigeria Teaching Hospital, Enugu over a nine-year period was carried out. The hospital is the only teaching hospital in the State of six million people and serves a dual role of tertiary and primary care centre. Between January 1976 and December 1984 there were 55 cases of destructive operation out of 46 719 deliveries, an incidence of 0.12%. Taken over three-year intervals there was a fall in the incidence from 0.29% in the first interval to 0.06% and 0.05% in the second and third intervals respectively. Over 85% of the patients were referred from peripheral health units. Most of the patients were aged 25 years or less and 36% were primigravidae, compared with 19% of the total hospital deliveries. The most common indication for destructive operation was obstructed labour due to cephalopelvic disproportion (43 cases or 78% of the total). There were three maternal deaths, a fatality rate of 5.5%. Vesicovaginal fistulae occurred in five cases and rectovaginal fistulae in a further two cases.

St. George, J. Factors in the prediction of successful vaginal repair of vesicovaginal fistulae. *Journal of Obstetrics and Gynaecology of the British Commonwealth* 1969; 76: 741-745. WHE 0952

Based on his experience in the course of treating 134 women with obstetric fistulae in northern Nigeria over three-and-a-half years, the author describes factors involved in successful repair of vesicovaginal fistulae, aimed at the inexperienced surgeon. Puerperal sepsis is mentioned as a major contributing factor to complicating fistulae, and details are given of how this can be prevented in hospital. Whenever secondary amenorrhea was found, there was also evidence of vaginal stenosis, dense fibrosis round the fistula and minimal tissue for repair, showing that extensive infection must have been present. Fistula patients are described as invariably in a poor state of health, with excoriation of the vulva.

Tahzib, F. Epidemiological determinants of vesicovaginal fistulas. *British Journal of Obstetrics and Gynaecology* 1983; 90: 387-391. WHE 0686

A study of 1443 patients with vesico-vaginal fistulae who were operated on between 1969 and 1980 at the Ahmadu Bello University Hospital in Zaria, Nigeria, is presented. Prolonged, obstructed labour was responsible for 84% of the fistulae, and the traditional gishiri cut for 13%. (The gishiri cut is a traditional operation performed throughout Northern Nigeria. It consists of cutting the anterior (and rarely the posterior) aspect of the vagina with a razor blade. It is used to treat a wide variety of conditions including obstructed labour, infertility, dyspareunia, amenorrhea, goitre, backache, dysuria and a number of other complaints. Vesicovaginal fistulae, haemorrhage and sepsis may result.)

Four hundred and seventy-five women (33%) were aged 16 and under, and 80 (5.5%) of these were 13

years or under. The vast majority (83%) were under 30. Fifty-two percent of the women were primiparous. Only three fistula patients had received some rudimentary conventional education compared with 7% of all the women who gave birth in the area. Of the 1209 women whose fistula was caused by labour, 778 (64%) gave birth at home.

With increasing use of hospital deliveries between 1970 and 1978, the number of patients with vesicovaginal fistulae treated in Zaria doubled. But by 1978 the number of such patients coming from Zaria and the immediate environs had decreased to zero. This seemed to indicate that the women from Zaria were more readily using the hospital services, thus avoiding prolonged, obstructed labour. The author proposes that reducing early marriages and eradicating harmful traditional practices are key preventive measures.

Tahzib, F. Vesicovaginal fistula in Nigerian children. *Lancet 1985;* December: 1291-1293. WHE 1618

Of 80 cases of vesico-vaginal fistula in children under 13 years of age in Northern Nigeria, 48 (60%) were due to labour, 12 to the traditional practice of gishiri cutting, and 20 to other causes including congenital abnormalities, coitus, infections, and trauma. Preventive measures proposed include improved socioeconomic status of the community, education, and reevaluation of the role of women in society.

Tahzib, F. *What of those injured mothers who did not die? Obstetric fistulae – a cause for concern.* Sokoto, (1988). 19p. Unpublished. WHE 2149

Demonstrating that historically the problem of obstetric fistula in Europe and America had the same underlying causes - poverty, malnutrition and inadequate health services - as the problem in developing countries today, the author argues that implementing programmes to answer the needs of fistula sufferers could have an important impact on increasing the acceptability of health services. If positive, human services can be offered, women with successfully repaired fistulae could be important health agents on their return to their isolated villages. A detailed study of the epidemiology of these wounded survivors from childbirth could also provide insights into the aetiology and prevention of obstructed labour. Programmes geared to reaching the thousands of women waiting for fistula repair should be set in place urgently.

8. FURTHER READING

Adelusi, A. et al. Acquired gynaestresia in Ibadan. *Nigerian Medical Journal* 1976; 6(2): 198-200. WHE 1861

Adetoro, O.O. Septic induced abortion at Ilorin, Nigeria: an increasing gynaecological problem in developing countries. *Asia-Oceania Journal of Obstetrics and Gynaecology* 1986; 12(2): 201-205. WHE 1480

Adetoro, O.O. Issues of concern in prevention and better management of postpartum haemorrhage: needs for action and issues for research. (unpublished document) 1989. WHE 2226

Ahnaimugan, S. and Asuen, M.I. Acquired gynaestresia in Nigeria. *Tropical Doctor* 1978; 8(4): 201-204. WHE 1011

Akesode, F.A. Factors affecting the use of primary health care clinics for children. *Journal of Epidemiology and Community Health* 1982; 36: 310-314. WHE 0193

Apenasami, Iwese, F.A. Taboos of childbearing and childrearing in Bendel State of Nigeria. *Journal of Nurse-Midwifery* 1983; 28(3): 31-33. WHE 0039

Ayeni, O. Causes of mortality in an African city. *African Journal of Medicine and Medical Science* 1980; 9(3-4): 139-149. WHE 0050

Bademosi, O. et al. Obstetric neuropraxia in the Nigerian African. *International Journal of Gynaecology and Obstetrics* 1980; 17: 611-614. WHE 1807

Brennan, M. *Training traditional birth attendants reduces maternal mortality and morbidity.* Paper presented at the Third International Conference of Obstetrics and Gynaecology, Enugu, Nigeria 1986. WHE 1827

Egwuatu, V.E. and Agugua, N.E.N. Complications of female circumcision in Nigerian Ibos. *British Journal of Obstetrics and Gynaecology* 1981; 88: 1090-1093. WHE 1614

Egwuatu, V.E. and Ozumba, B.S. Unexpectedly low ratio and falling incidence rate of ectopic pregnancy in Enugu, Nigeria, 1978-81. *International Journal of Fertility* 1987; 32(2): 113-121. WHE 1725

Ekwempu, C.C. and Harrison, K.A. Endometriosis among the Hausa-Fulani population of Nigeria. *Tropical and Geographical Medicine* 1979; 31: 201-205. WHE 1065

Fleming, A.F. et al. The prevention of megoblastic anaemia in pregnancy in Nigeria. *Journal of Obstetrics and Gynaecology of the British Commonwealth* 1968; 75: 425-432. WHE 0263

Fleming, A.F. Anaemia in pregnancy in tropical Africa. *Transactions of the Royal Society of Tropical Medicine and Hygiene* 1989; 83: 441-448. WHE 2499

Groen, G.P. Uterine rupture in rural Nigeria. *Obstetrics and Gynecology* 1974; 44: 682-687. WHE 1074

Harrington, J.A. Nutritional stress and economic responsibility: a study of Nigerian women. In: Buvinic, M. (ed.) *Women and poverty in the third world.* Baltimore, Johns Hopkins University Press, 1983

Harrison, K.A. Approaches to reducing maternal and perinatal mortality in Africa. In: Philpott, R.H. (ed.) *Maternity services in the developing world – what the community needs.* London, Royal College of Obstetricians and Gynaecologists, 1980. WHE 1105

Harrison, K.A. Maternal problems in the community. *Bulletin of the International Pediatric Association* 1984; 5(7): 45-51. WHE 1123

Ifabumuyi, O.I. and Akindele, M.O. Postpartum mental illness in northern Nigeria. *Acta Pediatrica Scandinavica* 1985; 72(1): 63-68. WHE 1245

Itavyer, D.A. A traditional midwife practice, Sokoto State, Nigeria. *Social Science and Medicine* 1984; 18(6): 497-501. WHE 0572

Iyun, F. An assessment of a rural health programme on child and maternal care: the Ogbomoso Community Health Care Programme (CHCP), Oyo State, Nigeria. *Social Science and Medicine* 1989; 29(8): 933-938. WHE 2466

Kelly, J.V. The influences of native customs on obstetrics in Nigeria. *Obstetrics and Gynecology* 1967; 30(4): 608-612. WHE 1135

Mtimavalye, L.A.R. Reproductive health care among women in Africa: current trends and the future. *Journal of Obstetrics and Gynaecology of Eastern and Central Africa* 1982; 1(2): 48-53. WHE 0468

Murphy, M. *Education and health; the place of education in the prevention of a health problem.* Zaria (unpublished) 1989. WHE 2304

Odejide, A.O. et al Infertility among Nigerian women: a study of related psychological factors. *Journal of Obstetrics and Gynaecology of Eastern and Central Africa* 1986; 5: 61-63. WHE 1517

Ogunbode, O. and Aimakja, V.E. Uterine prolapse during pregnancy in Ibadan. *American Journal of Obstetrics and Gynecology* 1975; 116: 622-625. WHE 1196

Ombuloye, I.O. and Oyeneye, O.Y. Primary health care in developing countries: the case of Nigeria, Sri Lanka and Tanzania. *Social Science and Medicine* 1982; 16(6): 675-686. WHE 0507

Osefo, N.J. and Okeke, B.C. Endometriosis: incidence among the Ibos of Nigeria. *International Journal of Gynecology and Obstetrics* 1989; 30: 349-353. WHE 2468

Osinusi, B.O. and Adeleve, J.A. Symptomatology and clinical presentation of uterovaginal prolapse in Ibadan. *Nigerian Medical Journal* 1976; 6: 451-454. WHE 1199

Osinusi, B.O. The role of previous abortions on secondary infertility in Ibadan, Nigeria. *Journal of Obstetrics and Gynaecology of Eastern and Central Africa* 1986; 5: 37-38. WHE 1518

Otubu, J.A. and Ezem, B.U. Genital prolapse in the Hausa-Fulani of northern Nigeria. *The East African Medical Journal* 1982; 59(9): 605-609. WHE 1200

Oyakhire, G.K. Environmental factors influencing maternal mortality in Zaria, Nigeria. *Royal Society of Health Journal* 1980; 100(2): 72-74. WHE 0516

Ozumba, B.C. Abruptio placentae at the University of Nigeria Teaching Hospital, Enugu: a 3-year study. *Australia New Zealand Journal of Obstetrics and Gynaecology* 1989; 29: 117-120. WHE 2489

Sogbanmu, M.O. Perinatal mortality and maternal mortality in General Hospital, Ondo, Nigeria: Use of high risk pregnancy prediction scoring index. *Nigerian Medical Journal* 1979; 9(1): 123-127. WHE 0663

Sogunro, G.O. Traditional obstetrics: a Nigerian experience of a traditional birth attendant training program. *International Journal of Gynaecology and Obstetrics* 1987; 25: 375-379. WHE 1855

Tahzib, F. An initiative on vesicovaginal fistula. *Lancet* June 10 1989: 1316-1317. WHE 2124

Trevitt, L. Attitudes and customs among the Hausa in Zaria City. *Savanna* 1973; 2: 223-226. WHE 1810

Watts, S.J. Guinea worm: an in-depth study of what happens to mothers, families and communities. *Social Science and Medicine* 1989; 29(9): 1043-1049. WHE 2465

9. DATA SOURCES

WHE 0014   Agbolla, A. Rupture of the uterus. *Nigerian Medical Journal* 1972; 2: 19-21

WHE 0023   Akingba, J.B. Abortion, maternity and other health problems in Nigeria. *Nigerian Medical Journal* 1977; 7(4): 465-471

WHE 0049   Ayangade, S.O. Maternal mortality in a semi-urban Nigerian community. *Journal of the National Medical Association* 1981; 73(2): 137-140

WHE 0057   Balachandran, V. Maternal mortality in Kaduna 1964-72 *Nigerian Medical Journal* 1975; 5: 366-370

WHE 0117   Caffrey, K.Y. Maternal mortality: a continuing challenge in tropical practice. A report from Kaduna, Northern Nigeria. *East African Medical Journal* 1979; 56(6): 274-277

WHE 0164   Courtney, L.D. Maternal parity, haemoglobin level, mortality rate, labour and complications in a tropical centre. *Journal of the Irish Medical Association* 1974; 67(6): 159-161

WHE 0194   Efiong, E. The obstetric performance of Nigerian primigravidae aged 16 and under. *British Journal of Obstetrics and Gynaecology* 1975; 82: 228-233

WHE 0197   Ekempu, C.C. Maternal mortality in the Guinea Savannah region of Nigeria. *Clinical and Experimental Hypertension* 1982; 1(4): 531-537

WHE 0267   Alakija, W. Method of child delivery in Benin City and its environs. *Journal of Tropical Pediatrics* 1984; 30(1): 48-49

WHE 0313   Harrison, K.A. *Zaria maternity survey 1976-79:* I. Background information (unpublished paper) 1983

WHE 0314   Harrison, K.A. Lessons from a survey of 22 000 Nigerian births *Paul Hendrickse Memorial Lecture* 1983

WHE 0320   Hartfield, V.J. Maternal mortality in Nigeria compared with earlier international experience. *International Journal of Gynaecology and Obstetrics* 1980; 18(1): 70-75

WHE 0321   Hartfield, V.J. and Woodland, M. Prevention of maternal deaths in a Nigerian village. *International Journal of Gynaecology and Obstetrics* 1980; 18: 150-152

WHE 0426   Makinwa-Adebusoye, P.K. et al. *1980 Lagos contraception and breast-feeding study. Final report.* 1980

WHE 0449   Megafu, U. Jaundice in pregnancy aetiology, management and mortality at Enugu, Nigeria. *East African Medical Journal* 1981; 58(7): 501-509.

WHE 0467   Mott, F.L. Some aspects of health care in rural Nigeria. *Studies in Family Planning* 1976; 7(4): 109-114

WHE 0495   Nigeria, Ministry of Health. *Oyo State. Annual Statistical Bulletin 1978* Ibadan, Statistical Unit

WHE 0503   Ojo, O.A. and Savage, V.Y. A ten-year review of maternal mortality rates in the University Hospital, Ibadan, Nigeria. *American Journal of Obstetrics and Gynecology* 1974; 118(4): 517-522

WHE 0504   Okoisor, A.T. Maternal mortality in the Lagos University Teaching Hospital. A five-year survey, 1970-74. *Nigerian Medical Journal* 1978; 8(4): 349-354

WHE 0506   Olu Oduntan, S. and Olunlami, V.B. Maternal mortality in Western Nigeria. *Tropical and Geographic Medicine* 1975; 27(3): 313-316

WHE 0511   Omu, A.L. et al. Adolescent induced abortion in Benin City, Nigeria. *International Journal of Gynecology and Obstetrics* 1981; 19(6): 495-499

WHE 0514   Oronsaye, A.U. and Asuen, U.I. Obstructed labour – a four-year survey at the University of Benin Teaching Hospital, Benin City, Nigeria. *Tropical Doctor* 1980; 10: 113-116

WHE 0775   Waboso, M.F. The causes of maternal mortality in the Eastern States of Nigeria. *Nigerian Medical Journal* 1973; 3(2): 99

WHE 0793   World Health Organization. *Studies on measurement of coverage, effectiveness and efficiency of health care.* (unpublished papers discussed at a study group meeting) Geneva, 1982

WHE 0834   World Health Organization. *World Health Statistics annual - vital statistics and causes of death.* Geneva, various years

WHE 0908   World Health Organization. African Regional Office, *Training and supervision of traditional birth attendants.* Report of a study group, 1976

WHE 1112   Janowitz, B. et al. *Reproductive health in Africa: issues and options.* Family Health International, North Carolina, 1984

WHE 1217   Nigeria, Federal Ministry of Health, Statistics Division. *Statistical data in reply to an AFRO enquiry* (unpublished document) Lagos, August 9 1985

WHE 1227   Junker, T. Maternal mortality in developing countries. Letter. *International Journal of Epidemiology,* 1985; 14: 338.

WHE 1244   Harrison, K.A. *A review of maternal mortality in Nigeria with particular reference to the situation in Zaria, Northern Nigeria 1976-79* Paper presented to Interregional Meeting on Prevention of Maternal Mortality, Geneva, November 1985. Document No. FHE/PMM/85.9.12, 1985

WHE 1338   World Health Organization, African Regional Office. *Where are we in PHC? Countries take a close look at themselves through PHC reviews.* Part 2, 1985

WHE 1356   Harrison, K.A. Childbearing, health and social priorities: A survey of 22 774 consecutive births in Zaria, Northern Nigeria. *British Journal of Obstetrics and Gynecology* Supplement No. 5, 1985

WHE 1393   Lawson, J.B. Maternal mortality in West Africa *Ghana Medical Journal* 1962; 31-33

WHE 1519   Naghma-E-Rahan, and Sani, S. Obstetric behaviour of Hausa women. *Journal of Obstetrics and Gynaecology of Eastern and Central Africa* 1986; 5: 21-25

WHE 1658   Adewunmi, O.A. Maternal mortality in Ibadan City. *West African Journal of Medicine* 1986; 5(2): 121-127

WHE 1712   Mauldin W.P. and Segal, S.J. *Prevalence of contraceptive use in developing countries. A chart book.* Rockefeller Foundation, New York 1986

WHE 1728   Adetoro, O.O. Maternal mortality – a twenty-year survey at the University of Ilorin Teaching Hospital, Ilorin, Nigeria. *International Journal of Gynaecology and Obstetrics* 1987; 25: 93-98

WHE 1897   Adeoye, C.O. Maternal mortality at Ife University Teaching Hospital complex. In: *Primary health and neonatal health. A global concern.* New York and London, Plenum Press. 1983

WHE 1914   United Nations Children's Fund (UNICEF). *The state of the world's children,* various years, Oxford, Oxford University Press

WHE 1915   United Nations. Department of International Economic and Social Affairs. *World population prospects: estimates and projections as assessed in 1984.* Population Studies No. 98. New York 1986

WHE 1918   United Nations. Department of International Economic and Social Affairs. *First marriage: patterns and determinants.* New York 1988

WHE 2033   World Health Organization. *Global strategy for health for all by the year 2000. Second report on monitoring progress.* WHO document EB83/2 Add. 1, 1988

WHE 2152   Unuigbe, J.A. et al. Abortion-related morbidity and mortality in Benin City, Nigeria, 1973-85. *International Journal of Gynaecology and Obstetrics* 1988; 26: 435-439

WHE 2237   Chukudebelu, W.O. and Ozaumba, B.C. Maternal mortality in Anambra State of Nigeria *International Journal of Gynaecology and Obstetrics* 1988; 27: 365-370

WHE 2238   Ojo, V.A. et al. Characteristics of maternal deaths following caesarean section in a developing country. *International Journal of Gynaecology and Obstetrics* 1988; 27: 171-176

WHE 2244   Brennan, M. Training traditional birth attendants. *Postgraduate Doctor of Africa* 1988; 11(1): 16-18

WHE 2245 Adetoro, O.O. *Maternal mortality in pregnancy haemorrhage – analysis of a sixteen-year survey at the University of Ilorin Teaching Hospital* (unpublished document) 1989

WHE 2276   Adekolu-John, E.O. Maternal health care and outcome of pregnancies in Kainji Lake area of Nigeria. *Public Health* 1989; 103: 41-49

WHE 2310   Adetoro, O.O. and Agah, A. The implications of childbearing in postpubertal girls in Sokoto, Nigeria. *International Journal of Gynecology and Obstetrics* 1988; 27: 73-77

WHE 2371   Otolorin, E.O. et al. Maternity care monitoring: a contrast at two levels of health care delivery in Ibadan, Nigeria. *International Journal of Gynecology and Obstetrics* 1988; 26: 367-373

WHE 2404   Olusanya, O. and Amiegheme, N. Biosocial factors in maternal mortality – a study from a Nigerian Mission Hospital. *West African Journal of Medicine* 1989; 8(3): 160-165

WHE 2411   Adetoro, O.O. A sixteen-year survey of maternal mortality associated with eclampsia in Ilorin, Nigeria. *International Journal of Gynecology and Obstetrics* 1989; 30: 117-121

WHE 2413   Adetoro, O.O. A fifteen-year study of illegally induced abortion mortality at Ilorin, Nigeria. *International Journal of Gynecology and Obstetrics* 1989; 29: 65-72

WHE 2419   Tahzib, F. *Vesicovaginal fistulae in Nigeria.* Sokoto, Nigeria, University of Sokoto, College of Health Sciences 1989: 149

WHE 2457   Okafor, C.B. *Availability and use of services for maternal and child health care in rural Nigeria.* (unpublished document) 1989

WHE 2471   Osinusi, B.O. and Adeleye, J.A. Homozygous sickle cell anemia at the University College Hospital, Ibadan, revisited. *International Journal of Gynecology and Obstetrics* 1989; 30: 51-55

WHE 2478   Adetoro, O.O. The pattern of eclampsia at the University of Ilorin Teaching Hospital (U.I.T.H.) Ilorin, Nigeria. *International Journal of Gynecology and Obstetrics* 1990; 31: 221-226

WHE 2480   World Health Organization, African Regional Office. Nigeria country profile (personal communication) 1989

WHE 2488   Wright, E.A. and Disu, F.R. Maternal mortality in Jos University Teaching Hospital. *Nigerian Medical Practitioner* 1988; 15(3): 57-59

WHE 2491   Klitsch, M. Modern contraception is little known, rarely used in Ondo State, Nigeria. *International Family Planning Perspectives* 1989; 15(4): 155-157

REUNION

	Year	Source

1. BASIC INDICATORS

1.1 Population
		Year	Source
Size (millions)	0.6	1988	(1915)
Rate of growth (%)	1.7	1985-90	(1915)

1.1.2 Life expectancy
		Year	Source
Female	76	1985-90	(1915)
Male	67	1985-90	(1915)

1.1.3 Fertility
		Year	Source
Crude Birth Rate	23	1985-90	(1915)
Total Fertility Rate	2.4	1985-90	(1915)

1.1.4 Mortality
		Year	Source
Crude Death Rate	6	1985-90	(1915)
Infant Mortality Rate	19	1985-90	(1915)
Female			
Male			
1-4 years mortality rate			
Female			
Male			

1.2 Social and economic

1.2.1 Adult literacy rate (%)
		Year	Source
Female	81	1982	(2458)
Male	77	1982	(2458)

1.2.2 Primary school enrolment rate (%)
Female			
Male			

1.2.3 Female mean age at first marriage
		Year	Source
(years)	25.8	1980	(1918)

1.2.4 GNP/capita
		Year	Source
(US $)	3 830	1980	(2008)

1.2.5 Daily per capita calorie supply
(as a % of requirements)

2. HEALTH SERVICES

2.1 Health expenditure

2.1.1 Expenditure on health
(as % of GNP)

2.1.2 Expenditure on PHC
(as % of total health expenditure)

2.2 Primary Health Care
(Percentage of population covered by):

2.2.1 Health services
National			
Urban			
Rural			

2.2.2 Safe water
		Year	Source
National	80	1984	(2008)
Urban			
Rural			

2.2.3 Adequate sanitary facilities
National			
Urban			
Rural			

2.2.4 Contraceptive prevalence rate (%)

2.3   Coverage of maternity care (%)

Area	Prenatal care	Trained attendant	Institutional deliveries	Postnatal care	Sample size	Year	Source
National	–	–	96	–	–	1985	(2255)

3. COMMUNITY STUDIES

4. HOSPITAL STUDIES

5. CIVIL REGISTRATION DATA/GOVERNMENT ESTIMATES

5.1   National, 1985 [(2255)]

5.1.1   Rate
Live births	13 122
Maternal deaths	4
MMR (per 100 000 live births)	31

5.1.2   Causes of maternal deaths

5.1.3   Avoidable factors
During 1985, over 96% of all births occurred in a medical facility. However, 401 deliveries took place at home. There were two institutional deaths and two home deaths. The relative risk for a home delivery was 32.

	Hospital	Home
Births	12 879	393
Maternal deaths	2	2
MMR (per 100 000 births)	16	509

6. OTHER SOURCES/ ESTIMATES

7. SELECTED ANNOTATED BIBLIOGRAPHY

Combes, J.C. and Reynaud, B. Adolescence et maternité à la Reunion. *La Revue de Pediatrie* 1988; 24(6): 261-264. WHE 2282

The pregnancy rate for minors (under 17 years old) is 77 per 1000 in Reunion, twice that of metropolitan France. An analysis of 105 such pregnancies in 1985-87 found that 20 (19%) were less than 15 years old and 47% of the subjects abandoned their education as a result of the pregnancy. The girls are frequently from broken homes with sisters who are also single mothers. In comparison with the general population such pregnancies have an increased risk of toxaemia of pregnancy, delivery of low birth weight infants and neonatal complications.

8. FURTHER READING

9.   DATA SOURCES

WHE 0753   United Nations, *Demographic Yearbook.* New York, various years.

WHE 1915   United Nations. Department of International Economic and Social Affairs. *World population prospects: estimates and projections as assessed in 1984.* Population Studies No. 98. New York 1986

WHE 1918   United Nations. Department of International Economic and Social Affairs. *First marriage:patternsanddeterminants.*New York, 1988.

WHE 2008   World Health Organization. Regional Office for Africa. *Evaluation of the strategy for health for all by the year 2000. Seventh report on the world health situation*Vol 2, African region, Brazzaville1987

WHE 2255   Rochat, C. et al. A propos des accouchements à domicile. *La Revue de Pediatrie* 1988; 24(6): 241-252

WHE 2458   UNESCO. *Compendium of statistics on illiteracy.* Paris, Division of Statistics on Education, 1988.

RWANDA

		Year	Source

1. BASIC INDICATORS

1.1 Demographic

1.1.1 Population

		Year	Source
Size (millions)	6.8	1988	(1914)
Rate of growth (%)	3.4	1980-87	(1914)

1.1.2 Life expectancy

Female	48	1980-85	(1915)
Male	45	1980-85	(1915)

1.1.3 Fertility

Crude Birth Rate	51	1988	(1914)
Total Fertility Rate	8.3	1988	(1914)

1.1.4 Mortality

Crude Death Rate	17	1988	(1914)
Infant Mortality Rate	121	1988	(1914)
Female			
Male			
1-4 years mortality rate			
Female			
Male			

1.2 Social and economic

1.2.1 Adult literacy rate (%)

Female	33	1985	(1914)
Male	61	1985	(1914)

1.2.2 Primary school enrolment rate (%)

Female	66	1986-88	(1914)
Male	69	1986-88	(1914)

1.2.3 Female mean age at first marriage

(years)	21.2	1983	(1918)

		Year	Source

1.2.4 GNP/capita

(US $)	300	1987	(1914)

1.2.5 Daily per capita calorie supply

(as % of requirements)	81	1988	(1914)

2. HEALTH SERVICES

2.1 Health expenditure

2.1.1 Expenditure on health

(as % of GNP)	3	1984	(2033)

2.1.2 Expenditure on PHC

(as % of total health expenditure)	47	1984	(2033)

2.2 Primary Health Care
(Percentage of population covered by):

2.2.1 Health services

National			
Urban			
Rural			

2.2.2 Safe water

National	60	1983	(0834)
Urban	55	1983	(0834)
Rural	60	1983	(0834)

2.2.3 Adequate sanitary facilities

National	60	1983	(0834)
Urban	60	1983	(0834)
Rural	60	1983	(0834)

2.2.4 Contraceptive prevalence rate

(%)	10	1983	(0753)

2.3 Coverage of maternity care (%)

Area	Prenatal care	Trained attendant	Institutional deliveries	Postnatal care	Sample size	Year	Source
National		20				1981	(0764)
National	85	22				(1989)	(2033)
Three areas	96	48	45		445	1984	(1296)

3. COMMUNITY STUDIES

4. HOSPITAL STUDIES

4.1 All institutions, 1966-71 [(1906)]

4.1.1 Rate

	Live births	Maternal deaths	MMR (per 100 000 live births)
1966	18 771	369	1 966
1967	23 721	164	691
1968	23 814	126	529
1969	26 483	391	1 476
1970	28 747	152	529
1971	30 774	90	292
1966-71	152 310	1 292	848

4.2 Private and public hospitals and dispensaries, 1976 [(0627)]

4.2.1 Rate
Private hospitals

	Live births	Maternal deaths	MMR (per 100 000 live births)
Rutongo	251	1	398
Kabgayi	2 208	15	679
Remera Rukoma	977	0	–
Kigeme	390	6	1 538
Kilinda	1 189	5	421
Kibogora	522	0	–
Mugonero	262	1	382
Mibilizi	817	3	367
Shyira	220	3	1 364
Gahini	448	8	1 786
Rwinkwavu	114	15	13 158
Nemba	541	0	–
TOTAL	7 939	57	718

Dispensaries

	Live births	Maternal deaths	MMR (per 100 000 live births)
Byumba	1 459	0	–
Gikongoro	402	2	498
Kibungo	467	0	–
Gitarama	4 517	2	44
Butare	2 364	3	127
Kibuye	1 143	0	–
Kigali	2 915	2	69
Cyangugu	2 915	2	69
Gisenyi	2 332	0	–
Ruhengeri	2 050	0	–
TOTAL	18 830	10	53

Public hospitals

	Live births	Maternal deaths	MMR (per 100 000 live births)
Kigali	3 871	14	362
Butare	1 898	8	421
Nyanda	894	10	1 119
Muhororo	560	0	–
Rubengeri	2 381	3	126
Rwatagana	1 256	6	478
Kibuye	351	4	1 140
Buhhence	671	3	447
Byumba	519	9	1 734
Kibungo	628	10	1 592
Gisenyi	1 203	8	665
TOTAL	14 232	75	527

All institutions

	Private	Dispensaries	Public	TOTAL
Live births	7 939	18 830	14 232	41 001
Maternal deaths	57	10	75	142
MMR (per 100 000 live births)	718	53	527	346

4.3 Nyundo Maternity Hospital, 1979-82 [1112]

4.3.1 Rate

Live births	4 066
Maternal deaths*	0
MMR (per 100 000 live births)	–

* Deaths occurring in the hospital only

4.4 Seven major hospitals, 1971 [1906]

4.4.1 Rate

Hospital	Live births	Maternal deaths	MMR (per 100 000 live births)
Kabgayi	3 338	6	180
Ruhengiri	2 157	0	–
Kigali	2 055	4	195
Butare	1 667	3	180
Byumba	1 169	5	428
Mibirizi	1 164	3	258
Remera	1 073	7	652
TOTAL	12 670	28	221

The doctoral thesis quotes a study in Kabagayi hospital covering the period 1937-58, during which there were 21 777 deliveries and 198 maternal deaths, giving a maternal mortality rate of 909 per 100 000 deliveries. 56% of these deaths were from ruptured uterus. Pre- and postpartum haemorrhage and infectious diseases were the next most important causes of death.

A study at the Kigali Hospital in 1967 found a maternal mortality rate of 374 per 100 000 live births.

5. CIVIL REGISTRATION DATA/GOVERNMENT ESTIMATES

5.1 National, 1982 [1296]

5.1.1 Rate

A government report on the unmet needs in maternal health and family planning quotes a maternal mortality rate of 210 per 100 000 live births for 1982.

6. OTHER SOURCES/ ESTIMATES

7. SELECTED ANNOTATED BIBLIOGRAPHY

Vavdin, F. et al. Les ruptures utérines au Rwanda (à propos de 87 cas). *Médecine Tropicale* 1983; 43(1): 37-43. WHE 0767

Between 1978 and 1982 there were 9 994 births at the Ruhengeri Hospital in north Rwanda and 87 cases of uterine rupture, an incidence of 8.7 per 1000 births. There were 18 maternal deaths, a case fatality rate of 21%. The maternal mortality rate from uterine rupture alone was 180 per 100 000 births. There was one case of vesicovaginal fistula following a subtotal hysterectomy.

8. FURTHER READING

9. DATA SOURCES

WHE 0627   Rwanda, Ministère de la Santé Publique. *Rapport annuel 1976* Rwanda, 1976

WHE 0753   United Nations. *Demographic Yearbook.* New York, various years

WHE 0764   Van Sprindel, M. et al. Le poids à la naissance comme indicateur de santé. Example de Rwanda. *Médecine d'Afrique Noire* 1981; 28(2): 93-99

WHE 0834   World Health Organization. *World Health Statistics annual – vital statistics and causes of death.* Geneva, various years

WHE 1112   Janowitz, B. et al. *Reproductive health in Africa: issues and options.* Family Health International, North Carolina, 1984

WHE 1296   Rwanda, Office de la Population. *Etude sur les besoins non satisfaits en santé maternelle et planification familiale.* (unpublished document) 1985

WHE 1906   Nsengumuremyi, F. *Les problèmes de protection de la mère et de l'enfant au Rwanda* (Doctoral thesis) Rwanda, 1974

WHE 1914   United Nations Children's Fund (UNICEF). *The state of the world's children,* various years, Oxford, Oxford University Press

WHE 1915   United Nations. Department of International Economic and Social Affairs. *World population prospects: estimates and projections as assessed in 1984.* Population Studies No. 98. New York 1986

WHE 1918   United Nations. Department of International Economic and Social Affairs. *First marriage: patterns and determinants.* New York 1988

WHE 2033   World Health Organization. *Global strategy for health for all by the year 2000. Second report on monitoring progress.* WHO document EB83/2 Add. 1, 1988

SENEGAL

		Year	Source

1. BASIC INDICATORS

1.1 Demographic

1.1.1 Population
		Year	Source
Size (millions)	7.0	1988	(1914)
Rate of growth (%)	2.6	1980-87	(1914)

1.1.2 Life expectancy
		Year	Source
Female	45	1980-85	(1915)
Male	42	1980-85	(1915)

1.1.3 Fertility
		Year	Source
Crude Birth Rate	46	1988	(1914)
Total Fertility Rate	6.4	1988	(1914)

1.1.4 Mortality
		Year	Source
Crude Death Rate	19	1988	(1914)
Infant Mortality Rate	80	1988	(1914)
Female	81	1981-86	(2657)
Male	92	1981-86	(2657)
1-4 years mortality rate			
Female	112	1981-86	(2657)
Male	117	1981-86	(2657)

1.2 Social and economic

1.2.1 Adult literacy rate (%)
		Year	Source
Female	19	1985	(1914)
Male	37	1985	(1914)

1.2.2 Primary school enrolment rate (%)
		Year	Source
Female	49	1986-88	(1914)
Male	71	1986-88	(1914)

1.2.3 Female mean age at first marriage
		Year	Source
(years)	18.3	1978	(1918)

1.2.4 GNP/capita
		Year	Source
(US $)	520	1987	(1914)

1.2.5 Daily per capita calorie supply
		Year	Source
(as % of requirements)	99	1984-86	(1914)

2. HEALTH SERVICES

2.1 Health expenditure

2.1.1 Expenditure on health
(% of GNP)

2.1.2 Expenditure on PHC
(as % of total health		Year	Source
expenditure)	70	1983	(2033)

2.2 Primary Health Care
(Percentage of population covered by):

2.2.1 Health services
		Year	Source
National	40	1984-86	(2033)
Urban			
Rural			

2.2.2 Safe water
		Year	Source
National	44	1983	(0834)
Urban	63	1983	(0834)
Rural	27	1983	(0834)

2.2.3 Adequate sanitary facilities
		Year	Source
National			
Urban	87	1984	(0834)
Rural	2	1980	(0834)

2.2.4 Contraceptive prevalence rate
		Year	Source
(%)	6	1986	(2657)

2.3   Coverage of maternity care (%)

Area	Prenatal care	Trained attendant	Institutional deliveries	Postnatal care	Sample size	Year	Source
National	30		85			(1981)	(1005)
National:	63	41			4 244	1981-86	(2657)
urban	95	82			1473	1981-86	(2657)
rural	46	20			2771	1981-86	(2657)
24 villages	66		38		290w	1988-89	(2459)
Sine-Saloum	45	20			1 894w	1982	(1002)
Sine-Saloum		46	21	17	1 250	1982	(1970)

3.   COMMUNITY STUDIES

3.1   Sine-Saloum Region, 1963-83 [0213, 1423]

3.1.1   Rate

A longitudinal study carried out over a period of two decades in the Sine-Saloum region found a maternal mortality rate of 700 per 100 000 live births. A subsequent study covering the Niakhar zone in the same region between 1983 and 1986 recorded 3 405 live births and 20 maternal deaths, giving a rate of 587 per 100 000 live births.

3.2   24 villages representing all regions, 1988-89 [2459]

This was a nationwide hospital and community study carried out in regional hospitals, health centres, health posts and in villages among women's groups and local health workers. (For details of the hospital survey see section 4.5). Twenty four villages were randomly selected. Within the villages interviews were conducted with village chiefs, leaders of women's groups, ten randomly selected households and the most recently delivered woman. Local civil registers were also examined.

3.2.1   Rate

Live births	1 371
Maternal deaths	13
MMR (per 100 000 live births)	948
MMR (per 100 000 women of reproductive age)	238

3.2.2   Causes of maternal deaths

3.2.3   Avoidable factors

Over one third of the women had had no prenatal care.

3.2.4   High risk groups

3.2.5   Other findings

- Only 7% of the women were literate.

- 69% of the women were aged less than 17 years old at their first pregnancy.

- 36% of the women had between 7 and 17 previous pregnancies.

- In nearly half the women the birth interval was under two years.

- 47% of the women had experienced a difficult labour, in 60% due to p rolonged labour, 19% excessive pain and 13% excessive bleeding.

- 70% maintained their normal (heavy) workload throughout pregnancy.

- 25% of the women were unable to cite any sign of a complicated pregnancy. Nearly one third were unable to cite any sign of a difficult labour.

- The decision to refer women in labour to a health centre or hospital was either the responsibility of the husband (52%) or another member of the family (44%). None of the women were themselves able to take the decision to seek hospital assistance.

4. HOSPITAL STUDIES

4.1 L'Hôpital Aristide Le Dantec, 1971-75 [0160, 0706, 1391]

4.1.1 Rate

	1971-75	1986-87
Live births	62 020	6 217
Maternal deaths	498	100
MMR (per 100 000 live births)	803	1 608

4.1.2 Causes of maternal deaths

A study of cases of dystocia encountered in the hospital in 1971 and 1975 found that 7-9% of the deaths were due to obstructed labour, including cases in which obstruction led to rupture of the uterus. More than 80% of the deaths from dystocia were during the rainy months between July and October.

4.1.3 High risk groups, 1971-75

Women who were above 30 years of age, and women of parity 1 or of parity 5 and above were at greater risk of death.

Age (years)

	% of obstetric population	% of maternal deaths
<19	28	24
20-24	20	21
25-29	21	16
30-34	10	18
35-39	5	15
40-44	1	5
45+	<1	<1
Unknown	14	<1
TOTAL	100	100

Parity

1	23	36
2	17	10
3	14	8
4	13	7
5+	34	39
TOTAL	100	100

4.1.5 Other findings

Maternal deaths were very high during two periods of the year, namely, January to March, and September to November, which coincide with the winter and rainy seasons respectively. The high number of maternal deaths in winter was due to an increase in the incidence of hypertensive disorders during this season, as well as the higher prevalence of viral hepatitis.

4.2 Centre Hospitalier Abasse N'Dao, 1980-81 [0551]

4.2.1 Rate

Births	8 769
Maternal deaths	32
MMR (per 100 000 births)	365

4.2.2 Causes of maternal deaths

43% of all deaths were due to haemorrhage and a further 7% due to obstructed labour.

4.2.3 Avoidable factors

4.2.4 High risk groups

Women who died were older, of higher parity, and had less education than the women who survived childbirth. The average age of women who died was 31.4 years, they had 3.8 living children on average and 93% of them were illiterate. The corresponding figures for those who survived was 25.3 years, 2.7 living children and 74% illiteracy rate.

4.3 L'Hôpital Principal de Dakar, 1978-81 [1041]

4.3.1 Rate

A maternal mortality rate of 200 per 100 000 live births was reported for the period 1978-81.

4.4 L'hôpital Aristide le Dantec, L'hôpital Principal, and Centre Hospitalier Abbas Ndao, 1986-87 [1878, 1925, 2017]

4.4.1 Rate

	CHU Aristide Dantec	Hôpital Principal	Centre Abbas Ndao	TOTAL
Live births	6 217	4 754	9 295	20 266
Maternal deaths	100	29	23	152
MMR (per 100 000 live births)	1 608	610	247	750

4.4.2   Causes of maternal deaths (for all 152 deaths)

	Number	%
Sepsis	37	24
Haemorrhage	32	21
Hypertensive disorders of pregnancy	29	19
Ruptured uterus	11	7
Transfusion shock	4	3
Embolisms	2	1
Complications of anaesthesia	1	1
DIRECT CAUSES	116	76
Anaemia	7	5
Hepatitis	5	3
Other infections	9	6
Others	15	10
INDIRECT CAUSES	36	24
TOTAL	152	100

The incidence of deaths from hypertensive disorders of pregnancy, sepsis, haemorrhage and rupture of the uterus was considerably higher during the four rainy months between July and October than during the remaining eight dry months. Thus over half of all maternal deaths occurred during the rainy season.

4.4.3   Avoidable factors

139 of the 152 deaths were considered preventable by the examining personnel. About 70% of the deaths were attributable to lack of equipment and facilities in the health centres.

4.4.4   High risk groups

Women who died were compared with two control groups. One consisted of women of the same age and parity who were admitted with the same complication as the women who died, but who had normal deliveries and live births. The second control group consisted of women of the same age and parity who came from the same residential areas as the women who died, but had normal deliveries and live births. This helped identify the risk factors involved other than age, parity, and residence.

Prenatal care

Women who did not have prenatal care were at a higher risk of death than those who did, and the number of prenatal visits was positively correlated to the chances of survival. 20% of women who died had had no prenatal care compared with 2% in each control group. Only 40% of those who died had made three or more prenatal visits compared to around three quarters of the women in the two control groups.

Problems during pregnancy

55% of the women who died had had problems during the prenatal period compared to 16% and 18% in the two control groups. The most significant health problems during the prenatal period were hypertensive disorders (19%) and haemorrhage (9%) .

Late referral and condition on admission

Almost half of the women who died had been admitted to hospital 24 hours or more after the onset of labour compared with only 3-5% of the control groups. Hypotension (systolic below 95mm Hg and diastolic below 50mm Hg) and hypertension (systolic above 140mm Hg and diastolic above 90mm Hg) on admission were significantly associated with maternal death. A body temperature above 37.5 degrees centigrade was found in 61% of the women who died compared with 15% and 21% of women in the control groups. Generalised oedema on admission was found to be another risk factor.

Marital status

14% of the women who died were single compared with 5% and 8% of the controls.

4.5   National, five hospitals, ten health centres and 28 health posts, 1988-89 [2459]

4.5.1   Rate

	MMR (per 100 000 live births)
Hospitals	3 232
Health Centres	407
Health Posts	459
Overall	933

Because most births take place at home, it is estimated that three out of four maternal deaths are not registered. In general, it was found that reporting was more complete for births than for maternal deaths. All hospitals and health centres kept record on births as did 89% of the health posts. Death records were maintained by all hospitals but only by 60% of health centres and 43% of health posts.

4.5.2   Causes of maternal deaths

	%
Haemorrhage	41
Sepsis	21
Hypertensive disorders of pregnancy	7
DIRECT CAUSES	69
Cardiopathies, anaemia, hepatitis malaria	23
Other	9
TOTAL	100

4.5.3   Avoidable factors

4.5.4   High risk groups

4.5.5 Other findings
Essential supplies

Not all hospitals and health centres had supplies of drugs and materials necessary for pregnancy surveillance. Single-use syringes are systematically reused in all hospitals, health centres and health posts.

	Percentage of availability		
	Hospitals	Health Centres	Health Posts
Sphygmomanometer	60	80	75
Stethoscope	60	90	75
Thermometer	60	90	86
Disinfectants	60	40	40
Oxytocics			
Syntocinon	20	10	11
Methergin	80	30	14
Antibiotics	40	50	54
I.V.solutes	80	90	71
Blood	60	10	0
Transport (in working order)	60	70	32

Although all the hospitals and 10% of the health centres had operative facilities, their functioning was frequently interrupted due to the absence of qualified medical personnel or lack of materials.

5. CIVIL REGISTRATION DATA/GOVERNMENT ESTIMATES

6. OTHER SOURCES/ ESTIMATES

6.1. National, 1981-85 [1745, 1746]

6.1.1 Rate
The maternal mortality rate for the country as a whole is estimated at 600 per 100 000 live births. However, there is considerable variation between different regions. The rate for Cap-Vert in Dakar is estimated to be less than 500 per 100 000, whereas rates for remote regions could be significantly above 600.

6.2. Bandafassi, 1975-87 [1928]

6.2.1 Rate
Live births	2 411
Maternal deaths	31
MMR (per 100 000 live births)	1 285

6.2.2 Causes of maternal deaths

6.2.3 Avoidable factors

6.2.4 High risk groups
Age

	Live births	Maternal deaths	MMR (per 100 000 live births)
10-14	22	2	9 091
15-19	476	7	1 471
20-24	656	5	762
25-29	585	3	513
30-34	340	8	2 353
35-39	214	3	1 402
40-44	89	3	3 371
45-49	22	0	–

7. SELECTED ANNOTATED BIBLIOGRAPHY

Sylla, S. et al. La place de la dystocie osseuse dans les fistules vésico-vaginales. *Bulletin de la Société de Médecine de l'Afrique Noire de Langue Française* 1975; 20(3): 315-322. WHE 2145

A study of the pelvic bones of 75 women with vesicovaginal fistulae in Dakar, Senegal, showed that pelvic distortion accounted for only 6% of the cases. The major cause of the fistula is thus attributed to neglected labour: lack of qualified birth attendants, lack of roads and means of transport, clinging to traditional practices, Islamic fatalism, and incorrect use of forceps. The authors suggest that the Ministry of Health must give priority to the setting up of maternity centres, the appropriate training of personnel, an adequate referral system, and free welfare services.

8. FURTHER READING

Correa, P. et al. Le syndrome de Sheehan chez l'africaine. *Afrique Médicale* 1975; 14(126): 27-32. WHE 1873

Dano, P. et al. Le syndrome de Sheehan. *Dakar Médical* 1982; 27(3): 323-330. WHE 1061

Ducloux, M. et al. Pan-hypopituitarisme du post partum chez une Sénégalaise (syndrome de Sheehan). *Bulletin de la Societé Médicale d'Afrique Noire de langue Française* 1976; 21(3): 307-309. WHE 1874

Kimball, A.M. et al. Preliminary report of an identification mission for safe motherhood, Senegal: putting the M back in M.C.H. *International Journal of Gynaecology and Obstetrics* 1988; 26. WHE 1987

Papiernik, E. Principales causes de morts maternelles, quotient de mortalité, fréquence dans la population des accouchées, une meta-analyse. In: Bouyer, J. et al (eds) *Réduire la mortalité maternelle dans les pays en développement.* INSERM, Paris, 1988

Sankale, M. et al. Le syndrome de Sheehan en Afrique noire (à propos de neuf cas, dont cinq personnels). *African Journal of Medicine and Medical Science* 1978; 7: 65-69. WHE 0944

9. DATA SOURCES

WHE 0160   Correa, P. Mortalité maternelle au cours de la parturition à la Clinique Gynécologique et Obstétrique de Dakar. *Afrique Médicale* 1978; 17(162): 489-495

WHE 0213   Family Health International. Study of maternal mortality in Senegal planned. *Network* 1983; 5(1): 2

WHE 0551   Lauroy, J. Quelques characteristiques obstetricales de la population d'une maternité de la banlieue de Dakar. *Afrique Médicale* 1983; 22(212): 383-390

WHE 0706   Traore, M. *Contribution à l'étude de la dystocie en milieu africain à Dakar.* Université de Dakar (thesis) 1980

WHE 0834   World Health Organization. *World Health Statistics annual – vital statistics and causes of death.* Geneva, various years

WHE 1002   Goldberg, H.I. et al. *Sine-Saloum family health survey - final report.* Dakar, United States Agency for International Development, 1982

WHE 1005   Garenne, M. et al. *Politique de santé et mortalité au Senegal, 1960-80.* 1981

WHE 1041   Breda, Y. et al. Obstetrical activities at the Dakar Principal Hospital (a four-year retrospective study 1978-81). *Médecine Tropicale* 1983; 41(1): 15-18

WHE 1391   Correa, P. et al. La mortalité maternelle au cours de la dystocie en milieu africain à Dakar. *Dakar Médical* 1982; 331-338

WHE 1423   Garenne, M. *Maternal mortality in Niakhar* (personal communication), 1986 ORSTROM, Dakar, Senegal

WHE 1745   Senegal, Government of, and United Nations Development Programme. *Rapport de la mission d'identification pour la reduction de la mortalité maternelle au Sénégal* Dakar, 1987

WHE 1746   Kimball, A.M. Personal communication, 1987

WHE 1878   Mbaye, K. and Garenne, M. *Determinants de la mortalité maternelle à Dakar. Analyse et principaux résultats d'une étude hospitalière.* (unpublished document) 1987

WHE 1914   United Nations Children's Fund (UNICEF). *The state of the world's children,* various years, Oxford, Oxford University Press

WHE 1915   United Nations. Department of International Economic and Social Affairs. *World population prospects: estimates and projections as assessed in 1984.* Population Studies No. 98. New York 1986

WHE 1918 United Nations. Department of International Economic and Social Affairs. *First marriage: patterns and determinants.* New York 1988

WHE 1925   Correa, P. et al. *Rapport final de l'étude sur la mortalité maternelle à Dakar (Senegal): Causes et mesures à prendre pour l'ameliorer* 1987

WHE 1928   Pison, G. *La mortalité maternelle à Bandafossi (Senegal)* (unpublished document) 1987

WHE 1970   USAID, Dakar. *Sine-Saloum family health survey* 1982, Georgia, 1984

WHE 2017   Diadhiou, F. Expérience sénégalaise sur la mortalité maternelle dans les pays en developpement. In: Bouyer, J. et al. *Réduire la mortalité maternelle dans les pays en développement.* Paris, INSERM/Centre Internationale de l'enfance. 1988

WHE 2033   World Health Organization. *Global strategy for health for all by the year 2000. Second report on monitoring progress.* WHO document EB83/2 Add. 1, 1988

WHE 2459   Gueye, A. et al. *Rapport de la deuxième mission d'identification pour la reduction de la mortalité maternelle au Senegal* Gouvernement de la République du Senegal, UNDP, WHO, University of Columbia. 1989

WHE 2657   Demographic and Health Surveys. *Enquête démographique et de santé au Sénégal 1986,* Ministère de l'Economie et des Finances/ Institute for Resource Development/ Westinghouse, 1988

NOTES

SIERRA LEONE

		Year	Source

1. BASIC INDICATORS

1.1 Demographic

1.1.1 Population

		Year	Source
Size (millions)	3.9	1988	(1914)
Rate of growth (%)	2.4	1980-87	(1914)

1.1.2 Life expectancy

		Year	Source
Female	36	1980-85	(1915)
Male	33	1980-85	(1915)

1.1.3 Fertility

		Year	Source
Crude Birth Rate	48	1988	(1914)
Total Fertility Rate	6.5	1988	(1914)

1.1.4 Mortality

		Year	Source
Crude Death Rate	23	1988	(1914)
Infant Mortality Rate	153	1988	(1914)
Female			
Male			
1-4 years mortality rate			
Female			
Male			

1.2 Social and economic

1.2.1 Adult literacy rate (%)

		Year	Source
Female	21	1985	(1914)
Male	38	1985	(1914)

1.2.2 Primary school enrolment rate (%)

		Year	Source
Female	48	1982	(1914)
Male	68	1982	(1914)

1.2.3 Female mean age at first marriage
(years)

1.2.4 GNP/capita

		Year	Source
(US $)	300	1987	(1914)

1.2.5 Daily per capita calorie supply

		Year	Source
(as % of requirements)	81	1984-86	(1914)

2. HEALTH SERVICES

2.1 Health expenditure

2.1.1 Expenditure on health

		Year	Source
(as % of GNP)	7	1984	(0800)

2.1.2 Expenditure on PHC

		Year	Source
(as % of total health expenditure)	15	1984	(0800)

2.2 Primary Health Care
(Percentage of population covered by):

2.2.1 Health services

		Year	Source
National	36	1984	(0834)
Urban			
Rural			

2.2.2 Safe water

		Year	Source
National	24	1984	(0834)
Urban	58	1984	(0834)
Rural	8	1984	(0834)

2.2.3 Adequate sanitary facilities

		Year	Source
National	21	1984	(0834)
Urban	43	1984	(0834)
Rural	10	1984	(0834)

2.2.4 Contraceptive prevalence rate

		Year	Source
(%)	4	1982	(1712)

2.3 Coverage of maternity care (%)

Area	Prenatal care	Trained attendant	Institutional deliveries	Postnatal care	Sample size	Year	Source
National	30	25				1984	(0834)
rural	50	26	5		2 189w	1977	(1845)
urban	80	80	27		2 189w	1977	(1845)

3. COMMUNITY STUDIES

4. HOSPITAL STUDIES

4.1 All hospitals, 1976 [0781]

4.1.1 Rate

Region	Live births	Maternal deaths	MMR (per 100 000 live births)
Western Province	8 058	48	596
Southern Province	1 954	13	665
Eastern Province	3 137	381	211
Northern Province	1 344	24	1 785
TOTAL	14 493	123	849

4.1.2 Causes of maternal deaths

The study gives causes of death for 86 maternal deaths of which 40 occurred in the Western Province, 3 in the Southern Province, 19 in the Eastern and 29 in the Northern Province.

	Number	%
Haemorrhage	24	28
Rupture of the uterus	15	17
Sepsis	8	9
Hypertensive disorders of pregnancy	8	9
Obstructed labour	2	2
DIRECT CAUSES	57	66
Anaemia	7	8
Infections	4	5
INDIRECT CAUSES	11	13
Others/unknown	18	21
TOTAL	86	100

4.2 Connaught Hospital, Freetown, 1970-72 [0782]

4.2.1 Rate

Deliveries	17 494
Maternal deaths	134
MMR (per 100 000 deliveries)	766

4.2.2 Causes of maternal deaths

10% of the maternal deaths were related to abortions. There were 13 deaths out of 670 abortion admissions to the hospital.

4.3 Princess Christian Maternity Hospital, Freetown, 1969-76 and 1980-81 [0781, 1112]

4.3.1 Rate

	1969-76	1980-81
Live births	51 257	5 788
Maternal deaths	302	8
MMR (per 100 000 live births)	589	140

4.3.2 Causes of maternal deaths, 1976

	Number	%
Hypertensive disorders of pregnancy	10	21
Haemorrhage	7	15
Uterine rupture	5	10
Sepsis	3	6
Obstructed labour	2	4
DIRECT CAUSES	27	56
Cardiac disease	6	13
Anaemia	2	4
Malaria	2	4
INDIRECT CAUSES	10	21
Others/unknown	11	23
TOTAL	48	100

In 1972, 50% of all deaths were from postpartum haemorrhage, uterine rupture and abruptio placentae. The same pattern continued in 1974 when the same three causes accounted for 22 of the 44 maternal deaths.

5. CIVIL REGISTRATION DATA/GOVERNMENT ESTIMATES

6. OTHER ESTIMATES

6.1 National, 1980 [0032]

6.1.1 Rate
A review of the health sector published by UNDP and WHO quotes a maternal mortality rate of 450 per 100 000 deliveries.

6.2 National [0273]

6.2.1 Rate
Based on various mean levels of maternal mortality proposed or calculated for Sierra Leone, and assuming a birth rate of 50 per 1 000 population, a maternal mortality rate of 650 per 100 000 live births has been estimated.

7. SELECTED ANNOTATED BIBLIOGRAPHY

Edwards, N.C. Payment for deliveries in Sierra Leone. *Bulletin of the World Health Organization* 1989; 67(2): 163-169. WHE 2162

Theoretically, deliveries in government peripheral health units and in district and provincial hospitals are provided free or at minimal cost. The results of this study indicate, however, that this is not the case. The type and amount of payment for deliveries were investigated in 1982 during a survey on health status in two districts. Data on the payments made for 83.5% of the 2 591 deliveries in 535 randomly selected study villages showed that the most common method of payment was in cash only. Payments in kind were mostly given to traditional birth attendants (for 38.1% of their deliveries) and rare for professional staff (2.9% of deliveries).

The total amount paid for a delivery differed significantly with the type of birth attendant (hospital, peripheral health unit or home). The total average payment for a delivery was highest for professional birth attendants and lowest for untrained TBAs.

The outcome of a delivery had a significant effect on the amount paid. Payments were significantly higher for stillbirths than for live births among professional and auxiliary birth attendants.

However, the trained and untrained TBAs received less payment for stillbirths than for live births. The results show that there are several levels of financial disincentives for pregnant women requiring the services of trained auxiliary or professional health workers at the time of delivery.

Leigh, B. The use of partograms by maternal and child health aides. *Journal of Tropical Pediatrics* 1986; 32: 107-110. WHE 1587

Thirty Maternal and Child Health Aides (MCH-Aide) working in various villages in the Southern Province of Sierra Leone, identified by random selection, were trained in the use of partograms to monitor primigravid labour. The performances of these Aides in the effective use of the partogram was compared with that of midwives chosen by random selection from all government hospitals and similarly trained.

Of 74 patients referred by the MCH-Aides over a 12-month period following their training, 35 were primigravidae. 20% of those whose labours were monitored on the partogram were delivered by caesarean section, while 55% of those where no partogram was used required a caesarean section. This difference is statistically significant.

Though the MCH-Aides promptly instituted the patient's transfer to hospital, these could not benefit from timely intervention because of infrastructural difficulties such as transportation and problems of resources such as the non-availability of blood for transfusion.

Thus the extensive use of the partogram by the MCH-Aides brought to light the complex interrelationship between obstetric, social and environmental factors in determining the outcome of pregnancy among the rural population of Sierra Leone.

Sevali, B. *Vesico-vaginal fistula – yet another health problem fast emerging.* Serabu, 1989. 3p. (Unpublished). WHE 2299

In Serabu Hospital, Sierra Leone, 28 cases of vesico-vaginal fistulae were admitted from all over the country between 1987 and 1988. Most patients were aged 18-25. Women with fistulae are said to risk losing their husbands.

8. FURTHER READING

Aitken, I.W. et al. Planning a community-oriented midwifery service for Sierra Leone. *World Health Forum* 1985; 6: 110-114. WHE 1018

Karbo, T.K. Certain practices related to delivery. Paper prepared for seminar on *Traditional Practices Affecting the Health of Women and Children in Africa.* 6-10 February 1984, Dakar, Senegal. WHE 0557

Simpson-Herbert, M. et al. Traditional midwives and family planning. *Population Reports* 1980; Series J, 22. WHE 0655

Wright, M.L. Some aspects of the paediatric situation in Sierra Leone. *Bulletin of the International Pediatric Association* 1984; 5(7): 4-10. WHE 0921

9. DATA SOURCES

WHE 0032   Amonoo-Lartson, R. and Olu Williams, A.E. *Health sector review.* Freetown, United Nations Development Programme and World Health Organization. 1981

WHE 0273   Aitken, I.W. *Screening for antenatal risk factors in pregnant women in Sierra Leone.* (Unpublished document), 1983

WHE 0781   Williams, B. *Maternal mortality in Sierra Leone.* Freetown, Ministry of Health, 1979

WHE 0782   Williams, B. Data on four problem areas to be discussed. On: WHO *Regional Multidisciplinary Meeting on Human Reproduction,* Yaoundé, 4-7 December 1978. (Unpublished WHO document No. HRP/RMC/78.1), 1978

WHE 0800   World Health Organization. *Country reports to regional offices of the progress in implementing Health for All by the Year 2000.* (Unpublished documents) 1983

WHE 0834   World Health Organization. *World Health Statistics annual – vital statistics and causes of death.* Geneva, various years

WHE 1112   Janowitz, B. et al. *Reproductive health in Africa: issues and options.* Family Health International, North Carolina, 1984

WHE 1712   Mauldin W.P. and Segal, S.J. *Prevalence of contraceptive use in developing countries. A chart book.* Rockefeller Foundation, New York 1986

WHE 1845   Hardiman M.G.W. and Midgley, J.O. Planning and the health of mothers and children in the rural area of Sierra Leone. *Journal of Tropical Pediatrics* 1981; 27: 83-87

WHE 1914   United Nations Children's Fund (UNICEF). *The state of the world's children,* various years, Oxford, Oxford University Press

WHE 1915   United Nations. Department of International Economic and Social Affairs. *World population prospects: estimates and projections as assessed in 1984.* Population Studies No. 98. New York 1986

SOMALIA

		Year	Source

1. BASIC INDICATORS

1.1 Demographic

1.1.1 Population

Size (millions)	7.1	1988	(1914)
Rate of growth (%)	3.5	1980-87	(1914)

1.1.2 Life expectancy

Female	43	1980-85	(1915)
Male	39	1980-85	(1915)

1.1.3 Fertility

Crude Birth Rate	51	1988	(1914)
Total Fertility Rate	6.6	1988	(1914)

1.1.4 Mortality

Crude Death Rate	20	1988	(1914)
Infant Mortality Rate	131	1988	(1914)
Female			
Male			
1-4 years mortality rate			
Female			
Male			

1.2 Social and economic

1.2.1 Adult literacy rate (%)

Female	6	1985	(1914)
Male	18	1985	(1914)

1.2.2 Primary school enrolment rate* (%)

Female	10	1986-88	(1914)
Male	19	1986-88	(1914)

* Net

1.2.3 Female mean age at first marriage

(years)	20.1	1980-81	(1918)

1.2.4 GNP/capita

(US$)	290	1987	(1914)

1.2.5 Daily per capita calorie supply

(as % of requirements)	90	1984-86	(1914)

2. HEALTH SERVICES

2.1 Health expenditure

2.1.1 Expenditure on health
(as % of GNP)

2.1.2 Expenditure on PHC

(as % of total health expenditure)	43	1984	(2033)

2.2 Primary Health Care
(Percentage of population covered by):

2.2.1 Health services

National	27	1985-87	(1914)
Urban	50	1985-87	(1914)
Rural	15	1985-87	(1914)

2.2.2 Safe water

National	33	1985	(0834)
Urban	60	1985	(0834)
Rural	20	1985	(0834)

2.2.3 Adequate sanitary facilities

National	17	1985	(0834)
Urban	60	1985	(0834)
Rural	5	1985	(0834)

2.2.4 Contraceptive prevalence rate

(%)	2	1982	(1712)

2.3   Coverage of maternity care (%)

Area	Prenatal care	Trained attendant	Institutional deliveries	Postnatal care	Sample size	Year	Source
National		11			5 781	1981	(0813)
National		2				(1983)	(0800)
National	2	2				1988	(2033)
Hargeisa	44-72	58-85				1981	(0816)
Merca, Johar, Mogadishu			55			1981	(0816)

3. COMMUNITY STUDIES

4. HOSPITAL STUDIES

5. CIVIL REGISTRATION DATA/GOVERNMENT ESTIMATES

6. OTHER SOURCES/ ESTIMATES

6.1   National [(0816)]

6.1.1   Rate

A WHO report on Expanded Programme of Immunisation and Maternal and Child Health published in 1981, quotes a maternal mortality rate of 1 100 per 100 000 live births.

7. SELECTED ANNOTATED BIBLIOGRAPHY

8. FURTHER READING

Ahmed, F. *The role of the traditional birth attendants in the nomadic communities: An investigation in Borama District, Awdal Region, North West Somalia.* (Unpublished document), Centre of Adult and Higher Education, University of Manchester, 1986. WHE 1684

Cook, R. *Damage to physical health from pharaonic circumcision (infibulation) of females.* Paper prepared for Seminar on Traditional Practices Affecting the Health of Women and Children in Africa, 1984, 6-10 February, Dakar, Senegal. WHE 1911

El Sherbini, A. *Risk approach, maternal and child health, Somalia* (Assignment report), Geneva, 1989. WHE 2344

Faour, M. Fertility policy and family planning in the Arab countries. *Studies in Family Planning* 1989; 20(5): 254-263. WHE 2367

9. DATA SOURCES

WHE 0800   World Health Organization. *Country reports to regional offices of the progress in implementing Health for All by the Year 2000.* (Unpublished documents) 1983

WHE 0813   World Health Organization, Eastern Mediterranean Regional Office. *Report of the EMR/SEAR meeting on prevention of neonatal tetanus.* (WHO document No. EM/IMZ/27, EM/BD/14, EM-SEAR/MTG.PREV.NNL.TTN/8) Lahore, 1982

WHE 0816   World Health Organization, Eastern Mediterranean Regional Office. *Report on the expanded programme of immunization and maternal and child health in Somali Democratic Republic.* (unpublished WHO document no. EM/IMZ/20, EM/MCH/159, EM/SOM/EPI/001), 1981

WHE 0834   World Health Organization. *World Health Statistics annual – vital statistics and causes of death.* Geneva, various years

WHE 1712   Mauldin W.P. and Segal, S.J. *Prevalence of contraceptive use in developing countries. A chart book.* Rockefeller Foundation, New York 1986

WHE 1914   United Nations Children's Fund (UNICEF). *The state of the world's children,* various years, Oxford, Oxford University Press

WHE 1915   United Nations. Department of International Economic and Social Affairs. *World population prospects: estimates and projections as assessed in 1984.* Population Studies No. 98. New York 1986

WHE 1918   United Nations. Department of International Economic and Social Affairs. *First marriage: patterns and determinants.* New York 1988

WHE 2033   World Health Organization. *Global strategy for health for all by the year 2000. Second report on monitoring progress.* WHO document EB83/2 Add. 1, 1988

NOTES

SOUTH AFRICA

		Year	Source

1. BASIC INDICATORS

1.1 Demographic

1.1.1 Population

		Year	Source
Size (millions)	33.7	1988	(1914)
Rate of growth (%)	2.2	1980-87	(1914)

1.1.2 Life expectancy

Female	55	1980-85	(1915)
Male	52	1980-85	(1915)

1.1.3 Fertility

Crude Birth Rate	32	1988	(1914)
Total Fertility Rate	4.4	1988	(1914)

1.1.4 Mortality

Crude Death Rate	10	1988	(1914)
Infant Mortality Rate	71	1988	(1914)
Female			
Male			
1-4 years mortality rate			
Female			
Male			

1.2 Social and economic

1.2.1 Adult literacy rate (%)
Female
Male

1.2.2 Primary school enrolment rate (%)
Female
Male

1.2.3 Female mean age at first marriage

(years)	22.8	1960	(1918)

1.2.4 GNP/capita

(US $)	1 890	1987	(1914)

1.2.5 Daily per capita calorie supply

(as % of requirements)	120	1984-86	(1914)

2. HEALTH SERVICES

2.1 Health expenditure

2.1.1 Expenditure on health
(as % of GNP)

2.1.2 Expenditure on PHC
(as % of total health expenditure)

2.2 Primary Health Care
(Percentage of population covered by):

2.2.1 Health services
National
Urban
Rural

2.2.2 Safe water
National
Urban
Rural

2.2.3 Adequate sanitary facilities
National
Urban
Rural

2.2.4 Contraceptive prevalence rate

(%)	37-50	1976	(1712)

2.3 Coverage of maternity care (%)

Area	Prenatal care	Trained attendant	Institutional deliveries	Postnatal care	Sample size	Year	Source
Cape Town		98	73			1981	(0664)
Kwazulu, rural			8		364	1983	(0406)
Mosvold, rural			54		212	1987	(2330)

3. COMMUNITY STUDIES

3.1 Umphambinyoni Valley, Dudulu district, Kwazulu rural area, 1972-82 [(0406)]

This is a rural area, some 3-4 hours' walk from the nearest clinic. There is no bus service. The clinic is equipped with a "waiting mothers' area" which can accommodate six women. However its catchment area covers the domain of three chiefs and women are reluctant to use the waiting home if they come from a domain outside that on which the clinic is built. 92% of the women in the area deliver at home with the assistance of a traditional birth attendant.

A community survey was carried out as part of a pilot project for training traditional birth attendants in rural areas. With the permission of the local chief a house-to-house survey of women was conducted in a sample of 100 representative households scattered across the valley.

The interviewer (a man) was able to obtain interviews with only 85 parous women. There were two maternal deaths, both of haemorrhage, and a total of 364 deliveries.

3.1.1 Rate
Deliveries	364
Maternal deaths	2
MMR (per 100 000 deliveries)	550

4. HOSPITAL STUDIES

4.1 267 hospitals throughout the country, 1980-82 [(1520)]

4.1.1 Rate
Births	971 791
Maternal deaths	812
MMR (per 100 000 births)	84

4.1.2 Causes of maternal deaths (available for 737 cases)

	Number	%
Hypertensive disorders of pregnancy	224	30
Haemorrhage	125	18
Sepsis	106	14
Ruptured uterus	56	8
Embolism	48	7
Abortion	36	5
Complications of anaesthesia	35	5
Ectopic pregnancy	5	1
Other direct obstetric causes	25	3
DIRECT CAUSES	660	90
INDIRECT CAUSES	61	8
Unrelated causes	13	2
Unknown	3	-
TOTAL	737	100

4.1.3 Avoidable factors

Avoidable factors involving medical attendants were present in 261 cases, whereas in 109 cases responsibility was ascribed to the patient.

Avoidable factor	Number	%
Treatment given "too little, too late"	87	11
Delay in consultation or transfer	25	3
Technical problems (surgical and anaesthetic)	24	3
Delay in diagnosis	11	1
Errors in diagnosis	11	1
Inadequate hospital facilities	5	0.5
Inadequate nursing care	5	0.5
TOTAL	261	20

4.2 Peninsula Maternal and Neonatal Services, Cape Town, 1953-83 (0762, 0763, 2153)

4.2.1 Rate

Year	Deliveries	Maternal deaths*	MMR (per 100 000 deliveries)
1953	7 315	22	301
1954-59	40 354	58	143
1960-65	56 091	49	87
1966-71	85 831	50	58
1972-77	102 209	50	49
1953-77	291 800	223	76

* Includes deaths occurring up to one year after the termination of pregnancy.

By racial origin, 1975-77, 1978-80, 1981-83

	Deliveries	Maternal deaths	MMR (per 100 000 deliveries)
Blacks			
1975-77	11 554	8	69
1978-80	15 405	12	78
1981-83	21 159	11	52
Coloureds			
1975-77	39 684	16	40
1978-80	42 291	14	33
1981-83	47 044	18	38
Whites			
1975-77	3 708	1	27
1978-80	2 975	2	70
1981-83	2 514	0	–

4.2.2 Causes of maternal deaths

There is remarkable consistency in the major obstetric causes of death throughout the 25 year period. The most common cause of maternal death was hypertension followed by haemorrhage, cardiac disease, sepsis and pulmonary embolism in that order.

	1953	1954-59*	1960-65*	1966-71	1972-77	% 1978-83
Hypertensive disorders of pregnancy	23	38	27	18	15	26
Haemorrhage	32	16	20	12	10	11
Sepsis	4	3	10	16	12	11
Uterine rupture	4	7	10	4	2	2
Embolisms	0	12	12	8	10	2
Complications of anaesthesia	0	0	6	14	6	2
Obstructed labour	9	3	0	0	0	0
DIRECT CAUSES	72	79	85	72	55	54

	1953	1954-59*	1960-65*	1966-71	1972-77	% 1978-83
Cardiac diseases	4	10	10	12	8	7
Hepatitis	0	2	0	0	0	2
Other infections	0	0	0	4	8	4
Other causes	18	7	6	8	22	28
Unknown	4	2	0	4	0	7
TOTAL	100	100	100	100	100	100
(N)	22	58	49	50	50	57

* Data for two years only.

The rank order of the commonest causes of death during the period 1978-83 was as follows:

	Blacks	Coloureds
Sepsis	1	3
Haemorrhage	2	2
Hypertensive disorders of pregnancy	3	1
Embolism/uterine rupture/ complications of anaesthesia	4	4

4.2.3 Avoidable factors, 1978-83

In approximately 55% of cases the deaths were judged unavoidable. A number of deaths so classified nevertheless involved patient and/or staff-avoidable factors, but at the time these were not thought to have had a major influence on the final outcome. Important patient- and staff-avoidable factors were each identified in around 30% of maternal deaths. Those attributed to patients included failure to book, default from the prenatal clinic, embarking on a pregnancy against medical advice, grand multiparity, advanced age and refusal of contraception. Avoidable factors contributed by medical and nursing staff centre on poor perinatal management. A specific area of concern during the prenatal period was inadequate history-taking in regard to diabetes and pulmonary tuberculosis. A recurring factor was a failure to appreciate the seriousness of anaemia, antepartum haemorrhage, severe asthma, proteinuric hypertensions and imminent eclampsia and urinary tract infections. In labour poor monitoring of blood pressure and progress led to several deaths. In one case delay in supplying transport was a major factor.

4.2.4 High risk groups
Age and parity specific maternal mortality rates and relative risk

	Blacks		Coloureds	
	MMR*	RR**	MMR*	RR**
Age				
<20	41	0.7	30	0.8
20-34	51	0.8	21	0.6
34+	136	2.2	179	5.0
39+	155	2.5	194	5.4
all ages	63	1.0	36	1.0
Parity				
1	39	0.6	36	1.0
2-4	68	1.1	26	0.7
4+	86	1.4	82	2.3
All parities	63	1.0	36	1.0

*   MMR (per 100 000 deliveries)
**   Calculated by dividing age specific by overall MMR

Maternal mortality rates by age and parity

For blacks the lowest risk category (RR 0.6) consisted of patients aged 20-34 and of parity 1. Those of parity 2-4 and aged over 34 years had a RR of 4.1 and those older than 39 years an RR of 5.5.

Coloured patients at lowest risk for maternal death were aged 20-34 years and of parity 2-4 with an RR of 0.5. There was a marked decrease in the RR with increasing parity in patients aged >34 and <39 years. The RRs for older primiparous patients were very high. Their numbers were, however, very small.

Age and parity specific MMR

	Parity		
	1	2-4	4+
Blacks			
<20	45	0	0
20-34	35	48	103
34+	0	258	72
39+	0	346	103
Coloureds			
<20	32	0	0
20-34	24	17	37
34+	885	155	145
39+	1 471	169	155

4.3 King Edward VIII Hospital, Durban, 1953-71 and 1975-82 [0165, 0581]

4.3.1 Rate**

	Deliveries	Maternal deaths	MMR (per 100 000 deliveries)
1953-71	316 053	538*	170
1975-82	134 661	258	192

*   Excluding abortions.
**   The population consisted exclusively of Bantu and Indians.

4.3.2 Causes of maternal deaths

The incidence of deaths from haemorrhage fell during the second period but sepsis became a serious problem due to overcrowding, and non-adherence to aseptic and antiseptic principles during, for example, vaginal examinations. Deaths from ameobiasis declined from 5% of the total in 1953-60 to 0.8% in 1961-71 because all pregnant women with chronic diarrhea or blood and mucus in stools were treated empirically as cases of ameobiasis.

	1953-60	1961-71	% 1975-82
Hypertensive disorders of pregnancy	28	21	19
Abortion	n.a.	n.a.	18
Sepsis	8	17	12
Haemorrhage	23	7	10
Ruptured uterus	6	13	n.a.
Embolisms	n.a.	4	3
Complications of anaesthesia	3	5	2
Associated medical and surgical conditions	17	8	n.a.
Liver disease	n.a.	n.a.	9
Other infections	5	n.a.	5
Cardiac diseases	4	7	5
Malignancies	0	0	7
Others	6	18	11
TOTAL	100	100	100
(N)	n.a.	n.a.	258

Ruptured uterus [1847]

A detailed analysis of 129 cases of rupture of the uterus between 1980 and 1983 is presented and compared with previous reports from the same hospital. The 129 patients with uterine rupture during the 42 months, January 1980 – June 1983 were all multigravid Black women. No ruptures occurred in primigravidae. The total number of deliveries over the period was 90 362, giving a hospital incidence of uterine rupture of 1.4 per 1000. 64 cases had a previously scarred uterus and 65 an unscarred uterus. There were four maternal deaths, a case fatality rate of 3.1%. In 1973, the incidence of uterine rupture was 2.7 per 1000 deliveries and the case fatality rate was 12%. This decline in incidence and mortality is thought to be due to an improvement in obstetric services following the establishment of a community-based health service. The authors observe that in 1973 the incidence of cephalopelvic disproportion in the patients with uterine rupture was 38% compared with only 9% of the unscarred group in 1980-82.

4.4 Edendale Hospital, Pietermaritzburg, 1973-75 [(0066)]

4.4.1 Rate (Black population only)

Deliveries	26 018
Maternal deaths	118
MMR (per 100 000 deliveries)	454

4.4.2 Causes of maternal deaths

	Number	%
Sepsis	30	24
Abortion	15	12
Hypertensive disorders of pregnancy	14	12
Haemorrhage	7	6
Embolisms	5	4
Ruptured uterus	4	4
Complications of anaesthesia	4	4
Ectopic pregnancy	1	1
DIRECT CAUSES	80	68
Hepatitis	25	21
Cardiac diseases	2	2
Other infections	4	4
Others	7	6
TOTAL	118	100

4.4.3 Avoidable factors

Avoidable factors were found to be present in a number of cases and were grouped by causes of death.

Cause of death	Avoidable factor	Number
Sepsis	Delayed laparotomy	7
	Undiagnosed uterine rupture	1
Abortion	Inadequate monitoring in theatre	2
	Evacuation performed too late	2
	Inadequate fluid and blood replacement	1
Haemorrhage		
	Inadequate fluid and blood replacement	3
	Undiagnosed uterine rupture	2
	Undiagnosed retroperitoneal haemorrhage	2
	Over transfusion	1
	Undiagnosed vaginal laceration	1
	Laparotomy delayed	1

4.5 Pelonomi Hospital, Bloemfontein, 1980-85, [(2331)]

Pelonomi Hospital is the main referral centre for the southern two-thirds of the Orange Free State, south-western Transkei, QwaQwa and the Kingdom of Lesotho. A retrospective analysis of all maternal deaths from 1 January 1980 to 31 December 1985 was carried out.

4.5.1 Rate

Deliveries	27 896
Maternal deaths*	81
MMR (per 100 000 births)**	287**

*   Including deaths occurring up to one year after the termination of pregnancy.

** Births defined as births of babies, alive or dead, with a birth weight of 1000g or more.

4.5.2 Causes of maternal deaths

	Number	%
Sepsis	25	31
Hypertensive disorders of pregnancy	17	21
Abortion	12	15
Haemorrhage	11	14
Embolism	3	4
Obstetric shock	2	3
Complications of anaesthesia	1	1
Other direct causes	3	4
DIRECT CAUSES	74	91
Cardiac diseases	2	2
Liver disease	1	1
Other indirect causes	3	4
INDIRECT CAUSES	6	7
Fortuitous	1	1
TOTAL	81	100

4.5.3 Avoidable factors

Avoidable factors were identified in 65 patients (80%). In some patients more than one factor was identified. Factors attributable to the patient included late presentation, refusal of treatment and being unbooked, resulting in a total of 39 deaths or 48% of all deaths. Factors attributable to the peripheral hospital or to Pelonomi Hospital included failure or delay in diagnosis or in instituting appropriate treatment and poor operative technique, accounting for 51 deaths (62% of the total). In six patients no avoidable factor could be identified and a further ten deaths were classified as unknown in respect of preventable factors.

Avoidable factor	Number of deaths*
Attributable to patient	39
Late presentation	22
Unbooked status	14
Refusal of treatment	3
Attributable to the peripheral hospital	23
Failure to institute appropriate treatment	11
Delay in transfer	9
Failure in diagnosis	3
Attributable to Pelonomi Hospital	28
Failure or delay in surgery	8
Failure or delay in diagnosis	6
Failure to institute appropriate treatment	6
Poor operative technique	3
Over transfusion	3
Blocked endotracheal tube	1
Complications of anaesthesia	1
Unknown	10
No avoidable factor identified	6

*   In several cases more than one factor was identified.

Booking status

	MMR (per 100 000 deliveries)
Booked	32
Unbooked	1 113

4.5.4 High risk groups

4.5.5 Other findings

5. CIVIL REGISTRATION DATA/GOVERNMENT ESTIMATES

5.1 Cape Town, 1971-81 [(0664)]

5.1.1 Rate (Black, Asiatic and coloured populations only)

	MMR (per 100 000 births)
1977	31
1978	24
1979	23
1980	34
1981	10

5.2 Durban, 1978 [(0664)]

5.2.1 Rate

According to Government statistics, in 1978 the maternal mortality rate for Durban was 20 per 100 000 live births.

6. OTHER SOURCES/ ESTIMATES

7. SELECTED ANNOTATED BIBLIOGRAPHY

Bieler, E.U. and Schnabel, T. Pituitary and ovarian function in women with vesicovaginal fistulae after obstructed and prolonged labour. *South African Medical Journal* 1976; 50: 257-266. WHE 2134

Approximately 25% of women suffering from vesicovaginal fistulae experience amenorrhea after their pregnancies. Sixteen Black women who had vesicovaginal fistulae due to obstructed labour were studied at the University of Pretoria, South Africa (in 1975) for causes of such amenorrhea. Five of the patients had normal menstrual cycles, five had secondary amenorrhea, one polymenorrhea and five oligomenorrhea Various pituitary stimulatory tests were carried out, and are described. The study suggests that menstrual disorders after obstructed labour are associated with derangement of different hypophyseotrophic areas of the hypothalamus.

Coetzee, T. and Lithgow, D.M. Obstetric fistulae of the urinary tract. *Journal of Obstetrics and Gynaecology of the British Commonwealth* 1966; 73: 837-844. WHE 1609

A retrospective study carried out at the Edendale Hospital in Pietermaritzburg, Natal, South Africa from 1954 to 1963 showed that 309 fistulae of the urinary tract were treated, 248 (80%) of which resulted from labour complications. Obstetric fistulae accounted for 2.2% of all cases admitted to the gynaecology wards.

Although the age of the women varied from 16 to 75 years, 80% were in the age group 17-30 years. In more than 75% of cases the fistula complicated a first or second confinement. Most patients were young primiparae who had lost a baby, who were unlikely to bear a live child unattended, who often found sexual intercourse impossible, and whose social existence was difficult because of the continuous urinary leak. The average interval between fistula formation and first consultation was eight months.

The authors present a classification of fistulae into three groups, and a description of surgical techniques, with detailed discussion on 25 difficult cases. The total cure rate was 54%, with 16% having stress incontinence, 21% with a residual pin-hole, and 7% with no change after surgery. Among postoperative conditions were dyspareunia or apareunia due to contracture of the vulval introitus or shortening of the vagina; vaginal stenosis, traumatic amenorrhea, and bladder calculus.

Fisk, N.M. and Shweni, P.M. Labor outcome of juvenile primiparae in a population with a high incidence of contracted pelvis. *International Journal of Gynecology and Obstetrics* 1989; 28: 5-7. WHE 2277

Labour outcome of primiparae less than 17 years old was compared with non-juvenile primiparae in a population with a high incidence of contracted pelvis. Juvenile primiparae were referred to hospital on the basis of age alone, whereas non-juveniles were referred on the basis of risk of obstetric complications. It was found that the frequency of obstetric interventions (Ventouse, forceps, caesarean section, symphysiotomy) was no lower in this unselected group of juvenile primiparae than in a high-risk group of non-juvenile primiparae referred for prenatal or intrapartum complications. Symphysiotomy rates were significantly higher in the juvenile group whereas caesarean rates were slightly lower. This might be expected if symphysiotomy were favoured over abdominal delivery by obstetric attendants anxious to avoid uterine scar in very young women. It is concluded that the practice of referral for juveniles on the basis of age alone should continue.

8. FURTHER READING

Hamilton R.A. et al. The unbooked patient. Part I. Reasons for failure to attend antenatal clinics. *South African Medical Journal* 1987; 71: 28-31. WHE 1478

Larsen, J.V. and Muller, E.J. Obstetric care in a rural population. *South African Medical Journal* 1978; 54(27): 1137-1140. WHE 0405

9. DATA SOURCES

WHE 0066   Barford, D.A. and Parkes, J.R. Maternal mortality: a survey of 118 maternal deaths and the avoidable factors involved. *South African Medical Journal* 1977; 51(4): 101-105

WHE 0165   Crichton, D.A. and Parkes, J.R. The principals of prevention of avoidable maternal death. *South African Medical Journal* 1973; 47(42): 2005-2010

WHE 0406   Larsen, J.V. et al. The fate of women who deliver at home in rural Kwazulu. *South African Medical Journal* 1984; 65(4): 161-165

WHE 0581   Melrose, S.B. Maternal deaths at King Edward VIII Hospital, Durban. *South African Medical Journal* 1984; 65(4): 161-165

WHE 0664   South Africa, City of Cape Town, Medical Officer of Health. *Annual Report 1981* Printing Division of the Town Clerk's Department 1981

WHE 0762   Van Coeverden de Groot, H.A. Trends in maternal mortality in Cape Town 1953-77. *South African Medical Journal* 1979; 56: 547-552

WHE 0763   Van Coeverden de Groot, H.A. Maternal mortality (letter) *South African Medical Journal* 1977; 51(15): 491.

WHE 1520   Boes, E.G.M. Maternal mortality in Southern Africa 1980-82. *South African Medical Journal* 1987; 71: 158-161

WHE 1712   Mauldin W.P. and Segal, S.J. *Prevalence of contraceptive use in developing countries. A chart book.* Rockefeller Foundation, New York 1986

WHE 1847   Lachman, E. et al. Rupture of the gravid uterus. *South African Medical Journal* 1985; 67: 333-335.

WHE 1914   United Nations Children's Fund (UNICEF). *The state of the world's children,* various years, Oxford, Oxford University Press

WHE 1915   United Nations. Department of International Economic and Social Affairs. *World population prospects: estimates and projections as assessed in 1984.* Population Studies No. 98. New York 1986

WHE 1918   United Nations. Department of International Economic and Social Affairs. *First marriage: patterns and determinants.* New York 1988

WHE 2153   Van Coeverden de Groot, H.A. Maternal mortality in Cape Town 1978-83. *South African Medical Journal* 1986; 69: 797-802

WHE 2330   Buchmann, E. et al. Home births in the Mosvold health ward of Kwazulu. *South African Medical Journal* 1989; 76: 29-31

WHE 2331   Cooreman, B.F. et al. Maternal deaths at Pelonomi Hospital, Bloemfontein, 1980-1985. *South African Medical Journal* 1989; 76: 24-26

NOTES

SUDAN

	Year	Source

1. BASIC INDICATORS

1.1 Demographic

1.1.1 Population
		Year	Source
Size (millions)	23.8	1988	(1914)
Rate of growth (%)	3.0	1988	(1914)

1.1.2 Life expectancy
		Year	Source
Female	49	1980-85	(1915)
Male	47	1980-85	(1915)

1.1.3 Fertility
		Year	Source
Crude Birth Rate	44	1988	(1914)
Total Fertility Rate	6.4	1988	(1914)

1.1.4 Mortality
		Year	Source
Crude Death Rate	16	1988	(1914)
Infant Mortality Rate	107	1988	(1914)
Female			
Male			
1-4 years mortality rate			
Female			
Male			

1.2 Social and economic

1.2.1 Adult literacy rate (%)
		Year	Source
Female	14	1986	(1914)
Male	33	1986	(1914)

1.2.2 Primary school enrolment rate (%)
		Year	Source
Female	41	1986-88	(1914)
Male	59	1986-88	(1914)

1.2.3 Female mean age at first marriage
		Year	Source
(years)	18.7	1973	(1918)

1.2.4 GNP/capita
		Year	Source
(US $)	330	1987	(1914)

1.2.5 Daily per capita calorie supply
		Year	Source
(as % of requirements)	88	1984-86	(1914)

2. HEALTH SERVICES

2.1 Health expenditure

2.1.1 Expenditure on health
		Year	Source
(as % of GNP)	4	1985	(1888)

2.1.2 Expenditure on PHC
(as % of total health expenditure)

2.2 Primary Health Care
(Percentage of population covered by):

2.2.1 Health services
		Year	Source
National	70	1984	(0834)
Urban			
Rural			

2.2.2 Safe water
		Year	Source
National	40	1984	(0834)
Urban			
Rural			

2.2.3 Adequate sanitary facilities
		Year	Source
National	5	1984	(0834)
Urban	20	1984	(0834)
Rural	1	1984	(0834)

2.2.4 Contraceptive prevalence rate
		Year	Source
(%)	5	1978-79	(1712)

2.3   Coverage of maternity care (%)

Area	Prenatal care	Trained attendant	Institutional deliveries	Postnatal care	Sample size	Year	Source
National	20	20				1984	(1888)
National	40	60				1988	(2033)
Khartoum Province	54					1976	(0201)
Khartoum: urban			25			1983	(0892)
Omdurman			29			(1983)	(1660)
Wad Medani			10			1988	(2406)

3. COMMUNITY STUDIES

3.1   Khartoum, 1985 [2405]

Data were collected from a variety of catchment areas and sources including hospital records, death certificates, operating theatre case notes, postmortem room records and the community midwives and health visitors.

3.1.1   Rate
MMR (per 100 000 live births)   522

3.2   Gezira Province, 1987 [2407]

A 10% random sample was taken of the population in the area. The total population is some 2 millions, and the crude birth rate is estimated at 41 per 1000, giving an expected number of live births of around 83 000. Households were asked about deaths of pregnant women during the previous year.

3.2.1   Rate
MMR (per 100 000 live births)   319

4. HOSPITAL STUDIES

4.1   All Hospitals, 1958-68 [0381]

4.1.1   Rate
Deliveries   25 484
Maternal deaths   160
MMR (per 100 000 deliveries)   628

4.1.2   Causes of maternal deaths (Kassala, Port Sudan and Khartoum hospitals)
The most serious complication of pregnancy was infective hepatitis. This accounted for eight of the fifteen deaths at Kassala Hospital, four of the eight maternal deaths at Port Sudan Hospital and four of the eight deaths at Khartoum North Hospital.

4.2   Khartoum Teaching Hospital, 1968-82 [0004, 0552]

4.2.1   Rate

	1968-72	1973-77	1978-82
Deliveries	8 447	13 517	18 165
Maternal deaths	108	142	140
MMR (per 100 000 deliveries)	1 279	1 050	771

4.2.2   Causes of maternal deaths (available for 256 of a total of 390 cases)
Deaths from haemorrhage fell while sepsis became a more frequent cause of death after 1978. Infective hepatitis is endemic in several areas of the country and claims many maternal lives.

	1968-72		1973-77		1978-82	
	No.	%	No.	%	No.	%
Sepsis	10	19	8	14	46	32
Hypertensive disorders of pregnancy	6	11	5	8	23	16
Haemorrhage	12	22	8	14	20	16
Complications of anaesthesia	1	2	1	2	4	3
DIRECT CAUSES	29	54	22	37	93	65
Hepatitis	11	20	16	27	24	17
Cardiac disease	2	4	1	2	8	6
Respiratory diseases	3	6	6	10	1	1
Vascular diseases	1	2	6	10	2	1
Others	8	15	8	13	15	10
INDIRECT CAUSES	25	46	37	63	50	35
TOTAL	54	100	59	100	143	100

4.2.3 Avoidable factors [0004]

A study of all caesarean sections carried out in the hospital between 1978 and 1982 found 24 maternal deaths following caesarean section of a total of 140 maternal deaths. There were 1 624 caesarean sections in all, giving a mortality rate of 14.7 per 1000. Only six of the 24 deaths could be attributed to the underlying causes, while in the remaining 18 cases the death was a direct result of the caesarean section itself.

4.3 Khartoum North Hospital, Khartoum, 1979-81 [1112]

4.3.1 Rate

Live births	2 222
Maternal deaths	2
MMR (per 100 000 live births)	90

4.4 Soba University Teaching Hospital, Khartoum, 1976-81 [0198]

4.4.1 Rate

Births	7 512
Maternal deaths	12
MMR (per 100 000 births)	160

4.4.2 Causes of maternal deaths

	Number
Complications of anaesthesia	3
Hypoplastic anaemia	2
Haemorrhage	2
Ectopic pregnancy	1
Abortion	1
Sepsis	18
Ruptured uterus	1
Hypertensive disorders of pregnancy	1
TOTAL	12

The maternal mortality rate for caesarean sections was 328 per 100 000 births compared to 67 per 100 000 for vaginal deliveries.

4.5 All Hospitals, Omdurman, 1962-70 [0056]

4.5.1 Rate

	1962-67	1968-70
MMR (per 100 000 births)	881	523

The fall in the maternal mortality rates was attributable to the introduction of a blood bank in the area in 1968.

4.6 Omdurman Hospital, Omdurman, 1975-84 [0217, 1112, 1263]

4.6.1 Rate

	1975-80	1979-81	1980-84*
Deliveries	27 045	1 429	28 136
Maternal deaths	96	2	86
MMR (per 100 000 deliveries)	355	140	306

* Live births.

4.6.2 Causes of maternal deaths

Cause of death is available for 107 cases during 1970-79 and for 102 cases in 1980-85.

	1970-79		1980-85	
	Number	%	Number	%
Haemorrhage	24	22	21	21
Hypertensive disorders of pregnancy	16	15	17	17
Complications of anaesthesia	2	2	15	15
Sepsis	10	9	8	7
Ruptured uterus	7	7	7	7
Obstructed labour	18	17	4	4
Ectopic pregnancy	–	–	1	1
DIRECT CAUSES	77	72	73	72
Hepatitis	17	16	19	19
Malaria	–	–	1	1
Anaemia	1	1	–	–
Others	12	11	9	8
INDIRECT CAUSES	30	28	29	28
TOTAL	107	100	102	100

4.7 El Fashir Civic Hospital, Northern Darfur, 1980-82 [0272]

4.7.1 Rate

Live births	1 592
Maternal deaths *	24
MMR (per 100 000 live births)	1 508

* Abortion and ectopic pregnancies excluded.

4.7.2 Causes of maternal deaths

	Number	%
Sepsis	13	54
Hypertensive disorders of pregnancy	5	21
Ruptured uterus	3	13
Haemorrhage	2	8
Others	1	4
TOTAL	24	100

4.8 Wad Medani Hospital, Wad Medani, 1979-81 and 1988 [1112, 2406]

4.8.1 Rate

	1979-81	1988
Live births	1 500	3 102
Maternal deaths	9	47
MMR (per 100 000 live births)	600	1 515

4.8.2 Causes of maternal deaths, 1988

	Number	%
Haemorrhage	11	23
Hepatitis	10	21
Sepsis following caesarean section	8	17
Hypertensive disorders of pregnancy	5	11
Anaesthetic death	4	9
Cardiac arrest	4	9
Tetanus	1	2
Enteric fever	1	2
Unknown	3	6
TOTAL	47	100

4.8.3 Avoidable factors, 1988

Seventeen of the women who died had had no prenatal care. A further twelve were attended in labour only by the village midwife. Over 90% of all deliveries take place at home.

4.9 El Obeid Hospital, West Country, 1974-76 [0323]

4.9.1 Rate

Live births	2 243
Maternal deaths	51
MMR (per 100 000 live births)	2 270

5. CIVIL REGISTRATION DATA/GOVERNMENT ESTIMATES

5.1 Khartoum Province, 1972 [0073]

5.1.1 Rate

The Annual Statistical Report of the Ministry of Health gives a domiciliary rate of 320 per 100 000 live births in Khartoum Province, and an institutional rate of 420 per 100 000 live births.

6. OTHER SOURCES/ ESTIMATES

6.1 National, 1983 [1735]

6.1.1 Rate

An article published in the Arab Medical Journal in 1983 gave a maternal mortality rate for Sudan of 655 per 100 000 live births.

7. SELECTED ANNOTATED BIBLIOGRAPHY

Abbo, A.H. and Mukhtar, M. New trends in the operative management of urinary fistulae. *Sudan Medical Journal* 1975; 13(4): 126-132. WHE 2147

An analysis of 70 cases of urinary fistulae treated from April to December 1974 is presented. Thirty of the cases were operated in Addis Ababa, Ethiopia and 40 in Khartoum Civil Hospital, Sudan. Sixty-two (88%) of the fistulae were caused by prolonged labour, and eight (12%) by hysterectomy. Four of the post hysterectomy cases were obstetrical in origin because they followed ruptured uteri for which a hysterectomy was done.

Nearly all of the women were between ages 12 and 30 and were primiparae. 34 of the women had undergone previous unsuccessful attempts at fistula repair. Most patients were extremely poor and malnourished and many were suffering from malaria, dysentery, helminthic diseases and anaemia. Associated conditions included bladder calculus in 4 cases.

Surgical techniques are described. Of the eight cases with urethrovaginal fistulae, all were successfully repaired, with complete restoration of function in five cases and partial restoration of function in three cases. Of the 60 cases of vesicovaginal fistulae, 57 were successfully repaired, with 50 cases of restoration of continence and seven cases with stress incontinence. In three cases the repair failed.

Mustafa, A.Z. and Rushwan, H.M.E. Acquired genito-urinary fistulae in the Sudan. *Journal of Obstetrics and Gynaecology of the British Commonwealth* 1971; 78: 1039-1043. WHE 1191

A review of 122 cases of fistula treated in Khartoum Teaching Hospital, Sudan, between January 1966 and October 1968 is presented. They comprised 16.4% of all major gynaecological conditions seen during that period. Ninety-one (75%) of the women had fistulae caused by prolonged obstructed labour, 25 (21%) from instrumental delivery – mainly forceps – and six (4.7%) from gynaecological operations. Over half (55%) of the women were below 25 years of age, and 86 (70%) were primiparae, whose labour ended in stillbirth.

Associated conditions included anaemia, malaria, parametritis, bilharzia and vesical calculi. Excoriation of the vulva and perineum was present in 73% of patients. Fourteen (11.6%) had both vesico-vaginal and rectovaginal fistula. Repair was successful in 90 women (74%). Almost all were operated via the vaginal route. Inadequate postoperative bladder drainage and postoperative infection were responsible for 80% of failures in the series - factors which are said to be avoidable with a high standard of nursing care.

Rushwan, H. Etiological factors in pelvic inflammatory disease in Sudanese women. *American Journal of Obstetrics and Gynecology* 1980; 138(7): 877-879. WHEØ0942

An analysis of women attending the gynaecological clinic of Khartoum Hospital found that only 1.4% of those complaining of vaginal discharge had gonorrhea and 0.4% had had abortions. The author concludes that female circumcision, widely practised in the Sudan, is an important cause of pelvic inflammatory disease in the Sudan.

8. FURTHER READING

Aziz, F.A. Pregnancy and labor of grand multiparous Sudanese women. *International Journal of Gynecology and Obstetrics* 1980; 18(2): 144-146. WHE 0288

Cook, R. *Damage to physical health from pharaonic circumcision (infibulation) of females.* Paper prepared for Seminar on Traditional Practices Affecting the Health of Women and Children in Africa, 1984, 6-10 February, Dakar, Senegal. WHE 1911

Faour, M. Fertility policy and family planning in the Arab countries. *Studies in Family Planning* 1989; 20(5): 254-263. WHE 2367

Rahman, T.A. (ed.) *Proceedings of the congress on on-going studies of the Obstetrical and Gynaecological Society of the Sudan.* 26-28 February 1980. WHE 0600

9. DATA SOURCES

WHE 0004   Abbo, A.H. Preventable factors in maternal mortality in Khartoum Teaching Hospital. *Arab Medical Journal* 1982; 4(11/12): 23-28

WHE 0056   Bakr, S.A. *Maternal mortality Workshop.* Khartoum, Sudan (mimeographed document) 1982

WHE 0073   Bayoumi, A. The training and activity of village midwives in the Sudan. *Tropical Doctor* 1976; 6: 118-125

WHE 0198   El Fadil, S. Maternal mortality in Soba University Hospital. *Arab Medical Bulletin.* 1982; 4(11/12): 47-48

WHE 0201   El Hakim, S.Y. Village midwives in the Sudan. In: Philpott, R.H. (ed.) *Maternity services in the developing world – what the community needs.* London, Royal College of Obstetricians and Gynaecologists, 1980

WHE 0217   Fathalla, M.F. *Maternal health – Sudan* (unpublished WHO document No. EM/MCH/ 161) 1981

WHE 0272   Ahmed, G.M. A review of maternal mortality in El Fashire Hospital. *Arab Medical Bulletin,* 1983: 4(11/12): 38-43

WHE 0323   Hassanein, O.M. Maternal mortality in El Obeid Hospital, 1974-1976. *Arab Medical Bulletin* 1982; 4(11/12): 4-13

WHE 0381   Karoum, H.O. Observations on maternal mortality in the Sudan. *Sudan Medical Journal* 1972; 10(2): 102-107

WHE 0552   Mudawi, O. Maternal mortality in Khartoum Teaching Hospital. *Arab Medical Bulletin* 1983; 5(1/2): 1-5

WHE 0834   World Health Organization. *World Health Statistics annual – vital statistics and causes of death.* Geneva, various years

WHE 0892   Sudan Women's Union. *Maternity wards in health centres* (unpublished paper), 1984

WHE 1112   Janowitz, B. et al. *Reproductive health in Africa: issues and options.* North Carolina, Family Health International, 1984

WHE 1263   Baldo, M.H. Maternal mortality in the Sudan. In: *Interregional meeting on the prevention of maternal mortality* Geneva, 11-15 November 1985 (unpublished WHO document No. FHE/PMM/85.9.5)

WHE 1660   Al-Hasani, A.M. *The role of the village midwives in postnatal care in Sudan,* 1983 (unpublished document)

WHE 1712   Mauldin W.P. and Segal, S.J. *Prevalence of contraceptive use in developing countries. A chart book. Rockefeller Foundation, New York 1986*

WHE 1735   Rushwan, H. and Farah, A.A. *Towards safe motherhood: policies and strategies* Paper presented to the Third National Population Conference (unpublished document) 1987

WHE 1888 World Health Organization, Eastern Mediterranean Regional Office. *Evaluation of the strategy for Health for All by the year 2000. Seventh report of the world health situation.* Alexandria, EMRO 1987

WHE 1914   United Nations Children's Fund (UNICEF). *The state of the world's children,* various years, Oxford, Oxford University Press

WHE 1915   United Nations. Department of International Economic and Social Affairs. *World population prospects: estimates and projections as assessed in 1984.* Population Studies No. 98. New York 1986

WHE 1918   United Nations. Department of International Economic and Social Affairs. *First marriage: patterns and determinants.* New York 1988

WHE 2033   World Health Organization. *Global strategy for health for all by the year 2000. Second report on monitoring progress.* WHO document EB83/2 Add. 1, 1988

WHE 2405   Rahman, T.A. The trap method for accurate data base in the collection of maternal deaths. *Arab Medical Bulletin* 1989; 10(7/8): 12-17

WHE 2406   Ahmed, A.M. Maternal mortality in Wad Medani Hospital. *Arab Medical Bulletin* 1989; 10(7/8): 18-20

WHE 2407   Marghany, O.A. The epidemiological study to estimate the maternal mortality rate in Gezira Province. *Arab Medical Bulletin* 1989; 10(7/8): 21-29

SWAZILAND

	Year	Source

1. BASIC INDICATORS

1.1 Demographic

1.1.1 Population

Size (millions)	0.7	1987	(1915)
Rate of growth (%)	3.0	1980-85	(1915)

1.1.2 Life expectancy

Female	50	1980-85	(1915)
Male	47	1980-85	(1915)

1.1.3 Fertility

Crude Birth Rate	47	1980-85	(1915)
Total Fertility Rate	6.5	1980-85	(1915)

1.1.4 Mortality

Crude Death Rate	17	1980-85	(1915)
Infant Mortality Rate	117	1988	(1914)
Female			
Male			
1-4 years mortality rate			
Female			
Male			

1.2 Social and economic

1.2.1 Adult literacy rate (%)

Female	66	1985	(1914)
Male	70	1985	(1914)

1.2.2 Primary school enrolment rate (%)

Female	103	1986-88	(1914)
Male	105	1986-88	(1914)

1.2.3 Female mean age at first marriage
(years)

	Year	Source

1.2.4 GNP/capita

(US $)	700	1987	(1914)

1.2.5 Daily per capita calorie supply
(as % of requirements)

2. HEALTH SERVICES

2.1 Health expenditure

2.1.1 Expenditure on health

(as % of GNP)	3	1983-84	(0800)

2.1.2 Expenditure on PHC

(as % of total health expenditure)	12	1983-84	(0800)

2.2 Primary Health Care
(Percentage of population covered by):

2.2.1 Health services
National
Urban
Rural

2.2.2 Safe water

National	38	1984	(0834)
Urban			
Rural			

2.2.3 Adequate sanitary facilities

National			
Urban	62	1980	(0834)
Rural	10	1984	(0834)

2.2.4 Contraceptive prevalence rate
(%)

2.3   Coverage of maternity care (%)

Area	Prenatal care	Trained attendant	Institutional deliveries	Postnatal care	Sample size	Year	Source
National	80		25			1977-78	(0745)
National		52				1983	(1338)
National		50				1984	(0834)
National			30-40			(1988)	(2008)
National			50			1987	(1980)

3.   COMMUNITY STUDIES

4.   HOSPITAL STUDIES

4.1   All health institutions, 1986 and 1987 [(1980)]

4.1.1   Rate

	1986**	1987
Deliveries	14 792	7 785
Maternal deaths*	11	10
MMR (per 100 000 deliveries)	74	129

*   Excluding abortions and deaths occurring subsequent to the discharge of the mother.
**   January-June

4.1.2   Causes of maternal deaths, 1987

	Number
Sepsis	5
Haemorrhage	2
Ruptured uterus	1
Hypertensive disorders of pregnancy	1
Cardiac arrest during caesarean section	1
TOTAL	10

4.1.3   Avoidable factors, 1987
In seven of the ten maternal deaths the women had had no prenatal care. Four of the women who died had had a home delivery or had attempted one. All four had risk factors for which home delivery was contraindicated.

5.   CIVIL REGISTRATION DATA/GOVERNMENT ESTIMATES

6.   OTHER SOURCES/ ESTIMATES

6.1   National, 1982 [(1338)]

6.1.1   Rate
A WHO report quotes an institutional maternal mortality rate (estimate) of 120 per 100 000 births for 1982.

7.   SELECTED ANNOTATED BIBLIOGRAPHY

8.   FURTHER READING

9. DATA SOURCES

WHE 0745   United Nations Fund for Population Activities. *Report of a mission on needs assessment for population assistance – Swaziland.* New York, UNFPA, 1981

WHE 0800   World Health Organization. *Country reports to regional offices of the progress in implementing Health for All by the Year 2000.* (Unpublished documents) 1983

WHE 0834   World Health Organization. *World Health Statistics annual – vital statistics and causes of death.* Geneva, various years

WHE 1338   World Health Organization, Regional Office for Africa. *Where are we in PHC? Countries take a close look at themselves through PHC reviews.* Swaziland, 7-15 October 1985

WHE 1914   United Nations Children's Fund (UNICEF). *The state of the world's children,* various years, Oxford, Oxford University Press

WHE 1915   United Nations. Department of International Economic and Social Affairs. *World population prospects: estimates and projections as assessed in 1984.* Population Studies No. 98. New York 1986

WHE 1980   McDermott, J. *Report of the proceedings of the national maternal and perinatal mortality meeting of Swaziland* Manzizni, 2 September 1987

WHE 2008   World Health Organization. Regional Office for Africa *Evaluation of the strategy for health for all by the year 2000. Seventh report on the world health situation* Vol 2, African region, Brazzaville 1987

NOTES

TOGO

		Year	Source

1. BASIC INDICATORS

1.1 Demographic

1.1.1 Population

		Year	Source
Size (millions)	3.2	1988	(1914)
Rate of growth (%)	3.0	1980-87	(1914)

1.1.2 Life expectancy

Female	52	1980-85	(1915)
Male	49	1980-85	(1915)

1.1.3 Fertility

Crude Birth Rate	45	1988	(1914)
Total Fertility Rate	6.1	1988	(1914)

1.1.4 Mortality

Crude Death Rate	14	1988	(1914)
Infant Mortality Rate	93	1988	(1914)
Female	79	1978-88	(2123)
Male	88	1978-88	(2123)
1-4 years mortality rate			
Female	90	1978-88	(2123)
Male	75	1978-88	(2123)

1.2 Social and economic

1.2.1 Adult literacy rate (%)

Female	28	1985	(1914)
Male	53	1985	(1914)

1.2.2 Primary school enrolment rate (%)

Female	59	1986-88	(1914)
Male	87	1986-88	(1914)

1.2.3 Female mean age at first marriage

(years)	18.5	1971	(1918)

1.2.4 GNP/capita

		Year	Source
(US $)	290	1987	(1914)

1.2.5 Daily per capita calorie supply

(as % of requirements)	97	1985	(1914)

2. HEALTH SERVICES

2.1 Health expenditure

2.1.1 Expenditure on health

(as % of GNP)	5	1983-84	(2008)

2.1.2 Expenditure on PHC

(as % of total health expenditure)	50	1982	(0800)

2.2 Primary Health Care
(Percentage of population covered by):

2.2.1 Health services

National
Urban
Rural

2.2.2 Safe water

National	35	1983	(0834)
Urban	68	1983	(0834)
Rural	26	1983	(0834)

2.2.3 Adequate sanitary facilities

National	14	1983	(0834)
Urban	34	1983	(0834)
Rural	8	1983	(0834)

2.2.4 Contraceptive prevalence rate

(%)	12	1983-88	(2123)

2.3   Coverage of maternity care (%)

Area	Prenatal care	Trained attendant	Institutional deliveries	Postnatal care	Sample size	Year	Source
National			50			1978	(0858)
National:	81	54			3 095	1983-88	(2123)
urban	97	89			810	1983-88	(2123)
rural	75	42			2 285	1983-88	(2123)

3. COMMUNITY STUDIES

4. HOSPITAL STUDIES

4.1   Centre Hospitalier Universitaire, Lomé, 1974 and 1982-86 [0774, 1189, 2490]

4.1.1   Rate

	1974	1982-86
Live births	8 608*	52 785
Maternal deaths	41	259
MMR (per 100 000 live births)	476	491

*   Deliveries

4.1.2   Causes of maternal deaths, 1974 and 1982-86 (210 deaths)

	1974 Number	1974 %	1982-86 Number	1982-86 %
Sepsis	n.a.	n.a.	57	27
Haemorrhage	6	15	41	20
Abortion	n.a.	n.a.	35	17
Hypertensive disorders of pregnancy	3	7	25	12
Postoperative shock	n.a.	n.a.	6	3
Embolisms	2	5	4	2
Complications of anaesthesia	1	2	5	2
Ruptured uterus	7	17	n.a.	n.a.
Unregistered emergency cases	20	49	n.a.	n.a.
Others	2	5	21	10
Unknown	–	–	16	8
TOTAL	41	100	210	100

4.1.3   Avoidable factors

4.1.4   High risk groups

4.1.5   Other findings

There was a caesarean section rate of 4.4% in 1974 and 4.1 % in the first 9 months of 1975. About 55% of the caesareans were performed for cephalopelvic disproportion.

There was a high incidence of uterine rupture:1 in 225 admissions. Most were emergency admissions.

A study of uterine rupture during the period 1978-1982 (1164) found 165 cases of ruptured uterus and 52 331 deliveries, an incidence of 1 per 317 deliveries or 3.1 per 1000. Nearly half of the women (80 cases) were transferred to the C.H.U. Lomé from peripheral health centres and private hospitals. Some had had to travel for over 100 kilometers. In 101 cases the rupture occurred at home, in 58 cases on the way to the hospital and in six cases at the hospital itself. 48 patients had previous caesarean scars, the remainder of the ruptures occurred among women with unscarred uteri. Among the latter there were 35 cases of dystocia and the same number of cases of cephalopelvic disproportion. In ten cases the rupture was caused by medical or surgical intervention. There were seven maternal deaths, a mortality rate of 4.2%. One women developed a vesicovaginal fistula.

Vesicovaginal fistulae resulting from obstructed labour were common. Between January and September 1975, 37 cases of vesicovaginal fistulae and three cases of vesicocervical fistulae were operated on in the hospital.

According to a paper presented at a WHO seminar (0774), cases referred to the hospital in 1977 included :

– 97 severe haemorrhages associated with malposition of the placenta, premature detachment of the placenta, retained placenta etc.;

– 47 impending ruptures of the uterus;

– 16 completed ruptures of the uterus, some of which had occurred several days earlier;

– 24 cases of shoulder dystocia.

4.2 Eight hospitals, including the C.H.U. Lomé, 1985 [2490]

4.2.1 Rate

	MMR (per 100 000 births)
C.H.U. Lomé	420
Seven hospitals	1 025
Total	718

5. CIVIL REGISTRATION DATA/GOVERNMENT ESTIMATES

6. OTHER SOURCES/ESTIMATES

6.1 National, 1977 [0774]

6.1.1 Rate

Live births	51 551
Maternal deaths	45
MMR (per 100 000 live births)	87

6.1.2 Causes of maternal death

The main causes of maternal deaths in decreasing order of frequency were:

– postoperative complications (infectious states and septicemia, cardiorespiratory disorders, etc.);

– haemorrhage occurring before or after delivery, including complications of blood coagulation;

– eclampsia;

6.1.3 Avoidable factors

6.1.4 High risk groups

6.1.5 Other findings

About 60% of the women attending prenatal consultations in the medical and welfare centres of Lomé were found to be suffering from anaemia caused by nutritional deficiency and intestinal parasites. Proteinuria and eclampsia were also common.

7. SELECTED ANNOTATED BIBLIOGRAPHY

Hodonou, A.S.K. et al. Sur la néphropathie gravidique en milieu Africain: à propos de 1733 cas traités à la Maternité du C.H.U. de Lomé. *Médecine d'Afrique Noire* 1988; 30(12). WHE 1896

Between 1978 and 1980, 1,733 cases of renal disease (representing 3.2% of all admissions) complicating the third trimester of pregnancy were analyzed at the Maternité C.H.U. in Lomé. Young, primiparous women of low socioeconomic status were more likely to suffer from pregnancy-related nephrotic syndromes. Although it is provided free of charge only 7% of the patients had received prenatal care. The outcome for the patients was often poor. There were 99 cases of eclampsia (8.5%), 49 cases of abruptio placentae and 23 maternal deaths. The importance of prenatal care and improvement of socioeconomic conditions, especially for young women having their first pregnancy, is stressed.

8. FURTHER READING

9. DATA SOURCES

WHE 0774   Vovor, M. and Hodonou, T. Togo. In: WHO *Regional Multidisciplinary Consultative Meeting on Human Reproduction,* Yaoundé 4-7 December 1978 (unpublished WHO document).

WHE 0800   World Health Organization. *Country reports to regional offices of the progress in implementing Health for All by the Year 2000.* (Unpublished documents) 1983

WHE 0834   World Health Organization. *World Health Statistics annual – vital statistics and causes of death.* Geneva, various years

WHE 0858   United Nations Fund for Population Activities. *Rapport de mission sur l'évaluation des besoins d'aide en matière de population.* New York, UNFPA, 1983

WHE 1164   Hodonou, A.K.S. et al. Les ruptures utérines en milieu africain au C.H.U. de Lomé. *Médecine d'Afrique Noire* 1983; 30(2): 507-517

WHE 1189   Muller-Holve, W. and Muller-Holve, D. Aspects cliniques concernant le bassin de la femme en obstétrique au Togo. *Afrique Médicale* 1979; 18(173): 607-610

WHE 1914   United Nations Children's Fund (UNICEF). *The state of the world's children,* various years, Oxford, Oxford University Press

WHE 1915   United Nations. Department of International Economic and Social Affairs. *World population prospects: estimates and projections as assessed in 1984.* Population Studies No. 98. New York 1986

WHE 1918   United Nations. Department of International Economic and Social Affairs. *First marriage: patterns and determinants.* New York 1988

WHE 2008   World Health Organization, Regional Office for Africa. *Evaluation of the strategy for health for all by the year 2000. Seventh report on the world health situation* Vol 2, African region, Brazzaville 1987

WHE 2123   Demographic and Health Surveys. *Enquête démographique et de santé au Togo 1988* Unité de Recherche Démographique/Institute for Resource Development/Westinghouse, 1989

WHE 2490   World Health Organization. Mortalité et morbidité maternelles. *Séminaire-Atelier INFOSEC* Cotonou, 28 November - 4 December 1989

TUNISIA

		Year	Source

1. BASIC INDICATORS

1.1 Demographic

1.1.1 Population

Size (millions)	3.8	1988	(1914)
Rate of growth (%)	2.5	1980-87	(1914)

1.1.2 Life expectancy

Female	61	1980-85	(1915)
Male	60	1980-85	(1915)

1.1.3 Fertility

Crude Birth Rate	30	1988	(1914)
Total Fertility Rate	4.0	1988	(1914)

1.1.4 Mortality

Crude Death Rate	7	1988	(1914)
Infant mortality rate	58	1988	(1914)
Female	45	1983-87	(2074)
Male	55	1983-87	(2074)
1-4 years mortality rate			
Female	14	1983-87	(2074)
Male	18	1983-87	(2074)

1.2 Social and economic

1.2.1 Adult literacy rate (%)

Female	41	1986	(1914)
Male	68	1986	(1914)

1.2.2 Primary school enrolment rate (%)

Female	89	1986-88	(1914)
Male	100	1986-88	(1914)

1.2.3 Female mean age at first marriage

(years)	24.3	1984	(1918)

		Year	Source

1.2.4 GNP/capita

(US $)	1 180	1987	(1914)

1.2.5 Daily per capita calorie supply

(as % of requirements)	123	1984-86	(1914)

2. HEALTH SERVICES

2.1 Health expenditure

2.1.1 Expenditure on health

(as % of GNP)	5	1982	(1888)

2.1.2 Expenditure on PHC
(as % of total health
 expenditure)

	23	1984	(1888)

2.2 Primary Health Care
(Percentage of population covered by):

2.2.1 Health services

National	91	1984	(0834)
Urban			
Rural			

2.2.2 Safe water

National	89	1984	(0834)
Urban	98	1984	(0834)
Rural	79	1984	(0834)

2.2.3 Adequate sanitary facilities

National	46	1984	(0834)
Urban	66	1984	(0834)
Rural	29	1984	(0834)

2.2.4 Contraceptive prevalence rate

(%)	50	1983-88	(2074)

2.3   Coverage of maternity care (%)

Area	Prenatal care	Trained attendant	Institutional deliveries	Postnatal care	Sample size	Year	Source
National			53			1980	(1497)
National	60	60				1984	(1888)
National:	57	68			4 417	1983-88	(2074)
rural	42	49			2 182	1983-88	(2074)
urban	71	86			2 235	1983-88	(2074)
Kairouan	2		11		13 000b	1976	(0309)
Kasserine	0		5		9 000b	1976	(0309)
Ksar-Hellah		84	9		324b	1982	(0047)
Medenine	5		9		1 200b	1976	(0309)
Sfax			75			1989	(2438)
Sousse	12		39		22 700b	1976	(0309)
Tunis	15		53		37 000b	1976	(0309)
Tunis	81	93			682	1983-88	(2074)

3. COMMUNITY STUDIES

4. HOSPITAL STUDIES

4.1   All hospitals, 1971 and 1989 [0309, 2562]

4.1.1   Rate

Governorate	MMR (per 100 000 hospital births) 1971	1989
Ariana	–	267
Beja	373	251
Bizerte	261	277
Gabes	390	17
Gafsa	472	40
Jendouba	239	14
Kairouan	300	27
Kasserine	398	134
Kebili	–	145
Le Kef	594	149
Mahdia	–	89
Medenine	1 001	44
Monastir	–	31
Nabeul	118	30

4.1.1   Rate (continued)

Governorate	MMR (per 100 000 hospital births) 1971	1989
Sfax	235	343
Sidi Bouzid	–	226
Siliana	–	54
Sousse	205	20
Tataouine	–	92
Tozeur	–	800
Tunis	72	119
Zaghouan	–	61
Total	–	127

4.2   Charles Nicolle Hospital ,Tunis, 1951-81 [0079, 0199, 0814, 2487]

4.2.1   Rate

	Births	Maternal deaths	MMR (per 100 000 deliveries)
1951-59	25 774	124	481
1965-71	40 043	37	92
1972-75	21 917*	11	50
1976-81	–	–	50

*   Excluding abortions

4.2.2 Causes of maternal deaths

Haemorrhage and ruptured uterus were the most frequent causes of death during 1951-71 and continued to be a significant cause of death between 1972-75. Although there was a fall in the proportion of deaths from hypertensive disorders of pregnancy, they continued to occupy the second place in order of frequency. There was a reduction in deaths from tuberculosis – from 12 deaths between 1951-64 to no deaths between 1965-71. Infective hepatitis was an important associated cause of death in the first period, but did not feature as a cause over 1972-75.

	1951-71		1972-75	
	Number	%	Number	%
Haemorrhage	59	30	5	39
Ruptured uterus	37	18	2	15
Hypertensive disorders of pregnancy	17	8	2	15
Sepsis	7	3	1	8
Anaesthetic, operative or postoperative shock	29	15	1	8
DIRECT CAUSES	149	74	11	85
Infectious hepatitis	12	6	–	–
Tuberculosis	12	6	–	–
Cardiac diseases	14	7	–	–
Others	15	7	2	15
INDIRECT CAUSES	53	26	2	15
TOTAL	202	100	13	100

4.3 Aziza Othmana Hospital, Tunis, 1963-724 [0102, 0814]

4.3.1 Rate
Deliveries	59 831
Maternal deaths	100
MMR (per 100 000 deliveries)	167

4.3.2 Causes of maternal deaths

	Number
Hypertensive disorders of pregnancy	22
Ruptured uterus	10
Haemorrhage	28
Embolisms	9
Sepsis	4
Anesthesia	2
Other direct causes	4
DIRECT CAUSES	79
Cardiac diseases	7
Hepatitis	4
Other indirect causes	10
INDIRECT	21
TOTAL	100

4.4 La Rabta Hospital, Tunis, 1975-89 [2487]

4.4.1 Rate
MMR (per 100 000 deliveries) 1975-84	160
MMR (per 100 000 live births) 1985-89	69

4.5 Habib Thameur Hospital, Tunis, 1970 and 1980 [0414]

4.5.1 Rate

	1970	1980
MMR (per 100 000 deliveries)	183	67

4.6 Regional Hospital, Beja Governorate, 1971-72 [0844]

4.6.1 Rate
Live births	3 026
Maternal deaths	14
MMR (per 100 000 live births)	463

4.6.2 Cause of maternal deaths

	Number
Haemorrhage	4
Ruptured uterus	4
Hypertensive disorders of pregnancy	1
Associated with caesarean section	1
Embolisms	1
Others	3
Total	14

4.7 Regional Hospital, Sfax Governorate, 1976-83 [0553, 2487]

4.7.1 Rate

	Deliveries	Maternal deaths	MMR (per 100 000 deliveries)
1976-78	20 546	34	165
1979-83	–	–	55

4.7.2   Causes of maternal deaths

	Number	%
Haemorrhage	8	24
Sepsis	4	12
Associated with caesarean section	4	12
Hypertensive disorders of pregnancy	4	12
Embolisms	4	12
Ruptured uterus	2	5
DIRECT CAUSES	26	76
Hepatitis	6	18
Other	2	5
INDIRECT CAUSES	8	24
TOTAL	34	100

Uterine rupture [2236]

A study of uterine rupture from 1980-1984 found 72 cases of ruptured uterus for 44 628 deliveries, an incidence of 1/620 deliveries. There were three maternal deaths, a mortality rate of 4%. Another three women developed vesicovaginal fistulae.

4.8   Bizerte Maternity Hospital, 1971-82 [2487]

4.8.1   Rate
MMR (per 100 000 live births)   104

4.9   Kasserine Maternity Hospital, 1979-80 [2487]

4.9.1   Rate
MMR (per 100 000 live births)   698

5. CIVIL REGISTRATION DATA/GOVERNMENT ESTIMATES

6. OTHER SOURCES/ ESTIMATES

6.1   Tunis, 1975 [0748]

6.1.1   Rate
The UNFPA report of Mission on Needs Assessment for Population Assistance quotes an institutional maternal mortality rate of 54 per 100 000 deliveries for Tunis in 1975. The rate for rural Tunisia is estimated at around 1 000 per 100 000 deliveries.

6.2   National, 1971 [0817]

6.2.1   Rate
According to a WHO report the maternal mortality rate for Tunisia was 310 per 100 000 live births in 1971.

6.3   National and by region, 1966-82 [2487]
Maternal mortality ratios were estimated on the basis of death rates for women of reproductive age and the estimated relationship to maternal deaths.

6.3.1   Rate

Governorate	MMR (per 100 000 live births)			
	1966	1975	1978	1982
Tunis	71	69	46	27
Sahel	76	68	41	28
North-East	120	86	51	37
Sfax	109	38	46	41
North-West	191	109	90	43
Centre-West	159	130	86	61
South	254	92	59	41
Tunisia	134	88	61	39

7. SELECTED ANNOTATED BIBLIOGRAPHY

8. FURTHER READING

Baldwin, C.S. Policies and realities of delayed marriages: the cases of Tunisia, Sri Lanka, Malaysia and Bangladesh *Population Reference Bureau Report* 1977; 3(4): 1-11. WHE 0058

Faour, M. Fertility policy and family planning in the Arab countries. *Studies in Family Planning* 1988; 20(5): 254-263. WHE 2367

Nazer, I. The Tunisian Experience in legal abortion. *International Journal of Gynaecology and Obstetrics* 1980; 17: 488-492. WHE 2231

9. DATA SOURCES

WHE 0047   Auerbach, L.S. Childbirth in Tunisia. *Social Science and Medicine* 1982; 16(16): 1499-1506

WHE 0079   Ben Zineb, T. et al. La mortalité maternelle à la Maternité de l'Hôpital Charles Nicolle pendant les deux dernières décades. *Journal de Gynécologie et Obstétrique* 1972; 1(5): 449-450

WHE 0102   Boudjemaa, S. et al. Etude de la mortalité maternelle à la maternité de l'Hôpital Aziza Othmana, Tunis. Analyse statistique– Action médicale – Résultats. *Tunisie Médicale* 1974; 52(2): 97-99

WHE 0199   El Goulli, M. et al. La mortalité maternelle à la maternité de l'Hôpital Charles Nicolle à Tunis de 1972 à 1975. *Journal de Gynécologie Obstétrique et Biologie de la Réproduction* 1978; 7: 779-784

WHE 0309   Hamza, B. et al. *La santé mère-enfant.* Tunis, Maison Tunisienne de l'édition, 1976

WHE 0414   Lewin, D. *Mise en place d'un système d'enquêtes confidentielles sur la mortalité maternelle en Tunisie.* (unpublished WHO document No. EM/MCH/169) 1982

WHE 0553   Milliez, J. et al. Activité de la maternité de Sfax: à propos de 20 000 accouchements. *Journal de Gynécologie Obstétrique et Biologie de la Réproduction* 1980; 9: 741-749

WHE 0748   United Nations Fund for Population Activities. *Report of a mission on needs assessment for population assistance - Tunisia.* New York, UNFPA, 1981

WHE 0814   World Health Organization, Regional Office for the Eastern Mediterranean. *Studies of maternal mortality in the WHO Region* University of Assiut, Faculty of Medicine, 1980

WHE 0817   World Health Organization, Eastern Mediterranean Regional Office. Basic country information - Tunisia (unpublished WHO document) 1974.

WHE 0834   World Health Organization. *World Health Statistics annual – vital statistics and causes of death.* Geneva, various years

WHE 0844   Zatuchni, G.I. *WHO Beja project* (undated, mimeographed document).

WHE 1497   Bouraoui, A. Structure et évolution de l'accouchement (1979-1982). *Famille et Population* 1986; 3: 10-22

WHE 1888   World Health Organization, Eastern Mediterranean Regional Office. *Evaluation of the strategy for Health for All by the year 2000. Seventh report of the world health situation.* Alexandria, EMRO 1987

WHE 1914   United Nations Children's Fund (UNICEF). *The state of the world's children,* various years, Oxford, Oxford University Press

WHE 1915   United Nations. Department of International Economic and Social Affairs. *World population prospects: estimates and projections as assessed in 1984.* Population Studies No. 98. New York 1986

WHE 1918   United Nations. Department of International Economic and Social Affairs. *First marriage: patterns and determinants.* New York 1988

WHE 2074   Demographic and Health Surveys. *Enquête démographique et de santé en Tunis* 1988, Tunis, Office National de la Famille et de la Population/Institute for Resource Development/ Westinghouse

WHE 2236   Rekik, S. et al. Les rupture utérines à la Maternité de Sfax. *La Tunisie Médicale* 1987; 65(4): 243-246

WHE 2438   Coeytaux, F. Celebrating mother and child on the fortieth day: the Sfax, Tunisia postpartum program. The Population Council *Quality/ Calidad/Qualité* 1989;1:

WHE 2487   Tunisia, Ministère de la Santé publique. *Etude des principaux facteurs de risque de décéder d'une femme au cours de la grossesse, de l'issue d'une grossesse et dans les 42 jours suivant l'issue d'une grossesse.* (unpublished personal communication) 1990

WHE 2562   Ministère de la Santé Publique. *Annuaire Nationale des Statistiques Sanitaires 1989.* Tunis, 1990

NOTES

UGANDA

		Year	Source

1. BASIC INDICATORS

1.1 Demographic

1.1.1 Population
Size (millions)	17.2	1988	(1914)
Rate of growth (%)	3.4	1980-87	(1914)

1.1.2 Life expectancy
Female	51	1980-85	(1915)
Male	47	1980-85	(1915)

1.1.3 Fertility
Crude Birth Rate	50	1988	(1914)
Total Fertility Rate	6.9	1988	(1914)

1.1.4 Mortality
Crude Death Rate	15	1988	(1914)
Infant Mortality Rate	102	1988	(1914)
Female	102	1978-88	(2132)
Male	111	1978-88	(2132)
1-4 years mortality rate			
Female	86	1978-88	(2132)
Male	97	1978-88	(2132)

1.2 Social and economic

1.2.1 Adult literacy rate (%)
Female	45	1985	(1914)
Male	70	1985	(1914)

1.2.2 Primary school enrolment rate (%)
Female	63	1986-88	(1914)
Male	76	1986-88	(1914)

1.2.3 Female mean age at first marriage
(years)	17.7	1969	(1918)

1.2.4 GNP/capita
(US $)	260	1985	(1914)

1.2.5 Daily per capita calorie supply
(as % of requirements)	95	1984-86	(1914)

2. HEALTH SERVICES

2.1 Health expenditure

2.1.1 Expenditure on health
(as % of GNP)

2.1.2 Expenditure on PHC
(as % of total health expenditure)	27	1982	(0800)

2.2 Primary Health Care
(Percentage of population covered by):

2.2.1 Health services
National	42	1984	(0834)
Urban			
Rural			

2.2.2 Safe water
National	16	1983	(0834)
Urban	45	1983	(0834)
Rural	12	1983	(0834)

2.2.3 Adequate sanitary facilities
National	13	1983	(0834)
Urban	40	1983	(0834)
Rural	10	1983	(0834)

2.2.4 Contraceptive prevalence rate
(%)	5	1983-88	(2132)

2.3   Coverage of maternity care (%)

Area	Prenatal care	Trained attendant	Institutional deliveries	Postnatal care	Sample size	Year	Source
National	86					1988	(2033)
National:	87	38			5 048	1988	(2132)
urban	90	85				1987	(1943)
urban	95	80			491	1983-88	(2132)
rural		40				1987	(1943)
rural	86	34			4 557	1983-88	(2132)
West Nile	67	18			279	1983-88	(2132)
East	95	47			1 394	1983-88	(2132)
Central	91	51			1 275	1983-88	(2132)
West	74	18			625	1983-88	(2132)
South West	82	18			1 207	1983-88	(2132)
Kampala	95	86			269	1983-88	(2132)

3. COMMUNITY STUDIES

4. HOSPITAL STUDIES

4.1   All institutions, by region, 1966-67 (0241, 0242)

4.1.1   Rate

	Deliveries	Maternal deaths	MMR (per 100 000 births)
Eastern	40 367	134	332
Central	34 953	126	360
Western	17 323	104	600
Northern	13 192	56	425
All	105 835	420	397

4.1.2   Causes of maternal deaths

Ruptured uterus was the main cause of maternal deaths and was more frequent in the southern, predominantly Bantu speaking districts. Bantu women were found to have a generally contracted and shallow pelvis. Another factor that seemed to play a role in causing uterine rupture was the use of traditional medicine with oxytocic properties. Almost all case records in this series mentioned such medicines. Haemorrhage was the next most common cause of death.

	Number	%
Ruptured uterus	78	19
Haemorrhage	61	15
Associated with caesarean section	50	12
Obstructed labour	49	12
Hypertensive disorders of pregnancy	21	5
Abortions	15	4
Sepsis	14	3
Ectopic pregnancy	12	3
DIRECT CAUSES	300	71
Anaemia	15	4
Hepatitis	7	2
Others	21	5
INDIRECT CAUSES	43	10
Unknown	77	18
TOTAL	420	100

4.2 Government hospitals, 1972-76 [0115]

4.2.1 Rate

Live births	484 676
Maternal deaths	1 580
MMR (per 100 000 live births)	326

4.3 Mulago, Nsambya, Old Kampala, Rubaga and Mengo hospitals, Kampala 1980-86 [1577]

4.3.1 Rate

Live births	167 044
Maternal deaths*	580
MMR (per 100 000 live births)	347

* It is thought that this represents an underestimate because records for two hospitals for the years 1980 and 1981 were not complete; records on abortion-related deaths were not complete for the year 1983 in another hospital; deaths which occurred in the casualty departments immediately on arrival may have been missed; and record keeping was not complete in all the hospitals.

4.3.2 Causes of maternal deaths
(available for 372 of the 580 deaths)

	Number	%
Sepsis	115	31
Haemorrhage	57	15
Abortions	41	11
Ruptured uterus	22	6
Complications of anaesthesia	20	5
Embolisms	11	3
Hypertensive disorders of pregnancy	8	2
Ectopic pregnancy	3	1
DIRECT CAUSES	277	75
Cardiopathies	12	3
Anaemia	10	3
Sickle cell disease	5	1
Hepatitis	3	1
Malaria	3	1
INDIRECT CAUSES	33	9
AIDS	3	1
Others	42	11
Unknown	17	5
TOTAL	372	100

4.3.3 Avoidable factors

4.3.4 High risk groups

According to a case control study carried out, women who were above 45 years of age, who were pregnant for the 11th time or more, and were residing more than 20 kilometers from the hospital faced a higher risk of death than other women.

	Maternal deaths		Case controls	
	Number	%	Number	%
Age				
10-14	2	1	2	1
15-19	127	34	120	32
20-24	103	28	129	35
25-29	50	13	50	13
30-34	46	12	35	9
35-39	15	4	20	5
40-44	10	3	8	2
45+	19	5	8	2
Total	372	100	372	100
Gravidity				
1-2	158	42	175	47
3-4	68	18	80	22
5-6	41	11	35	9
7-8	30	8	33	9
9-1	17	5	21	6
11+	58	16	28	8
Total	372	100	372	100
Residential distance from hospital				
1-9 kilometers	109	29	137	37
10-19	127	34	167	45
20-29	24	7	12	3
30-39	9	2	5	1
40-49	14	4	4	1
50+	89	24	47*	13
Total	372	100	372	100

* Most of these patients came from the then disturbed areas and had taken refuge in Kampala.

4.4 Mbale Referral General hospital, Mbale, 1971-80 [0841]

4.4.1 Rate

Deliveries	67 876
Maternal deaths	256
MMR (per 100 000 deliveries)	377

4.4.2 Causes of maternal deaths

	Number	%
Sepsis	81	32
Haemorrhage	66	26
Ruptured uterus	46	18
Complications of anaesthesia	17	7
Hypertensive disorders of pregnancy	9	4
Ectopic pregnancy	6	2
Embolisms	5	2
Others	26	9
Total	256	100

5. CIVIL REGISTRATION DATA/GOVERNMENT ESTIMATES

5.1 National, 1984 (0900)

5.1.1 Rate
According to the response sent by the government to the UN Review and Appraisal of the Decade for Women, the maternal mortality rate for Uganda was 300 per 100 000 live births in 1984.

6. OTHER SOURCES/ ESTIMATES

6.1 National, 1989 (2216)
A report by Family Care International gives a maternal mortality rate of 400-700 per 100 000 live births.

7. SELECTED ANNOTATED BIBLIOGRAPHY

Kampikaho, A. Puerperal sepsis in some health institutions in and around Kampala. (unpublished results of a pilot study) 1989. WHE 2353

Between 5 May and 30 June 1989 165 women delivered at the Kawempe Maternity Clinic in Kampala. The incidence of puerperal sepsis was 44.6%. The administration of Procaine Penicillin Fortified intramuscularly on admission appeared to reduce the incidence by about 20%. In view of the importance of puerperal sepsis as a cause of maternal deaths, a randomised control trial will be carried out in order to evaluate the influence of antibiotics on the incidence of puerperal sepsis.

Ndugwa, C.M. Pregnancy in sickle cell anaemia in Uganda (1971-1980). *East African Medical Journal* 1982; 59(5): 320-326. WHE 0488

Sickle cell anaemia has become one of the foremost inherited genetic diseases in Uganda. Many patients are now surviving into adulthood and childbearing age. Between 1971 and 1980, 60 patients with sickle cell anaemia were observed during the course of 71 pregnancies. 51 pregnancies went to term, there were two premature deliveries, eight caesarean sections and ten abortions. There were six maternal deaths, a mortality rate of 84.5 per 1000 pregnancies.

8. FURTHER READING

Grech, E.S. et al. Epidemiological aspects of acute pelvic inflammatory disease in Uganda. *Tropical Doctor* 1973; 3(3): 123-127. WHE 1073

Lwanga, C. Abortion in Mulago Hospital, Kampala. *East African Medical Journal* 1977; 54(3): 142-148. WHE 2064

9. DATA SOURCES

WHE 0115   Bulwa, F. *Maternity services in Uganda.* In: WHO Regional Multidisciplinary Consultative Meeting on Human Reproduction. Yaoundé, 4-7 December 1978 (unpublished WHO document).

WHE 0241   Grech, E.S. Maternal mortality in Uganda. *International Journal of Gynaecology and Obstetrics* 1969; 7(6): 263-277

WHE 0242   Grech, E.S. Maternal mortality. In: Hall, S.A. *Uganda atlas of disease distribution.* Nairobi, East Africa Publishing House, 1975

WHE 0800   World Health Organization. *Country reports to regional offices of the progress in implementing Health for All by the Year 2000.* (Unpublished documents) 1983

WHE 0841   Zake, E.Z. A ten-year review of maternal mortality in an upcountry regional and referral general hospital. *Singapore Journal of Obstetrics and Gynaecology* 1982; 13(1): 55-59

WHE 0834   World Health Organization. *World Health Statistics annual – vital statistics and causes of death.* Geneva, various years

WHE 0900 United Nations, Secretariat of the Decade for Women. *Country responses to the questionnaire on the Review and Appraisal of the UN Decade for women: equality, development and peace:* part II (B) Health and nutrition (unpublished documents) 1984.

WHE 1577   Kampikaho, A. *Maternal mortality in hospitals of Kampala* (unpublished document) 1987

WHE 1914   United Nations Children's Fund (UNICEF). *The state of the world's children,* various years, Oxford, Oxford University Press

WHE 1915   United Nations, Department of International Economic and Social Affairs. *World population prospects: estimates and projections as assessed in 1984.* Population Studies No. 98. New York 1986

WHE 1918   United Nations, Department of International Economic and Social Affairs. *First marriage: patterns and determinants.* New York 1988

WHE 1943   World Health Organization, EPI Programme review: Uganda. *Weekly Epidemiological Record* 1988; 63: 114-117

WHE 2033   World Health Organization. *Global strategy for health for all by the year 2000. Second report on monitoring progress.* WHO document EB83/2 Add. 1, 1988

WHE 2132   Demographic and Health Surveys, Ministry of Health. *Uganda demographic and health survey.* Ministry of Health/ Institute for Resource Development/Westinghouse, 1989

WHE 2216   Sheffield, J.W. *Women's reproductive health in Uganda and Zimbabwe.* Family Care International (unpublished report on Safe Motherhood activities) 1989

NOTES

UNITED REPUBLIC OF TANZANIA

		Year	Source

1. BASIC INDICATORS

1.1 Demographic

1.1.1 Population

		Year	Source
Size (millions)	25.4	1988	(1914)
Rate of growth (%)	3.7	1980-87	(1914)

1.1.2 Life expectancy

Female	53	1980-85	(1915)
Male	49	1980-85	(1915)

1.1.3 Fertility

Crude Birth Rate	50	1988	(1914)
Total Fertility Rate	7.1	1988	(1914)

1.1.4 Mortality

Crude Death Rate	14	1988	(1914)
Infant Mortality Rate	105	1988	(1914)
Female			
Male			
1-4 years mortality rate			
Female			
Male			

1.2 Social and economic

1.2.1 Adult literacy rate (%)

Female	88	1986	(1914)
Male	93	1986	(1914)

1.2.2 Primary school enrolment rate (%)

Female	66	1986-88	(1914)
Male	67	1986-88	(1914)

1.2.3 Female mean age at first marriage

(years)	18.6	1973	(1918)

1.2.4 GNP/capita

(US $)	180	1987	(1914)

1.2.5 Daily per capita calorie supply

(as % of requirements)	96	1984-86	(1914)

2. HEALTH SERVICES

2.1 Health expenditure

2.1.1 Expenditure on health

(as % of GNP)	5	1982	(2033)

2.1.2 Expenditure on PHC

(as % of total health expenditure)	30	1978-79	(0800)

2.2 Primary Health Care
(Percentage of population covered by):

2.2.1 Health services

National	73	1983	(0834)
Urban			
Rural			

2.2.2 Safe water

National	52	1984	(0834)
Urban	85	1984	(0834)
Rural	47	1984	(0834)

2.2.3 Adequate sanitary facilities

National	78	1984	(0834)
Urban	91	1984	(0834)
Rural	76	1984	(0834)

2.2.4 Contraceptive prevalence rate

(%)	1	1977	(1712)

2.3 Coverage of maternity care (%)

Area	Prenatal care	Trained attendant	Institutional deliveries	Postnatal care	Sample size	Year	Source
National	98	74				1983	(0834)
National	95		60			1984	(2008)
National		33				1986	(1798)

National
  rural
  urban
		
		27
		68
						
						1986
						1986
							
							(1798)
							(1798)

Dar es-Salaam	98	80	79			1984	(1495)
Kilimanjaro region			15			1979	(0042)
Sthrn. Highlands			34			1983	(1229)

3. COMMUNITY STUDIES

3.1 Southern Highlands Zone, 1983 [1229]

3.1.1 Rate

A study in the Southern Highlands Zone comprising Mbeya, Iringa and Rukwa, found 115 maternal deaths for a total of 147 000 'expected' births during 1983, giving a maternal mortality rate of 78 per 100 000 live births. The deaths were identified by questionnaires to hospitals and health centres. Information on deaths occurring outside health institutions was obtained by hearsay. Two-thirds of the births in the zone took place at home. The low number of births identified in the villages coupled with the low maternal mortality rate indicate substantial undercounting.

3.1.2 Causes of maternal deaths

	Number	%
Haemorrhage	25	22
Abortion	20	17
Sepsis	17	15
Anaemia	6	5
Obstructed labour	6	5
Ruptured uterus	6	5
Hypertensive disorders of pregnancy	4	4
Ectopic pregnancy	1	1
Other direct causes	6	5
DIRECT CAUSES	91	79
Hepatitis	1	1
Herbal Medicine	2	2
Others	21	18
TOTAL	115	100

3.1.3 Avoidable factors

	Number	%
In hospital		
Risk factor noted but not acted upon	30	34
Lack of blood	17	19
No partogram in labour	16	18
Other factors	26	29
Total	89	100
Outside the hospital		
Risk factor not acted upon after detection in:		
– village	10	38
– health centre	4	15
– dispensary	3	12
Delay in referral	3	12
Other factors	6	23
Total	26	100

3.1.4 High risk groups

3.1.5 Other findings

89 of the 115 reported deaths took place in hospitals, four in health centres, seven in dispensaries and 15 in villages. Twelve deaths occurred in women who had travelled more than 10 kilometers to seek help. Two had walked 15 and 70 kilometers after the onset of labour.

3.2. Isere and Mtua villages, Ilula Ward, Iringa District, Southern Highlands, June 1983 - November 1985. [2093, 2410]

A total of 707 women registered for prenatal care at the village dispensary. The relatively good communications and higher than average female literacy encouraged attendance at prenatal clinics and it is thought that nearly all pregnant women (97%) attended at some stage of pregnancy.

3.2.1 Rate

Live births	701
Maternal deaths	4
MMR (per 100 000 live births)	571

3.2.2 Causes of maternal deaths

Two deaths were from postpartum haemorrhage. A third death was due to uterine rupture in a woman who had previously had a caesarean section and the fourth from septic complications after a caesarean section.

3.2.3 Avoidable factors

No relationship was found between the number of prenatal visits and pregnancy outcome. Even with a mean attendance of six visits and full coverage of prenatal care both maternal and perinatal mortality remained high.

3.2.4. High risk groups

One of the four deaths was in a primiparous woman aged 18 years. The other three deaths were of women aged over 34 years who had five or more children.

Age	Parity	Cause of death
18	0	Postpartum haemorrhage
34	7	Uterine rupture , previous caesarean section
34	5	Caesarean section, postoperative sepsis
40	9	Postpartum haemorrhage

3.2.5 Other findings

Place of death

The case of postoperative sepsis occurred at the regional hospital; the two cases of postpartum haemorrhage occurred at home and in the village dispensary.

Prenatal visits

The four women who died had all visited the prenatal clinic eight or nine times during the pregnancy.

4. HOSPITAL STUDIES

4.1 All institutional deliveries, 1970 and 1977 [0319, 1495]

4.1.1 Rate

	1970	1977
Deliveries	212 000	n.a.
Maternal deaths	572	n.a.
MMR (per 100 000 deliveries)	270	250

4.2 48 hospitals throughout the country, 1986 [1798]

4.2.1 Rate

Deliveries	81 264
Maternal deaths	278
MMR (per 100 000 live births)	342

4.2.2 Causes of maternal deaths

	Number	%
Sepsis	61	22
Haemorrhage	49	18
Ruptured uterus	48	17
Abortion	23	8
Hypertensive disorders of pregnancy	16	6
Embolisms	10	4
Use of traditional medicines	9	3
Complications of anaesthesia	8	3
Ectopic pregnancy	1	0
DIRECT CAUSES	225	81
Anaemia	14	5
Other non-obstetric causes	39	14
INDIRECT CAUSES	64	23
TOTAL	278	100

4.2.3 Avoidable factors

4.2.4 High risk groups

4.2.5   Other findings

Transport problems were among the most important constraints causing delays or making it impossible for women at risk to deliver in hospitals even if they wanted to. Of the 247 maternal deaths for which information was available, 63% of the women lived more than 10 kilometers away from the hospital in which they died and 37% lived more than 30 kilometers away.

Other problems mentioned by the health personnel in the hospitals studied as contributing to high maternal mortality were:

– scarcity of medical and para-medical trained personnel, especially in the rural areas;

– insufficient on the job training and supervision of health staff at all levels;

– low salaries and poor working conditions for health workers leading to lack of motivation.

4.3   45 rural hospitals, 1972-73 [0212]

4.3.1   Rates

Deliveries	56 217
Maternal deaths	270
MMR (per 100 000 deliveries)	480

4.3.2   Causes of maternal deaths

	Number	%
Haemorrhage	75	28
Ruptured uterus	61	23
Sepsis	30	11
Anaemia	23	9
Hypertensive disorders of pregnancy	17	6
Other difficulties in labour	9	3
Complications of anaesthesia	9	3
DIRECT CAUSES	224	83
Others/unknown	46	17
TOTAL	270	100

4.3.3   Avoidable factors

4.3.4   High risk groups

4.3.5   Other findings

Anaemia, eclampsia and abruptio placenta were more common in the coastal areas, while preeclampsia and eclampsia were very rare in the inland regions.

4.4   Iringa, Mbeya, Moshi and Mwanza regions, 1984 [0995]

4.4.1   Rate

	Iringa	Mbeya	Moshi	Mwanza
Deliveries	15 056	12 071	11 295	10 077
Maternal deaths	39	30	27	46
MMR (per 100 000 deliveries)	259	249	239	457

A more detailed breakdown of maternal deaths by district and by month is also given.

4.5   Dar es-Salaam, Kilimanjaro, Mbeya and Mwanza Regions, July 1983-December 1984 [1243]

4.5.1   Rate

	Live births	Maternal deaths	MMR (per 100 000 births)
Dar es-Salaam	44 601	149	334
Kilimanjaro	21 343	52	243
Mbeya	19 342	79	408
Mwanza	22 900	129	563
Total	108 186	409	378

4.5.2   Causes of maternal deaths
(available for 294 of the 409 deaths)

	Number	%
Haemorrhage	52	18
Abortion	49	17
Sepsis	45	15
Ruptured uterus	19	7
Hypertensive disorders of pregnancy	10	2
Ectopic pregnancy	6	1
Other direct obstetric causes	25	9
DIRECT CAUSES	206	70
Anaemia	31	11
Other indirect obstetric causes	34	12
INDIRECT CAUSES	65	22
Fortuitous	23	8
TOTAL	294	100

4.5.3   Avoidable factors

Avoidable factors were associated with maternal death in 367 cases and in several instances several avoidable factors were present. As a result 183 of the deaths (64%) were classified as definitely preventable and a further 98 as probably or possibly preventable.

	Number of cases
Patient unbooked	30
Patient noncompliance	34
Use of inappropriate traditional medicines	35
Action delayed or incorrect	80
Lack of drugs/blood/equipment	188
Total	367

4.5.4 High risk groups

Women who died were compared with women who survived (the controls were the next patients entered in the labour ward registry - no other matching criteria were used). No significant differences in age or parity were found between the deaths and the controls.

	% of maternal deaths	% of controls
Age		
< 15	<1	0
15-19	24	21
20-24	29	33
25-29	20	20
30-34	16	17
35-39	5	7
40-44	5	2
Parity		
1	29	30
2-5	47	47
6-10	23	23
> 10	1	0

4.5.5 Other findings

Place of death

Region	Number of deaths in: Health centres	Non-specialist hospitals	Specialist hospitals	Total
Dar es-Salaam	1	2	146	149
Kilimanjaro	1	31	20	52
Mbeya	10	47	22	79
Mwanza	29	59	41	129
Total	41	139	229	409

4.6 Ocean Road Hospital, Dar es-Salaam, 1972-73 [0212]

4.6.1 Rate
Deliveries	43 356
Maternal deaths	79
MMR (per 100 000 deliveries)	182

4.6.2 Causes of maternal deaths

	Number	%
Haemorrhage	23	29
Hypertensive disorders of pregnancy	13	17
Ruptured uterus	11	14
Sepsis	9	11
Complications of anaesthesia	1	1
DIRECT CAUSES	57	72
Anaemia	12	15
Others/unknown	10	13
TOTAL	79	100

4.7 Muhimbili Medical Centre, Dar es-Salaam, 1974-77 and 1983-84 [0471, 1322]

4.7.1 Rate

	1974-77	1983-84
Deliveries	105 311	12 509
Maternal deaths	224	85
MMR (per 100 000 deliveries)	213	680

4.7.2 Causes of maternal deaths

	1974-77 Number	%	1983-84 Number	%
Haemorrhage	22	10	12	14
Abortion	28	13	11	13
Sepsis	26	12	11	13
Hypertensive disorders of pregnancy	43	19	6	7
Ruptured uterus	17	8	4	5
Ectopic pregnancy	8	4	3	3
Associated with caesarean section	31	14	0	0
DIRECT CAUSES	175	78	47	55
Anaemia	28	13	18	21
Others	21	9	20	24
INDIRECT CAUSES	49	22	38	45
TOTAL	224	100	85	100

4.7.3 Avoidable factors, 1983-84*

Case notes for 81 cases were examined for avoidable factors.

	Number	%
Patient factors		
Delay in arrival in hospital	11	
Interference with pregnancy	2	
Late booking	1	
Total	14	16
Peripheral hospital or clinic factors		
Late referral	23	
Insufficient prenatal care	7	
Insufficient information on transfer	6	
Other	2	
Total	38	47
Factors in the Muhimbili Medical centre		
Delay in instituting treatment	18	
Insufficient examination, observation or investigation	15	
Wrong treatment	8	
Wrong diagnosis	5	
Others	1	
Total	47	58

*   Categories not mutually exclusive.

4.8 Ocean Road Hospital and Muhimbili Medical centre, Dar es-Salaam 1976-77 [0287]

4.8.1 Rate

Deliveries	13 027
Maternal deaths	8
MMR (per 100 000 deliveries)	61

4.8.2 Causes of maternal death

	Number
Hypertensive disorders of pregnancy	4
Severe anaemia	2
Poisoning	1
Unexpected postpartum collapse	1
Total	8

4.8.3 Avoidable factors

4.8.4 High risk groups
Seven of the eight deaths occurred in women aged less than 20 years old.

4.9. Kilimanjaro Christian Medical Centre, Moshi, 1971-77 and 1980-81 [0043, 1112]

4.9.1 Rate

	1971-77	1980-81
Deliveries	24 292	1 956
Maternal deaths	80	5
MMR (per 100 000 deliveries)	329	256

4.9.2 Causes of maternal deaths, 1971-77

	Number	%
Ruptured uterus	10	13
Hypertensive disorders of pregnancy	7	9
Sepsis	7	9
Haemorrhage	6	8
Ectopic pregnancy	4	5
Abortion	4	5
Other direct causes	7	9
DIRECT CAUSES	45	56
Enterocolitis	12	15
Anaemia	2	2
Malaria	2	2
Meningitis	2	2
Cardiac disease	2	2
Renal and hypertensive disease	4	5
Others	11	14
INDIRECT CAUSES	35	44
TOTAL	80	100

4.10 Bugando Hill Hospital, Mwanza, 1975-76 and 1981-82 [0469, 1112]

4.10.1 Rate

	1975-76	1981-82
Deliveries	9 328	3 986
Maternal deaths	36	9
MMR (per 100 000 deliveries)	386	230

4.10.2 Causes of maternal deaths

	Number	%
Haemorrhage	12	34
Sepsis	7	19
Abortion	4	11
Liver failure	4	12
Ruptured uterus	2	6
Others	7	18
Total	36	100

4.11 Lugarwa Mission Hospital, Ludewa district, 1976-79 [1578]

4.11.1 Rate

Live births	2 271
Maternal deaths	11*
MMR (per 100 000 live births)	484

* One additional maternal death took place at home in a woman who left hospital for fear of having a repeat caesarean section.

4.11.2 Causes of maternal deaths

	Number
Ruptured uterus	2
Obstructed labour	2
Abortion	1
Sepsis	1
Haemorrhage	1
Anaemia	1
Others	3
Total	11

4.11.3 Avoidable factors
Eight of the deaths occurred among women admitted as emergencies. Only three women were not in a desperate condition on admission. In three women the mode of treatment contributed to mortality: augmentation with oxytocin instead of awaiting spontaneous delivery; delivery by caesarean section when the fetus had already died in utero instead of destructive operation; non-availability of blood.

4.12 Mbozi Designated Hospital, Mbeya region, 1976-79 [1578]

4.12.1 Rate

Live births	5 165
Maternal deaths	34*
MMR (per 100 000 live births)	660

* Includes five deaths which occurred on the way to the hospital.

4.12.2 Causes of maternal deaths

	Number	%
Sepsis	7	20
Obstructed labour	6	18
Abortion	3	9
Haemorrhage	3	9
Ruptured uterus	3	9
Hypertensive disorders of pregnancy	2	6
Ectopic pregnancy	1	2
Others/unknown	9	27
Total	34	100

5. CIVIL REGISTRATION DATA/GOVERNMENT ESTIMATES

5.1 National, 1979-89 [2332]

A Ministry of Health report quotes a maternal mortality rate of 185 per 100 000 deliveries overall, ranging in different regions from 44 per 100 000 to 436 per 100 000 deliveries. The rate is said to have remained stable for a decade.

6. OTHER SOURCES/ ESTIMATES

6.1 National, 1984-86 [1627]

An article on the health and reproductive situation in Tanzania quotes an estimated maternal mortality rate of 200 per 100 000 live births for 1984-86.

7. SELECTED ANNOTATED BIBLIOGRAPHY

8. FURTHER READING

Mtimavalye, L.A.R. Reproductive health care among women in Africa: current trends and the future. *Journal of Obstetrics and Gynaecology in Eastern and Central Africa* 1982; 1: 48-52. WHE 0468

Ombuloye, I.O. and Oyeneye, O.Y. Primary health care in developing countries: the case of Nigeria, Sri Lanka and Tanzania. *Social Science and Medicine* 1982; 16(6): 675-686. WHE 0507

Raikes, A. Women's health in East Africa. *Social Science and Medicine* 1989; 28(5): 447-459. WHE 2220

9. DATA SOURCES

WHE 0042   Armon, P.J. Rupture of the uterus in Malawi and Tanzania. *East African Medical Journal* 1977; 54(9): 462-471

WHE 0043   Armon, P.J. Maternal deaths in the Kilimanjaro region of Tanzania. *Transactions of the Royal Society of Tropical Medicine and Hygiene* 1979; 73(3): 284-288

WHE 0212   Everett, V.J. Maternal mortality in Tanzania. *Dar es-Salaam Medical Journal* 1974; 6: 7-8

WHE 0287   Arkutu, A.A. A clinical study of maternal age and parturition in 2791 Tanzanian primiparae. *International Journal of Gynaecology and Obstetrics* 1978; 16(1): 20-23

WHE 0319   Hart, R.H. Maternal and child health services in Tanzania. *Tropical Doctor* 1977; 7: 179-185

WHE 0469   Mtimavalye, L.A.R. *Maternal mortality in Tanzania.* In: WHO Multidisciplinary Consultative Meeting on Human Reproduction, Yaoundé, 4-7 December 1978

WHE 0471   Mtimavalye, L.A. et al. Maternal mortality in Dar es-Salaam, Tanzania 1974-77. *East African Medical Journal* 1980; 57(2): 111-118

WHE 0800   World Health Organization. *Country reports to regional offices of the progress in implementing Health for All by the Year 2000.* (Unpublished documents) 1983

WHE 0834   World Health Organization. *World Health Statistics annual – vital statistics and causes of death.* Geneva, various years

WHE 0995   United Republic of Tanzania, Government of. *Statistical tables* Principal secretary of MCH/NUT Unit (unpublished private communication) 1985

WHE 1112   Janowitz, B. et al. *Reproductive health in Africa: issues and options.* North Carolina, Family Health International, 1984

WHE 1229   Price, T.G. Preliminary report on maternal deaths in the Southern Highlands of Tanzania in 1983. *Journal of Obstetrics and Gynaecology of Eastern and Central Africa* 1984; 3: 103-110

WHE 1243   Mtimavalye, L.A.R. et al. Survey on institutional maternal deaths in four regions of Tanzania, July 1983-December 1984, preliminary report. In: *Interregional Meeting on the Prevention of Maternal Mortality,* 11-15 November 1985

WHE 1322   Justesen, A. An analysis of maternal mortality in Muhimbili Medical Centre, Dar es-Salaam, July 1983-June 1984, preliminary report. *Journal of Obstetrics and Gynaecology of Eastern and Central Africa* 1985; 4: 5-8

WHE 1495   United Republic of Tanzania, Government of. *Analysis of the situation of children and women* Dar es-Salaam, Government of Tanzania and United Nations Children's Fund 1985

WHE 1578   Van Roosmalen, J. *Maternal health care in the South Western Highlands of Tanzania.* (unpublished doctoral thesis) 1987

WHE 1627   Kimaryo, S. Women and current reproduction: related health problems in Tanzania. In: *Women and Reproduction.* Report of a seminar in Visby, Stockholm, SAREC/SIDA, 1983

WHE 1712   Mauldin W.P. and Segal, S.J. *Prevalence of contraceptive use in developing countries. A chart book.* Rockefeller Foundation, New York 1986

WHE 1798   Murru, M. *Hospital maternal mortality in Tanzania.* (unpublished dissertation) 1987

WHE 1914   United Nations Children's Fund (UNICEF). *The state of the world's children,* various years, Oxford, Oxford University Press

WHE 1915   United Nations. Department of International Economic and Social Affairs. *World population prospects: estimates and projections as assessed in 1984.* Population Studies No. 98. New York 1986

WHE 1918   United Nations. Department of International Economic and Social Affairs. *First marriage: patterns and determinants.* New York 1988

WHE 2008   World Health Organization. Regional Office for Africa. *Evaluation of the strategy for health for all by the year 2000. Seventh report on the world health situation* Vol 2, African region, Brazzaville 1987

WHE 2033   World Health Organization. *Global strategy for health for all by the year 2000. Second report on monitoring progress.* WHO document EB83/2 Add. 1, 1988

WHE 2093   Moller, B. *The outcome of pregnancy and antenatal care in rural Tanzania.* (Doctoral thesis) Uppsala University, Uppsala, 1988

WHE 2332   United Republic of Tanzania, Ministry of Health. *The National family planning programme in Tanzania* 1989

WHE 2410   Boller, B. et al. A study of antenatal care at village level in rural Tanzania. *International Journal of Gynecology and Obstetrics* 1989; 30: 123-131

ZAÏRE

		Year	Source

1. BASIC INDICATORS

1.1 Demographic

1.1.1 Population

		Year	Source
Size (millions)	33.8	1988	(1914)
Rate of growth (%)	3.1	1980-87	(1914)

1.1.2 Life expectancy

Female	52	1980-85	(1915)
Male	48	1980-85	(1915)

1.1.3 Fertility

Crude Birth Rate	46	1988	(1914)
Total Fertility Rate	6.1	1988	(1914)

1.1.4 Mortality

Crude Death Rate	14	1988	(1914)
Infant Mortality Rate	83	1988	(1914)
Female			
Male			
1-4 years mortality rate			
Female			
Male			

1.2 Social and economic

1.2.1 Adult literacy rate (%)

Female	45	1985	(1914)
Male	79	1985	(1914)

1.2.2 Primary school enrolment rate (%)

Female	68	1986-88	(1914)
Male	84	1986-88	(1914)

1.2.3 Female mean age at first marriage

(years)	20.1	1975-76	(1918)

1.2.4 GNP/capita

(US $)	150	1987	(1914)

1.2.5 Daily per capita calorie supply

(as % of requirements)	98	1984-86	(1914)

2. HEALTH SERVICES

2.1 Health expenditure

2.1.1 Expenditure on health

(as % of GNP)	3	1985	(0800)

2.1.2 Expenditure on PHC

(as % of total health expenditure)	15	1987	(2008)

2.2 Primary Health Care
(Percentage of population covered by):

2.2.1 Health services

National	33	1984	(0834)
Urban			
Rural			

2.2.2 Safe water

National	33	1985-87	(1914)
Urban	54	1986	(2033)
Rural	20	1986	(2033)

2.2.3 Adequate sanitary facilities

National			
Urban	8	1980	(0834)
Rural	10	1983	(0834)

2.2.4 Contraceptive prevalence rate

(%)	1	1977	(0834)

2.3   Coverage of maternity care (%)

Area	Prenatal care	Trained attendant	Institutional deliveries	Postnatal care	Sample size	Year	Source
	–	–	–	–	–	–	–

3. COMMUNITY STUDIES

4. HOSPITAL STUDIES

4.1 All Hospitals, 1980 [0496]

4.1.1 Rate

A government report quotes an institutional maternal mortality rate of 200-800 per 100 000 live births for 1980.

4.2 Hôpital de la Communauté Evangélique en Ubangi-Mongala, Karawa, 1981-83 [0924, 1112]

Live births	3 175
Maternal deaths	20
MMR (per 100 000 live births)	630

4.2.2 Cause of maternal deaths

	Number
Sepsis	10
Haemorrhage	6
Complications of anaesthesia	2
Others	2
Total	20

4.2.3 Avoidable factors

4.2.4 High risk groups

Maternal mortality rates were higher among women more than 35 years of age, primiparae and among women with five or more previous pregnancies. Mortality risk was also related to educational status, prenatal visits and to thyroid status of the women.

MMR (per 100 000 deliveries)

Age

<15	0
15-17	410
18-35	520
35-40	1 170
40+	1 020

Parity

1	600
2-4	430
4+	790

Educational status

none	720
some	130

Prenatal care

none	3 770
1-3 visits	270
4+ visits	250

Thyroid status

Diet in the region is iodine deficient, and can result in hypothyroidism, and cretinism in the infant. The probability of conception and successful maintenance of pregnancy is reduced for cretin women because of their reduced stature and contracted pelvis. Maternal mortality rates were considerably higher in women with goiter and with cretinism.

(MMR per 100 000 deliveries)

no goiter	0
goiter	550
cretin	2 520

Length of labour

All but two of the women who died were admitted in a critical condition. The most common complication was prolonged labour (18 hours+) due to fetopelvic disproportion or malpresentation. 16 of the 20 who died had been in labour for more than 18 hours and nine of these had been in labour for more than 48 hours. The longer the labour, the greater the risk of death. For women in labour for more than 48 hours the risk was more than 400 times greater than for those who laboured 12 hours or less. Prolonged labour resulted in ruptured uterus in 14 cases which increased the risk of death more than 100 fold.

4.2.5 Other findings

13 of the 20 maternal deaths occurred during the five months of planting and harvest, seasons when the need for women's work in the fields can render them reluctant to go to hospital.

4.3 Centre Medical Evangélique (CME)-Nyakunde, Aba and Aru Hospitals, Upper Zaïre region, 1981-84 [1461]

4.3.1 Rate

	CME-Nyakunde 1981-82	Aba Hospital 1981-84	Aru Hospital 1982-84
Live births	3 665	729	2 252
Maternal deaths	17	3	4
MMR (per 100 000 live births)	464	412	178

4.3.2 Causes of maternal deaths (all three hospitals)

	Number
Obstructed labour	3
Ruptured uterus	2
Haemorrhage	2
Sepsis	1
Hypertensive disorders of pregnancy	1
Shock	1
Embolism	1
Anaemia	1
Unknown	12
TOTAL	24

4.3.3 Avoidable factors

4.3.4 High risk groups

4.3.5 Other findings

All three hospitals have nurse practitioner surgeons (NPS) trained in surgical skills. The study found them capable of delivering all types of labour, normal or dystocic.

4.4 General Hospital, Kinshasa, 1969 [1381]

4.4.1 Rate
MMR (per 100 000 births) 2 000

4.5 Cliniques Universitaires du Mont Amba, Kinshasa, 1961-80 and 1986 [1909, 2021]

4.5.1 Rate

	1961-80	1986*
Live births	87 482	2 125
Maternal deaths	60	5
MMR (per 100 000 live births)	69	236

*   April – September

4.5.2 Causes of maternal deaths 1961-80 *(for 40 cases)*

	Number	%
Haemorrhage	14	35
Sepsis	6	15
Cardiovascular accidents	6	15
Hypertensive disorders of pregnancy	5	13
Complications of anaesthesia	4	10
Other	5	13
TOTAL	40	100

Twelve maternal deaths followed caesarean section. Over the 20-year period there were 2 394 caesarean sections, an incidence of 2.7%. The mortality rate for caesarean section was 5/1000.

Abortion [1290]

A study of abortion complications treated between 1978 and 1979 found a total of 1 084 admissions for complications of abortion, of which 248 were induced and 836 spontaneous. The majority of the patients with induced abortion were young and unmarried. There were two maternal deaths among the spontaneous abortions (a death-to-case ratio of 2.4/1000) and 13 deaths among the induced abortions (a death-to-case ratio of 52/1000).

4.6 Vanga Mission Hospital, Kinshasa, 1972-81 [1774]

4.6.1 Rate
Births	8 815
Maternal deaths	23
MMR (per 100 000 live births)	261

4.7 Bonzola Hospital, April-September 1986 [2021]

4.7.1 Rate
Deliveries	2 756
Maternal deaths	1
MMR (per 100 000 deliveries)	36

5. CIVIL REGISTRATION DATA/GOVERNMENT ESTIMATES

6. OTHER SOURCES/ ESTIMATES

7. SELECTED ANNOTATED BIBLIOGRAPHY

Bongwele, O. et al. *Determinants and consequences of pregnancy wastage in Zaïre. A study of patients with complications requiring hospital treatment in Kinshasa, Matadi and Bukavu.* Family Health International, North Carolina, 1986. WHE 1443

A hospital-based study of the determinants and consequences of abortions was initiated in 1982 in ten centres located in three regions of Zaïre. Between November 1982 and March 1984 a total of 2 465 women were admitted to the participating centres for complications resulting from abortion. Of the total, 617 (25%) were diagnosed by the attending medical personnel as illegally induced and 1848 (75%) as spontaneous. Women aged less than 18 years old represented only 7.6% of the total admissions but accounted for 57.5% of the induced abortions. Unmarried women accounted for 16.8% of admissions and 67.8% of induced abortions. Thirteen of the women with complications following induced abortion died in the hospital, a death-to-case ratio of 21/1000. All were young and unmarried.

Duale, S. *A case control follow-up study of pregnancy outcome in women with symphysiotomy versus caesarean section* (unpublished paper) Family Health International, North Carolina, 1989. WHE 2327

The report presents findings of a study to compare the immediate and longer-term effects of symphysiotomy versus caesarean section for obstructed labour due to cephalopelvic dispropor-tion at the Hôpital de la Communauté Evangélique en Ubangi-Mongala, near the town of Karawa. Data were collected from 91 women who had under-gone symphysiotomy and from 80 women who had had caesarean section. Fistulae were the most commonly reported complications associated with

symphysiotomy with five women reporting vesicovaginal or urethrovaginal fistulae. Higher initial rates of symptoms associated with certain physical activities were reported by women with symphysiotomy but that rates decreased over time so that no significant differences between the two groups remained in the longer term. A significant proportion of both groups suffered social and psychological effects.

Lufuma, L.N. and Tshipeta. L'incidence de l'infection urinaire dans la cure des fistules vésico-vaginales obstétricales. A propos de 60 cas. *Médecine d'Afrique Noire* 1978; 25(2): 107-110. WHE 1181

A urine examination of 60 women with vesicovaginal fistula repair in Kinshasa showed that nearly all cases had some kind of urinary infection (an itemized description of bacteria found is given). However, since the cure rate was 85%, it is concluded that these bacteria do not play a significant role in the cure of vesicovaginal fistulae. It was found that the site, size and type of fistula was more significant.

Monseur, J. Le remplacement du vagin par un greffon sigmoïdien pour la cure des grandes nécroses uro-génitales post partum africaines. *Journal d'Urologie* 1980; 86(3): 159-166. WHE 2265

Of 100 cases of extensive urogenital necrosis following obstructed labour, treated at the National University in Lubumbashi, Zaïre, from 1966-1976, 17 cases are analysed and a description of sigmoidovaginoplasty surgery presented.

The major causes of the fistulae and other damage was labour lasting several days, far from any health services, with no prenatal care, and the fact that the women were malnourished, had very narrow pelves, and frequently suffered from bilharzia. 80% of the women in this series were under 25 years old, and 40% under 20. Nine women had rectal tearing, all had secondary amenorrhea, and most had already undergone unsuccessful surgery elsewhere.

Given the importance of bearing children (over and above the importance of being continent) for the women in the rural areas of Zaïre, the author carried out surgery, which he describes, to replace the vagina with a sigmoid graft. There was one death. In eight women total continence was achieved, and five suffered stress incontinence; 13 were subsequently able to have normal sexual intercourse.

Sitolo, Y. *Prognostic foeto-maternel de l'hypertension gravidique à la Maternité des Cliniques Universitaires de Kisangani.* Mémoire, Université de Kisangani, Faculté de Médecine, 1989. WHE 2485

A study of hypertensive disorders of pregnancy from 1986-87, found 48 cases in a total of 832 deliveries, an incidence of 5.8%. There were two maternal deaths, a case fatality rate of 41 per 1000 cases and a maternal mortality rate from eclampsia of 240 per 100 000 deliveries.

8. FURTHER READING

Duale, S. Maternal care breakthrough in Zaïre. *People* 1987; 14(3): 16-17. WHE 1567

Kalungwe, K. Etude multicentrique de l'accouchement au Zaïre. *Memoire presented to the University of Kinshasa* 1988. WHE 2020

Kayembe, T.B. Traditional structures clash with new imperatives. *Draper Fund Report* 1983; 12: 3-5. WHE 1708

Manshande, J.P. et al. Rest versus heavy work during the last weeks of pregnancy: influence on fetal growth. *British Journal of Obstetrics and Gynaecology* 1987; 94: 1059-1067. WHE 1974

Tandu-Umba, N.F. et al. Profil obstetrical de la maternité précoce à Kinshasa. *Journal de Gynécologie et Biologie de la Réproduction* 1988; 12(8): 873-877. WHE 2103

VandenBroek, N. et al. Cesarean sections for maternal indications in Kasongo, (Zaïre). *International Journal of Gynecology and Obstetrics* 1989; 28: 337-342. WHE 2381

White, S.M. et al. Emergency obstetric surgery performed by nurses in Zaïre. *Lancet* 1987: 612-613. WHE 1726

Moens, F. Design, implementation and evaluation of a community financing scheme for hospital care in developing countries: a pre-paid health plan in the Bwemanda health zone, Zaïre. *Social Science and Medicine* 1990; 30(12): 1319-1327. WHE 2517

9. DATA SOURCES

WHE 0496   Nkamany, K. *Resumé de l'énoncé de la philosophie du développement de la stratégie "Nutrition et soins de Santé Primaires" en vue de la santé pour tous les Zaïrois d'ici à l'an 2000.* Centre National de Planification de Nutrition Humaine, N'sele 1982

WHE 0800   World Health Organization. *Country reports to regional offices of the progress in implementing Health for All by the Year 2000.* (Unpublished documents) 1983

WHE 0834   World Health Organization. *World Health Statistics annual – vital statistics and causes of death.* Geneva, various years

WHE 0924   Smith, J.B. et al. *Hospital deaths in a high risk obstetric population, Kawara, Zaïre.* (unpublished document) Family Health International, North Carolina, 1984

WHE 1112   Janowitz, B. et al. *Reproductive health in Africa: issues and options* Family Health International, North Carolina, 1984

WHE 1290   Tshibangu, K. et al. Avortement clandestin, problème de santé publique à Kinshasa (Zaïre). *Journal de Gynécologie Obstétrique et Biologie de la Réproduction* 1984; 13: 759-763

WHE 1381   Van der Berghe, H. *Nutritional and other risk factors for the outcome of pregnancy* Leuven, University of Leuven, 1985

WHE 1461   Monoja, L.T. *The role of medical auxiliaries in operative obstetrics in rural Zaïre* (unpublished dissertation), London, Institute of Child Health 1984

WHE 1774   Fallis, G.B. Obstetrics in a rural African population. *East African Medical Journal* 1986; 63(1): 54-62

WHE 1909   Kinkeda, K.N. et al. Mortalité maternelle en obstétrique aux Cliniques Universitaires du Mont Amba, Kinshasa. *Afrique Médicale* 1985; 24(234): 495-500

WHE 1914   United Nations Children's Fund (UNICEF). *The state of the world's children,* various years, Oxford, Oxford University Press

WHE 1915   United Nations. Department of International Economic and Social Affairs. *World population prospects: estimates and projections as assessed in 1984.* Population Studies No. 98. New York 1986

WHE 1918   United Nations. Department of International Economic and Social Affairs. *First marriage: patterns and determinants.* New York 1988

WHE 2008   World Health Organization, Regional Office for Africa. *Evaluation of the strategy for health for all by the year 2000. Seventh report on the world health situation* Vol 2, African region, Brazzaville 1987

WHE 2021   Esimo, M. *Etude multicentrique de l'accouchement au Zaïre* Memoire to the University of Kinshasa 1988

WHE 2033   World Health Organization. *Global strategy for health for all by the year 2000. Second report on monitoring progress.* WHO document EB83/2 Add. 1, 1988

ZAMBIA

		Year	Source

1. BASIC INDICATORS

1.1 Demographic

1.1.1 Population

Size (millions)	7.9	1988	(1914)
Rate of growth (%)	3.9	1980-87	(1914)

1.1.2 Life expectancy

Female	53	1980-85	(1915)
Male	50	1980-85	(1915)

1.1.3 Fertility

Crude Birth Rate	51	1988	(1914)
Total Fertility Rate	7.2	1988	(1914)

1.1.4 Mortality

Crude Death Rate	14	1988	(1914)
Infant Mortality Rate	79	1988	(1914)
Female			
Male			
1-4 years mortality rate			
Female			

1.2 Social and economic

1.2.1 Adult literacy rate (%)

Female	67	1985	(1914)
Male	84	1985	(1914)

1.2.2 Primary school enrolment rate (%)

Female	92	1986-88	(1914)
Male	102	1986-88	(1914)

1.2.3 Female mean age at first marriage

(years)	19.4	1980	(1918)

1.2.4 GNP/capita

(US $)	250	1987	(1914)

1.2.5 Daily per capita calorie supply

(as % of requirements)	92	1984-86	(1914)

2. HEALTH SERVICES

2.1 Health expenditure

2.1.1 Expenditure on health

(as % of GNP)	5	1987	(2033)

2.1.2 Expenditure on PHC

(as % of total health expenditure)	35	1987	(2033)

2.2 Primary Health Care
(Percentage of population covered by):

2.2.1 Health services

National	70	1984	(0834)
Urban			
Rural			

2.2.2 Safe water

National	48	1984	(0834)
Urban	70	1984	(0834)
Rural	32	1984	(0834)

2.2.3 Adequate sanitary facilities

National	47	1987	(2008)
Urban	70	1987	(2008)
Rural	56	1987	(2008)

2.2.4 Contraceptive prevalence rate

(%)	1	1977	(0834)

2.3 Coverage of maternity care (%)

Area	Prenatal care	Trained attendant	Institutional deliveries	Postnatal care	Sample size	Year	Source
National	88					1984	(0834)
National	74					1986	(2033)
Lusaka			86		23 100	1976	(0240)
Luampungu		47		22	111	(1984)	(1647)
Kabinga		46		10	101	(1984)	(1647)

3. COMMUNITY STUDIES

4. HOSPITAL STUDIES

4.1 All hospitals, 1977 [0842]

4.1.1 Rate

Deliveries	75 630
Maternal deaths	173
MMR (per 100 000 deliveries)	229

4.2 University Teaching Hospital, Lusaka, 1974-76 and 1980-83 [0325, 0382, 1792]

4.2.1 Rate

	1974-76	1980-81	1982-83
Total births	51 386	n.a.	50 779*
Maternal deaths	80	n.a.	60
MMR (per 100 000 births)	156	106-109	118

* Live births

4.2.2 Causes of maternal deaths

	1974-76		1982-83	
	Number	%	Number*	%
Hypertensive disorders of pregnancy	23	29	12	19
Sepsis	14	18	12	19
Abortion	6	7	10	16
Haemorrhage	12	15	6	9
Ruptured uterus	11	14	4	6
Ectopic pregnancy	6	7	4	6
Embolism	–	–	3	5
DIRECT CAUSES	72	90	51	80
Cerebral malaria	–	–	3	5
Anaemia	1	1	2	3
Sickle cell disease	–	–	1	2
Hepatitis	1	1	1	2
Others	6	8	9	13
INDIRECT CAUSES	8	10	13	20
TOTAL	80	100	64	100

* Including 4 patients who died later than 42 days following termination of the pregnancy.

Rupture of the uterus [1053]

A five-year retrospective study of ruptured uterus over the period 1970-74 found 72 523 deliveries and 125 ruptured uteri, an incidence of 1 per 580 deliveries, or 1.7 per 1000. The rupture was spontaneous in 59 cases, traumatic in eleven cases and through a previous scar in 55 cases. 51 of the women had had no prenatal care. Eight patients died, a mortality rate of 6.4%. There were four cases of vesicovaginal fistula, four of stress incontinence and two cases of drop foot.

Eclampsia [(0128)]

During 1975 and 1976 there were 35 024 deliveries and 79 cases of eclampsia, an incidence of 1 per 443 deliveries. Thirteen of the patients died, a mortality rate of 16.5%. Although eclampsia was more common among young primigravidae, multiparous women above 35 years of age had the highest mortality rates.

Abortions [(1842)]

Over the four-year period 1977-1980 there were 13 350 admissions for complications of abortion, representing nearly 60% of all gynaecological admissions. The author estimates that 2.5% of these (334 cases) were septic/illegal abortions and resulted in 15 maternal deaths, a mortality rate of 4.5%.

4.2.3 Avoidable factors

Avoidable factors were present in 64 of the 80 deaths (80%) which occurred during 1974-76.

	Number of deaths	%
In the hospital		
Poor intrapartum assessment	13	
Failure to correct anaemia	10	
Undiagnosed ruptured ectopic pregnancy	5	
Delay taking patient to theatre	4	
Inadequate antibiotic therapy	4	
Discharged home too soon	3	
Anaesthetic accident	2	
Anaesthetist not available	1	
Total	42	(66%)
Outside the hospital		
Delay in coming to the hospital	8	
No prenatal care	5	
Failure of clinics to refer patients at risk	4	
Failure to seek legal abortion	3	
Failure to obtain transport	1	
Failure of patient to accept treatment	1	
Total	22	(34%)

Of the 64 maternal deaths during 1982-83, avoidable factors were found in 51 cases.

	Number	%
Inappropriate/inadequate management in hospital	25	49
Failure to seek legal abortion	9	18
Home delivery	6	12
Inappropriate/inadequate management in referral unit	5	10
Failure to seek other available treatment	4	8
Failure by facility to provide blood transfusion	1	2
Community failure to provide accessible facility	1	2
Total	51	100

4.2.4 High risk groups

An analysis of maternal deaths during 1982-83 by age and parity shows significantly higher maternal mortality rates for women over 35 years of age, women of parity 5 or more, and to a lesser extent, nulliparous women.

Age

	Deliveries	Maternal deaths	MMR (per 100 000 births)
15-24	31 280	28	90
25-34	16 960	16	94
35-44	2 285	12	525
45 and above	254	1	394
Unknown	–	3	–
Total	50 779	60	118

Parity

	Deliveries	Maternal deaths	MMR (per 100 000 births)
Nulliparous	12 850	14	109
1-4	28 280	24	85
5+	9 650	22	228
Total	50 780	60	118

4.3 Six hospitals*, 1983-88 [(2463)]

* University Teaching Hospital, Lusaka; Livingstone General Hospital; Choma District Hospital; Lewanika General Hospital; Senanga District Hospital; Kaoma District Hospital.

4.3.1 Rate

Deliveries	137 869
Maternal deaths	145
MMR (per 100 000 deliveries)	105

4.3.2 Causes of maternal deaths

	Number	%
Sepsis	37	26
Hypertensive disorders of pregnancy	26	18
Haemorrhage	22	15
Ruptured uterus	11	8
Abortions	5	3
Ectopic pregnancy	2	1
Embolism	2	1
Cardiac arrest	1	1
DIRECT CAUSES	106	73
Malaria	11	8
Anaemia	7	5
Use of herbal medicines	4	3
Meningitis	3	2
INDIRECT CAUSES	25	17
Other	9	6
Unknown	5	3
TOTAL	145	100

4.4 General Hospital, rural health centres and mission hospitals, Luapula Province, 1983-87 [2495]

4.4.1 Rate

	Deliveries	Maternal deaths	MMR (per 100 000 births)
Mansa District	11 773	32	272
Kawamba District	4 770	14	294
Mwense District	3 791	5	132
Nchelenge District	8 238	38	461
Samfya District	2 601	15	577
Luapula Province	31 173	104	334

4.4.2 Causes of maternal deaths *(for 91 cases)*

	Number
Haemorrhage	21
Ruptured uterus	17
Sepsis	12
Anaemia	6
Hypertensive disorders of pregnancy	4
Other	31

4.4.3 Avoidable factors

4.4.4 High risk groups

4.4.5 Other findings

The majority of the patients were admitted in a moribund condition. Of the 86 cases for which the dates of admission and death are available, 32 died on the day of admission and a further 24 on the following day.

5. CIVIL REGISTRATION DATA/GOVERNMENT ESTIMATES

5.1 National, 1975-80 [1143, 1792]

5.1.1 Rate

A government report quotes a rate of between 100 and 140 per 100 000 live births during 1974-79 and 106-109 per 100 000 live births in 1980. The report also states that these figures are likely to be underestimates.

6. OTHER ESTIMATES

6.1 National, 1982 [1339]

6.1.1 Rate

A WHO report quotes an institutional maternal mortality rate of 100 per 100 000 live births for 1982.

6.2 National, 1980-83 [1421]

6.2.1 Rate

Year	MMR (per 100 000 live births)
1980	122
1981	151
1982	142
1983	151

7. SELECTED ANNOTATED BIBLIOGRAPHY

Fleming, A.F. The aetiology of severe anaemia in pregnancy in Ndola, Zambia. *Annals of Tropical Medicine and Parasitology* 1989; 83(1): 37-49. WHE 2464

The aetiology of severe anaemia was studied in 37 pregnant women. Aetiology was usually multiple; 31 had *Plasmodium falciparum* malaria, 23 were folate deficient, 13 were iron deficient, one had sickle cell anaemia and one had AIDS. Folate deficiency was most often secondary to malarial haemolysis; iron deficiency was nutritional but hookworm was contributory in about one third of the patients. The anaemia of malaria and folate deficiency was both more common and more severe than anaemia due to iron deficiency. Vigorous antimalarial treatment and prophylaxis are essential in the management and prevention of anaemia in pregnancy. Total dose iron infusion is indicated only when severe iron deficiency anaemia has been proven and must be accompanied by antimalarial therapy and folic acid supplements. Because of the risk of transmission of HIV it is of particular importance to prevent anaemia and malaria in pregnancy and to give blood transfusion only as a lifesaving treatment.

Hassim, A.M. and Lucas, C. Reduction in the incidence of stress incontinence complicating fistula repair. *British Journal of Surgery* 1974; 61: 461-465. WHE 2168

During the period July 1966 to October 1972 there were 161 consecutive cases of urinary tract fistulae seen at the University of Zambia School of Medicine, Lusaka, Zambia. Of these, 150 (93%) were obstetric fistulae, mostly caused by prolonged obstructed labour. The rest were gynaecological fistulae caused by trauma, operations or cervical cancer. During the first two years of the study, 72% of the fistulae were closed and 64% of the patients were totally continent, as compared with 91% and 82% respectively after primary repair during the following four years of the study. This improved functional cure rate was due to an operative technique which included reinforcement of the bladder neck, as well as increased experience of the surgeons and the nursing staff. Surgical techniques are described. Of the 150 women with obstetric fistulae, 131 were functionally cured, and 11 had stress incontinence. It is concluded that a positive surgical approach to the prevention of stress incontinence at the initial repair of vesicovaginal fistulae and enlargement in the bladder capacity in cases of gross vesical contraction result in an improved functional cure rate.

Ransjo-Arvidson, et al. Maternity care routines in a teaching hospital in Zambia. *East African Medical Journal* 1989; 66(7): 427-437. WHE 2479

At the University Teaching Hospital, Lusaka, 59 uncomplicated vaginally delivered mothers were studied with regard to maternity care during the prenatal period and delivery. Information was collected from prenatal cards, labour records, observations during delivery and interviews with the mothers themselves. The results indicate that many recommended routines were applied in fewer than half the cases. The average of more than five prenatal visits suggests that there was sufficient demand for health care on the part of the mothers. All women had blood pressure checked and urine examination but only one-third received full tetanus immunization coverage. Half the mothers were anaemic but only one-third were

offered iron supplementation. During labour, procedures such as hand-washing, measurement of blood loss, and examination of the perineum for tears and placenta for completeness, were not routinely applied. There was a positive correlation between the application of maternity care and the mother's educational level. These findings suggest a need for systematic critical review and modification of current maternal care technologies and improved general and health education of women.

Wadhawan, W. and Wacha, D.S.O. A review of urinary fistulae in a university teaching hospital. *International Journal of Gynaecology and Obstetrics* 1983; 21: 381-385. WHE 1837

An eight-year study of urinary fistulae from 1974 to 1981 was carried out in the University Teaching Hospital, Lusaka, Zambia. A total of 163 cases of urinary fistulae were registered, and 82 operations were performed. Complete records were available for 61 of these cases. Fifty-four fistulae (88.5%) were caused by prolonged obstructed labour, and seven by gynaecological surgery. Of the 54 women with obstetric fistulae, 26% were aged 19 and under, and 55% aged 30 and under. The highest percentage (38%) were primiparous women. Of the 44 cases operated, 27 (61%) were successfully closed, and seven women suffered stress incontinence. Operative management is discussed.

8. FURTHER READING

Arnold, G. Urban maternity services in Lusaka. *Africa Health* October/November 1987. WHE 2252

Bhagwandeen, S.B. and Patel, B.G. Chronic endometritis: a clinical and histopathological study. *Medical Journal of Zambia* 1976; 10: 99-102. WHE 1036

Kwofie, K. et al. Malnutrition and pregnancy wastage in Zambia. *Social Science and Medicine* 1983; 17(9): 539-543. WHE 0402

9. DATA SOURCES

WHE 0128   Chatterjee, T.K. et al. A review of 79 cases of eclampsia at the University Teaching Hospital, Lusaka. *Medical Journal of Zambia* 1980; 12(3): 77-80

WHE 0240   Grech, E.S. *Obstetric deaths in Lusaka.* (unpublished document) 1976

WHE 0325   Hickey, M.U. and Kasonde, J.M. Maternal mortality at the University Teaching Hospital, Lusaka. *Medical Journal of Zambia* 1977; 11(3): 74-78

WHE 0382   Kasonde, J.M. Problems of human reproduction in Zambia. in: *WHO Regional Multidisciplinary Meeting on Human Reproduction,* Yaoundé 4-7 December 1978 (unpublished document).

WHE 0834   World Health Organization. *World Health Statistics annual – vital statistics and causes of death.* Geneva, various years

WHE 0842   Zambia, Ministry of Health. *Reports for the years 1973-77* Lusaka, 1980

WHE 1053   Chatterjee, T.K. and Patel, B.G. Rupture of the uterus. *Medical Journal of Zambia* 1979; 12(6): 130-133

WHE 1143   Osborne, C.M. Health care of children in Zambia. In: *Proceedings of a symposium on health care of children in African countries.* African-Finnish workshop for Pediatricians. Kaduna, Nigeria 11-15 January 1982

WHE 1339   World Health Organization, Regional Office for Africa. *Where are we in PHC? Countries take a close look at themselves through PHC reviews.* 17-25 June 1985

WHE 1421   Mwanza, F. Drive to cut maternal deaths. *People* 1986; 13(4): 32

WHE 1647   Freund, P.J. and Kalumba, K. Maternal health and child survival rates in Zambia: a comparative study. *Medical Journal of Zambia* 1984; 18(2): 12-17

WHE 1792   Mhango, C. et al. Reproductive mortality in Lusaka, Zambia, 1982-1983. *Studies in Family Planning* 1987; 17(5): 243-251

WHE 1842   Narone, J.N. et al. Criminal abortions as seen in the University Teaching Hospital, Lusaka. *Medical Journal of Zambia* 1981; 15(3): 80-84

WHE 1914   United Nations Children's Fund (UNICEF). *The state of the world's children,* various years, Oxford, Oxford University Press

WHE 1915   United Nations. Department of International Economic and Social Affairs. *World population prospects: estimates and projections as assessed in 1984.* Population Studies No. 98. New York 1986

WHE 1918   United Nations. Department of International Economic and Social Affairs. *First marriage: patterns and determinants.* New York 1988

WHE 2008   World Health Organization. Regional Office for Africa *Evaluation of the strategy for health for all by the year 2000. Seventh report on the world health situation* Vol 2, African region, Brazzaville 1987

WHE 2033   World Health Organization. *Global strategy for health for all by the year 2000. Second report on monitoring progress.* WHO document EB83/2 Add. 1, 1988

WHE 2463   Zambia, Ministry of Health. *Family Health Programme: Maternal mortality.* Paper presented at the preliminary workshop on the UNFPA funded family health programme reformulation exercise. 18-19 August 1988

WHE 2495   Zambia. *Maternal mortality in Luapula Province from 1983.* (unpublished document) 1987

ZIMBABWE

	Year	Source

1. BASIC INDICATORS

1.1 Demographic

1.1.1 Population

		Year	Source
Size (millions)	9.1	1988	(1914)
Rate of growth (%)	3.1	1980-87	(1914)

1.1.2 Life expectancy

Female	58	1980-85	(1915)
Male	54	1980-85	(1915)

1.1.3 Fertility

Crude Birth Rate	42	1988	(1914)
Total Fertility Rate	5.8	1988	(1914)

1.1.4 Mortality

Crude Death Rate	10	1988	(1914)
Infant mortality rate	71	1988	(1914)
Female	65	1978-88	(2516)
Male	30	1978-88	(2516)
1-4 years mortality rate			
Female	33	1978-88	(2516)
Male	30	1978-88	(2516)

1.2 Social and economic

1.2.1 Adult literacy rate (%)

Female	67	1985	(1914)
Male	81	1985	(1914)

1.2.2 Primary school enrolment rate* (%)

Female	126	1986-88	(1914)
Male	130	1986-88	(1914)

1.2.3 Female mean age at first marriage

(years)	20.4	1982	(1918)

1.2.4 GNP/capita

		Year	Source
(US $)	580	1987	(1914)

1.2.5 Daily per capita calorie supply

(as % of requirements)	89	1984-86	(1914)

2. HEALTH SERVICES

2.1 Health expenditure

2.1.1 Expenditure on health

(as % of GNP)	6	1986-87	(2033)

2.1.2 Expenditure on PHC

(as % of total health expenditure)	50	1986-87	(2033)

2.2 Primary Health Care

(Percentage of population covered by):

2.2.1 Health services

National	71	1984	(0834)
Urban			
Rural			

2.2.2 Safe water

National	52	1984	(0834)
Urban	100	1984	(0834)
Rural	10	1984	(0834)

2.2.3 Adequate sanitary facilities

National	26	1984	(0834)
Urban	100	1984	(0834)
Rural	5	1984	(0834)

2.2.4 Contraceptive prevalence rate

(%)	43	1983-88	(2516)

2.3   Coverage of maternity care (%)

Area	Prenatal care	Trained attendant	Institutional deliveries	Postnatal care	Sample size	Year	Source
National	89	69				1984	(0834)
National	90	60				1986	(2033)
National: rural		73	49		217	1982	(0798)
National: urban	92	70			3 334	1983-88	(2516)
urban	96	91			886	1983-88	(2516)
rural	90	62			2 448	1983-88	(2516)
Bulawayo		91	87		214	1982	(0798)
Chitungwiza		91	80		210	1982	(0798)
Harare		88	85		206	1982	(0798)
Manicaland			40			1985	(1255)

3.   COMMUNITY STUDIES

4.   HOSPITAL STUDIES

4.1   All hospitals, 1979 [0845]

4.1.1   Rate
Live births	68 127
Maternal deaths	99
MMR (per 100 000 live births)	145

4.2   Harare Maternity Hospital, 1976 and 1981 [0110, 1307, 1389]

4.2.1   Rate
There were 56 maternal deaths (defined as deaths occurring during pregnancy, delivery or labour or as a consequence of pregnancy, within one year of delivery) in the hospital in 1976, and 51 maternal deaths in 1983. Of the 51 deaths in 1983, 26 were of women referred from peripheral hospitals as emergency cases. The total number of live births to women thus referred is not known. The maternal mortality rates for 1983 therefore relate to the 25 maternal deaths from within the hospital.

	1976	1983
Deliveries	16 947	44 519
Maternal deaths	56	25*
MMR (per 100 000 deliveries)	330	56

*   Including 3 deaths which occurred after 42 days following the termination of the pregnancy.

4.2.2   Causes of maternal deaths
(in 1983 includes deaths of 26 women referred from peripheral clinics or hospitals who did not deliver at the hospital)

	1976 Number	1976 %	1983 Number	1983 %
Sepsis	19	34	12	24
Haemorrhage	0	–	11	22
Abortion	18	32	9	18
Hypertensive disorders of pregnancy	2	4	8	16
Ectopic pregnancy	1	2	0	–
Hepatitis	–	–	1	2
Cerebral malaria	–	–	1	2
Cardiac disease	3	5	2	4
Others	13	23	7	12
TOTAL	56	100	51	100

4.2.3 Avoidable factors

Booking status

In 1976 the maternal mortality rate for booked patients was 59 per 100 000 live births. In 1983 the maternal mortality rate for booked patients was 29 per 100 000.

1983	Booked	Unbooked
Live births	41 525	2 994
Maternal deaths	12	13
MMR (per 100 000 live births)	29	430

Analysis of maternal deaths in 1983 found that avoidable factors were equally attributable to the patient and to treatment at the hospital.

Factors attributable to:	Number	%
Patient		
Late presentation	8	
Refusal of treatment	2	
Unbooked	5	
Took traditional medicine "muti"	1	
TOTAL	16	47
Peripheral Hospital		
Delay in transfer	1	
Poor operative technique	1	
TOTAL	2	6
Harare Maternity Hospital		
Failure to diagnose or delay in diagnosis	4	
Failure to operate or delay in operating	5	
Failure of appropriate treatment	2	
Poor operative technique	2	
Over transfusion	2	
Anaesthetic problem	1	
TOTAL	16	47

4.2.4 High risk groups, 1983

A comparison of those who died with the general obstetric population at the hospital showed a significant association between maternal death and advancing maternal age and increasing parity.

	% of those who died	% of obstetric population
Age		
<15	0	0
15-19	10	18
20-24	39	40
25-29	20	23
30-34	10	12
35-39	16	5
40+	5	2
Parity		
0	18	20
1-3	52	57
4+	30	23

4.3 Gweru General Hospital, 1982-84, 1984-86 (1976, 2481)

4.3.1 Rate

	1982-84	1984-86
Total births	5 162	5 273*
Maternal deaths	10	30
MMR (per 100 000 births)	194	57

* Deliveries

In September 1984, in an attempt to reduce the caesarean section rate without an adverse effect on the obstetrical outcome, new guidelines for the management of dystocia, previous caesarean delivery, fetal distress and breech presentation were introduced. In essence, these consisted of allowing trial of labour, the administration of oxytocin and Ventouse extraction whenever possible. Comparison of the two-year period prior to September 1984 with the two years following, found that the caesarean section rate dropped from 16.8% to 8%, the perinatal mortality from 71.9% to 56.2% and the maternal mortality from 194 per 100 000 to 57 per 100 000.

4.3.2 Causes of death

Maternal death was seven times more frequent in cases of caesarean section compared to vaginal delivery. Booking status did not significantly influence the maternal mortality rate.

	Number
Sepsis	3
Hypertensive disorders of pregnancy	2
Cardiovascular conditions	2
Abortion	1
Haemorrhage	1
Ruptured uterus	1
Embolism	1
TOTAL	10

5. CIVIL REGISTRATION DATA/GOVERNMENT ESTIMATES

5.1   National, 1979 [(0845)]

5.1.1   Rate

Live births	18 856
Maternal deaths	91
MMR (per 100 000 live births)	483

5.2   National and by Province, 1988 [(2561)]

5.2.1   Rate

	Live Births	Maternal deaths	MMR (per 100 000 live births)
Manicaland	24 847	36	145
Mash. Central	13 538	19	140
Mash. East	15 695	8	51
Mas. West	20 126	12	60
Masvingo	28 126	14	50
Mat. North	9 650	5	52
Mat. South	9 314	12	129
Midlands	28 388	27	95
Bulawayo City	20 707	11	53
Chitungxiza City	4 379	0	–
Harare City	13 510	1	7
National	188 280	145	77

6. OTHER SOURCES/ ESTIMATES

7. SELECTED ANNOTATED BIBLIOGRAPHY

Clegg, D.R. Vaginal repair of obstetric vesicovaginal fistulae. *Central African Journal of Medicine* 1979; 25(4): 67-71. WHE 1057

A description of the management, including operative technique, of 29 consecutive patients with vesicovaginal fistulae in Harare Central Hospital, Zimbabwe in 1977, is presented. All fistulae were due to obstructed labour, and were repaired by the vaginal route. Closure was obtained in 26 (90%), with a 34% functional cure rate, 34% with stress incontinence, and one death.

De Muylder, X. Vaginal delivery after caesarean section: is it safe in a developing country. *Australia and New Zealand Journal of Obstetrics and Gynaecology* 1988; 28: 99-102. WHE 2359

At Gweru Hospital, 401 patients with scarred uteri were managed according to a standard protocol and 288 were allowed to have a trial of scar. The latter was restricted to patients who had only one previous lower segment caesarean section, whose current pregnancy was a singleton occipital presentation and whose pelvis was clinically normal. When these circumstances were not fulfilled the patient was booked for an elective lower segment caesarean section. Of the 288 women who were allowed a trial of scar this was successful in 235 mothers (82%). There were no maternal deaths in this series but there were two uterine ruptures (0.7%), both requiring hysterectomy. The author suggests that both could have been avoided with better monitoring of labour. Postpartum morbidity was higher after caesarean section than after vaginal delivery. Apart from the two cases of uterine rupture, no fetus died as a result of the trial of scar. It is concluded that even in developing countries where, in most cases, there is no electronic fetal heart rate monitoring , no information about the prior section and no X-ray pelvimetry, trial of scar can be a safe alternative to repeated caesarean section when certain criteria are fulfilled.

De Muylder, X. and De Wals, P. Poor acceptance of caesarean section in Zimbabwe. *Tropical and Geographical Medicine* 1989; 41: 230-233. WHE 2408

A survey was carried out in a maternity hospital in Gweru, Zimbabwe, in order to analyse the acceptance of caesarean section. The behaviour of 210 pregnant women who had had a previous caesarean section was compared with that of a control group of 278 women with no history of caesarean section. More frequently the former failed to attend the prenatal clinic and came to the maternity hospital in an advanced stage of labour. The majority did not wish to have a further caesarean section and did not know they were at high risk of complications.

The authors suggest that these findings have important implications for medical training and public health policies. The medical indications for caesarean section should be restricted to the safest minimum and other procedures such as symphysiotomy, oxytocin use for dysfunctional labour, instrumental extraction and external cephalic version for breech presentation should be considered. Educational programmes targeted at pregnant women should be devised and tested in order to increase health care compliance when caesarean section is required.

Dick, J.S. and Strover, R.M. Vaginoplasty following vesicovaginal fistula repair: a preliminary report. *South African Medical Journal* 1971; June: 617-620. WHE 2129

From 1968-1969 there were 4 418 patients discharged from the gynaecological wards of Harare Hospital, Harare, Zimbabwe. Of these, 127 women developed a vesicovaginal fistula as a result of obstetrical trauma, usually in their first pregnancy. The authors have found that vaginal stenosis with severe dyspareunia or apareunia often remains following repair of a vesicovaginal fistula caused by obstructed labour. They therefore carried out vaginoplasty operation – insertion of full-thickness flaps of labia minora into the incised fibrous wall of the vagina – on five women to correct vaginal stenosis following fistula repair. Details of the operation are described. In four cases the grafts had taken satisfactorily at a six month follow-up exam. The vagina in each case was soft and pliable and coitus was reported to be satisfactory. The repaired fistulae also remained intact.

Linke, C.A. et al. Bladder and urethral injuries following prolonged labor. *Journal of Urology* 1971; 105: 679-682. WHE 2169

During a one-year period (1967-68) ten women who survived prolonged labour but sustained injury to the bladder or urethra were evaluated at the Willis F. Pierce Memorial Hospital, Mt. Selinka, Zimbabwe. Seven of the women were primiparous. Closure of the fistula was accomplished in all patients in whom it was attempted, but stress incontinence persisted in three. Preoperative evaluation is discussed.

8. FURTHER READING

Brown, I. and Cruickshank, J.G. Aetiological factors in pelvic inflammatory disease in urban blacks in Rhodesia. *South African Medical Journal* 1976; 50: 1342-1344. WHE 1042

Mahomed, K. et al. The young pregnant teenager - why the poor outcome? *Central African Journal of Medicine* 1989; 35(5): 403-406. WHE 2281

Mason, P.R. and Patterson, B. Epidemiology and clinical diagnosis of Trichomonas Vaginalis infection in Zimbabwe.

Mutambirwa, J. Pregnancy, childbirth, mother and child care among the indigenous people of Zimbabwe. *International Journal of Gynecology and Obstetrics* 1985; 23(4): 275-285. WHE 1324

Mutambirwa, J. Health problems in rural communities, Zimbabwe. *Social Science and Medicine* 1989; 29(8): 927-932. WHE 2473

9. DATA SOURCES

WHE 0110   Brown, I. Maternal mortality: a survey of maternal deaths occurring during 1976. *Central African Journal of Medicine* 1978; 24(10): 212-214

WHE 0798   World Health Organization, Extended Programme of Immunization. Coverage evaluation Zimbabwe. *Weekly Epidemiological Record* 1983; 58: 45

WHE 0834   World Health Organization. *World Health Statistics annual – vital statistics and causes of death.* Geneva, various years

WHE 0845   Zimbabwe, Ministry of Health. *Report of the Secretary for Health for the year ended 31 December 1979.* 1980

WHE 1255   Egullion, C. Training traditional midwives in Manicaland, Zimbabwe. *International Journal of Gynecology and Obstetrics* 1985; 23: 287-290

WHE 1307   Crowther, C.A. Maternal deaths at Harare Maternity Hospital during 1983. *South African Medical Journal* 1986; 69: 180-182

WHE 1389   Crowther, C. Prevention of maternal deaths: a continuing challenge. *Central African Journal of Medicine* 1986; 32(1): 11-14

WHE 1914   United Nations Children's Fund (UNICEF). *The state of the world's children,* various years, Oxford, Oxford University Press

WHE 1915   United Nations. Department of International Economic and Social Affairs. *World population prospects: estimates and projections as assessed in 1984.* Population Studies No. 98. New York 1986

WHE 1918   United Nations. Department of International Economic and Social Affairs. *First marriage: patterns and determinants.* New York 1988

WHE 1976   De Muylder, X. Maternity services in a general hospital. Part I: Obstetrical data. *Central African Journal of Medicine* 1987;

WHE 2033   World Health Organization. *Global strategy for health for all by the year 2000. Second report on monitoring progress.* WHO document EB83/2 Add. 1, 1988

WHE 2481   De Muylder, X. and Thiery, M. L'impact d'une nouvelle stratégie obstetricale stricte sur la mortalité maternelle et les résultats obstetricaux. *Archives Belges* 1989; 47(1-4): 67-69

WHE 2516   Demographic and Health Surveys. *Zimbabwe demographic and health survey 1988.* Ministry of Health/Institute for Resource Development/Westinghouse 1989.

WHE 2561   Department of Census and Statistics. *Health Statistics Annual Report 1988.* Harare 1989

LATIN AMERICA

ARGENTINA

	Year	Source

1. BASIC INDICATORS

1.1 Demographic

1.1.1 Population
Size (millions)	32.3	1990	(1915)
Rate of growth (%)	1.3	1985-90	(1915)

1.1.2 Life expectancy
Female	74	1985-90	(1915)
Male	67	1985-90	(1915)

1.1.3 Fertility
Crude Birth Rate	21	1985-90	(1915)
Total Fertility Rate	3.0	1985-90	(1915)

1.1.4 Mortality
Crude Death Rate	9	1985-90	(1915)
Infant Mortality Rate	32	1985-90	(1915)
Female	24	1986	(2827)
Male	30	1986	(2827)
1-4 years mortality rate			
Female	1	1986	(2827)
Male	1	1986	(2827)

1.2 Social and economic

1.2.1 Adult literacy rate (%)
Female	95	1985	(1914)
Male	96	1985	(1914)

1.2.2 Primary school enrolment rate (%)
Female	110	1986-88	(1914)
Male	110	1986-88	(1914)

1.2.3 Female mean age at first marriage
(years)	22.9	1980	(1918)

	Year	Source

1.2.4 GNP/capita
(US $)	2 390	1987	(1914)

1.2.5 Daily per capita calorie supply
(as % of requirements)	136	1984-86	(1914)

2. HEALTH SERVICES

2.1 Health Expenditure

2.1.1 Expenditure on health
(as % of GNP)	8.2	1984	(2033)

2.1.2 Expenditure on PHC
(as % of total health expenditure)

2.2 Primary Health Care
(Percentage of population covered by):

2.2.1 Health services
National
Urban
Rural

2.2.2 Safe water
National	67	1983	(0834)
Urban	72	1983	(0834)
Rural	19	1983	(0834)

2.2.3 Adequate sanitary facilities
National	84	1983	(0834)
Urban	93	1983	(0834)
Rural	37	1983	(0834)

2.2.4 Contraceptive prevalence rate
(%)	74	1980-88	(1914)

2.3   Coverage of maternity care (%)

Area	Prenatal care	Trained attendant	Institutional deliveries	Postnatal care	Sample size	Year	Source
National			90			1985	(1372)
National			93			1987	(2713)
Buenos Aires	67				27 882	1989	(2760)
Cordoba			99			1979	(0515)
Salta, rural			20			1985	(2428)

3. COMMUNITY STUDIES

3.1   Greater Cordoba Metropolitan Area, 1987 [2316]

An analysis of death certificates for all women of reproductive age was carried out. Hospital records, for both public and private institutions were examined. A total of 17 maternal deaths had been registered as such. The investigators found a further 24 deaths which were most probably pregnancy related. The level of under-registration was over 58%. The quality of the case histories kept was substantially better in the public hospitals than in private institutions.

3.1.1   Rate

Live births	22 756
Maternal deaths registered	17
MMR (per 100 000 live births)	75
Total maternal deaths including under-registration	41
MMR (per 100 000 live births)	180

3.1.2   Causes of maternal deaths *(for all 41 deaths)*

	Number	%
Complications of surgical intervention	9	22
Abortion	7	17
Hypertensive disorders of pregnancy	4	10
Embolisms	4	10
Haemorrhage	4	10
Fetal death/disseminated intravascular coagulation	4	10
Premature rupture of the membranes	1	2
Coriocarcinoma	1	2
Other complications of pregnancy	7	17
TOTAL	41	100

3.1.3   Avoidable factors

Of the 41 deaths 32 (78%) were considered by the investigators to have been avoidable.

4. HOSPITAL STUDIES

5. CIVIL REGISTRATION DATA/GOVERNMENT ESTIMATES

5.1   National, 1960-86 and by region, 1980-81
(0825, 0827, 1625, 1960, 2713, 2722, 2827)

5.1.1   Rate
National

	Maternal deaths	MMR (per 100 000 live births)
1960	512	108
1965	688	143
1970	757	154
1980	485	70
1981	472	69
1982	464	70
1983	395	60
1984	386	61
1985	386	59
1986	369	55

By region, 1980

Region	MMR (per 100 000 live births)
Buenos Aires	50
Capital Federal	31
Catamarca	86
Chaco	125
Chubut	99
Cordoba	52
Corrientes	102

Region	MMR (per 100 000 live births)
Entre Rios	39
Formosa	170
Ignorada	35
Jujuy	161
La Pampa	50
La Rioja	57
Mendoza	68
Misiones	108
Neuquén	50
Rio Negro	26
Salta	160
San Juan	108
San Luis	112
Santa Cruz	46
Santa Fé	66
Santiago del Estero	97
Tierra del Fuego	–
Tucuman	104
Total	70

5.1.2 Causes of maternal deaths, 1981 and 1986.

	% 1981	1986
Abortion	32	35
Hypertensive disorders of pregnancy	16	–
Haemorrhage	14	14
Sepsis	8	n.a.
Embolisms	3	n.a.
Complications of the puerperium	3	16
Ectopic pregnancy	2	n.a.
Hydatidiform mole	<1	n.a.
Other direct obstetric causes	21	35
TOTAL	100	100

5.1.3 Avoidable factors

5.1.4 High risk groups, 1968-70 and 1978-80
Age

	MMR (per 100 000 live births)		Relative risk (20-24=1)	
	1968-70	1978-80	1968-70	1978-80
<20	135	66	1.69	1.47
20-24	81	45	1.00	1.00
25-29	100	56	1.24	1.25
30-34	167	89	2.08	2.16
35-39	271	170	3.39	3.80
40-44	357	201	4.41	4.44
45+	236	171	2.93	3.81

Age and cause specific mortality rates (1978-80) show that abortion and haemorrhage mortality rates are highest among older women.

	MMR (per 100 000 live births)							
	<20	20-24	25-29	30-34	35-39	40-44	45+	Total
Abortion	20	18	21	29	41	48	57	24
Hypertensive disorders of pregnancy	25	7	6	14	29	37	29	13
Haemorrhage	7	3	8	15	39	48	29	12
Sepsis	8	6	5	9	11	26	29	8
Other causes	8	11	15	23	50	42	29	18
Total	66	45	56	89	170	201	171	75

5.2 Salta Province, 1981-1989 [2793]

5.2.1 Rate

	Live births	Maternal deaths	MMR (per 100 000 live births)
1981	23 473	35	149
1982	23 472	52	222
1983	22 695	34	150
1984	23 457	25	107
1985	24 112	27	112
1986*	25 873	27	104
1987*	25 007	28	112
1988*	24 707	28	113
1989*	23 470	23	98

*   Provisional

6. OTHER SOURCES/ ESTIMATES

6.1 National, 1990 [2713]

National maternal mortality rates were recalculated by PAHO adjusting for underreporting of deaths as observed in the Cordoba study. Half of all maternal deaths were not registered as such.

6.1.1 Rate
Births	669 000
Maternal deaths	936
MMR (per 100 000 births)	140

7. SELECTED ANNOTATED BIBLIOGRAPHY

De la Fuente, M. Maternal mortality and morbidity: a call to women for action. *Women's Global Network for Reproductive Rights Newsletter* 30, July – September 1989. WHE 2338

An extract from the report of the Second National Women's Conference on Health and Development states that given the low fertility rate the level of maternal mortality is surprisingly high, all the more so as the rate of institutional delivery is approaching 95%. Maternal death is one of the five most important causes of death among women of reproductive age and mortality rates are particularly high in the north of the country. Abortion accounts for over a third of the maternal deaths followed by eclampsia and haemorrhage (around 15%).

8. FURTHER READING

Chackiel, J. *Medicion indirecta de la mortalidad materna*. Unpublished document presented at the Reunion regional sobre prevencion de la mortalidad materna, Sao Paulo, 12-15 April 1988. WHE 2387

9. DATA SOURCES

WHE 0515   Ortiz, M.E.A. *Cordoba developmental program for mother and child care.* (unpublished research proposal prepared for the Meeting of the Steering Committee of the Task Force on the Risk Approach and Programme Research in MCH/FP Care, Geneva 1983.

WHE 0825   World Health Organization. Pan American Health Organization. *Health conditions in the Americas. 1969-72.* (PAHO scientific publication no. 306) PAHO, Washington, 1975.

WHE 0827   World Health Organization. Pan American Health Organization. *Health conditions in the Americas. 1977-1980.* (PAHO scientific publication no. 427) PAHO, Washington, 1982.

WHE 0834   World Health Organization. *World Health Statistics Annual – vital statistics and causes of death.* Geneva, various years.

WHE 1372   World Health Organization. Pan American Health Organization. *Documento de referencia sobre estudio y prevención de la mortalidad materna.* (unpublished document no. HRM/HST.) March 1986.

WHE 1625   World Health Organization, Pan American Health Organization. *Health conditions in the Americas.* 1981-84. Vol. I (PAHO Scientific Publication no. 500). PAHO, Washington, 1986.

WHE 1914   United Nations Children's Fund (UNICEF). *The state of the world's children*, Oxford University Press,Oxford, various years.

WHE 1915   United Nations. Department of International Economic and Social Affairs. *World population prospects: estimates and projections as assessed in 1984.* Population Studies No. 98. New York 1986.

WHE 1918   United Nations. Department of International Economic and Social Affairs. *First marriage: patterns and determinants.* New York 1988.

WHE 1960   Argentina, Ministerio de Salud y Acción Social. *La mortalidad materna en la Argentina.* Analisis de datos serie 8, numero 4, Buenos Aires, Republica Argentina 1987.

WHE 2033   World Health Organization. *Global strategy for health for all by the year 2000. Second report on monitoring progress.* WHO document EB83/2 Add. 1, 1988.

WHE 2316   Molina Morey de Illia, M. et al. *Resumen de la metodologia y resultados de la investigacion sobre mortalidad materna en la provincia de Cordoba, Argentina* (unpublished document) 1989.

WHE 2428   Casares de Vergara, M.A. *Affective learning for non-risk motherhood* (unpublished document) Salta, Argentina, 1990.

WHE 2713   World Health Organization, Pan American Health Organization *Regional plan of action for the reduction of maternal mortality in the Americas,* Document No. CSP23/10, XXIII Pan American Sanitary Conference, Washington 1990.

WHE 2722   World Health Organization, *Maternal deaths and maternal mortality rates* (unpublished) 1990.

WHE 2760   Cattaneo, M. et al. *Programa educativo para una maternidad sin riesgo.* (unpublished), Buenos Aires, 1990.

WHE 2793   Casares, M.A. et al. *Hacia una maternidad sin riesgo.* Grupo NACE, WHO/PAHO, Salta, 1990.

WHE 2827   World Health Organization. Pan American Health Organization. *Health conditions in the Americas,* Scientific Publication No. 524, Washington, 1990.

BAHAMAS

	Year	Source

1. BASIC INDICATORS

1.1 Demographic

1.1.1 Population

Size (millions)	0.2	1989	(2827)
Rate of growth (%)	1.3	1980-85	(1625)

1.1.2 Life expectancy
Female
Male

1.1.3 Fertility

Crude Birth Rate	20	1988	(2827)
Total Fertility Rate			

1.1.4 Mortality

Crude Death Rate	5	1988	(2827)
Infant Mortality Rate	29	1987	(2827)
Female	28	1987	(2827)
Male	30	1987	(2827)
1-4 years mortality rate			
Female	2	1987	(2827)
Male	1	1987	(2827)

1.2 Social and economic

1.2.1 Adult literacy rate (%)

Female	89	1963	(2458)
Male	90	1963	(2458)

1.2.2 Primary school enrolment rate (%)
Female
Male

1.2.3 Female mean age at first marriage
(years)

	Year	Source

1.2.4 GNP/capita

(US $)	10 700	1988	(1914)

1.2.5 Daily per capita calorie supply
(as % of requirements)

2. HEALTH SERVICES

2.1 Health Expenditure

2.1.1 Expenditure on health

(as % of GNP)	6.5	1984	(2033)

2.1.2 Expenditure on PHC

(as % of total health expenditure)	8	1980	(1942)

2.2 Primary Health Care
(Percentage of population covered by):

2.2.1 Health services

National	100	1984	(1625)
Urban			
Rural			

2.2.2 Safe water

National	100	1985	(2033)
Urban	100	1985	(2033)
Rural			

2.2.3 Adequate sanitary facilities

National	100	1985	(2033)
Urban	100	1985	(2033)
Rural			

2.2.4 Contraceptive prevalence rate
(%)

2.3   Coverage of maternity care (%)

Area	Prenatal care	Trained attendant	Institutional deliveries	Postnatal care	Sample size	Year	Source
National			98			1981	(2334)
National	99	99				1984	(0834)
National	100	100				1987	(2033)

3. COMMUNITY STUDIES

4. HOSPITAL STUDIES

5. CIVIL REGISTRATION DATA/GOVERNMENT ESTIMATES

5.1   National, 1970-87 (0825, 0826, 0827, 0834, 1625, 2722)

5.1.1   Rate

	Maternal deaths	MMR (per 100 000 live births)
1970	4	94
1975	2	50
1980	0	–
1985	1	18
1987	3	69

6. OTHER SOURCES/ ESTIMATES

7. SELECTED ANNOTATED BIBLIOGRAPHY

8. FURTHER READING

9. DATA SOURCES

WHE 0825   World Health Organization. Pan American Health Organization. *Health conditions in the Americas. 1969-72.* (PAHO scientific publication no. 306) PAHO, Washington, 1975.

WHE 0826   World Health Organization. Pan American Health Organization. *Health conditions in the Americas. 1973-1976.* (PAHO scientific publication no. 364) PAHO, Washington, 1982.

WHE 0827   World Health Organization. Pan American Health Organization. *Health conditions in the Americas. 1977-1980.* (PAHO scientific publication no. 427) PAHO, Washington 1982.

WHE 0834   World Health Organization *World Health Statistics annual – vital statistics and causes of death.* Geneva, various years.

WHE 1625   World Health Organization, Pan American Health Organization. *Health conditions in the Americas.* 1981-84. Vol. I (PAHO Scientific Publication no. 500). PAHO, Washington, 1986.

WHE 1914   United Nations Children's Fund (UNICEF). *The state of the world's children*, Oxford University Press, Oxford, various years.

WHE 1942   World Health Organization. Pan American Health Organization. *Evaluation of the strategy for Health for All by the Year 2000.* Seventh Report on the World Health Situation. Vol.3. Region of the Americas. PAHO, Washington, 1986.

WHE 2033   World Health Organization. *Global strategy for health for all by the year 2000. Second report on monitoring progress.* WHO document EB83/2 Add. 1, 1988.

WHE 2334   Sinha, D.P. *Children of the Caribbean* Caribbean Food and Nutrition Institute/Pan American Health Organization 1988.

WHE 2458   United Nations Educational, Social and Cultural Organization, UNESCO, *Compendium of statistics of illiteracy.* Division of Statistics on Education, Paris 1988.

WHE 2722   World Health Organization, *Maternal deaths and maternal mortality rates* (unpublished) 1990.

WHE 2827   World Health Organization. Pan American Health Organization. *Health conditions in the Americas*, Scientific Publication No. 524, Washington, 1990.

BARBADOS

		Year	Source

1. BASIC INDICATORS

1.1 Demographic

1.1.1 Population

Size (millions)	0.3	1990	(1915)
Rate of growth (%)	0.2	1985-90	(1915)

1.1.2 Life expectancy

Female	77	1985-90	(1915)
Male	72	1985-90	(1915)

1.1.3 Fertility

Crude Birth Rate	16	1985-90	(1915)
Total Fertility Rate	1.8	1985-90	(1915)

1.1.4 Mortality

Crude Death Rate	9	1985-90	(1915)
Infant Mortality Rate	11	1985-90	(1915)
Female	15	1984	(1625)
Male	19	1984	(1625)
1-4 years mortality rate			
Female	1	1984	(1625)
Male	1	1984	(1625)

1.2 Social and economic

1.2.1 Adult literacy rate (%)

Female	99	1970	(2458)
Male	99	1970	(2458)

1.2.2 Primary school enrolment rate (%)

Female	108	1983-86	(1914)
Male	113	1983-86	(1914)

1.2.3 Female mean age at first marriage
(years)

1.2.4 GNP/capita
(US $)   6 010   1988   (1914)

1.2.5 Daily per capita calorie supply
(as % of requirements)

2. HEALTH SERVICES

2.1 Health Expenditure

2.1.1 Expenditure on health
(as % of GNP)   4.3   1984   (2033)

2.1.2 Expenditure on PHC

(as % of total health			
expenditure)	13	1984	(1942)

2.2 Primary Health Care
(Percentage of population covered by):

2.2.1 Health services

National	100	1983	(0834)
Urban			
Rural			

2.2.2 Safe water

National	100	1985	(2033)
Urban	100	1985	(2033)
Rural	100	1985	(2033)

2.2.3 Adequate sanitary facilities

National	100	1985	(2033)
Urban	100	1985	(2033)
Rural	100	1985	(2033)

2.2.4 Contraceptive prevalence rate
(%)

2.3   Coverage of maternity care (%)

Area	Prenatal care	Trained attendant	Institutional deliveries	Postnatal care	Sample size	Year	Source
National	98	98				1984	(0834)

3. COMMUNITY STUDIES

4. HOSPITAL STUDIES

5. CIVIL REGISTRATION DATA/GOVERNMENT ESTIMATES

5.1   National, 1960-88 (0825, 0826, 0827, 1625, 2722)

5.1.1   Rate

	Maternal deaths	MMR (per 100 000 live births)
1960	17	217
1965	7	110
1970	7	143
1975	1	21
1980	1	24
1986	1	24
1988	1	27

6. OTHER SOURCES/ ESTIMATES

7. SELECTED ANNOTATED BIBLIOGRAPHY

8. FURTHER READING

9. DATA SOURCES

WHE 0825   World Health Organization. Pan American Health Organization. *Health conditions in the Americas. 1969-72.* (PAHO scientific publication no. 306) Washington, PAHO 1975.

WHE 0826   World Health Organization. Pan American Health Organization. *Health conditions in the Americas. 1973-1976.* (PAHO scientific publication no. 364) Washington, PAHO, 1982.

WHE 0827   World Health Organization. Pan American Health Organization. *Health conditions in the Americas. 1977-1980.* (PAHO scientific publication no. 427) Washington, PAHO, 1982.

WHE 0834   World Health Organization *World Health Statistics annual – vital statistics and causes of death.* Geneva, various years.

WHE 1625   World Health Organization, Pan American Health Organization. *Health conditions in the Americas.* 1981-84. Vol. I (PAHO Scientific Publication no. 500). Washington, PAHO 1986.

WHE 1914   United Nations Children's Fund (UNICEF). *The state of the world's children*, Oxford University Press, Oxford, various years.

WHE 1915   United Nations. Department of International Economic and Social Affairs. *World population prospects: estimates and projections as assessed in 1984.* Population Studies No. 98. New York 1986.

WHE 1942   World Health Organization. Pan American Health Organization. *Evaluation of the strategy for Health for All by the Year 2000.* Seventh Report on the World Health Situation. Vol.3. Region of the Americas. PAHO, Washington, 1986.

WHE 2033   World Health Organization. *Global strategy for health for all by the year 2000. Second report on monitoring progress.* WHO document EB83/2 Add. 1, 1988.

WHE 2458   United Nations Educational, Social and Cultural Organization, *Compendium of statistics of illiteracy.* Division of Statistics on Education, UNESCO, Paris 1988.

WHE 2722   World Health Organization, *Maternal deaths and maternal mortality rates* (unpublished) 1990.

BOLIVIA

	Year	Source

1. BASIC INDICATORS

1.1 Demographic

1.1.1 Population

		Year	Source
Size (millions)	7.3	1990	(1915)
Rate of growth (%)	2.8	1985-90	(1915)

1.1.2 Life expectancy

		Year	Source
Female	55	1985-90	(1915)
Male	51	1985-90	(1915)

1.1.3 Fertility

		Year	Source
Crude Birth Rate	43	1985-90	(1915)
Total Fertility Rate	6.1	1985-90	(1915)

1.1.4 Mortality

		Year	Source
Crude Death Rate	14	1985-90	(1915)
Infant Mortality Rate	110	1985-90	(1915)
Female	86	1979-89	(2839)
Male	106	1979-89	(2839)
1-4 years mortality rate			
Female	51	1979-89	(2839)
Male	51	1979-89	(2839)

1.2 Social and economic

1.2.1 Adult literacy rate (%)

		Year	Source
Female	65	1985	(1914)
Male	84	1985	(1914)

1.2.2 Primary school enrolment rate (%)

		Year	Source
Female	85	1986-88	(1914)
Male	97	1986-88	(1914)

1.2.3 Female mean age at first marriage

		Year	Source
(years)	22.1	1976	(1918)

1.2.4 GNP/capita

		Year	Source
(US $)	580	1987	(1914)

1.2.5 Daily per capita calorie supply

		Year	Source
(as % of requirements)	89	1984-86	(1914)

2. HEALTH SERVICES

2.1 Health Expenditure

2.1.1 Expenditure on health

		Year	Source
(as % of GNP)	0.4	1984	(2033)

2.1.2 Expenditure on PHC
(as % of total health expenditure)

2.2 Primary Health Care
(Percentage of population covered by):

2.2.1 Health services
National
Urban
Rural

2.2.2 Safe water

		Year	Source
National	43	1983	(0834)
Urban	81	1985	(2033)
Rural	27	1985	(2033)

2.2.3 Adequate sanitary facilities

		Year	Source
National	24	1983	(0834)
Urban	51	1985	(2033)
Rural	22	1985	(2033)

2.2.4 Contraceptive prevalence rate

		Year	Source
(%)	30*	1987	(2713)

* Married or cohabiting women aged 15-49 years.

2.3   Coverage of maternity care (%)

Area	Prenatal care	Trained attendant	Institutional deliveries	Postnatal care	Sample size	Year	Source
National			20			1984	(2038)
National	17	17				1983-87	(2033)
National			30			1985-88	(3013)
National	50		38			1989	(2713)
National:	45	42			5 764	1985-89	(2839)
urban	62	63			2 779	1985-89	(2839)
rural	29	23			2 985	1985-89	(2839)
Altiplano	39	34			2 874	1985-89	(2839)
Valles	46	44			1 615	1985-89	(2839)
Llanos	58	58			1 274	1985-89	(2839)

3.   COMMUNITY STUDIES

3.1   National, 1989 [2565, 2585]

An application of the "sisterhood method" was undertaken in connection with a demographic and health survey. Respondents were all women aged 15-49 years and information was sought about sisters ever married or cohabiting. The total sample size was 7,454 and there were 116 maternal deaths. The lifetime risk for women aged between 15 and 49 years was calculated as one in 44.

3.1.1   Rate
MMR (per 100 000 live births)   371

3.2   Province of Avaroa, 1988 [2565]

A survey was carried out among a rural population where the female life expectancy was 42.5 years and the total fertility rate was 7.5 children per woman. The "sisterhood method" was used to estimate maternal mortality rates. The weighted sample size was 5,784 adults and there were an estimated 386 maternal deaths. The lifetime risk of dying from pregnancy related causes was estimated at one in ten.

3.2.1   Rate*
MMR (per 100 000 live births)   1 379

*   Based on data from respondents aged 25-39 years.

4.   HOSPITAL STUDIES

4.1   National, hospital data 1985-88 [3013]

4.1.1   Rate

MMR (per 100 000 live births)

1985	200
1986	154
1987	210
1988	247

5.   CIVIL REGISTRATION DATA/GOVERNMENT ESTIMATES

5.1   National, 1973-77 [0791, 2713]

5.1.1   Rate
MMR (per 100 000 live births)   480

6. OTHER SOURCES/ ESTIMATES

6.1 National, 1990 [2713]

An adjusted rate was estimated by PAHO on the basis of information from the Ministry of Social Welfare and Public Health on the degree of underreporting of maternal deaths.

6.1.1 Rate
Births	293 000
Maternal deaths	1 758
MMR (per 100 000 live births)	600

6.2 National, (1990) [2809]

A study was carried out by MEDICON SRL which estimated the degree of under reporting of maternal deaths at 80%.

6.2.1 Rate
Maternal deaths	1 530
MMR (per 100 000 live births)	770

7. SELECTED ANNOTATED BIBLIOGRAPHY

Bailey, P.E. et al. A hospital study of illegal abortion in Bolivia. *PAHO Bulletin* 1988; 22(1): 27-41. WHE 2061

Over the twelve-month period, July 1983-84, data were collected at eleven hospitals in five Bolivian cities on 4 371 women admitted for medical treatment following spontaneous or illegally induced abortions. The abortion was illegally induced in 23% of the cases, of which 65% were induced by medically trained persons and 35% by people without medical training or by the women themselves. Seven of the hospitalized women died, a mortality rate of 160 per 100 000 admissions. Twenty women had to have total hysterectomies as a result of abortion-induced complications.

World Health Organization. Pan American Health Organization. *Health conditions in the Americas*, Scientific Publication No. 524, Washington, 1990. WHE 2827

A report of the Pan American Health Organization quotes a study of four hospitals in Bolivia which found an institutional maternal mortality rate of 90 per 100 000 live births coupled with a rate of caesarean delivery of 19%. It is noted that there is considerable variation in rates of caesarean delivery in different countries of the region, from under 10% in Honduras to over 30% in Mexico. An epidemiological study of caesarean delivery, undertaken by the Centro Latino Americano de Perinatology y Desarrollo Humano (CLAP) and PAHO in 1985 in 17 countries indicated that the frequency of caesarean delivery explains only 5% of the variations in perinatal mortality and that there is no correlation between frequency of operative delivery and reduction in maternal mortality. Indeed, caesarean delivery is associated with higher rates of mortality and morbidity than vaginal delivery and is a bigger strain on the human and financial resources of the health service.

8. FURTHER READING

Chackiel, J. *Medicion indirecta de la mortalidad materna*. Unpublished document presented at the Reunion regional sobre prevencion de la mortalidad materna, Sao Paulo, 12-15 April 1988. WHE 2387

Frerichs, R.R. et al. A household survey of health and illness in rural Bolivia *Bulletin of the Pan American Health Organization* 1980; 14(4): 343-355. WHE 2202

9. DATA SOURCES

WHE 0791   World Health Organization. *Sixth Report on the World Health Situation* 1973-77. Part II: review by country and area. Geneva, 1980.

WHE 0834   World Health Organization *World Health Statistics annual – vital statistics and causes of death.* Geneva, various years.

WHE 1914   United Nations Children's Fund (UNICEF). *The state of the world's children*, Oxford University Press, Oxford, various years.

WHE 1915   United Nations. Department of International Economic and Social Affairs. *World population prospects: estimates and projections as assessed in 1984.* Population Studies No. 98. New York 1986.

WHE 1918   United Nations. Department of International Economic and Social Affairs. *First marriage: patterns and determinants.* New York 1988.

WHE 2033   World Health Organization. *Global strategy for health for all by the year 2000. Second report on monitoring progress.* WHO document EB83/2 Add. 1, 1988.

WHE 2038   World Health Organization, Pan American Health Organization. *Regional Committee document* no. CE101/9. 1988.

WHE 2565   Maine, D. *Results of applications of the sisterhood method for estimating maternal mortality* London School of Hygiene and Tropical Medicine, 1990 (unpublished document).

WHE 2585   Rutenberg, N. et al. *Direct and indirect estimates of maternal mortality with data on the survivorship of sisters: results from the Bolivia demographic and health survey.* Paper prepared for presentation at the Annual Meeting of the Population Association of America, Toronto, Ontario, 3-5 May 1990.

WHE 2713   World Health Organization, Pan American Health Organization *Regional plan of action for the reduction of maternal mortality in the Americas,* Document No. CSP23/10, XXIII Pan American Sanitary Conference, Washington 1990.

WHE 2809   Bolivia, Ministry of Health. *Mortalidad materna total y especifica, tendencias. Subregistro estimado.* (unpublished), 1990.

WHE 2839   Demographic and Health Surveys. *Encuesta nacional de demografía y salud 1989.* Instituto Nacional de Estadística/Institute for Resource Development/Macro Systems Inc. 1990.

WHE 3013   Bolivia, Ministerio de Prevision Social y Salud Publica. *Fundamentos de la política nacional de salud.* La Paz, 1991.

BRAZIL

	Year	Source

1. BASIC INDICATORS

1.1 Demographic

1.1.1 Population

		Year	Source
Size (millions)	150	1990	(1915)
Rate of growth (%)	2.1	1985-90	(1915)

1.1.2 Life expectancy

		Year	Source
Female	68	1985-90	(1915)
Male	62	1985-90	(1915)

1.1.3 Fertility

		Year	Source
Crude Birth Rate	29	1985-90	(1915)
Total Fertility Rate	3.5	1985-90	(1915)

1.1.4 Mortality

		Year	Source
Crude Death Rate	8	1985-90	(1915)
Infant Mortality Rate	63	1985-90	(1915)
Female	54	1984	(0753)
Male	68	1984	(0753)
1-4 years mortality rate			
Female			
Male			

1.2 Social and economic

1.2.1 Adult literacy rate (%)

		Year	Source
Female	77	1985	(1914)
Male	80	1985	(1914)

1.2.2 Primary school enrolment rate (%)

Female			
Male			

1.2.3 Female mean age at first marriage

		Year	Source
(years)	22.6	1980	(1918)

1.2.4 GNP/capita

		Year	Source
(US $)	2 160	1988	(1914)

1.2.5 Daily per capita calorie supply

(as % of requirements)	111	1984-86	(1914)

2. HEALTH SERVICES

2.1 Health Expenditure

2.1.1 Expenditure on health

		Year	Source
(as % of GNP)	3.5	1984	(2033)

2.1.2 Expenditure on PHC
(as % of total health expenditure)

2.2 Primary Health Care
(Percentage of population covered by):

2.2.1 Health services

National
Urban
Rural

2.2.2 Safe water

		Year	Source
National	75	1983	(0834)
Urban	86	1986	(2033)
Rural	53	1986	(2033)

2.2.3 Adequate sanitary facilities

		Year	Source
National	24	1983	(0834)
Urban	33	1985	(2033)
Rural	2	1985	(2033)

2.2.4 Contraceptive prevalence rate

		Year	Source
(%)	52	1980	(1712)
	66*	1987	(2713)

* Married or cohabiting women aged 15-49 years.

2.3   Coverage of maternity care (%)

Area	Prenatal care	Trained attendant	Institutional deliveries	Postnatal care	Sample size	Year	Source
National:	74	95	81		3 463	1981-86	(1634)
urban	86	98	92		2 307	1981-86	(1634)
rural	51	89	58		1 156	1981-86	(1634)
Centro-Este	79	95	85		475	1981-86	(1634)
Nordeste	55	95	67		1 297	1981-86	(1634)
Norte-Centro-Oeste	74	95	78		199	1981-86	(1634)
Pelotas,	94				7 392	1982	(1599)
Pernambuco	54	72	22		1 300w	1980	(0045)
Rio-de-Janeiro	85	100	99		269	1981-86	(1634)
Sao Paulo	92	94	93		656	1981-86	(1634)
Sao Paulo:							
metropolitan area	85				381w	1987-88	(2762)
interior	90				288w	1987-88	(2762)
Sorocaba	82	98	98		361	1980	(1600)
Sul	86		84		475	1981-86	(1634)

3.   COMMUNITY STUDIES

3.1   Municipality of Sao Paulo, 1986 (1992, 2287, 2828)

The study evaluated the accuracy of death certification in a sample of 25% of all deaths of women of reproductive age resident in the municipality. For each death, further data were gathered by means of household interviews and from medical records and autopsy information where available. In all 953 deaths were analysed. There were discrepancies between *declared* maternal deaths and *total* maternal deaths as determined through the analysis of certificates. Analysis of the latter showed that as well as the 100 declared maternal deaths there were an additional 118 deaths which were related to pregnancy, childbirth or complications of the puerperium. The maternal mortality rate based on declared deaths was 42 (per 100 000 live births) compared with 97 (per 100 000 live births) when all maternal deaths were taken into account. Follow-up interviews with relatives, medical and social workers etc. were carried out in order to determine socioeconomic status and details of pregnancy.

3.1.1   Rate

Live births	224 850
Maternal deaths	218*
MMR (per 100 000 live births)	97

*   Excluding six deaths which occurred after 42 days following the termination of pregnancy.

3.1.2   Causes of maternal deaths

	%
Hypertensive disorders of pregnancy	15
Abortion	7
Haemorrhage	6
Embolisms	5
Normal delivery	5
Ectopic pregnancy	4
Other complications of pregnancy	4
Sepsis	4
Venous complications	2
Other complications of the puerperium	7
DIRECT CAUSES	59
Infective and parasitic conditions	9
Other maternal conditions	34
INDIRECT CAUSES	43
TOTAL	100

4. HOSPITAL STUDIES

4.1 Municipal Hospital Miguel Couto, Rio de Janeiro, 1978-87 [2493]

4.1.1 Rate

Live births	18 071
Maternal deaths	32
MMR (per 100 000 live births)	177

4.1.2 Causes of maternal deaths

	Number	%
Abortion	15	47
Hypertensive disorders of pregnancy	6	19
Haemorrhage	4	13
Sepsis	1	3
Accident of anaesthesia	1	3
DIRECT CAUSES	27	85
Cardiopathies	2	6
Respiratory illness	2	6
Diabetes	1	3
INDIRECT CAUSES	5	15
TOTAL	32	100

Cause specific mortality rates changed significantly over the two five-year periods, 1978-82 and 1983-87. The major contributor to the increase in overall maternal mortality rates was abortion-related death.

	Cause-specific MMR (per 100 000 live births)	
	1978-82	1983-87
Abortion	54	130
Haemorrhage	27	15
Hypertensive disorders of pregnancy	18	58
Total	135	250

From 1978-87, there were 7 633 admissions for complications due to abortion, constituting 40% of all admissions to the maternity ward. The abortion mortality rate was 197 per 100 000 admissions.

4.2 Maternity and general hospitals, Florianópolis, Santa Catarina State, 1975-79 [0666]

4.2.1 Rate

Live births	43 380
Maternal deaths	44
MMR (per 100 000 live births)	101

4.2.2 Causes of maternal deaths

4.2.3 Avoidable factors

4.2.4 High risk groups, 1978-79

MMR (per 100 000 live births)

Age	
15-19	77
20-24	65
25-29	95
30-34	109
35-39	115
40-50	205

4.2.5 Other findings, 1978-79

Mortality rates were higher for women residing outside the city and for those who were delivered by caesarean section.

MMR (per 100 000 live births)

Place of residence	
City	52
Other areas	181

Type of delivery*	
Normal	39
Caesarean section	93

* Excluding deaths due to abortion or ectopic pregnancy.

4.3 Servico de Obstetrica, Hospital Municipal Salgado Filho, 1977-83 [2055]

4.3.1 Rate

Live births	10 828
Maternal deaths	21
MMR (per 100 000 live births)	194

4.3.2 Causes of maternal deaths

	Number	%
Sepsis	6	29
Haemorrhage	5	24
Abortion	4	19
Hypertensive disorders of pregnancy	2	10
Complications of anaesthesia	1	5
DIRECT CAUSES	18	86
Cardiorespiratory complications	1	5
Other indirect causes	1	5
INDIRECT CAUSES	2	10
Other	2	10
TOTAL	21	100

4.3.3 Avoidable factors

4.3.4 High risk groups

4.4 Maternidade Nossa Senhora de Lourdes, Goiânia-GO, 1970-78 [2119]

4.4.1 Rate

Live births	19 988
Maternal deaths	36
MMR (per 100 000 live births)	180

4.4.2 Causes of maternal mortality *(34 cases)*

	Number	%
Haemorrhage	11	32
Hypertensive disorders of pregnancy	7	21
Sepsis	2	6
Abortion	2	6
Ruptured uterus	2	6
Complications of anesthesia	2	6
DIRECT CAUSES	26	77
Cardiopathies	4	12
Other indirect causes	2	6
INDIRECT CAUSES	6	18
Incidental	2	6
TOTAL	34	100

4.4.3 Avoidable factors

28 deaths were considered to have been avoidable; 16 were due to medical staff and two were due to administrative errors. A further ten deaths were ascribed to socioeconomic or cultural factors. Only six deaths were classified as inevitable.

4.4.4 High risk groups

Older women (36+ years) and grand multiparae (7+ deliveries) were the most vulnerable groups.

	% of maternal deaths	% of survivors
Age		
15-20	15	24
21-25	24	35
26-30	21	20
31-35	12	10
36-40	15	6
>40	15	5
Parity		
Primiparae	32	38
2-4	18	42
5-7	12	9
7-10	15	8
10+	24	3

4.5 Maternidade do Hospital Geral de Goiânia INAMPS, 1975-83 [2117]

4.5.1 Rate

Live births	n.a.
Maternal deaths	34
MMR (per 100 000 live births)	311

4.5.2 Causes of maternal deaths

	Number	%
Abortion	8	24
Hypertensive disorders of pregnancy	8	24
Haemorrhage	5	15
Sepsis	4	12
Ruptured uterus	2	6
DIRECT CAUSES	27	79
Cardiopathies	2	6
Hepatitis	1	3
INDIRECT CAUSES	3	9
Incidental	4	12
TOTAL	34	100

4.5.4 Avoidable factors

Of the 34 maternal deaths, 25 were considered inevitable and nine avoidable. Of the latter, five resulted from medical errors, three from administrative errors and one was due to socioeconomic factors.

4.5.4 High risk groups

Older women (40+ years) and adolescents were the most vulnerable groups.

4.6 Thirty seven hospitals, Fundaçao SESP, 1979-81 [2804]

4.6.1 Rate

Admissions	121 039
Maternal deaths	296
MMR (per 100 000 admissions)	245

4.6.2 Causes of maternal deaths

	Number	%
Haemorrhage	81	27
Hypertensive disorders of pregnancy	69	23
Sepsis	57	19
Complications of operative intervention	29	10
Abortion	8	3
Other direct causes	28	9
DIRECT CAUSES	272	92
INDIRECT CAUSES	17	6
Unknown	7	2
TOTAL	296	100

4.6.3 Avoidable factors

4.6.4 High risk groups

Analysis by cause and age group

	MMR (per 100 000 live births)				
Age (years)	< 20	20-29	30-39	40-49	All ages
Haemorrhage	20	40	130	180	70
Hypertensive disorders of pregnancy	120	40	40	90	60
Other causes	80	70	170	130	100
All direct causes	220	150	330	400	230

5. CIVIL REGISTRATION DATA/GOVERNMENT ESTIMATES

5.1 National and by region, 1984 [1999]

The study gives registered maternal deaths as well as an estimate of "probable" maternal deaths if some deaths classified as caused by "septicaemia" (most probably resulting from induced abortion) are included as maternal deaths.

5.1.1 Rate

| | MMR (per 100 000 live births) | |
	Registered	Probable
North	313	344
North East	155	193
South East	70	100
South	81	106
Centre East	121	151
National	120	152

5.1.2 Causes of maternal deaths (registered deaths)

	Number	%
Complications of pregnancy	1 710	44
Complications of delivery	780	20
Complications of the puerperium	595	15
Abortion	487	13
Indirect obstetric causes	143	4
Other	149	4
TOTAL	3 864	100

5.1.3 Avoidable factors

5.1.4 High risk groups (registered deaths)

Age

| | MMR (per 100 000 live births) | | | | |
	15-19	20-29	30-39	40-49	Total
North	311	210	520	954	313
North East	151	100	231	489	155
South East	52	46	116	293	70
South	47	61	125	291	81
Centre East	83	89	227	469	121
National	106	80	187	436	120

5.2 National, 1987 [2713]

5.2.1 Rate

MMR (per 100 000 live births)	140

5.3 State of Sao Paulo, 1980 and 1984 [2810]

5.3.1 Rate

	Maternal deaths	MMR (per 100 000 live births)
1980	397	55
1984	333	49

The authors estimate that the true maternal mortality rate is at least twice as high as the figures given due to under reporting.

5.3.2 Causes of maternal deaths, 1984

	Number	%
Hypertensive disorders of pregnancy	104	31
Haemorrhage	45	14
Abortion	28	8
Other complications of labour	22	7
Abnormal uterine contractions	20	6
Sepsis	26	8
Embolism	5	2
Placenta problems	4	1
Other direct causes	17	5
Indirect causes	31	9
TOTAL	333	100

5.3.3 Avoidable factors

The authors estimate that in 30% of the deaths there were serious shortcomings in health care provided at the hospital or health centre. The caesarean delivery rate was 46%. Only 16% of the pregnant women received prenatal care and although these women had an average of four visits the authors state that the prenatal care provided was of "doubtful" quality.

5.4 National, women aged 10-19 years, 1980 [2824]

An analysis of official statistics on deaths of adolescents found that complications of pregnancy, delivery and the puerperium were responsible for 4% of the deaths of women aged 10-19 years and for over 6% of women aged 15-19. Maternal mortality ranked in 6th place as a cause of death among adolescent women.

5.4.1 Rate *(15-19 year old women)*

Maternal deaths	288
MMR (per 100 000 live births)	64

5.4.2   Causes of maternal deaths *(10-19 year old women)*

	Number	%
Hypertensive disorders of pregnancy	145	47
Sepsis	50	16
Haemorrhage	26	8
Abortion	18	6
Other complications of delivery	15	5
Embolisms	7	2
Ectopic pregnancy	5	2
Other direct causes	18	6
Unknown	22	7
Total	306	100

5.5   National, reporting areas only, 1986 [(2713)]

It is not possible to calculate the maternal mortality rate as only numerator data are available.

5.5.2   Causes of maternal deaths

	%
Hypertensive disorders of pregnancy	29
Haemorrhage	16
Complications during the puerperium	16
Abortion	13
Other direct causes	19
Indirect causes	7
TOTAL (N=1 814)	100

6.   OTHER SOURCES/ ESTIMATES

6.1   National and by region, 1980 [(1299)]

The study calculated maternal deaths and maternal mortality rates on the basis of registered deaths, with estimations for the "probable" true number of maternal deaths. Data for live births were derived from the 1980 national census which is thought to give a more realistic estimate of actual births during the year than the registration figures.

6.1.1   Rate

	MMR (per 100 000 live births)	
	Registered	Probable
North	143	338
North East	55	229
South East	72	83
South	72	92
Centre East	69	144
Brazil	70	154

6.2   National, 1990 [(2713)]

The national maternal mortality rate was adjusted for underreporting by PAHO on the basis of the study undertaken in Sao Paulo mentioned in section 3.1 (1992).

Births	4 086 000
Maternal deaths	8 172
MMR (per 100 000 births)	200

6.3   City of Palmares, 1977-82 [(2803)]

Since the early 1980s the city has developed a comprehensive and efficient medical-sanitary service which is thought to have resulted in major improvements in public health, including maternal health.

6.3.1   Rate

	MMR (per 100 000 live births)
1970-79	290
1980-82	60

7.   SELECTED ANNOTATED BIBLIOGRAPHY

Araujo, G. et al. Improving obstetric care by training traditional birth attendants, Fortaleza, Brazil. In: Potts, M. et al. (eds.) *Childbirth in developing countries.* MTP Press, Lancaster, 1983. WHE 0564

An attempt was made to improve maternity care in a poor rural area in northeast Brazil. After discussions with community leaders their support was enlisted in recruiting local TBAs to participate in a programme to upgrade their skills. In addition, community leaders offered the use of a vacant building to serve as an obstetric unit. After a three-month practical and theoretical course, some of the newly trained TBAs were designated to work in the unit and the rest returned to continue their domiciliary work with instructions for referral of high risk pregnancies. Over a 10-month period from October 1980 to July 1981 data were obtained for 1 881 deliveries, of which 235 were cases referred for delivery from the local obstetric units to the teaching maternity hospital in the capital city of the region. It was found that the TBA training project achieved its primary goal of safer delivery and that TBAs with little formal education were able to identify and refer high-risk women while conducting safe deliveries in their own communities. The authors observe that community involvement is a vital ingredient in success of such programmes.

Beria, J.U. Back-street abortion in Brazil. *Lancet* 6 April 1983. WHE 0081

A study of registered maternal deaths in the southernmost state, Rio Grande do Sul, over the period 1974-78, found a total of 633 deaths registered as due to complications of pregnancy, childbirth and the puerperium. Abortion was the registered cause of death in 129 cases, 20% of the total. Only two were registered as induced for legal reasons and two others as spontaneous abortions.

Cecatti, J.G. et al. A experiência da Casa de Repouso do CAISM da Unicamp. *Revista Paulista de Medicina*, 1989, 107(4,5,6): 239-243. WHE 2960.

The Centre for Integral Women's Health Care (CAISM) of the State University of Campinas, has established a rest home which includes a maternity waiting area to accomodate women with a high risk of developing complications during pregnancy and delivery. The home also admits mothers in neonatal units who are required to breastfeed and women with gynaecological conditions. The conditions for admission are that the women need to make frequent visits to the hospital outpatient clinic but live far away and cannot afford rapid and easy transportation. The home offers lodging and food at a fraction of the cost of inpatient treatment. Between July 1986 and January 1989 a total of 2,130 women used the rest home. 55% of the cases were for care during pregnancy; 25% for neonatal care; the remaining 20% were cancer patients.

Demographic and Health Surveys. *Pesquisa nacional sobre saúde materno-infantil e planejamento familiar PNSMIPF-Brasil, 1986.* Sociedade Civil Bem-Estar Familiar no Brasil/Institute for Resource Development, Rio de Janeiro, 1987. WHE 1634.

A sample survey of hospital births in Brazil over the period 1981-86 found that of the 2,864 hospital births analysed, 32% were caesarean deliveries. There were wide regional variations, with the highest rates occurring in the two major cities, Rio de Janeiro and Sao Paulo where over 40% of the deliveries were by caesarean section. In urban areas in general the rate was 35% compared with 21% in rural areas. The lowest rate was in the North East of the country where only 19% of births were caesarean deliveries. The rates also varied with the educational status of the mother. Those with the highest educational level were the most likely to have had a caesarean delivery (43%) compared with 19% for those with little or no education. Rates of caesarean delivery appear to be related to the availability of private hospital care during delivery.

	% caesarean deliveries	% births in private hospitals
Region		
National:	32	19
urban	35	23
rural	21	11
Rio de Janeiro	43	26
Sao Paulo	43	25
Norte-Centro-Oeste	37	26
Centro-Leste	34	25
Sul	29	23
Nordeste	19	9
Educational level		
None	19	6
Less than primary level	20	8
Primary level education	27	16
More than primary level	43	33

Faundes, A. et al. Maternity care in developing countries: relevance of new technological advances. *International Journal of Gynecology and Obstetrics* 1988; 26: 349-354. WHE 2372

The authors suggest that improved maternity care in developing countries depends primarily on the increased provision of cost-effective, basic, easily accessible maternity care services. Expensive new technologies should be judged by their effectiveness, safety, technical feasibility, cost and local need. After identifying the major causes of morbidity and mortality, priority should be given to interventions applicable at the local level which do not require highly or specially trained personnel. The example is quoted in Brazil where the cost of electronic fetal monitoring during pregnancy to improve perinatal outcome was compared to the cost of increasing prenatal care coverage. It was concluded that for the same cost, an active prenatal care programme would have averted 8 times more perinatal deaths than electronic fetal monitoring.

Loffredo, L.C.M. and Simoes, M.J.S. Peso ao nascere e padroes de atendimento ao parto em Municipio do Estado de Sao Paulo, Brasil, 1986. *Revista Saúde Pública*, 1990; 24: 80-83. WHE 2829.

A survey was undertaken of delivery care in 4,776 live births at hospitals in the city of Araquara, S. Paulo State, Brazil. The incidence of caesarean delivery was 76% and was highest for deliveries with private medical care (92%) and lowest among women receiving free medical assistance (44%).

Merrick, T. *Financial implications of Brazil's high rate of cesarean section deliveries*. World Bank background paper, 1984. WHE 2979

A paper prepared for the World Bank found a very high rate of caesarean delivery in Brazil, ranging from 19% for women under 20 years old to over 30% for women aged 30-34 years. Rates were highest in major cities such as Sao Paulo where the rate varied between 33% and 53% depending on age. By contrast, in the Northeast of the country, where medical services are less developed, the ranges varied from 8% for the youngest age group to 15% for women aged 30-34.

Notzon, F.C. International differences in the use of obstetric interventions. *Journal of the American Medical Association*, 1990; 263(24): 3286-3291. WHE 2598.

A comparison of the levels and trends of caesarean delivery in 14 countries found the highest rate in Brazil where 32% of all hospital deliveries between 1981 and 1986 were by caesarean section. The authors question the appropriateness of the rise in caesarean deliveries and note the widespread national differences in obstetric practice. These cannot be explained by characteristics of the mother or complications of pregnancy and delivery.

World Health Organization. Pan American Health Organization. *Health conditions in the Americas*, Scientific Publication No. 524, Washington, 1990. WHE 2827

A report of the Pan American Health Organization quotes a study of 13 hospitals in Brazil which found an institutional maternal mortality rate of 70 per 100 000 live births coupled with a rate of caesarean delivery of 25%. It is noted that there is considerable variation in rates of caesarean delivery in different countries of the region, from under 10% in Honduras to over 30% in Mexico. An epidemiological study of caesarean delivery, undertaken by the Centro Latino Americano de Perinatologia y Desarrollo Humano (CLAP) and PAHO in 1985 in 17 countries indicated that the frequency of caesarean delivery explains only 5% of the variations in perinatal mortality and that there is no correlation between frequency of operative delivery and reduction in maternal mortality. Indeed, caesarean delivery is associated with higher rates of mortality and morbidity than vaginal delivery and is a bigger strain on the human and financial resources of the health service.

8. FURTHER READING

Araujo, G. et al. Improving obstetric care in northeast Brazil. *PAHO Bulletin* 1983; 17(3): 233-242. WHE 0265

Araujo, J.G. The Ceara experience. Traditional birth attendants and spiritual healers as partners in PHC. *Contact* 1984; 79: 1-10. WHE 1596

Caldeyro-Barcia, R. Problem of eclampsia and preeclampsia in Latin America. In: *WHO Meeting on Hypertensive Diseases of Pregnancy, Childbirth and the Puerperium*. Geneva, 1977 (unpublished WHO document no. MCH/TP/77.16). WHE 0118

Carvalheiro, C.D. Mortality patterns in the female population of the county of Ribeirao Preto, Sao Paulo, Brazil, from 1970 to 1974. *Revista Saúde Pública* 1977; 11(1): 65-72. WHE 0123

Chackiel, J. *Medicion indirecta de la mortalidad materna*. Unpublished document presented at the Reunion regional sobre prevencion de la mortalidad materna, Sao Paulo, 12-15 April 1988. WHE 2387

Edmunds, M. and Paxman, J.D. Early pregnancy and childbearing in Guatemala, Brazil, Nigeria and Indonesia. Addressing the consequences. *Pathpapers* no. 11, September 1984. WHE 1015

Faundes, A. et al. Intervençoes para a reduçao da mortalidade materna. *Revista Paulista de Medicina*, 1989; 107(1): 47-52. WHE 2679.

Fortney, J.A. The use of hospital resources to treat incomplete abortions: examples from Latin America. *Public Health Reports* 1981; 96(6): 574-579. WHE 2039

Goffi, P.S. Maternal mortality in the interior and in the capital of Sao Paulo. *Revista da Associaçao Medica Brasileira* 1966; 12(5): 220-223. WHE 0239

Herrick, T.W. Fertility and family planning in Brazil. *International Family Planning Perspectives* 1983; 9(4): 110-119. WHE 1104

International Fertility Research Program. *Abortion in Latin America*. Triangle Park, N.C. Research Report DDX 005, 1980. WHE 0348

Janowitz, B. et al. Sterilisation in the Northeast of Brazil. *Social Science and Medicine* 1985; 20(3): 215-221. WHE 1127

Janowitz, B. et al. Referrals by TBAs in Northwest Brazil. *American Journal of Public Health* 1985; 75(7): 745-748. WHE 1212

Janowitz, B. et al. TBAs in rural Northeast Brazil: referral patterns and perinatal mortality. *Health Policy and Planning* 1988; 3(1): 48-58. WHE 2339

Lacreta, O. and Maretti, M. Mortalidade materna. *Revista Brasileira de Medicina* 1982; 39(3): 89-106. WHE 0555

Pinotti, J.A. and Faundes, A. Obstetric and gynecological care for third world women. *International Journal of Gynaecology and Obstetrics* 1983; 21(5): 361-369. WHE 1102

Puffer, R.R. and Wynne Griffith, G. Patterns of urban mortality. *PAHO Scientific Publication* no. 151, Washington, PAHO 1967. WHE 0589

Reyes, E. et al. Atencion de parto distocico en el Hospital de Nueva Imperial (Novena Region). *Cuadernos Medico Sociales*, 1983; 24(1): 39-46. WHE 2805.

Shiroma, M. et al. Hepatite por vírus na gestaçao. *Revista do Hospital das Clinicas; Faculdade de Medicina da Universidade de Sao Paulo* 1969; 24: 249-360. WHE 1840

Singh, S. and Wulf, D. Estimating abortion levels in Brazil, Colombia and Peru, using hospital admissions and fertility survey data. *International Family Planning Perspectives*, 1991; 17(1): 9-13. WHE 2994.

Siqueira, de A.A.F. and Tanaka, A.C. d'A. Mortalidade na adolescencia com especial referência à mortalidade materna, Brasil, 1980 *Revista Saúde Pública* 1986; 20(4): 274-279. WHE 1723

Viggiano, M.G.C. and Ximenes, Y.R. Mortalidade materna: incidencia na Regiao Centro-Oeste. *Femina* June 1985; 499-503. WHE 2118

Yunes, J. et al. Assistência à infância, à adolescência e à maternidade no Brasil. *Boletín de la Oficina Sanitaria Panamericana* 1987; 103(1): 33-42. WHE 1793

9. DATA SOURCES

WHE 0045   Arruda, J.M. *Maternal and child health/family planning survey, Pernambuco State, Brazil, 1980.* Department of Health and Human Services, 1981.

WHE 0666   Souza, M. de L. Coeficiente de mortalidade materna segundo tipo de óbito, gruppo etario, paridade, local de residência e tipo de parto, obituario hospitalar, 1975 a 1979. Florianópolis, SC (Brasil). *Revista de Saúde Pública* 1983; 17: 279-289.

WHE 0753   United Nations, *Demographic Yearbook.* New York, various years.

WHE 0834   World Health Organization *World Health Statistics annual – vital statistics and causes of death.* Geneva, various years.

WHE 1299   Siqueira de A.A.F. et al. Mortalidade materna no Brasil, 1980. *Revista Saúde Pública* 1984; 18(6): 448-465.

WHE 1599   Barros, F.C. et al. Why so many caesarean births? The need for a further policy change in Brazil. *Health Policy and Planning* 1986; 1(1): 19-29.

WHE 1600   Cesar, C.L.G. and Walker, G.J.A. Diversity in provision and utilization of maternal and child health care in an urban area of Brazil. *Annals of Tropical Paediatrics* 1986; 6: 167-174.

WHE 1634   Demographic and Health Surveys *Brazil demographic and health survey* Washington, Sociedade Civil Bem-Estar Familiar no Brasil/Institute for Resource Development, 1986.

WHE 1712   Mauldin W.P. and Segal, S.J., *Prevalence of contraceptive use in developing countries. A chart book.* Rockefeller Foundation, New York 1986.

WHE 1914   United Nations Children's Fund (UNICEF). *The state of the world's children*, Oxford University Press, Oxford, various years.

WHE 1915   United Nations. Department of International Economic and Social Affairs. *World population prospects: estimates and projections as assessed in 1984.* Population Studies No. 98. New York 1986.

WHE 1918   United Nations. Department of International Economic and Social Affairs. *First marriage: patterns and determinants.* New York 1988.

WHE 1992   Laurenti, R. *Mortalidade de mulheres de 10 a 49 anos no município de Sao Paulo (com énfase à mortalidade materna).* (unpublished paper presented at the WHO/PAHO Workshop on maternal mortality) 12-15 April 1988.

WHE 1999   Becker, R.A. and Lechtig, A. *Brasil: aspectos da mortalidade infantil, pré-escolar e materna.* (unpublished paper) 1987.

WHE 2033   World Health Organization. *Global strategy for health for all by the year 2000. Second report on monitoring progress.* WHO document EB83/2 Add. 1, 1988.

WHE 2055   Arkader, J. Mortalidade materna no Hospital Municipal Salgado Filho. *Revista Brasiliana de Ginecologia y Obstetrica* 1988; 3: 44-46.

WHE 2117   Viggiano, M.G.C. et al. Mortalidade materna na Maternidade do Hospital Geral de Goiânia (1975-1983). *Jornal Brasiliero de Ginecologia* 1985; 95(3): 101-104.

WHE 2119   Viggiano, M.G.C. et al. Mortalidade materna na Maternidade Nossa Senhora de Lourdes: incidéncia, causas e responsabilidades. *Jornal Brasiliero de Ginecologia* 1979; 87(3): 137-141.

WHE 2287   Laurenti, R. Marcos referenciais para estudos e investigaçoes em mortalidade materna. *Revista Saúde Pública* 1988; 22(6): 507-512.

WHE 2493   A 10-year review of maternal mortality in a municipal hospital in Rio de Janeiro: a cause for concern. *Obstetrics and Gynecology* 1990; 75(!): 27-31.

WHE 2713   World Health Organization, Pan American Health Organization *Regional plan of action for the reduction of maternal mortality in the Americas,* Document No. CSP23/10, XXIII Pan American Sanitary Conference, Washington 1990.

WHE 2762   Hardy, E.E. et al. *Avaliaçao do programa de assistência integral à saúde da mulher no Estado de Sao Paulo,* Campinas, 1989.

WHE 2803   Lima, I.N. et al. Aspectos da mortalidade na cidade de Palmares, 1977 a 1982. *Revista da Fundaçao SESP,* 1984; 29(2): 221-231.

WHE 2804   Vieira Matos, et al. Mortalidade materna hospitalar nas unidades mistas da Fundaçao SESP 1979-1981. *Revista da Fundaçao SESP,* 1985; 30(1): 33-40.

WHE 2810   Tanaka, A.C.d'A. Situacao de saúde materna e perinatal no estado de Sao Paulo, Brasil. *Revista de Saúde Pública,* 1989; 23(1): 67-75.

WHE 2824   Siqueira, A.A.F. and Tanaka, A.C.d'A. Mortalidade na adolescencia com especial referencia a mortalidade materna, Brasil, 1980. *Revista Saúde Pública,* 1986; 20(4): 274-279.

WHE 2828   Laurenti, R. et al. Mortalidade de mulheres em idade fértil no Municipio de Sao Paulo (Brasil), 1986. I – Métodologia e resultados gerais. *Revista Saúde Pública,* 1990; 24(2): 128-133.

CHILE

	Year	Source

1. BASIC INDICATORS

1.1 Demographic

1.1.1 Population

Size (millions)	13.1	1990	(1915)
Rate of growth (%)	1.7	1985-90	(1915)

1.1.2 Life expectancy

Female	75	1985-90	(1915)
Male	68	1985-90	(1915)

1.1.3 Fertility

Crude Birth Rate	24	1985-90	(1915)
Total Fertility Rate	2.7	1985-90	(1915)

1.1.4 Mortality

Crude Death Rate	6	1985-90	(1915)
Infant Mortality Rate	20	1985-90	(1915)
Female	18	1987	(2827)
Male	21	1987	(2827)
1-4 years mortality rate			
Female	1	1987	(2827)
Male	1	1987	(2827)

1.2 Social and economic

1.2.1 Adult literacy rate (%)

Female	96	1984	(1914)
Male	97	1984	(1914)

1.2.2 Primary school enrolment rate (%)

Female	106	1983-86	(1914)
Male	108	1983-86	(1914)

1.2.3 Female mean age at first marriage

(years)	23.6	1982	(1918)

	Year	Source

1.2.4 GNP/capita

(US $)	1 510	1988	(1914)

1.2.5 Daily per capita calorie supply

(as % of requirements)	106	1985	(1914)

2. HEALTH SERVICES

2.1 Health Expenditure

2.1.1 Expenditure on health

(as % of GNP)	6.0	1983	(1942)

2.1.2 Expenditure on PHC

(as % of total health expenditure)	56	1984	(1942)

2.2 Primary Health Care.
(Percentage of population covered by):

2.2.1 Health services

National	95	1983	(0834)
Urban			
Rural			

2.2.2 Safe water

National	85	1983	(0834)
Urban	97	1985	(2033)
Rural	22	1985	(2033)

2.2.3 Adequate sanitary facilities

National	83	1983	(0834)
Urban	79	1985	(2033)
Rural	21	1985	(2033)

2.2.4 Contraceptive prevalence rate

(%)	43	1978	(1712)

2.3   Coverage of maternity care (%)

Area	Prenatal care	Trained attendant	Institutional deliveries	Postnatal care	Sample size	Year	Source
National	91	95				1983	(0834)
National		98				1986	(1989)
National		98				1987	(3152)

3. COMMUNITY STUDIES

3.1 Temuco, Province of Cautin, 1988 [2565]

This study was undertaken among a rural Indian population; female life expectancy was estimated at 58 years and total fertility was 4.4 children per woman. The study used the "sisterhood method" carried out in conjunction with the population census to calculate maternal mortality. Respondents were all adults and information was collected about all sisters. The weighted sample size was 8,714 and there were an estimated 253 maternal deaths. The lifetime risk was calculated as one in 53.

3.1.1 Rate*
MMR (per 100 000 live births)   414

*   Based on data from respondents aged 25-49 years.

4. HOSPITAL STUDIES

4.1 Hospital Felix Bulnes, Santiago de Chile, 1961-69 [1932]

4.1.1 Rate
Births   53 415
Maternal deaths   46
MMR (per 100 000 births)   86

4.1.2 Causes of maternal deaths (for 45 cases).

	Number
Haemorrhage	14
Sepsis	11
Complications of anaesthesia	5
Embolisms	5
Hypertensive disorders of pregnancy	5
Ruptured uterus	1
Indirect causes	4
Total	45

4.1.3 Avoidable factors

4.1.4 High risk groups
Parity

	Births	Maternal deaths	MMR (per 100 000 live births)
Primiparous	13 834	8	58
Multiparous	28 951	25	86
Grand multiparous (6+)	10 630	13	122

4.2 Hospital Gmo. Grant Benavente, Concepción 1975-79 [1875]

4.2.1 Rate
Live births   23 794
Maternal deaths   66
MMR (per 100 000 live births)   277

4.2.2 Causes of maternal deaths (for 64 cases)

	Number	%
Sepsis	45	70
Haemorrhage	9	14
Hypertensive disorders of pregnancy	5	8
Complications of anaesthesia	1	2
DIRECT CAUSES	60	94
INDIRECT CAUSES	4	6
TOTAL	64	100

5. CIVIL REGISTRATION DATA/GOVERNMENT ESTIMATES

5.1 National, 1960-86 (0283, 0825, 0826, 0827, 0834, 1625, 1881, 2116, 2713, 2722, 2811, 2827, 3152)

5.1.1 Rate

	Live births	Maternal deaths	MMR (per 100 000 live births)
1960	282 681	845	299
1965	308 014	860	279
1970	261 609	439	168
1975	256 543	336	131
1980	253 581	185	73
1981	260 273	173	66
1982	274 600	142	52
1983	260 655	105	41
1984	265 016	94	36
1985	261 978	132	50
1986	272 997	129	47
1987	279 909	135	48

5.1.2 Causes of maternal deaths, 1980-82 and 1987

	%	
	1980-82	1987
Abortions	37	35
Hypertensive disorders of pregnancy	9	12
Complications of the puerperium	19	24
Haemorrhage	8	8
Other direct obstetric causes	20	16
DIRECT CAUSES	93	95
INDIRECT CAUSES	7	5
TOTAL	100	100
	N=500	N=135

Abortion (0283)

Over the period 1973-83 the maternal mortality rate due to abortion fell from 43 per 100 000 live births to 15 per 100 000.

5.1.3 Avoidable factors (3152)

A government report carried out a detailed analysis of all registered maternal deaths during 1987 in order to determine the degree of avoidability and improve medical management. It found that over 64% of the deaths were probably avoidable, 10% were unavoidable and 16% were doubtful but possibly avoidable. In nearly 9% of the cases it was impossible to determine whether or not avoidable factors were present.

Of the 47 deaths related to complications of abortion (ICD 630-639), 43 were considered avoidable. In 36 cases, including five ectopic pregnancies diagnosis was made too late. The remaining cases presented too late at the hospital for successful intervention to be possible. Induced abortion was thought to have taken place in 22 cases and to have been a possibility in a further 11 cases.

Of the 88 deaths due to factors other than abortion, half were considered avoidable given better prenatal care, rapid diagnosis and adequate treatment.

Of the 35 deaths related to pregnancy (ICD 640-648) nine cases were considered avoidable and 13 possibly avoidable. Hypertensive disorders of pregnancy accounted for 16 of the deaths, of which six were considered avoidable, three unavoidable and four possibly avoidable. In particular, it was noted that there was inadequate prenatal care in eight cases and inadequate treatment in six cases. There were six deaths from antepartum haemorrhage, of which three were considered avoidable.

A large proportion of avoidable deaths occurred during labour and delivery (ICD 660-669). Of the 18 deaths in this group, 16 were considered definitely avoidable. In 11 cases there was a failure to correctly diagnose the complication and in ten cases there was inadequate treatment. Of the avoidable deaths, five were due to postpartum haemorrhage, four were due to trauma to the perineum and vulva during delivery, there were two cases of ruptured uterus and three instances of complications of anaesthesia.

Half of the deaths which occurred during the puerperium (ICD 670-676) were considered avoidable. There were 14 deaths from sepsis of which eight were avoidable, four possibly avoidable and in two cases there was insufficient information to determine the degree of avoidability. In most of the deaths from sepsis, the infection was probably iatrogenic. In ten cases of sepsis there was a failure to diagnose the problem. There were five avoidable deaths from complications of caesarean delivery, four of which were due to post operative haemorrhage.

	Total deaths	Avoidable deaths	Un-avoidable deaths	Possibly avoidable deaths	Insufficient information
Abortion (ICD 630-639)	47	43	0	1	3
Pregnancy (ICD 640-648)	35	9	9	13	4
Normal delivery (ICD 650-659)	2	2	0	0	0
Labour (ICD 660-669)	18	16	0	1	1
Puerperium (ICD 670-676)	33	17	5	7	4
Total (ICD 630-676)	135	87	14	22	12

5.1.4 High risk groups
Age

	MMR (per 100 000 live births)
< 15 years	–
15-19	54
20-24	39
25-29	77
30-34	84
35-39	143
40-44	175
45 +	159
All ages	67

5.1.5 Other findings [3152]

A government study found that in 1987 maternal mortality rates were higher among the unmarried. However, this was not uniformly true across all age groups. For women aged below 35 years mortality rates were higher among those who were unmarried. By contrast, rates for those aged 35 and over were higher among married women.

MMR (per 100 000 live births)

Age (years)	Unmarried	Married	Total
15-19	50	26	40
20-24	64	38	45
35+	73	90	86
Total	61	42	48

6. OTHER SOURCES/ ESTIMATES

6.1 National, 1987 [2713]

The maternal mortality rate was adjusted by PAHO to account for underreporting based on the estimated 39% under-registration observed in a study in the United States.

6.1.1 Rate
Births	301 000
Maternal deaths	202
MMR (per 100 000 births)	67

6.2 VIII Region Bio Bio, 1987 [2273]

6.2.1 Rate
MMR (per 100 000 live births)	78

7. SELECTED ANNOTATED BIBLIOGRAPHY

Guzman Serani, R. et al. Epidemiologia del aborto hospitalizado en Valdivia. *Revista Medica de Chile*, 1981; 109: 1099-1106. WHE 0251.

A family planning programme set up in Valdivia in 1964 resulted in the reduction in the numbers of abortions and in the abortion rate per 1,000 women of reproductive age. The rate stood at over 40 per 1,000 in 1964 and fell to 14.5 per 1,000 in 1980. However, the authors observe that more efforts need to be directed towards unmarried women who do not appear to have access to family planning information and services. In 1980 there were two maternal deaths resulting from complications of induced abortion. Both women were unmarried.

Mariano Requena, B. *Aborto inducido en Chile.* Edicion Sociedad Chilena de Salud Publica, Santiago de Chile, 1990. WHE 2980.

A study of induced abortion in Chile estimates that in 1987 there were 10.5 hospitalizations for complications of abortion per 1,000 women of reproductive age. This represented a decline compared with the 1960s when the equivalent figure was 30 per 1,000 women of reproductive age and coincides with an increase in contraceptive prevalence from 21 per 1,000 in 1965 to 242 per 1,000 in 1987. The study estimates that complications of abortion accounted for 33-42% of maternal deaths over the past two decades.

Roco, M.H. La operación cesarea en un hospital rural, Hospital de Lebu. *Revista Medica de Valparaiso*, 1987; 40(2): 93-98. WHE 2812.

A series of caesarean deliveries undertaken during 1984-85 at a rural hospital was analysed. The incidence of caesarean deliveries was 25%. The most common indications for caesarean delivery were previous caesarean, fetal distress and malpresentation. The incidence of complications was 18%, the most frequent being severe anaemia, headache and infections. There was one maternal death out of the 367 cases, a maternal mortality rate from caesarean delivery of 270 per 100 000 live births.

World Health Organization. Pan American Health Organization. *Health conditions in the Americas,* Scientific Publication No. 524, Washington, 1990. WHE 2827

A report of the Pan American Health Organization quotes a study of 58 hospitals in Chile which found an institutional maternal mortality rate of 40 per 100 000 live births coupled with a rate of caesarean delivery of 24%. It is noted that there is considerable variation in rates of caesarean delivery in different countries of the region, from under 10% in Honduras to over 30% in Mexico. An epidemiological study of caesarean delivery, undertaken by the Centro Latino Americano de Perinatologia y Desarrollo Humano (CLAP) and PAHO in 1985 in 17 countries indicated that the frequency of caesarean delivery explains only 5% of the variations in perinatal mortality and that there is no correlation between frequency of operative delivery and reduction in maternal mortality. Indeed, caesarean delivery is associated with higher rates of mortality and morbidity than vaginal delivery and is a bigger strain on the human and financial resources of the health service.

8. FURTHER READING

Chackiel, J. *Medicion indirecta de la mortalidad materna.* Unpublished document presented at the Reunion regional sobre prevencion de la mortalidad materna, Sao Paulo, 12-15 April 1988. WHE 2387

Guzman-Serani, R. et al. Epidemiología del aborto hospitalizado en Valdivia. *Revista Medica de Chile* 1981; 109(11): 1099-1106. WHE 0251.

International Fertility Research Program. *Abortion in Latin America.* Research Report DDX 005, Triangle Park, North Carolina, 1980. WHE 0348.

Molina Cartes, R. et al. Caracteristicas del aborto en Chile *Cuadernos Medico-Sociales* 1978; 19(1): 5-18. WHE 0460.

Monreal, T. Factores determinantes de la tendencia del aborto ilegal en Chile *Boletín de la Oficina Sanitaria Pana*ericana *1979; 86(3): 206-218. WHE 0584.*

Morales, M.A. and Montoya, G.M. *Analisis de la mortalidad materna en la region metropolitana de 1973 a 1977.* Revista Chilena de Obstetricia y Ginecología *1978; 43(6): 312-321. WHE 0464.*

Munoz-Aguero, W. et al. *Mortalidad materna* Revista Chilena de Obstetricia y Ginecología *1980; 45(3): 156-169. WHE 1875.*

Puffer, R.R. and Wynne Griffith, G. *Patterns of urban mortality.* PAHO Scientific Publication *No. 151, Washington, PAHO, 1967. WHE 0589.*

Rodriguez-Silva, F. *Natalidad, mortalidad infantil y mortalidad materna. Chile 1964-77.* Revista Chilena de Obstetrica y Ginecologia *1979; 44(4): 140-145. WHE 1931.*

Ugarte Avendano, J.M. *Evolución de algunos indicadores de salud, Chile 1960-80.* Cuadernos Medico-Sociales *1982; 23(3): 5-8. WHE 0721.*

Viel, B. *Illegal abortion in Latin America.* IPPF Medical Bulletin *1982; 16(4): 1-2. WHE 0770.*

9. DATA SOURCES

WHE 0283   Chile, Ministry of Health *Mortality in Chile,* Santiago, 1984.

WHE 0825   World Health Organization. Pan American Health Organization. *Health conditions in the Americas. 1969-72.* (PAHO scientific publication no. 306) PAHO, Washington, 1975.

WHE 0826   World Health Organization. Pan American Health Organization. *Health conditions in the Americas. 1973-1976.* (PAHO scientific publication no. 364) PAHO, Washington, 1982.

WHE 0827   World Health Organization. Pan American Health Organization. *Health conditions in the Americas. 1977-1980.* (PAHO scientific publication no. 427) PAHO, Washington,, 1982.

WHE 0834   World Health Organization. *World Health Statistics Annual – vital statistics and causes of death.* Geneva, various years.

WHE 1625   World Health Organization, Pan American Health Organization. *Health conditions in the Americas. 1981-84.* Vol. I (PAHO Scientific Publication no. 500). PAHO, Washington, 1986.

WHE 1712   Mauldin W.P. and Segal, S.J., *Prevalence of contraceptive use in developing countries. A chart book.* Rockefeller Foundation, New York 1986.

WHE 1875   Munoz-Aguero, W. et al. Maternal mortality. Review of cases for a period of 30 years, 1950-1979. *Revista Chilena de Obstetricia y Ginecología, 1*980; 45(3): 156-169.

WHE 1881   Orellna, M. et al. Analisis de la mortalidad materna Chile de 1981 y sus factores asociados segun el certificado de defuncion *Revista Chilena de Obstetrica y Ginecologia* 1984; 5(4): 195-210.

WHE 1914   United Nations Children's Fund (UNICEF). *The state of the world's children,* Oxford University Press, Oxford, various years.

WHE 1915   United Nations. Department of International Economic and Social Affairs. *World population prospects: estimates and projections as assessed in 1984.* Population Studies No. 98. New York 1986.

WHE 1918   United Nations. Department of International Economic and Social Affairs. *First marriage: patterns and determinants.* New York 1988.

WHE 1932   Lizana, L. et al. La mortalidad materna en la Maternidad del Hospital Felix Bulnes de Santiago de Chile. *Revista Chilena de Obstetricia y Ginecología, 1*971; 36(2): 122-126.

WHE 1942   World Health Organization. Pan American Health Organization. *Evaluation of the strategy for Health for All by the Year 2000.* Seventh Report on the World Health Situation. Vol.3. Region of the Americas. PAHO, Washington, 1986.

WHE 1989   Chile, République de. Caracteristicas de la mortalidad materna y rol de la attencion de salud en su prevencion. *Paper presented at WHO/PAHO workshop on maternal mortality research* Sao Paulo, 1988.

WHE 2033   World Health Organization. Global strategy for health for all by the year 2000. Second report on monitoring progress. WHO document EB83/2 Add. 1, 1988.

WHE 2116   Viel, B. and Campos, W. La experiencia Chilena de mortalidad infantil y materna, 1940-1985. *Perspectivas Internacionales en Planificación Familiar* 1987.

WHE 2713   World Health Organization, Pan American Health Organization *Regional plan of action for the reduction of maternal mortality in the Americas,* Document No. CSP23/10, XXIII Pan American Sanitary Conference, Washington 1990.

WHE 2273   Candia Llanos, M.E. Maternal mortality. (personal communication) 1989.

WHE 2565   Maine, D. *Results of applications of the sisterhood method for estimating maternal mortality.* London School of Hygiene and Tropical Medicine, 1990 (unpublished document).

WHE 2713   World Health Organization, Pan American Health Organization *Regional plan of action for the reduction of maternal mortality in the Americas,* Document No. CSP23/10, XXIII Pan American Sanitary Conference, Washington 1990.

WHE 2722   World Health Organization, *Maternal deaths and maternal mortality rates* (unpublished) 1990.

WHE 2811   Ristori, C. and Toro, J.A. Mortalidad general. infantil, materna y por grupos de causas. *Boletín Epidemiologico de Chile,* 1987; 14(4): 97-105.

WHE 2827   World Health Organization. Pan American Health Organization *Health conditions in the Americas 1990.* Scientific publication No. 524, PAHO, Washington, 1991.

WHE 3152   Chile, Ministerio de Salud. *La mortalidad materna en Chile,* Santiago, Chile, 1989.

COLOMBIA

		Year	Source

1. BASIC INDICATORS

1.1 Demographic

1.1.1 Population
Size (millions)	33.0	1990	(1915)
Rate of growth (%)	2.0	1985-90	(1915)

1.1.2 Life expectancy
Female	71	1985-90	(1915)
Male	66	1985-90	(1915)

1.1.3 Fertility
Crude Birth Rate	27	1985-90	(1915)
Total Fertility Rate	3.1	1985-90	(1915)

1.1.4 Mortality
Crude Death Rate	6	1985-90	(1915)
Infant Mortality Rate	40	1985-90	(1915)
Female	39	1976-86	(1635)
Male	41	1976-86	(1635)
1-4 years mortality rate			
Female	12	1976-86	(1635)
Male	13	1976-86	(1635)

1.2 Social and economic

1.2.1 Adult literacy rate (%)
Female	84	1981	(2458)
Male	86	1981	(2458)

1.2.2 Primary school enrolment rate (%)
Female	112	1986-88	(1914)
Male	115	1986-88	(1914)

1.2.3 Female mean age at first marriage
(years)	20.4	1985	(1918)

1.2.4 GNP/capita
(US $)	1 180	1988	(1914)

1.2.5 Daily per capita calorie supply
(as % of requirements)	110	1984-86	(1914)

2. HEALTH SERVICES

2.1 Health Expenditure

2.1.1 Expenditure on health
(as % of GNP)	4.1	1984	(2033)

2.1.2 Expenditure on PHC
(as % of total health expenditure)

2.2 Primary Health Care
(Percentage of population covered by):

2.2.1 Health services
National	87	1983-87	(2033)
Urban			
Rural			

2.2.2 Safe water
National	91	1985	(0834)
Urban	100	1985	(0834)
Rural	76	1985	(0834)

2.2.3 Adequate sanitary facilities
National	68	1985	(2033)
Urban	96	1985	(2033)
Rural	13	1985	(2033)

2.2.4 Contraceptive prevalence rate
(%)	65	1986	(2713)

2.3 Coverage of maternity care (%)

Area	Prenatal care	Trained attendant	Institutional deliveries	Postnatal care	Sample size	Year	Source
National	65	51				1984	(0834)
National	76		75			1987	(2713)
National:	80	71			3 713b	1986-90	(2765)
urban	86	81			2 470b	1986-90	(2765)
rural	68	52			1 242b	1986-90	(2765)
Atlantica	71	61			926b	1986-90	(2765)
Bogota	93	90			562b	1986-90	(2765)
Central	79	73			895b	1986-90	(2765)
Oriental	87	69			681b	1986-90	(2765)
Pacifica	75	67			645b	1986-90	(2765)

3. COMMUNITY STUDIES

4. HOSPITAL STUDIES

4.1 Instituto Materno-infantil "Concepcion Villaveces de Acosta", Bogota 1965-66, 1971-73 and 1976-80 [0632, 1825, 2816]

4.1.1 Rate

	Live births	Maternal deaths	MMR (per 100 000 live births)
1965-66	38 554	122	316
1971-73	68 930	209	303
1976-80	105 075	263	250

4.1.2 Causes of maternal deaths, 1976-80

	Number	%
Abortion	106	40
Sepsis	55	21
Hypertensive disorders of pregnancy	44	17
Haemorrhage	18	7
Embolisms	4	2
Ruptured uterus	4	2
DIRECT CAUSES	231	89
INDIRECT CAUSES	26	10
TOTAL	263	100

4.1.3 Avoidable factors

In 1973-74, 178 (85%) of the 209 maternal deaths were considered to have been avoidable; 54 resulted from medical or institutional errors and 80 were due to induced abortions. Over the period 1976-80 it was estimated that 27% of the deaths could have been prevented with better diagnosis and treatment in the hospital. Over one third of the women who died had been referred in a moribund condition from other hospitals. Sepsis was a serious problem and 34% of the deaths occurred during the puerperium.

4.2 Hospital Universitario San Vincente de Paul, Medellín, 1963-72 [0371]

4.2.1 Rate

Live births	39 323
Maternal deaths	104
MMR (per 100 000 live births)	264

The high rates are attributed to the fact that half the patients were referrals from other towns and most were in a poor condition at admission.

4.2.2 Causes of maternal deaths

Infection was the principal cause of death, and was associated with induced abortion in 91% of the cases. Haemorrhage as a cause of death moved from the second to the third rank due to better management and improved facilities.

	1963-67 No.	1963-67 %	1968-72 No.	1968-72 %
Abortion	20	40	20	37
Hypertensive disorders of pregnancy	6	12	14	26
Haemorrhage	10	20	5	9
Sepsis	5	10	2	4
Ruptured uterus	3	6	2	4
Complications of anaesthesia	0	0	2	4
Ectopic pregnancy	1	2	0	0
DIRECT CAUSES	45	90	45	83
Anaemia	0	0	1	2
Hepatitis	1	2	0	0
Other infections	1	2	1	2
Cerebrovascular accident	1	2	0	0
Others	2	4	7	12
INDIRECT CAUSES	5	10	9	17
TOTAL	50	100	54	100

5. CIVIL REGISTRATION DATA/ GOVERNMENT ESTIMATES

5.1 National, 1960-86 [0825, 0826, 0827, 1625, 2713, 2722, 2827]

5.1.1 Rate

	Maternal deaths	MMR (per 100 000 live births)
1960	1 553	259
1965	1 442	217
1970	1 556	230
1975	1 116	152
1981	969	126
1984	642	100
1985	720	86
1986	625	74

5.1.2 Causes of maternal deaths (1984)

	%
Abortion	23
Hypertensive disorders of pregnancy	20
Haemorrhage	17
Complications of the puerperium	9
Other direct causes	30
Indirect causes	1
TOTAL (N = 642)	100

5.2 Department of Valle del Cauca and Cali, 1970-84 [0996]

5.2.1 Rate

	MMR (per 100 000 live births)	
	Valle del Cauca excluding Cali	Cali
1970	196	151
1975	283	121
1980	165	103
1981	186	106
1982	99	123
1983	103	125
1984	115	89

5.2.2 Causes of maternal deaths (direct causes only)

	Number	%
Abortion	54	39
Hypertensive disorders of pregnancy	47	34
Haemorrhage	30	22
Other direct causes	8	6
TOTAL	139	100

5.2.3 Avoidable factors

The author estimates that 92% of the deaths were avoidable.

5.2.4 High risk groups

5.2.5 Other findings

In 1984 a Committee on Avoidable Mortality, comprising representatives from the Municipal Health Secretariat and several Departments of Obstetrics and Gynaecology was established. All death certificates of women of reproductive age were examined and the cause of death analysed. In cases of doubt a home visit was made and the attending physician was interviewed. In 115 cases there was agreement between the cause of death mentioned on the certificate and the analysis by the Committee. The Committee estimated that a maternal death had occurred in a further 24 cases which had not been classified as such. Eight of these deaths were thought to have resulted from complications of induced abortion. In two cases the death was wrongly classified as maternal on the certificate. The extent of underreporting of maternal mortality was, therefore, 17%.

5.3 Department of Antioquia, 1986 [2429]

5.3.1 Rate

Maternal deaths	98
MMR (per 100 000 live births)	110

6. OTHER SOURCES/ ESTIMATES

6.1 National, 1979 and 1981 [1415]

6.1.1 Rate

	Maternal deaths	MMR (per 100 000 live births)
1979	1 259	160
1981	965	126

6.1.2 Causes of maternal deaths

	1979 No.	1979 %	1981 No.	1981 %
Hypertensive disorders of pregnancy	279	22	227	24
Haemorrhage	227	18	181	19
Abortion	183	14	164	17
Complications of the puerperium	116	9	62	6
Other direct obstetric causes	437	35	303	31
DIRECT CAUSES	1 242	99	937	97
INDIRECT CAUSES	17	1	29	3
TOTAL	1 259	100	965	100

6.2 National, 1987 [2713]

The maternal mortality rate was recalculated by PAHO using estimates for underreporting based on a study carried out in Brazil. [1992]

6.2.1 Rate

Births	861 000
Maternal deaths	1 722
MMR (per 100 000 live births)	200

7. SELECTED ANNOTATED BIBLIOGRAPHY

Rodriguez, J. *Evaluation of the maternity waiting home, "Casa Hogar"* (unpublished document) WHE 2497

In 1982 a Committee on Avoidable Maternal Mortality was established in Cali. Realizing that geographical inaccessibility, transport difficulties and late referral or recourse were major factors in the inadequacy of maternal health care, it was decided to establish a maternity waiting home in order to fill the gap between the need for services and the supply, especially in rural areas. The waiting home is within easy access of a referral centre and provides educational materials for both users and community health workers as well as training of the latter. The waiting home is open to all women resident in rural areas who would like to deliver in a health institution, whether or not they are high risk cases. In addition, women in rural areas with a history of illness, gynaecological or obstetric surgery and other pathological conditions are encouraged, by local health workers, to attend the waiting home during the last weeks of pregnancy. Over the period March-August 1987 the strategy doubled the number of institutional deliveries among women from rural areas. Further evaluation of the project is continuing.

Velasco, A. and Barriga, H. Mortalidad materna y perinatal en los estados hipertensivos del embarazo. *Revista Colombiana de Obstetricia y Ginecologia*, 1984; 35(1): 13-35. WHE 2844.

A study analysed the maternal and perinatal outcomes of two groups of patients with hypertensive disorders of pregnancy who received different treatment regimens. Group A was systematically treated with diuretics, barbiturates and operative delivery was delayed in order to increase fetal maturity. Group B was treated with vessel dilators and active intervention supported by more careful fetal assessment. In group A the case fatality rate among hypertensive women was 5.2% compared with 0.3% in group B. Maternal mortality rates were 130 per 100 000 deliveries for the former compared with 9 per 100 000 for the latter.

World Health Organization. Pan American Health Organization. *Health conditions in the Americas*, Scientific Publication No. 524, Washington, 1990. WHE 2827

A report of the Pan American Health Organization quotes a study of five hospitals in Colombia which found an institutional maternal mortality rate of 60 per 100 000 live births coupled with a rate of caesarean delivery of 15%. It is noted that there is considerable variation in rates of caesarean delivery in different countries of the region, from under 10% in Honduras to over 30% in Mexico. An epidemiological study of caesarean delivery, undertaken by the Centro Latino Americano de Perinatologia y Desarrollo Humano (CLAP) and PAHO in 1985 in 17 countries indicated that the frequency of caesarean delivery explains only 5% of the variations in perinatal mortality and that there is no correlation between frequency of operative delivery and reduction in maternal mortality. Indeed, caesarean delivery is associated with higher rates of mortality and morbidity than vaginal delivery and is a bigger strain on the human and financial resources of the health service.

8. FURTHER READING

Browner, C.H. Women, household and health in Latin America. *Social Science and Medicine* 1989; 28(5): 461-473. WHE 2120

Caldeyro-Barcia, R. Problems of eclampsia and preeclampsia in Latin America. In: *WHO Meeting on Hypertensive Diseases of Pregnancy, Childbirth and the Puerperium*, Geneva, 1977 (unpublished WHO document no. MCH/TP/77.16). WHE 0118

Chackiel, J. *Medicion indirecta de la mortalidad materna*. Unpublished document presented at the Reunion regional sobre prevencion de la mortalidad materna, Sao Paulo, 12-15 April 1988. WHE 2387

Fortney, J.A. The use of hospital resources to treat incomplete abortions: examples from Latin America. *Public Health Reports* 1981; 96(6): 574-579. WHE 2039

Harrison, P. On the septic ward. *People* 1977; 4(3): 12-13. WHE 0318

International Fertility Research Programme. *Abortion in Latin America* 1980; IFRP Research Report DDX 005, Triangle Park, North Carolina. WHE 0348

Popline editorial. Abortions on the rise in Colombia. *Popline* 1986; 8(7): 2-4. WHE 1437

Puffer R.R. and Wynne Griffith, G. *Patterns of urban mortality.* PAHO Scientific Publication no. 151 Washington 1967. WHE 0589

Sanchez Torres, F. Illegal abortion in Latin America. *Draper Fund Report* 1980; 9: 14-15. WHE 0633

Silva Lorenzetti, L. Maternal health – desired pregnancies and spacing of children. *Paper prepared for the ICM/WHO/UNICEF pre-congress workshop on women's health and the midwife* 1987. WHE 1644

Singh, S. and Wulf, D. Estimating abortion levels in Brazil, Colombia and Peru, using hospital admissions and fertility survey data. *International Family Planning Perspectives*, 1991; 17(1): 9-13. WHE 2994.

Viel, B. Illegal abortion in Latin America. *IPPF Medical Bulletin* 1982; 16(4): 1-2. WHE 0770

World Health Organization, Pan American Health Organization. *Reference document on the study and prevention of maternal mortality.* Washington, 1987. WHE 1912

9. DATA SOURCES

WHE 0371   Jubiz Hasbún, A. and Sanchez, C.C. Mortalidad materna comparativa entre dos periodos 1963-1967, 1968-1972. *Revista Colombiana de Obstetricia y Ginecologia* 1976; 27(3): 129-136.

WHE 0632   Sanchez Torres, F. Mortalidad materna en el Instituto Materno Infantil, de Bogota (1971-1973). *Revista Colombiana de Obstetrica y Ginecología* 1974; 25(6): 395-401.

WHE 0825   World Health Organization. Pan American Health Organization. *Health conditions in the Americas. 1969-72.* (PAHO scientific publication no. 306) PAHO, Washington, 1975.

WHE 0826   World Health Organization. Pan American Health Organization. *Health conditions in the Americas. 1973-1976.* (PAHO scientific publication no. 364) PAHO, Washington, 1982.

WHE 0827   World Health Organization. Pan American Health Organization. *Health conditions in the Americas. 1977-1980.* (PAHO scientific publication no. 427) Washington, PAHO, 1982.

WHE 0834   World Health Organization. *World Health Statistics Annual – vital statistics and causes of death.* Geneva, various years.

WHE 0996   Rodriguez, J. et al. Avoidable mortality and maternal mortality in Cali, Colombia. In: *Interregional Meeting on the Prevention of Maternal Mortality,* Geneva, 11-15 November 1985. (unpublished WHO document no. FHE/PMM/85.9.1).

WHE 1415   Rodriguez, A.P. and Ruiz, M.S. *Analisis complementario de la mortalidad, Colombia, 1973-1983.* Instituto Nacional de Salud, 1986.

WHE 1625   World Health Organization, Pan American Health Organization. *Health conditions in the Americas.* 1981-84. Vol. I (PAHO Scientific Publication no. 500). PAHO, Washington, 1986.

WHE 1635   Demographic and Health Surveys. *Colombia. Tercera encuesta nacional de prevalencia del uso de anticonceptivos y primera de demografía y salud.* Corporación Centro Regional de Poblacion/ Ministerio de Salud de Colombia/Institute for Resource Development/Westinghouse. 1988.

WHE 1825   Morbilidad y mortalidad en el Instituto Materno-infantil "Concepción Villaveces de Acosta". *Revista Colombiana de Obstetricia y Ginecología* 1968; 19(4): 269-281.

WHE 1914   United Nations Children's Fund (UNICEF). *The state of the world's children*, Oxford University Press, Oxford, various years.

WHE 1915   United Nations. Department of International Economic and Social Affairs. *World population prospects: estimates and projections as assessed in 1984.* Population Studies No. 98. New York 1986.

WHE 1918   United Nations. Department of International Economic and Social Affairs. *First marriage: patterns and determinants.* New York 1988.

WHE 1992   Laurenti, R. *Mortalidade de mulheres de 10 a 49 anos no município de Sao Paulo (com énfase à mortalidade materna).* (unpublished paper presented at the WHO/PAHO Workshop on maternal mortality) 12-15 April 1988.

WHE 2033   World Health Organization. *Global strategy for health for all by the year 2000. Second report on monitoring progress.* WHO document EB83/2 Add. 1, 1988.

WHE 2429   Cataño Osorio, L.O. et al. *Maternal mortality and associated risk factors, Antioquia, Colombia, 1989, a case-control study.* (unpublished), 1990.

WHE 2458   United Nations Educational, Social and Cultural Organization, UNESCO, *Compendium of statistics of illiteracy.* Division of Statistics on Education, Paris 1988.

WHE 2713   World Health Organization, Pan American Health Organization *Regional plan of action for the reduction of maternal mortality in the Americas,* Document No. CSP23/10, XXIII Pan American Sanitary Conference, Washington 1990.

WHE 2765   Demographic and Health Surveys. *Colombia encuesta de prevalencia demografica y salud 1990.* PROFAMILIA/Institute for Resource Development/Macro Systems Inc. 1990.

WHE 2722   World Health Organization, *Maternal deaths and maternal mortality rates* (unpublished) 1990.

WHE 2816   Muñoz Gonzalez, L.A. et al. Mortalidad materna Instituto Materno Infantil 1976-1980. *Revista Colombiana de Obstetricia y Ginecología,* 1984; 36(4): 227-243.

WHE 2827   World Health Organization. Pan American Health Organization *Health conditions in the Americas 1990.* Scientific publication No. 524, PAHO, Washington, 1991.

COSTA RICA

		Year	Source

1. BASIC INDICATORS

1.1 Demographic

1.1.1 Population

		Year	Source
Size (millions)	3.0	1990	(1915)
Rate of growth (%)	2.6	1985-90	(1915)

1.1.2 Life expectancy

Female	77	1985-90	(1915)
Male	72	1985-90	(1915)

1.1.3 Fertility

Crude Birth Rate	28	1985-90	(1915)
Total Fertility Rate	3.3	1985-90	(1915)

1.1.4 Mortality

Crude Death Rate	4	1985-90	(1915)
Infant Mortality Rate	18	1985-90	(1915)
Female	12	1988	(2827)
Male	17	1988	(2827)
1-4 years mortality rate			
Female	1	1988	(2827)
Male	1	1988	(2827)

1.2 Social and economic

1.2.1 Adult literacy rate (%)

Female	92	1985	(1914)
Male	92	1985	(1914)

1.2.2 Primary school enrolment rate (%)

Female	97	1986-88	(1914)
Male	100	1986-88	(1914)

1.2.3 Female mean age at first marriage

(years)	22.2	1984	(2799)

1.2.4 GNP/capita

(US $)	1 690	1988	(1914)

1.2.5 Daily per capita calorie supply

(as % of requirements)	124	1984-86	(1914)

2. HEALTH SERVICES

2.1 Health Expenditure

2.1.1 Expenditure on health

(as % of GNP)	6.9	1984	(2033)

2.1.2 Expenditure on PHC

(as % of total health expenditure)	2	1983	(1942)

2.2 Primary Health Care

(Percentage of population covered by):

2.2.1 Health services

National	95	1983	(0834)
Urban			
Rural			

2.2.2 Safe water

National	88	1983	(0834)
Urban	93	1983	(0834)
Rural	86	1983	(0834)

2.2.3 Adequate sanitary facilities

National	76	1983	(0834)
Urban	100	1983	(0834)
Rural	40	1983	(0834)

2.2.4 Contraceptive prevalence rate

(%)	66	1981	(1712)

2.3   Coverage of maternity care (%)

Area	Prenatal care	Trained attendant	Institutional deliveries	Postnatal care	Sample size	Year	Source
National			93			1983	(1534)
National	54					1983	(0834)
National	40*		94			1986	(1945)
National	91	97				1983-87	(2033)

*   Ministry of Health prenatal care services.

3. COMMUNITY STUDIES

4. HOSPITAL STUDIES

5. CIVIL REGISTRATION DATA/GOVERNMENT ESTIMATES

5.1   National, 1960-88 (0753, 0825, 0826, 0827, 1625, 1945, 2713, 2722, 2827)

5.1.1   Rate

	Maternal deaths	MMR (per 100 000 live births)
1960	74	126
1965	92	146
1970	55	95
1975	41	69
1980	16	23
1985	29	34
1986	30	36
1987	16	20
1988	15	18

5.1.2   Causes of maternal deaths, 1985

	Number
Hypertensive disorders of pregnancy	6
Abortion	5
Complications of the puerperium	9
Other direct obstetric causes	9
TOTAL	29

6. OTHER SOURCES/ ESTIMATES

6.1   National, 1987 (2713)

The maternal mortality rate was recalculated by PAHO after adjusting for underreporting. The correction was based on the 39% under registration reported by a study in the United States of America.

6.1.1   Rate

Births	80 000
Maternal deaths	29
MMR (per 100 000 births)	36

7. SELECTED ANNOTATED BIBLIOGRAPHY

8. FURTHER READING

Chackiel, J. *Medicion indirecta de la mortalidad materna*. Unpublished document presented at the Reunion regional sobre prevencion de la mortalidad materna, Sao Paulo, 12-15 April 1988. WHE 2387

9. DATA SOURCES

WHE 0753   United Nations, *Demographic Yearbook.* New York, various years.

WHE 0825   World Health Organization. Pan American Health Organization. *Health conditions in the Americas. 1969-72.* (PAHO scientific publication no. 306) PAHO, Washington, 1975.

WHE 0826   World Health Organization. Pan American Health Organization. *Health conditions in the Americas. 1973-1976.* (PAHO scientific publication no. 364) PAHO, Washington, 1982.

WHE 0827   World Health Organization. Pan American Health Organization. *Health conditions in the Americas. 1977-1980.* (PAHO scientific publication no. 427) PAHO, Washington, 1982.

WHE 0834   World Health Organization *World Health Statistics annual – vital statistics and causes of death.* Geneva, various years.

WHE 1534   World Health Organization, Pan American Health Organization. Programa de salud materno-infantil. *Documento de referencia sobre estudio y prevención de la mortalidad materna* Fasiculo I, Washington, 1986.

WHE 1625   World Health Organization, Pan American Health Organization. *Health conditions in the Americas.* 1981-84. Vol. I (PAHO Scientific Publication no. 500). PAHO, Washington, 1986.

WHE 1712   Mauldin W.P. and Segal, S.J., *Prevalence of contraceptive use in developing countries. A chart book.* Rockefeller Foundation, New York, 1986.

WHE 1914   United Nations Children's Fund (UNICEF). *The state of the world's children*, Oxford University Press, Oxford, various years.

WHE 1915   United Nations. Department of International Economic and Social Affairs. *World population prospects: estimates and projections as assessed in 1984.* Population Studies No. 98. New York, 1986.

WHE 1942   World Health Organization. Pan American Health Organization. *Evaluation of the strategy for Health for All by the Year 2000.* Seventh Report on the World Health Situation. Vol.3. Region of the Americas. Washington, PAHO 1986

WHE 1945   Jimenez Gamboa, J. et al. *Mortalidad materna en Costa Rica.* (unpublished), Costa Rica, 1988.

WHE 2033   World Health Organization. *Global strategy for health for all by the year 2000. Second report on monitoring progress.* WHO document EB83/2 Add. 1, 1988

WHE 2713   World Health Organization, Pan American Health Organization *Regional plan of action for the reduction of maternal mortality in the Americas,* Document No. CSP23/10, XXIII Pan American Sanitary Conference, Washington 1990

WHE 2722   World Health Organization, *Maternal deaths and maternal mortality rates* (unpublished) 1990.

WHE 2799   United Nations. Department of International Economic and Social Affairs. *Patterns of first marriage: timing and prevalence.* New York, 1990.

WHE 2827   World Health Organization. Pan American Health Organization *Health conditions in the Americas 1990.* Scientific publication No. 524, PAHO, Washington, 1991.

NOTES

CUBA

		Year	Source

1. BASIC INDICATORS

1.1 Demographic

1.1.1 Population
Size (millions)	10.6	1990	(1915)
Rate of growth (%)	1.0	1985-90	(1915)

1.1.2 Life expectancy
Female	77	1985-90	(1915)
Male	74	1985-90	(1915)

1.1.3 Fertility
Crude Birth Rate	18	1985-90	(1915)
Total Fertility Rate	1.8	1985-90	(1915)

1.1.4 Mortality
Crude Death Rate	7	1985-90	(1915)
Infant Mortality Rate	15	1985-90	(1915)
Female	10	1988	(2827)
Male	13	1988	(2827)
1-4 years mortality rate			
Female	1	1988	(2827)
Male	1	1988	(2827)

1.2 Social and Economic

1.2.1 Adult literacy rate (%)
Female	96	1981	(1914)
Male	96	1981	(1914)

1.2.2 Primary school enrolment rate (%)
Female	100	1986-88	(1914)
Male	107	1986-88	(1914)

1.2.3 Female mean age at first marriage
(years)	19.9	1981	(1918)

		Year	Source

1.2.4 GNP/capita
(US $)	1 170	1988	(1914)

1.2.5 Daily per capita calorie supply
(as % of requirements)	135	1984-86	(1914)

2. HEALTH SERVICES

2.1 Health Expenditure

2.1.1 Expenditure on health
(as % of GNP)

2.1.2 Expenditure on PHC
(as % of total health expenditure)

2.2 Primary Health Care
(Percentage of population covered by):

2.2.1 Health services
National	100	1987	(2033)
Urban			
Rural			

2.2.2 Safe water
National	61	1983	(0834)
Urban			
Rural			

2.2.3 Adequate sanitary facilities
National	31	1982	(0834)
Urban			
Rural			

2.2.4 Contraceptive prevalence rate
(%)	60	1980	(1712)

2.3 Coverage of maternity care (%)

Area	Prenatal care	Trained attendant	Institutional deliveries	Postnatal care	Sample size	Year	Source
National			99			1985	(1534)
National	100	99				1987	(2033)

3. COMMUNITY STUDIES

4. HOSPITAL STUDIES

4.1 All health institutions, 1962-84 [1261]

4.1.1 Rate

	MMR (per 100 000 live births)
1962	118
1965	109
1970	70
1975	68
1980	53
1981	40
1982	48
1983	32
1984	31

4.1.2 Causes of maternal deaths (direct causes only).

	%				
	1960	1970	1975	1980	1984
Sepsis	8	11	17	17	19
Abortions	12	31	17	29	15
Hypertensive disorders of pregnancy	30	8	17	7	11
Haemorrhage	27	11	9	11	6
Other complications of pregnancy, childbirth and the puerperium	23	39	40	36	49
Total	100	100	100	100	100

4.1.3 Avoidable factors

4.1.4 High risk groups
Age

	Births	Maternal deaths	MMR (per 100 000 live births)
< 15	5 471	3	55
15-19	194 829	56	29
20-29	312 781	122	39
30-39	75 779	64	85
40+	5 751	11	191

Deaths to mothers under 15 were all from convulsive eclampsia. Among mothers over 40 mortality from haemorrhage was very high.

	Age (years)				
% of deaths from:	<15	15-19	20-29	30-39	40+
Abortion	0	27	21	22	18
Haemorrhage	0	14	17	13	36
Eclampsia	100	1	12	6	9
Ruptured uterus	0	2	7	5	9
Amniotic fluid embolism	0	11	11	25	18
Others	0	30	32	29	10
Total	100	100	100	100	100

Delivery by caesarean section constituted another risk factor. Of the 54 cases of death from sepsis between 1980 and 1984, 41 followed caesarean delivery. In addition, 13 cases of death from complications of anaesthesia were associated with caesarean section.

4.2 All health institutions, by province, 1980-84 [1261]

4.2.1 Rate

	Live births	Maternal deaths	MMR (per 100 000 live births)
Santiago de Cuba	86 016	48	56
Granma	71 532	36	50
Guantanamo	47 930	24	50
Havana city	124 125	54	44
Las Tunas	39 566	17	43
Holguin	73 828	32	43
Camaguey	53 774	21	39
Havana	42 256	15	36
Santi Spiritus	28 273	10	35
Matanzas	38 093	12	32
Cienfuegos	25 068	7	28
Ciego de Avila	25 415	7	28
Villa Clara	51 289	13	25
Pinar del Rio	51 336	11	21
Isla de la Juventud	5 934	1	17
Total	764 435	308	40

5. CIVIL REGISTRATION DATA/GOVERNMENT ESTIMATES

5.1 National, 1960-88 [0825, 0826, 0827, 0834, 1625, 2713, 2722]

5.1.1 Rate

	Maternal deaths	MMR (per 100 000 live births)
1960	250	116
1965	292	111
1970	173	76
1975	132	68
1980	82	60
1985	84	46
1986	87	52
1987	88	49
1988	73	39

5.1.2 Causes of maternal deaths, 1983, 1985 and 1987

	1983 No.	1983 %	1985 No.	1985 %	1987 No.	1987 %
Abortions	10	13	12	14	16	18
Complications of the puerperium	12	16	10	12	10	11
Haemorrhage	3	4	3	4	5	6
Hypertensive disorders of pregnancy	8	11	11	13	2	2
Other direct obstetric causes	19	25	20	24	28	32
DIRECT CAUSES	52	69	56	67	61	69
INDIRECT CAUSES	23	31	28	33	27	31
TOTAL	75	100	84	100	88	100

5.2 Havana City, Holguin and Cienfuegos, 1979-82 [2806]

5.2.1 Rate

	Live births	Maternal deaths	MMR (per 100 000 live births)
Havana City	92 801	42	45
Holguin	52 321	21	40
Cienfuegos	18 589	8	43
Total	163 711	71	43

5.2.2 Causes of maternal deaths (%)

	Havana	Holguin	Cienfuegos	Total
Abortion	31	24	13	27
Hypertensive disorders of pregnancy	7	24	38	15
Sepsis	10	19	38	15
Haemorrhage	2	5	-	3
Other causes	50	29	13	39
Total	100	100	100	100
(N)	42	21	8	71

5.2.3 Avoidable factors

5.2.4 High risk groups
Age

	MMR (per 100 000 live births)
15-19	20
20-24	29
25-29	52
30-34	83
35-39	122
40-44	440

Level of education

	MMR (per 100 000 live births)
Primary level only	69
Higher than primary	27

Marital status and abortion mortality

	MMR* (per 100 000 live births)
Married or cohabiting	7
Other	305

* Abortion deaths only.

6. OTHER SOURCES/ ESTIMATES

6.1 National, 1986-87 (1991)

6.1.1 Rate*

	MMR (per 100 000 live births)
1986	37
1987	34

* Direct causes only

6.1.2 Causes of maternal deaths, 1985-87

	Number	%
Associated with caesarean section	47	18
Abortion	28	11
Haemorrhage	21	8
Embolisms	20	8
Ectopic pregnancy	18	8
Hypertensive disorders of pregnancy	16	6
Sepsis	15	6
Complications of anaesthesia	12	5
Other direct causes	3	1
DIRECT CAUSES	180	70
Cardiopathies	28	11
Anaemia	10	4
Hepatitis	9	3
Other indirect causes	31	12
INDIRECT CAUSES	78	30
TOTAL	258	100

6.2 National, 1990 (2713)

The maternal mortality rate was adjusted by PAHO to take account of the estimated 39% under-registration observed in a study carried out in the United States of America.

6.2.1 Rate

Births	181 000
Maternal deaths	65
MMR (per 100 000 births)	36

7. SELECTED ANNOTATED BIBLIOGRAPHY

Cardoso, U.F. Giving birth is safer now. *World Health Forum* 1986; 7: 348-352. WHE 1465

The reasons for the large drop in Cuba's maternal mortality rate are examined. The author concludes that the establishment of maternity waiting homes in which women from outlying districts can be accommodated near hospitals during the last weeks of pregnancy has been an important contributory factor (see below). A substantial decrease in deaths from toxaemia is attributed to improved prenatal care and better socio-economic conditions. Deaths from haemorrhage were reduced as a result of the increasing proportion of deliveries which took place in hospitals. Other factors include the use of the risk approach as a guide for referral.

Gutiérrez Muñiz, J. *Contribución de los hogares maternos de Cuba a la maternidad sin riesgo.* (project proposal), Ministerio de Salud Publica/Instituto Superior de Ciencias Medicas de la Habana/ Facultad de Ciencias Medicas Julio Trigo. 1991. WHE 2831.

Maternity waiting homes are special institutions designed to encourage hospital delivery by providing accommodation during the last two weeks of pregnancy for women living in remote areas where rapid and easy access to hospitals is difficult. They are also used to supervise women with high risk of complications during pregnancy and delivery. Deliveries do not occur in the homes themselves, most of which are converted houses situated near the hospital. The first such maternity homes were opened on Government initiative in the early 1960s. In 1991 a total of 148 waiting homes with 2,424 rooms had been designated, covering all Cuba's provinces. Admissions have risen from 3,488 in 1968 to 45,462 in 1989. It is thought that the homes have made a significant contribution to the reduction in maternal mortality rates but a systematic appraisal and evaluation is not yet available.

8. FURTHER READING

Castell Moreno, J. Profilaxis de las muertes maternas por aborto. *Revista Cubana de Obstetricia y Ginecologia*, 1986; 12(1): 81-85. WHE 2832.

Chackiel, J. *Medicion indirecta de la mortalidad materna*. Unpublished document presented at the Reunion regional sobre prevencion de la mortalidad materna, Sao Paulo, 12-15 April 1988. WHE 2387

Steegers, E.L. Mortalidad materna en Cuba. Decenio 1970-1979. *Revista Cubana de Administración de Salud*, 1983; 9: 303-315. WHE 0705.

9. DATA SOURCES

WHE 0825   World Health Organization. Pan American Health Organization. *Health conditions in the Americas. 1969-72.* (PAHO scientific publication no. 306) PAHO, Washington, 1975.

WHE 0826   World Health Organization. Pan American Health Organization. *Health conditions in the Americas. 1973-1976.* (PAHO scientific publication no. 364) PAHO, Washington, 1982.

WHE 0827   World Health Organization. Pan American Health Organization. *Health conditions in the Americas. 1977-1980.* (PAHO scientific publication no. 427) PAHO, Washington, 1982.

WHE 0834   World Health Organization *World Health Statistics annual – vital statistics and causes of death.* Geneva, various years.

WHE 1261   Farnot, U.C. Maternal mortality in Cuba. In: *Interregional Meeting on the Prevention of Maternal Mortality* Geneva, 11-15 November 1985 (unpublished WHO document no. FHE/PMM/85.9.14).

WHE 1534   World Health Organization, Pan American Health Organization. Programa de salud materna infantil. *Documento de referencia sobre estudio y prevención de la mortalidad materna*, Fasciculo I. PAHO, Washington, 1986.

WHE 1625   World Health Organization, Pan American Health Organization. *Health conditions in the Americas.* 1981-84. Vol. I (PAHO Scientific Publication no. 500). PAHO, Washington, 1986.

WHE 1712   Mauldin W.P. and Segal, S.J., *Prevalence of contraceptive use in developing countries. A chart book.* Rockefeller Foundation, New York, 1986.

WHE 1914   United Nations Children's Fund (UNICEF). *The state of the world's children*, Oxford University Press, Oxford, various years.

WHE 1915   United Nations. Department of International Economic and Social Affairs. *World population prospects: estimates and projections as assessed in 1984.* Population Studies No. 98. New York 1986.

WHE 1918   United Nations. Department of International Economic and Social Affairs. *First marriage: patterns and determinants.* New York, 1988.

WHE 1991   Cabezas, E. *Mortalidad materna en Cuba.* Paper presented at WHO/PAHO Workshop on Maternal Mortality Research. Sao Paulo, April 1988.

WHE 2033   World Health Organization. *Global strategy for health for all by the year 2000. Second report on monitoring progress.* WHO document EB83/2 Add. 1, 1988.

WHE 2713   World Health Organization, Pan American Health Organization *Regional plan of action for the reduction of maternal mortality in the Americas,* Document No. CSP23/10, XXIII Pan American Sanitary Conference, Washington 1990.

WHE 2722   World Health Organization, *Maternal deaths and maternal mortality rates* (unpublished) 1990.

WHE 2806   Nebreda Moreno, M. and Avalos Triana, O. Aspectos sociodemograficos de la mortalidad materna en las provincias Cuidad de la Habana, Holguin y Cienfuegos, 1979-1982. *Revista Cubana de Administración de Salud*, 1985; 11(1): 43-54.

WHE 2827   World Health Organization. Pan American Health Organization. *Health conditions in the Americas*, Scientific Publication No. 524, Washington, 1990.

NOTES

DOMINICAN REPUBLIC

		Year	Source

1. BASIC INDICATORS

1.1 Demographic

1.1.1 Population

		Year	Source
Size (millions)	7.1	1990	(1915)
Rate of growth (%)	2.2	1985-90	(1915)

1.1.2 Life expectancy

Female	68	1985-90	(1915)
Male	64	1985-90	(1915)

1.1.3 Fertility

Crude Birth Rate	31	1985-90	(1915)
Total Fertility Rate	3.8	1985-90	(1915)

1.1.4 Mortality

Crude Death Rate	7	1985-90	(1915)
Infant Mortality Rate	65	1985-90	(1915)
Female	54	1985	(2827)
Male	59	1985	(2827)
1-4 years mortality rate			
Female	3	1985	(2827)
Male	3	1985	(2827)

1.2 Social and economic

1.2.1 Adult literacy rate (%)

Female	79	1985	(1914)
Male	82	1985	(1914)

1.2.2 Primary school enrolment rate (%)

Female	103	1986-88	(1914)
Male	99	1986-88	(1914)

1.2.3 Female mean age at first marriage

(years)	19.7	1970	(1918)

1.2.4 GNP/capita

		Year	Source
(US $)	720	1987	(1914)

1.2.5 Daily per capita calorie supply

(as % of requirements)	104	1984-86	(1914)

2. HEALTH SERVICES

2.1 Health Expenditure

2.1.1 Expenditure on health

(as % of GNP)	2.3	1984	(2033)

2.1.2 Expenditure on PHC
(as % of total health expenditure)

2.2 Primary Health Care
(Percentage of population covered by):

2.2.1 Health services
National
Urban
Rural

2.2.2 Safe water

National	62	1983	(0834)
Urban	72	1985	(2033)
Rural	24	1985	(2033)

2.2.3 Adequate sanitary facilities

National			
Urban	72	1985	(2033)
Rural	59	1985	(2033)

2.4 Contraceptive prevalence rate*

(%)	50	1986	(1636)

* Married and cohabiting women

2.3 Coverage of maternity care (%)

Area	Prenatal care	Trained attendant	Institutional deliveries	Postnatal care	Sample size	Year	Source
National			64			1980	(1534)
National:	95	90				1982-86	(1636)
urban	96	95				1982-86	(1636)
rural	93	83				1982-86	(1636)

3. COMMUNITY STUDIES

4. HOSPITAL STUDIES

5. CIVIL REGISTRATION DATA/GOVERNMENT ESTIMATES

5.1 National, 1960-85 (0825, 0826, 0827, 1625, 2713, 2722, 2827)

5.1.1 Rate

	Maternal deaths	MMR (per 100 000 live births)
1960	111	101
1965	106	99
1970	167	102
1975	151	94
1980	139	72
1981	127	65
1982	128	66
1983	114	65
1984	120	74
1985	106	94
1987	n.a.	100

5.1.2 Causes of maternal deaths, 1985

	Number	%
Hypertensive disorders of pregnancy	27	25
Abortions	18	17
Haemorrhage	17	16
Complications of the puerperium	0	–
Other direct obstetric causes	36	34
DIRECT CAUSES	98	92
Indirect causes	8	8
TOTAL	106	100

6. OTHER SOURCES/ ESTIMATES

6.1 National, 1985 (2713)

A Pan American Health Organization report estimated maternal deaths after adjusting for underreporting.

6.1.1 Rate
Births	213 000
Maternal deaths	639
MMR (per 100 000 births)	300

7. SELECTED ANNOTATED BIBLIOGRAPHY

World Health Organization. Pan American Health Organization. *Health conditions in the Americas*, Scientific Publication No. 524, Washington, 1990. WHE 2827

A report of the Pan American Health Organization quotes a hospital study in the Dominican Republic which found an institutional maternal mortality rate of 200 per 100 000 live births coupled with a rate of caesarean delivery of 26%. It is noted that there is considerable variation in rates of caesarean delivery in different countries of the region, from under 10% in Honduras to over 30% in Mexico. An epidemiological study of caesarean delivery, undertaken by the Centro Latino Americano de Perinatologia y Desarrollo Humano (CLAP) and PAHO in 1985 in 17 countries indicated that the frequency of caesarean delivery explains only 5% of the variations in perinatal mortality and that there is no correlation between frequency of operative delivery and reduction in maternal mortality.

Indeed, caesarean delivery is associated with higher rates of mortality and morbidity than vaginal delivery and is a bigger strain on the human and financial resources of the health service.

8. FURTHER READING

Chackiel, J. *Medicion indirecta de la mortalidad materna*. Unpublished document presented at the Reunion regional sobre prevencion de la mortalidad materna, Sao Paulo, 12-15 April 1988. WHE 2387

9. DATA SOURCES

WHE 0825   World Health Organization. Pan American Health Organization. *Health conditions in the Americas. 1969-72.* (PAHO scientific publication no. 306) PAHO, Washington, 1975.

WHE 0826   World Health Organization. Pan American Health Organization. *Health conditions in the Americas. 1973-1976.* (PAHO scientific publication no. 364) PAHO, Washington, 1982.

WHE 0827   World Health Organization. Pan American Health Organization. *Health conditions in the Americas. 1977-1980.* (PAHO scientific publication no. 427) PAHO, Washington, 1982.

WHE 0834   World Health Organization *World health statistics annual – vital statistics and causes of death.* Geneva, various years.

WHE 1534   World Health Organization. Pan American Health Organization. *Programa de salud materna infantil. Documento de referencia sobre estudio y prevencion de la mortalidad materna.* Fasciculo I. PAHO, Washington, 1986.

WHE 1625   World Health Organization, Pan American Health Organization. *Health conditions in the Americas.* 1981-84. Vol. I (PAHO Scientific Publication no. 500). PAHO, Washington, 1986.

WHE 1636   Demographic and Health Surveys. *Encuesta demografica y de salud*, Consejo Nacional de Poblacion y Familia/Institute for Resource Development/Westinghouse, 1987.

WHE 1914   United Nations Children's Fund (UNICEF). *The state of the world's children*, Oxford, Oxford University Press, various years.

WHE 1915   United Nations. Department of International Economic and Social Affairs. *World population prospects: estimates and projections*, Population Studies, New York, various years.

WHE 1918   United Nations. Department of International Economic and Social Affairs. *First marriage: patterns and determinants.* New York 1988.

WHE 2033   World Health Organization. *Global strategy for health for all by the year 2000. Second report on monitoring progress.* WHO document EB83/2 Add. 1, 1988.

WHE 2713   World Health Organization, Pan American Health Organization *Regional plan of action for the reduction of maternal mortality in the Americas,* Document No. CSP23/10, XXIII Pan American Sanitary Conference, Washington 1990.

WHE 2722   World Health Organization, *Maternal deaths and maternal mortality rates* (unpublished) 1990.

WHE 2827   World Health Organization. Pan American Health Organization. *Health conditions in the Americas*, Scientific Publication No. 524, Washington, 1990.

NOTES

ECUADOR

		Year	Source

1. BASIC INDICATORS

1.1 Demographic

1.1.1 Population
		Year	Source
Size (millions)	10.6	1990	(1915)
Rate of growth (%)	2.6	1985-90	(1915)

1.1.2 Life expectancy
		Year	Source
Female	68	1985-90	(1915)
Male	63	1985-90	(1915)

1.1.3 Fertility
		Year	Source
Crude Birth Rate	33	1985-90	(1915)
Total Fertility Rate	4.3	1985-90	(1915)

1.1.4 Mortality
		Year	Source
Crude Death Rate	7	1985-90	(1915)
Infant Mortality Rate	63	1985-90	(1915)
Female	52	1982-86	(1632)
Male	64	1982-86	(1632)
1-4 years mortality rate			
Female	26	1982-86	(1632)
Male	25	1982-86	(1632)

1.2 Social and economic

1.2.1 Adult literacy rate (%)
		Year	Source
Female	81	1985	(1914)
Male	86	1985	(1914)

1.2.2 Primary school enrolment rate (%)
		Year	Source
Female	116	1986-88	(1914)
Male	118	1986-88	(1914)

1.2.3 Female mean age at first marriage
		Year	Source
(years)	21.1	1981	(2799)

1.2.4 GNP/capita
		Year	Source
(US $)	1 120	1987	(1914)

1.2.5 Daily per capita calorie supply
		Year	Source
(as % of requirements)	89	1984-86	(1914)

2. HEALTH SERVICES

2.1 Health Expenditure

2.1.1 Expenditure on health
		Year	Source
(as % of GNP)	6.0	1984	(2033)

2.1.2 Expenditure on PHC
(as % of total health expenditure)

2.2 Primary Health Care
(Percentage of population covered by):

2.2.1 Health services
		Year	Source
National	80	1983-87	(2033)
Urban			
Rural			

2.2.2 Safe water
		Year	Source
National	59	1983	(0834)
Urban	83	1985	(2033)
Rural	33	1985	(2033)

2.2.3 Adequate sanitary facilities
		Year	Source
National	45	1983	(0834)
Urban	79	1985	(2033)
Rural	34	1985	(2033)

2.2.4 Contraceptive prevalence rate*
		Year	Source
(%)	44	1986	(1632)

* Married and cohabiting women.

2.3 Coverage of maternity care (%)

Area	Prenatal care	Trained attendant	Institutional deliveries	Postnatal care	Sample size	Year	Source
National	72	62	57	42	4 300	1982	(1535)
National	49	27				1983	(0834)
National	71	44				1983-87	(2033)
National		52				1986	(2390)
National:	70	62			3 032	1982-86	(1632)
urban	82	85			1 494	1982-86	(1632)
rural	58	40			1 538	1982-86	(1632)
Costa:							
Guayaquil	83	90			431	1982-86	(1632)
Resto Urbano	80	73			402	1982-86	(1632)
Rural	62	40			707	1982-86	(1632)
Sierra:							
Quito	84	89			332	1982-86	(1632)
Resto Urbano	82	90			329	1982-86	(1632)
Rural	54	40			831	1982-86	(1632)
Quito and Guayaquil		46	42		600	(1984)	(1536)

3. COMMUNITY STUDIES

4. HOSPITAL STUDIES

5. CIVIL REGISTRATION DATA/GOVERNMENT ESTIMATES

5.1 National, 1985 [1686]

5.1.1 Rate

Region	Live births	Maternal deaths	MMR (per 100 000 live births)
Sierra	108 725	220	202
Costa	92 404	164	177
Amazonica	8 670	12	138
Insular	175	1	571
Total	209 974	397	189

5.2 National, 1960-88 [0825, 0826, 0827, 0834, 1625, 1686, 2713, 2722, 2827]

5.2.1 Rate

	Live births	Maternal deaths	MMR (per 100 000 live births)
1960	206 178	557	270
1965	226 436	583	257
1970	230 184	529	230
1975	242 554	513	211
1980	262 778	426	162
1981	264 963	443	167
1982	262 102	394	150
1983	253 990	413	163
1984	257 044	384	149
1985	209 974	397	189
1986	n.a.	330	160
1987	n.a.	355	174
1988	n.a.	329	156

5.2.2 Causes of maternal deaths

	1980 No.	1980 %	1982 No.	1982 %	1984 No.	1984 %
Hypertensive disorders of pregnancy	87	20	108	27	107	28
Haemorrhage	71	17	84	21	82	21
Abortions	44	10	27	7	34	9
Complications of the puerperium	52	13	40	10	33	9
Other direct obstetric causes	172	40	124	32	123	32
Indirect obstetric causes	0	0	11	3	5	1
Total	426	100	394	100	384	100

6. OTHER SOURCES/ ESTIMATES

6.1 National, 1983 [(1912)]

6.1.1 Rate

A report of the Pan American Health Organization quotes a maternal mortality rate for Ecuador of 200 per 100 000 live births in 1983.

6.2 National [(2713)]

The rate was estimated by PAHO to be the same as that derived from a study in Peru.

6.2.1 Rate

Births	328 000
Maternal deaths	984
MMR (per 100 000 births)	300

7. SELECTED ANNOTATED BIBLIOGRAPHY

Calle, A. *Fistula de origen obstétrico.* (unpublished) Quito, 1989. WHE 2292

Obstetric fistula in Ecuador are found to occur in women who have poor access to health services. From 1985-88 at the Isidro Ayora Hospital in Quito, there were a total of eight cases of obstetric fistula, three of which were recto-vaginal and five of which were vesico-vaginal. Six patients were primigravidae. None of the women had had adequate prenatal care or appropriate care during birth.

Pino, A. *Obstetric fistulae.* (Personal communication), Quito, 1989. WHE 2291

An analysis of national data on hospital admissions in Ecuador from 1979-1987 showed that there were 673 cases of genital fistula, and 559 cases of trauma of the perineum and vulva during labour and birth. Of the fistula cases, 33 (4.9%) were in women under the age of 15, and 31% were in women aged 45 and over.

Pino, M. A. et al. Mortalidad materna en el Ecuador y aspectos culturales en la atención de la mujer embarazada. *Revista del Instituto Juan Cesar García*, 1991; 1(1): 33-56. Quito, Ecuador. WHE 3008.

An analysis of official data on maternal mortality found little change in rates over the past two decades. Rates are thought to be particularly high in rural areas although in the absence of systematic reporting of maternal deaths this is difficult to demonstrate. Of the 330 maternal deaths which occurred during 1986, over half of the women were residents of rural areas. The proportion of women receiving trained assistance during delivery was considerably lower in rural areas at 24% compared with 72% for women in urban areas. The major causes of maternal deaths are hypertensive disorders of pregnancy (24%) and haemorrhage (21%). Abortion is thought to account for over 8% of maternal deaths.

Interviews conducted with health service staff, traditional birth attendants and pregnant women indicated that a variety of cultural factors play an important role in the use (or nonuse) of modern health services, especially among rural populations. Both women and traditional birth attendants felt that prenatal visits were unnecessary as pregnancy is a natural condition. The only reason women sought prenatal care was to assess whether or not the fetus was in the correct position for natural childbirth. The formal prenatal care services worked to a fixed and rigid timetable and imposed a variety of restrictions which were perceived by the women themselves as an obstacle to health service utilization. For example, they did not permit husbands, friends or relatives to accompany the women during prenatal visits. The majority of the women refused treatment by male health service personnel.

All the women expressed a strong preference for home deliveries even though many were aware of the emergencies which can arise during delivery. This preference was further strengthened by the possibility of being assisted by relatives during home delivery, a possibility not given to women delivering in health centres.

Women observed a number of food restrictions during pregnancy, avoiding animal proteins and fats. Dietary information campaigns by health personnel had little effect given such strong cultural beliefs. In addition, many of the women were extremely poor and could ill afford the kinds of foods prescribed by the health services.

The study concludes that there is a need to further integrate traditional birth attendants into the formal health care system. Women prefer the flexibility and familiarity of home delivery with TBAs but the latter could greatly benefit from increased training, support and supervision by the formal sector.

World Health Organization. Pan American Health Organization. *Health conditions in the Americas*, Scientific Publication No. 524, Washington, 1990. WHE 2827

A report of the Pan American Health Organization quotes a study of four hospitals in Ecuador which found an institutional maternal mortality rate of 200 per 100 000 live births coupled with a rate of caesarean delivery of 25%. It is noted that there is considerable variation in rates of caesarean delivery in different countries of the region, from under 10% in Honduras to over 30% in Mexico. An epidemiological study of caesarean delivery, undertaken by the Centro Latino Americano de Perinatología y

Desarrollo Humano (CLAP) and PAHO in 1985 in 17 countries indicated that the frequency of caesarean delivery explains only 5% of the variations in perinatal mortality and that there is no correlation between frequency of operative delivery and reduction in maternal mortality. Indeed, caesarean delivery is associated with higher rates of mortality and morbidity than vaginal delivery and is a bigger strain on the human and financial resources of the health service.

8. FURTHER READING

Chackiel, J. *Medicion indirecta de la mortalidad materna*. Unpublished document presented at the Reunion regional sobre prevencion de la mortalidad materna, Sao Paulo, 12-15 April 1988. WHE 2387

Ruffing, K.L and Smith, H.L. Maternal and child health care in Ecuador: obstacles and solutions. *Issues in Health Care for Women*, 1984; 5(4): 195-210. WHE 0933.

Weigel, M. Calcio y hipertensión inducida por el embarazo. *Revista de la Facultad de Ciencias Médicas (Quito)*, 1987; 12:13-26. WHE 2815.

9. DATA SOURCES

WHE 0825   World Health Organization. Pan American Health Organization. *Health conditions in the Americas. 1969-72.* (PAHO scientific publication no. 306) PAHO, Washington, 1975.

WHE 0826   World Health Organization. Pan American Health Organization. *Health conditions in the Americas. 1973-1976.* (PAHO scientific publication no. 364) PAHO, Washington, 1982.

WHE 0827   World Health Organization. Pan American Health Organization. *Health conditions in the Americas. 1977-1980.* (PAHO scientific publication no. 427) PAHO, Washington, 1982.

WHE 0834   World Health Organization *World health statistics annual – vital statistics and causes of death.* Geneva, various years.

WHE 1535   Centro de estudios de población y paternidad responsable. *Fecundidad en el Ecuador, 1979 y 1982.* CEPAR, Quito, 1984.

WHE 1536   Centro de estudios de población y paternidad responsable. *Encuesta sobre las repercusiones de un nuevo nacimiento.* CEPAR, Quito, 1984.

WHE 1625   World Health Organization, Pan American Health Organization. *Health conditions in the Americas. 1981-84.* Vol. I (PAHO Scientific Publication no. 500). PAHO, Washington, 1986.

WHE 1632   Demographic and Health Surveys. *Encuesta nacional de demografía y salud familiar 1987.* CEPAR/INIMS/Institute for Resource Development, 1987.

WHE 1686   Ecuador, Ministerio de Salud Pública. *Indicadores de salud.* Division Nacional de Estadística, 1986.

WHE 1912   World Health Organization. Pan American Health Organization. *Reference document on study and prevention of maternal mortality.* Washington D.C. 1987.

WHE 1914   United Nations Children's Fund
(UNICEF). *The state of the world's children*, Oxford,
Oxford University Press, various years.

WHE 1915   United Nations. Department of
International Economic and Social Affairs. *World
population prospects: estimates and projections*,
Population Studies, New York, various years.

WHE 2033   World Health Organization. *Global
strategy for health for all by the year 2000. Second
report on monitoring progress.* WHO document
EB83/2 Add. 1, 1988.

WHE 2390   Pino, M.A. et al. *Mortalidad materna y
servicios de salud en el Ecuador.* Instituto Juan
García, Quito, 1989.

WHE 2713   World Health Organization, Pan
American Health Organization *Regional plan of
action for the reduction of maternal mortality in the
Americas,* Document No. CSP23/10, XXIII Pan
American Sanitary Conference, Washington 1990.

WHE 2722   World Health Organization, *Maternal
deaths and maternal mortality rates* (unpublished)
1990.

WHE 2799   United Nations. Department of
International Economic and Social Affairs. *Patterns
of first marriage: timing and prevalence.* New York,
1990.

WHE 2827   World Health Organization. Pan
American Health Organization. *Health conditions
in the Americas*, Scientific Publication No. 524,
Washington, 1990.

NOTES

EL SALVADOR

	Year	Source

1. BASIC INDICATORS

1.1 Demographic

1.1.1 Population

		Year	Source
Size (millions)	5.3	1990	(1915)
Rate of growth (%)	1.9	1985-90	(1915)

1.1.2 Life expectancy

		Year	Source
Female	67	1985-90	(1915)
Male	58	1985-90	(1915)

1.1.3 Fertility

		Year	Source
Crude Birth Rate	36	1985-90	(1915)
Total Fertility Rate	4.9	1985-90	(1915)

1.1.4 Mortality

		Year	Source
Crude Death Rate	9	1985-90	(1915)
Infant Mortality Rate	64	1985-90	(1915)
Female	32	1984	(2827)
Male	37	1984	(2827)
1-4 years mortality rate			
Female	3	1984	(2827)
Male	3	1984	(2827)

1.2 Social and economic

1.2.1 Adult literacy rate (%)

		Year	Source
Female	65	1985	(1914)
Male	73	1985	(1914)

1.2.2 Primary school enrolment rate (%)

		Year	Source
Female	81	1986-88	(1914)
Male	77	1986-88	(1914)

1.2.3 Female mean age at first marriage

		Year	Source
(years)	19.4	1971	(2799)

1.2.4 GNP/capita

		Year	Source
(US $)	940	1987	(1914)

1.2.5 Daily per capita calorie supply

		Year	Source
(as % of requirements)	94	1984-86	(1914)

2. HEALTH SERVICES

2.1 Health expenditure

2.1.1 Expenditure on health

		Year	Source
(as % of GNP)	2.1	1983	(1942)

2.1.2 Expenditure on PHC

		Year	Source
(as % of total health expenditure)	100	1983	(1942)

2.2 Primary Health Care
(Percentage of population covered by):

2.2.1 Health services

		Year	Source
National			
Urban			
Rural			

2.2.2 Safe water

		Year	Source
National	58	1985	(2033)
Urban	76	1985	(2033)
Rural	47	1985	(2033)

2.2.3 Adequate sanitary facilities

		Year	Source
National	41	1983	(0834)
Urban	89	1983	(2033)
Rural	35	1983	(2033)

2.2.4 Contraceptive prevalence rate

		Year	Source
(%)	47	1985	(3009)

2.3 Coverage of maternity care (%)

Area	Prenatal care	Trained attendant	Institutional deliveries	Postnatal care	Sample size	Year	Source
National			50			1982	(1534)
National	23	35				1984	(1534)
National			28		142 202	1984	(2830)
National	34	50				(1987)	(2713)
National:		51			3 491	1981-85	(3009)
urban		59			886	1981-85	(3009)
rural		28			1 667	1981-851	(3009)
metropolitan		84			928	1981-85	(3009)

3. COMMUNITY STUDIES

4. HOSPITAL STUDIES

4.1 22 public hospitals throughout the country, 1983-87 [2830]

A study was carried out in a number of public hospitals in order to compare numbers of registered maternal deaths and numbers estimated following a detailed examination and analysis of hospital records.

4.1.1 Rate

Live births	250 801
Maternal deaths	372
MMR (per 100 000 live births)	148

Over the same period, only 277 maternal deaths were registered as such.

4.1.2 Causes of maternal deaths *(for 315 deaths)*

The study found that in 71% of the registered maternal deaths the cause of death given on the certificate was "ill defined causes". Half of these deaths were, on examination of the medical records, found to have been due to sepsis and the other half to indirect causes.

	Number	%
Hypertensive disorders of pregnancy	81	26
Sepsis	79	25
Haemorrhage	66	21
Abortion	24	8
Complications of anaesthesia	7	2
Obstructed labour	1	<1
DIRECT CAUSES	258	82
Hepatitis	9	3
Cardiopathies	6	2
Meningitis	6	2
Malaria	2	1
Other indirect causes	22	7
INDIRECT CAUSES	45	14
Fortuitous	12	4
TOTAL	315	100

4.1.3 Avoidable factors

	Number	%
Definitely avoidable	107	34
Potentially avoidable	189	60
Probably unavoidable	18	6

Prenatal care

	Definitely avoidable deaths %	Potentially avoidable deaths %	Probably unavoidable deaths %
No prenatal care	64	76	75
1-3 prenatal visits	33	19	8
4-6 prenatal visits	2	5	8
More than 6 visits	1	0	8

Place of delivery

	Definitely avoidable deaths %	Potentially avoidable deaths %	Probably unavoidable deaths %
Hospital delivery	83	64	71
Home delivery	17	36	29

4.1.4 High risk groups

4.1.5 Other findings

Most of the deaths occurred among women who were not legally married but cohabiting. Over 70% of the deaths were in rural areas where access to the hospitals was difficult.

Over half the women who died did so within 24 hours of admission to the hospital. In the Eastern region of the country this figure was 70%.

In 38% of the deaths, a caesarean delivery had been performed. In at least half of these cases, the death was considered definitely or potentially preventable.

Registration of deaths and of the circumstances surrounding them was inadequate. In 55% of the cases, no information on the fate of the infant was noted on the certificate. Records on previous obstetric history of the women who died were inadequate.

5. CIVIL REGISTRATION DATA/GOVERNMENT ESTIMATES

5.1 National, 1960-85 (0753, 0825, 0826, 0834, 1625, 2713, 2722, 2827)

5.1.1 Rate

	Maternal deaths	MMR (per 100 000) live births)
1960	210	173
1965	155	113
1970	143	101
1975	148	93
1980	118	71
1981	101	62
1982	133	85
1983	107	74
1984	99	70
1985	82	59

5.1.2 Causes of maternal deaths, 1984

	%
Abortion	7
Haemorrhage	7
Hypertensive disorders of pregnancy	5
Complications of the puerperium	8
Other direct causes	72
Indirect causes	1
Total	100

6. OTHER SOURCES/ESTIMATES

6.1 National, 1984 (2713)

The rate was estimated by PAHO to be the same as that derived from a study in Peru.

6.1.1 Rate

Live births	182 000
Maternal deaths	546
MMR (per 100 000 live births)	300

7. SELECTED ANNOTATED BIBLIOGRAPHY

8. FURTHER READING

Chackiel, J. *Medicion indirecta de la mortalidad materna*. Unpublished document presented at the Reunion regional sobre prevencion de la mortalidad materna, Sao Paulo, 12-15 April 1988. WHE 2387

9. DATA SOURCES

WHE 0753   United Nations, *Demographic Yearbook.* New York, various years.

WHE 0825   World Health Organization. Pan American Health Organization. *Health conditions in the Americas. 1969-72.* (PAHO scientific publication no. 306) PAHO, Washington, 1975.

WHE 0826   World Health Organization. Pan American Health Organization. *Health conditions in the Americas. 1973-1976.* (PAHO scientific publication no. 364) PAHO, Washington, 1982.

WHE 0834   World Health Organization. *World health statistics annual – vital statistics and causes of death.* Geneva, various years.

WHE 1534   World Health Organization, Pan American Health Organization. *Programa de salud materna infantil.* Documento de referencia sobre estudio y prevención de la mortalidad materna, Fasciculo I. PAHO, Washington, 1986.

WHE 1625   World Health Organization, Pan American Health Organization. *Health conditions in the Americas.* 1981-84. Vol. I (PAHO Scientific Publication no. 500). PAHO, Washington, 1986.

WHE 1914   United Nations Children's Fund (UNICEF). *The state of the world's children*, Oxford, Oxford University Press, various years.

WHE 1915   United Nations. Department of International Economic and Social Affairs. *World population prospects: estimates and projections*, Population Studies, New York, various years.

WHE 1942   World Health Organization. Pan American Health Organization. *Evaluation of the strategy for Health for All by the Year 2000.* Seventh Report on the World Health Situation. Vol.3. Region of the Americas. PAHO, Washington, 1986.

WHE 2033   World Health Organization. *Global strategy for health for all by the year 2000. Second report on monitoring progress.* WHO document EB83/2 Add. 1, 1988.

WHE 2713   World Health Organization, Pan American Health Organization *Regional plan of action for the reduction of maternal mortality in the Americas,* Document No. CSP23/10, XXIII Pan American Sanitary Conference, Washington 1990.

WHE 2722   World Health Organization, *Maternal deaths and maternal mortality rates* (unpublished) 1990.

WHE 2799   United Nations. Department of International Economic and Social Affairs. *Patterns of first marriage: timing and prevalence.* New York, 1990.

WHE 2827   World Health Organization. Pan American Health Organization. *Health conditions in the Americas*, Scientific Publication No. 524, Washington, 1990.

WHE 2830   Jarquin, J.D. and Rocuts, F.K. *Epidemiología y prevención de la muerte materna institucional en El Salvador – 1983-1987.* (unpublished), San Salvador, 1989.

WHE 3009   Demographic and Health Surveys. *Encuesta nacional de salud familiar FESAL-85.* Asociación Demografica Salvadoreña/Institute for Resource Development/Westinghouse, 1987.

GUATEMALA

		Year	Source

1. BASIC INDICATORS

1.1 Demographic

1.1.1 Population
		Year	Source
Size (millions)	9.2	1990	(1915)
Rate of growth (%)	2.9	1985-90	(1915)

1.1.2 Life expectancy
		Year	Source
Female	64	1985-90	(1915)
Male	60	1985-90	(1915)

1.1.3 Fertility
		Year	Source
Crude Birth Rate	41	1985-90	(1915)
Total Fertility Rate	5.8	1985-90	(1915)

1.1.4 Mortality
		Year	Source
Crude Death Rate	9	1985-90	(1915)
Infant Mortality Rate	59	1985-90	(1915)
Female	68	1977-87	(3010)
Male	90	1977-87	(3010)
1-4 years mortality rate			
Female	47	1977-87	(3010)
Male	44	1977-87	(3010)

1.2 Social and economic

1.2.1 Adult literacy rate (%)
		Year	Source
Female	44	1985	(1914)
Male	60	1985	(1914)

1.2.2 Primary school enrolment rate (%)
		Year	Source
Female	70	1986-88	(1914)
Male	82	1986-88	(1914)

1.2.3 Female mean age at first marriage
		Year	Source
(years)	20.5	1981	(1918)

1.2.4 GNP/capita
		Year	Source
(US $)	900	1987	(1914)

1.2.5 Daily per capita calorie supply
		Year	Source
(as % of requirements)	105	1984-86	(1914)

2. HEALTH SERVICES

2.1 Health Expenditure

2.1.1 Expenditure on health
		Year	Source
(as % of GNP)	3.7	1984	(1942)

2.1.2 Expenditure on PHC
		Year	Source
(as % of total health expenditure)	17	1985	(1942)

2.2 Primary Health Care
(Percentage of population covered by):

2.2.1 Health services
		Year	Source
National	59	1984	(0834)
Urban			
Rural			

2.2.2 Safe water
		Year	Source
National	51	1983	(0834)
Urban	89	1985	(2033)
Rural	39	1985	(2033)

2.2.3 Adequate sanitary facilities
		Year	Source
National	36	1983	(0834)
Urban	73	1985	(2033)
Rural	42	1985	(2033)

2.4 Contraceptive prevalence rate
		Year	Source
(%)*	23	1987	(3010)

* Married and cohabiting women.

2.3   Coverage of maternity care (%)

Area	Prenatal care	Trained attendant	Institutional deliveries	Postnatal care	Sample size	Year	Source
National			22			1983	(1534)
National	59					1984	(0834)
National	62			26	3 670	1983-84	(1666)
National:	34	29			4 581	1982-87	(3010)
urban	58	60			1 245	1982-87	(3010)
rural	26	18			3 336	1982-87	(3010)
Central	26				557	1982-87	(3010)
Guatemala	63	67			854	1982-87	(3010)
Norte	22	17			386	1982-87	(3010)
N. Occidental	15	7			682	1982-87	(3010)
S. Occidental	23	19			1 161	1982-87	(3010)
N. Oriental	42	30			453	1982-87	(3010)
S. Oriental	49	31			488	1982-87	(3010)
Indigenes	16	9			1 947	1982-87	(3010)
Latinos	47	44			2 634	1982-87	(3010)

3.   COMMUNITY STUDIES

4.   HOSPITAL STUDIES

5. CIVIL REGISTRATION DATA/GOVERNMENT ESTIMATES

5.1 National, 1960-84 [0245, 0753, 0825, 0826, 0827, 0834, 1625, 2827]

5.1.1 Rate

	Maternal deaths	MMR (per 100 000 live births)
1960	433	232
1965	392	195
1970	333	157
1975	352	145
1980	276	91
1981	326	107
1982	387	124
1983	355	123
1984	236	79
1985	365	112
1986	360	113
1987	352*	111*
1988	315*	92*

*   Provisional

5.1.2 Causes of maternal deaths

	1980-81		1984	
	No.	%	No.	%
Abortions	54	9	40	17
Haemorrhage	16	3	4	2
Hypertensive disorders of pregnancy	13	2	24	10
Complications of the puerperium	39	6	36	15
Other direct obstetric causes	480	80	124	53
Indirect obstetric causes	–	–	8	3
Total	602	100	236	100

5.2 National and by region, 1986 [3011]

5.2.1 Rate

	MMR (per 100 000 deliveries)
Alta Verapaz	214
Baja Verapaz	210
Huehuetenango	207
Peten	178
Solola	176
Totonicapan	175
Sacatepequez	155
Jalapa	130
Escuintla	130
San Marcos	130
Chiquimula	126
Quezaltenango	122
Jutiapa	117
Izabal	112
Suchitepequez	111
Chimaltenango	108
Santa Rosa	105
Quiche	95
Guatemala	85
Zacapa	76
Retalhuleu	75
Progreso	54
Total	132

6. OTHER SOURCES/ ESTIMATES

6.1 National, 1984 [2713]

The rate was estimated by PAHO to be the same as that derived from a study in Peru.

6.1.1 Rate

Live births	350 000
Maternal deaths	1 050
MMR (per 100 000 live births)	300

7. SELECTED ANNOTATED BIBLIOGRAPHY

8. FURTHER READING

9. DATA SOURCES

WHE 0245   Guatemala, Direccion General de Estadística. *Annuario estadística*, 1978.

WHE 0753   United Nations, *Demographic Yearbook*. New York, various years.

WHE 0825   World Health Organization. Pan American Health Organization. *Health conditions in the Americas. 1969-72*. (PAHO scientific publication no. 306) PAHO, Washington, 1975.

WHE 0826   World Health Organization. Pan American Health Organization. *Health conditions in the Americas. 1973-1976*. (PAHO scientific publication no. 364) PAHO, Washington, 1982.

WHE 0827   World Health Organization. Pan American Health Organization. *Health conditions in the Americas. 1977-1980*. (PAHO scientific publication no. 427) PAHO, Washington, 1982.

WHE 0834   World Health Organization *World health statistics annual – vital statistics and causes of death*. Geneva, various years.

WHE 1534   World Health Organization, Pan American Health Organization. *Programa de salud materna infantil*. Documento de referencia sobre estudio y prevención de la mortalidad materna, Fasciculo I. PAHO, Washington, 1986.

WHE 1625   World Health Organization, Pan American Health Organization. *Health conditions in the Americas*. 1981-84. Vol. I (PAHO Scientific Publication no. 500). PAHO, Washington, 1986.

WHE 1666   Monteith, R.S. et al. Use of maternal and child health services and immunization coverage in Panama and Guatemala. *Bulletin of the Pan American Health Organization*, 1987; 21(1): 1-15.

WHE 1914   United Nations Children's Fund (UNICEF). *The state of the world's children*, Oxford, Oxford University Press, various years.

WHE 1915   United Nations. Department of International Economic and Social Affairs. *World population prospects: estimates and projections*, Population Studies, New York, various years.

WHE 1918   United Nations. Department of International Economic and Social Affairs. *First marriage: patterns and determinants*. New York 1988.

WHE 1942   World Health Organization. Pan American Health Organization. *Evaluation of the strategy for Health for All by the Year 2000*. Seventh Report on the World Health Situation. Vol.3. Region of the Americas. PAHO, Washington, 1986.

WHE 2033   World Health Organization. *Global strategy for health for all by the year 2000. Second report on monitoring progress*. WHO document EB83/2 Add. 1, 1988.

WHE 2713   World Health Organization, Pan American Health Organization *Regional plan of action for the reduction of maternal mortality in the Americas,* Document No. CSP23/10, XXIII Pan American Sanitary Conference, Washington 1990.

WHE 2827   World Health Organization. Pan American Health Organization. *Health conditions in the Americas*, Scientific Publication No. 524, Washington, 1990.

WHE 3010   Demographic and Health Surveys. *Encuesta nacional de salud materno infantil 1987*. Ministerio de Salud Pública y Asistencia Social/ Institute for Resource Development/ Westinghouse, 1989.

WHE 3011   Kestler, E. *Maternal mortality rate by department of death: Guatemala 1986*. (unpublished preliminary tabulations), 1990.

GUYANA

		Year	Source

1. BASIC INDICATORS

1.1 Demographic

1.1.1 Population

Size (millions)	0.8	1990	(1915)
Rate of growth (%)	0.2	1985-90	(1915)

1.1.2 Life expectancy

Female	66	1985-90	(1915)
Male	60	1985-90	(1915)

1.1.3 Fertility

Crude Birth Rate	27	1985-90	(1915)
Total Fertility Rate	2.8	1985-90	(1915)

1.1.4 Mortality

Crude Death Rate	8	1985-90	(1915)
Infant Mortality Rate	56	1985-90	(1915)
Female	33	1984	(2827)
Male	39	1984	(2827)
1-4 years mortality rate			
Female	2	1984	(2827)
Male	2	1984	(2827)

1.2 Social and economic

1.2.1 Adult literacy rate (%)

Female	95	1985	(1914)
Male	97	1985	(1914)

1.2.2 Primary school enrolment rate (%)

Female			
Male			

1.2.3 Female mean age at first marriage

(years)	23.7	1980	(2799)

1.2.4 GNP/capita

(US $)	420	1987	(1914)

1.2.5 Daily per capita calorie supply
(as % of requirements)

2. HEALTH SERVICES

2.1 Health expenditure

2.1.1 Expenditure on health

(as % of GNP)	5.2	1984	(2033)

2.1.2 Expenditure on PHC
(as % of total health expenditure)

2.2 Primary Health Care
(Percentage of population covered by):

2.2.1 Health services

National	96	1983-87	(2033)
Urban			
Rural			

2.2.2 Safe water

National	80	1983	(0834)
Urban	100	1983	(0834)
Rural	61	1983	(0834)

2.2.3 Adequate sanitary facilities

National	90	1983	(0834)
Urban	54	1983	(0834)
Rural	81	1983	(0834)

2.2.4 Contraceptive prevalence rate

(%)	35	1975	(1712)

2.3   Coverage of maternity care (%)

Area	Prenatal care	Trained attendant	Institutional deliveries	Postnatal care	Sample size	Year	Source
National			72	20		1979	(2334)
National	100	93				1984	(0834)
National			96			1985	(1692)
National	95	93				1983-97	(2033)

3.   COMMUNITY STUDIES

4.   HOSPITAL STUDIES

5.   CIVIL REGISTRATION DATA/GOVERNMENT ESTIMATES

5.1   National, 1976-79 and 1984[0827, 1625, 2713, 2827]

5.1.1   Rate

	Maternal deaths	MMR (per 100 000 live births)
1976	32	153
1977	24	104
1978	10	44
1979	8	35
1984	17	11

5.1.2   Causes of maternal deaths, 1984

	%
Haemorrhage	7
Abortion	5
Hypertensive disorders of pregnancy	3
Complications of the puerperium	1
Other direct causes	1
Indirect causes	—
TOTAL	17

6.   OTHER SOURCES/ ESTIMATES

6.1   National, 1984 [2713]

6.1.1   Rate

The maternal mortality rate was recalculated by PAHO using estimates for underreporting based on a study carried out in Brazil.

Births	26 000
Maternal deaths	52
MMR (per 100 000 births)	200

7.   SELECTED ANNOTATED BIBLIOGRAPHY

8.   FURTHER READING

9. DATA SOURCES

WHE 0827　World Health Organization. Pan American Health Organization. *Health conditions in the Americas. 1977-1980.* (PAHO scientific publication no. 427) PAHO, Washington, 1982.

WHE 0834　World Health Organization *World health statistics annual – vital statistics and causes of death.* Geneva, various years.

WHE 1625　World Health Organization, Pan American Health Organization. *Health conditions in the Americas.* 1981-84. Vol. I (PAHO Scientific Publication no. 500). PAHO, Washington, 1986.

WHE 1692　Observatoire Régional de la Santé de Guyane. *Surveillance et issue des grossesses en Guyane. Résultats 1984-85.* Cayenne, 1986.

WHE 1712　Mauldin W.P. and Segal, S.J., *Prevalence of contraceptive use in developing countries. A chart book.* Rockefeller Foundation, New York 1986.

WHE 1914　United Nations Children's Fund (UNICEF). *The state of the world's children*, Oxford, Oxford University Press, various years.

WHE 1915　United Nations. Department of International Economic and Social Affairs. *World population prospects: estimates and projections*, Population Studies, New York, various years.

WHE 2033　World Health Organization. *Global strategy for health for all by the year 2000. Second report on monitoring progress.* WHO document EB83/2 Add. 1, 1988.

WHE 2334　Sinha, D.P. *Children of the Caribbean.* Caribbean Food and Nutrition Institute/Pan American Health Organization, 1988.

WHE 2713　World Health Organization, Pan American Health Organization *Regional plan of action for the reduction of maternal mortality in the Americas,* Document No. CSP23/10, XXIII Pan American Sanitary Conference, Washington 1990.

WHE 2799　United Nations. Department of International Economic and Social Affairs. *Patterns of first marriage: timing and prevalence.* New York, 1990.

WHE 2827　World Health Organization. Pan American Health Organization. *Health conditions in the Americas*, Scientific Publication No. 524, Washington, 1990.

NOTES

HAITI

	Year	Source

1. BASIC INDICATORS

1.1 Demographic

1.1.1 Population

		Year	Source
Size (millions)	6.5	1990	(1915)
Rate of growth (%)	2.0	1985-90	(1915)

1.1.2 Life expectancy

		Year	Source
Female	56	1985-90	(1915)
Male	53	1985-90	(1915)

1.1.3 Fertility

		Year	Source
Crude Birth Rate	36	1985-90	(1915)
Total Fertility Rate	5.0	1985-90	(1915)

1.1.4 Mortality

		Year	Source
Crude Death Rate	13	1985-90	(1915)
Infant Mortality Rate	97	1985-90	(1915)
Female	16	1972	(0753)
Male	21	1972	(0753)
1-4 years mortality rate			
Female	30	1972	(0753)
Male	30	1972	(0753)

1.2 Social and economic

1.2.1 Adult literacy rate (%)

		Year	Source
Female	42	1985	(1914)
Male	54	1985	(1914)

1.2.2 Primary school enrolment rate (%)

		Year	Source
Female	72	1986-88	(1914)
Male	83	1986-88	(1914)

1.2.3 Female mean age at first marriage

		Year	Source
(years)	29.7	1982	(2799)

1.2.4 GNP/capita

		Year	Source
(US $)	380	1985	(1914)

1.2.5 Daily per capita calorie supply

		Year	Source
(as % of requirements)	84	1984-86	(1914)

2. HEALTH SERVICES

2.1 Health expenditure

2.1.1 Expenditure on health

		Year	Source
(as % of GNP)	3.5	1984	(2033)

2.1.2 Expenditure on PHC
(as % of total health expenditure)

2.2 Primary Health Care.
(Percentage of population covered by):

2.2.1 Health services

		Year	Source
National	96	1983-87	(2033)
Urban			
Rural			

2.2.2 Safe water

		Year	Source
National			
Urban	59	1985	(2033)
Rural	32	1985	(2033)

2.2.3 Adequate sanitary facilities

		Year	Source
National			
Urban	42	1985	(2033)
Rural	14	1985	(2033)

2.2.4 Contraceptive prevalence rate

		Year	Source
(%)	7	1983	(0834)

2.3   Coverage of maternity care (%)

Area	Prenatal care	Trained attendant	Institutional deliveries	Postnatal care	Sample size	Year	Source
National		12				(1983)	(0796)
National	45	20				1983	(0834)
National			25			(1984)	(1013)
National	63		23	22		(1987)	(1824)
National	41	40				1988	(2033)
National: rural		20				1983	(0207)

3. COMMUNITY STUDIES

4. HOSPITAL STUDIES

4.1 All hospitals, 1981 [0304]

4.1.1 Rate
Live births	34 856
Maternal deaths	57
MMR (per 100 000 live births)	164

5. CIVIL REGISTRATION DATA/GOVERNMENT ESTIMATES

5.1 National, 1974-78 [0207]

5.1.1 Rate
According to a report on the Integrated Project of Health and Population published by the Department of Public Health, the maternal mortality rate for the years 1974-78 was 367 per 100,000 live births.

6. OTHER SOURCES/ ESTIMATES

6.1 National [0271]

6.1.1 Rate
According to a consultant report submitted to the UNFPA in 1978, the maternal mortality rate for Haiti was estimated to be 1 370 per 100,000 live births.

6.2 National, 1984 [1912]

6.2.1 Rate
The Pan American Health Organization reported a maternal mortality rate for Haiti of 230 per 100,000 live births in 1984.

6.3 National, (1990) [2713]

6.3.1 Rate
An adjusted rate was estimated by PAHO on the basis of information from the Bolivian Ministry of Social Welfare and Public Health on the degree of underreporting of maternal deaths.

Births	213 000
Maternal deaths	1 278
MMR (per 100 000 births)	600

7. SELECTED ANNOTATED BIBLIOGRAPHY

8. FURTHER READING

9. DATA SOURCES

WHE 0207   Berggren, G.G. et al. Traditional mid-wives, tetanus immunization and infant mortality in rural Haiti. *Tropical Doctor*, 1983; 13(2): 79-87.

WHE 0271   Adamson, H. *Country background review: Haiti*. Unpublished paper submitted to United Nations Fund for Population Activities, UNFPA, 1978.

WHE 0304   Haiti, Section Centrale de Statistique. *Rapport annuel d'activités hospitalières: année 1981*. Port au Prince, 1981.

WHE 0753   United Nations, *Demographic Yearbook*. New York, various years.

WHE 0796   World Health Organization. *Global strategy for health for all by the year 2000*. Thirty-sixth World Health Assembly. Provisional agenda item 21. (WHO document no. A36/INF.DOC/1). Geneva, 1983.

WHE 0834   World Health Organization. *World health statistics annual – vital statistics and causes of death*. Geneva, various years.

WHE 1013   Family Health International. Maternity care monitoring to be undertaken in Haiti. *Network*, 1984; 6(1): 1.

WHE 1824   Population Reference Bureau. Haiti – survey report. *Population Today*, 1987; 15(10): 5.

WHE 1912   World Health Organization. Pan American Health Organization. *Reference document on study and prevention of maternal mortality*, PAHO, Washington, 1987.

WHE 1914   United Nations Children's Fund (UNICEF). *The state of the world's children*, Oxford, Oxford University Press, various years.

WHE 1915   United Nations. Department of International Economic and Social Affairs. *World population prospects: estimates and projections*, Population Studies, New York, various years.

WHE 2033   World Health Organization. *Global strategy for health for all by the year 2000. Second report on monitoring progress*. WHO document EB83/2 Add. 1, 1988.

WHE 2713   World Health Organization, Pan American Health Organization *Regional plan of action for the reduction of maternal mortality in the Americas,* Document No. CSP23/10, XXIII Pan American Sanitary Conference, Washington 1990.

WHE 2799   United Nations. Department of International Economic and Social Affairs. *Patterns of first marriage: timing and prevalence*. New York, 1990.

NOTES

HONDURAS

		Year	Source

1. BASIC INDICATORS

1.1 Demographic

1.1.1 Population

		Year	Source
Size (millions)	5.1	1990	(1915)
Rate of growth (%)	3.2	1985-90	(1915)

1.1.2 Life expectancy

		Year	Source
Female	66	1985-90	(1915)
Male	62	1985-90	(1915)

1.1.3 Fertility

		Year	Source
Crude Birth Rate	40	1985-90	(1915)
Total Fertility Rate	5.6	1985-90	(1915)

1.1.4 Mortality

		Year	Source
Crude Death Rate	8	1985-90	(1915)
Infant Mortality Rate	69	1985-90	(1915)
Female	21	1981	(2827)
Male	25	1981	(2827)
1-4 years mortality rate			
Female	4	1981	(2827)
Male	5	1981	(2827)

1.2 Social and economic

1.2.1 Adult literacy rate (%)

		Year	Source
Female	65	1985	(1914)
Male	71	1985	(1914)

1.2.2 Primary school enrolment rate (%)

		Year	Source
Female	108	1986-88	(1914)
Male	104	1986-88	(1914)

1.2.3 Female mean age at first marriage

		Year	Source
(years)	20.0	1974	(1918)

1.2.4 GNP/capita

		Year	Source
(US $)	860	1987	(1914)

1.2.5 Daily per capita calorie supply

		Year	Source
(as % of requirements)	92	1984-86	(1914)

2. HEALTH SERVICES

2.1 Health Expenditure

2.1.1 Expenditure on health

		Year	Source
(as % of GNP)	12.2	1984	(2033)

2.1.2 Expenditure on PHC
(as % of total health expenditure)

2.2 Primary Health Care
(Percentage of population covered by):

2.2.1 Health services

		Year	Source
National	62	1983-87	(2033)
Urban			
Rural			

2.2.2 Safe water

		Year	Source
National	50	1985	(2033)
Urban	51	1985	(2033)
Rural	49	1985	(2033)

2.2.3 Adequate sanitary facilities

		Year	Source
National			
Urban	22	1985	(2033)
Rural	38	1985	(2033)

2.4 Contraceptive prevalence rate

		Year	Source
(%)	27	1981	(1712)

2.3   Coverage of maternity care (%)

Area	Prenatal care	Trained attendant	Institutional deliveries	Postnatal care	Sample size	Year	Source
National		50				1983	(0834)
National			24			1983	(1534)
National	65	90				1983-87	(2033)
National	21	66				(1987)	(2713)
National			41			1989-90	(2776)

3.   COMMUNITY STUDIES

3.1   National and by region, 1989-90 [2776]

All deaths of women of reproductive age occurring over the period April 1989 to April 1990 were examined retrospectively. The analysis included all institutional deaths, whether in government, private or social security hospitals, as well as those which occurred outside the health system, at home or on the way to the hospital. The latter were obtained by collating information from a variety of sources including local health personnel, administrative officials, priests, undertakers, cemetery officials, local leaders, employers, leaders of cooperatives etc.

Data on numbers of live births, female population of reproductive age, educational and socio-economic levels, residence and labour force participation were obtained from the 1988 national census and from the 1987 epidemiological and family health survey.

A supervising committee, composed of representatives of the Ministry of Health, the University and international agencies was established to oversee data collection and analysis.

3.1.1   Rate
National

Live births	172 442
Maternal deaths	381
MMR (per 100 000 live births)	221

Maternal deaths accounted for one fifth of all deaths of women of reproductive age. The lifetime risk of dying from pregnancy related causes was estimated as 1 in 67. The maternal mortality rate thus calculated is 4.5 times higher than the officially registered rate.

The study was able to calculate the maternal mortality rate separately for hospital deaths and for those which occurred outside the hospital.

	Hospital	Extra-hospital
Live births	71 252	101 190
Maternal deaths	125	256
MMR (per 100 000 live births)	175	253

By region (all deaths)

	Live births	Maternal deaths	MMR (per 100 000 live births)
Atlantida	9 284	24	259
Colón	5 834	15	257
Comayagua	9 339	21	225
Copan	8 559	31	362
Cortés	25 603	38	148
Choluteca	11 520	17	148
El Paraíso	9 918	20	202
Fco Morazan	31 724	46	145
Grazias a Dios	1 367	12	878
Intibuca	4 867	26	534
Islas de la Bahía	861	1	116
La Paz	4 133	19	460
Lempira	6 919	25	361
Ocotepeque	2 899	8	276
Olancho	11 071	19	172
Santa Barbara	10 875	22	202
Valle	4 677	9	192
Yoro	12 991	24	185
Total	172 442	381	221

3.1.2   Causes of maternal deaths*

	Total deaths No.	%	Hospital deaths %	Extra-hospital deaths %
Haemorrhage	125	33	15	41
Sepsis	79	21	30	16
Hypertensive disorders of pregnancy	47	12	19	9
Obstructed labour	16	4	1	6
DIRECT CAUSES	267	70	65	72
INDIRECT CAUSES	47	12	17	10
Fortuitous	67	18	18	18
TOTAL	381	100	100 N=125	100 N=256

*   Abortion was found to be implicated in at least 33 deaths (9%) but the authors estimated that this figure greatly underestimated the true number of abortion deaths. A comparison of the social and demographic profiles of the women who died as a result of abortion with maternal deaths in general found that women who died from abortion were more likely to be unmarried, employed outside the home and nulliparous.

3.1.3   Avoidable factors

An analysis of the 256 cases of maternal deaths which occurred outside hospital found that distance from the hospital and transport problems were the main contributory cause of death.

	% of deaths
Distance from the hospital	16
Transport problems	26
Patient thought she would recover at home	12
TBA delayed seeking help	15
Medical personnel delayed seeking help	4
Patient and/or family refusal	20
Shortage of money	16
Other	6

3.1.4   High risk groups

Age over 35 years, nulliparity and parity of 5 or over together with poor housing conditions were significant risk factors. The most important risk factor, however, was marital status with unmarried women facing a relative risk of death over 14 times that for married women or women living in consensual unions. It should be noted, however, that this very high figure may, in part, reflect under-registration of pregnancy among unmarried women. The authors conclude that marital status is, nonetheless, a major risk factor.

	Relative risk	Degree of significance
Age (18-34=1)		
15-17	1.1	NS
35+	1.9	p<0.05
Parity (1-4=1)		
0	1.6	p<0.05
5	1.9	p<0.05
6	2.0	p<0.05

	Relative risk	Degree of significance
Residence (urban=1)		
rural	1.2	NS
Marital status (other=1)		
unmarried	14.5	p<0.05
Housing (other=1)		
earth floor	2.0	p<0.05
Educational level (other=1)		
none	3.1	p<0.05

3.1.5   Other findings

The study compared risk factors for deaths occurring within and outside the hospitals. The average age of women who died in hospital was slightly lower than that of women who died outside, 27.5 years compared with 29.3 years. The difference was not statistically significant. More unmarried women died in hospital, probably due to the fact that the proportion of unmarried women was considerably higher in urban areas where access to hospital was easier. The most noteworthy differences in hospital and extra-hospital deaths concerned educational level and type of housing. Prenatal care was not significantly related to place of death.

	Hospital death %	Extra-hospital deaths %
Educational level		
none	35	47
failed to complete primary	35	38
completed primary	25	12
secondary	4	2
tertiary	1	1
Literacy		
illiterate	36	46
Type of housing		
earth floor	56	78
cement floor	21	10
Prenatal care		
none	50	50
Distance from hospital		
<1 hour	62	20
<3 hours	81	42

4. HOSPITAL STUDIES

4.1 National, 1989-90 [2776]

As part of the analysis of the data collected in study 3.1 above, a case control study was undertaken for the hospital deaths. Matching criteria included the type of pregnancy termination (abortion, ectopic pregnancy, caesarean delivery, vaginal delivery etc.) as well as the place of delivery. Two controls were taken for each maternal death. In order to ensure that the type of care given was similar for cases and for controls, the latter were selected from matched cases admitted prior to the maternal death.

	Odds ratio	Degree of significance
Socio-demographic characteristics		
residence in rural area	1.9	p<0.05
earth floor only	2.5	p<0.05
age 15-17	0.9	NS
age 35+	2.1	p<0.05
Obstetric history		
nulliparity	0.6	NS
parity 4 or higher	1.9	p<0.05
birth interval <12 months	2.1	p<0.05
Medical care		
no prenatal care	2.0	p<0.05
fewer than 3 prenatal visits	0.7	NS

Caesarean delivery

An analysis of rates of caesarean delivery by type of hospital found that rates were highest in private institutions.

	% of total deliveries	% of deliveries by caesarean section
National/State hospitals	23	11
Regional hospitals	37	11
Area hospitals	17	8
IHSS (Tegucigalpa)*	14	17
IHSS (San Pedro Sula)*	5	14
Private hospitals	4	29
Total	100	12

*   Social security hospitals

5. CIVIL REGISTRATION DATA/GOVERNMENT ESTIMATES

5.1 National, 1960-84 [0825, 0826, 0827, 1625, 2827]

5.1.1 Rate

	Maternal deaths	MMR (per 100 000 live births)
1960	255	310
1965	256	256
1970	186	174
1975	128	99
1980	147	94
1981	28	17*
1982	149	92
1983	79	50

*   There is no explanation in the text for the fluctuations in numbers and rates.

6. OTHER ESTIMATES/ SOURCES

6.1 National, 1983 [2713]

The rate was estimated by PAHO to be the same as that derived from a study in Peru.

6.1.1 Rate

Births	189 000
Maternal deaths	567
MMR (per 100 000 births)	300

7. SELECTED ANNOTATED BIBLIOGRAPHY

8. FURTHER READING

Chackiel, J. *Medicion indirecta de la mortalidad materna*. Unpublished document presented at the Reunion regional sobre prevencion de la mortalidad materna, Sao Paulo, 12-15 April 1988. WHE 2387

9. DATA SOURCES

WHE 0825   World Health Organization. Pan American Health Organization. *Health conditions in the Americas. 1969-72.* (PAHO scientific publication no. 306) PAHO, Washington, 1975.

WHE 0826   World Health Organization. Pan American Health Organization. *Health conditions in the Americas. 1973-1976.* (PAHO scientific publication no. 364) PAHO, Washington, 1982.

WHE 0827   World Health Organization. Pan American Health Organization. *Health conditions in the Americas. 1977-1980.* (PAHO scientific publication no. 427) PAHO, Washington, 1982.

WHE 0834   World Health Organization *World health statistics annual – vital statistics and causes of death.* Geneva, various years.

WHE 1534   World Health Organization, Pan American Health Organization. *Programa de salud materna infantil.* Documento de referencia sobre estudio y prevención de la mortalidad materna, Fasciculo I. PAHO, Washington, 1986.

WHE 1625   World Health Organization, Pan American Health Organization. *Health conditions in the Americas.* 1981-84. Vol. I (PAHO Scientific Publication no. 500). PAHO, Washington, 1986.

WHE 1712   Mauldin W.P. and Segal, S.J., *Prevalence of contraceptive use in developing countries. A chart book.* Rockefeller Foundation, New York 1986.

WHE 1914   United Nations Children's Fund (UNICEF). *The state of the world's children*, Oxford, Oxford University Press, various years.

WHE 1915   United Nations. Department of International Economic and Social Affairs. *World population prospects: estimates and projections*, Population Studies, New York, various years.

WHE 1918   United Nations. Department of International Economic and Social Affairs. *First marriage: patterns and determinants.* New York 1988.

WHE 2033   World Health Organization. *Global strategy for health for all by the year 2000. Second report on monitoring progress.* WHO document EB83/2 Add. 1, 1988.

WHE 2713   World Health Organization, Pan American Health Organization *Regional plan of action for the reduction of maternal mortality in the Americas,* Document No. CSP23/10, XXIII Pan American Sanitary Conference, Washington 1990.

WHE 2776   Castellanos, M. et al. *Mortalidad materna*, Investigación sobre mortalidad de mujeres en edad reproductiva con énfasis en mortalidad materna, Honduras, 1990.

WHE 2827   World Health Organization. Pan American Health Organization. *Health conditions in the Americas*, Scientific Publication No. 524, Washington, 1990.

NOTES

JAMAICA

		Year	Source

1. BASIC INDICATORS

1.1 Demographic

1.1.1 Population

		Year	Source
Size (millions)	2.5	1990	(1915)
Rate of growth (%)	1.2	1985-90	(1915)

1.1.2 Life expectancy

Female	75	1985-90	(1915)
Male	70	1985-90	(1915)

1.1.3 Fertility

Crude Birth Rate	24	1985-90	(1915)
Total Fertility Rate	2.7	1985-90	(1915)

1.1.4 Mortality

Crude Death Rate	7	1985-90	(1915)
Infant Mortality Rate	17	1985-90	(1915)
Female	14	1984	(2827)
Male	19	1984	(2827)
1-4 years. mortality rate			
Female	2	1984	(2827)
Male	2	1984	(2827)

1.2 Social and economic

1.2.1 Adult literacy rate (%)

Female	98	1985	(1914)
Male	98	1985	(1914)

1.2.2 Primary school enrolment rate (%)

Female	106	1986-88	(1914)
Male	104	1986-88	(1914)

1.2.3 Female mean age at first marriage

(years)	29.7	1982	(2799)

1.2.4 GNP/capita

(US $)	1 070	1987	(1914)

1.2.5 Daily per capita calorie supply

(as % of requirements)	116	1984-86	(1914)

2. HEALTH SERVICES

2.1 Health expenditure

2.1.1 Expenditure on health

(as % of GNP)	2.5	1984	(2033)

2.1.2 Expenditure on PHC
(as % of total health expenditure)

2.2 Primary Health Care
(Percentage of population covered by):

2.2.1 Health services
National
Urban
Rural

2.2.2 Safe water

National	96	1985	(2033)
Urban	99	1985	(2033)
Rural	93	1985	(2033)

2.2.3 Adequate sanitary facilities

National	91	1985	(2033)
Urban	92	1985	(2033)
Rural	90	1985	(2033)

2.2.4 Contraceptive prevalence rate

(%)	52	1983	(1712)

2.3   Coverage of maternity care (%)

Area	Prenatal care	Trained attendant	Institutional deliveries	Postnatal care	Sample size	Year	Source
National	78	86	73	37		1981	(0360)
National			72			1982	(1372)
National	72	89				1983	(0834)
National			89			1987	(1534)
National		87	82		10 428w	1986-87	(2437)
National	98	90	79			1982-89	(2996)
Kingston and St.Andrew	78		83	32	67 700	(1983)	(0046)

3. COMMUNITY STUDIES

3.1 National, 1981-83 [0991, 1343, 2934, 2977]

Multiple sources were used to identify maternal deaths occurring over the period 1981-83 and their causes. These sources included a review of all deaths of women of reproductive age and included those occurring in hospitals (on maternity, surgical and medical wards and in casualty departments); those reported to the police and coroner's courts; those on whom postmortems were carried out at hospitals, public morgues and for the Ministry of National Security; and those obtained from discussions with public health staff. It was found that no single source of information independently identified all the maternal deaths. Hospital records yielded 133 deaths (69%) and death certificates 74 (38%). In all, 193 maternal deaths were identified, giving a maternal mortality rate over twice as high as as the official rate.

3.1.1 Rate

Births	178 544
Maternal deaths*	193
MMR (per 100 000 births)	108

*   Includes deaths occurring up to one year after termination of pregnancy.

3.1.2 Causes of maternal deaths

	Number	%
Hypertensive disorders of pregnancy	49	25
Haemorrhage	38	20
Ectopic pregnancy	20	10
Embolisms	16	8
Sepsis	15	8
Abortion	9	5
Ruptured uterus	4	2
Complications of anaesthesia	4	2
Cerebrovascular accident	2	1
Obstructed labour	1	1
Incompatible blood transfusion	1	1
Other direct causes	3	2
DIRECT CAUSES	162	84
Sickle cell disease	8	4
Cardiac diseases	2	1
Other indirect causes	12	6
INDIRECT CAUSES	22	11
Fortuitous	3	2
Unknown	6	3
TOTAL	193	100

3.1.3 Avoidable factors

Hypertensive disorders of pregnancy

One or more avoidable factors were considered to be present in 79% of the women who died as a result of hypertensive disorders of pregnancy. The types of avoidable factors fell into two groups; those related to patient and extra-hospital factors; and those related to in-hospital factors. The former were mainly associated with nonattendance for prenatal care or, when patients were in contact with the prenatal care services, delay in returning for care when complications developed. There were also delays by midwives in referring to hospitals patients with signs and symptoms of incipient severe preeclampsia.

In-hospital factors included:

- absence of relevant information on antenatal surveillance of symptoms and signs for example, weight gain, blood pressure readings, at time of admission to hospital; inadequate monitoring of patient's blood pressure and urine particularly on admission and immediately after delivery;
- delay by nurses in contacting a doctor when signs of pre-eclampsia were found or a patient had had a fit, but more often and importantly, delay in doctors responding to a telephone contact by a midwife regarding a patient in this condition;
- lack of clear-cut clinical-therapeutic strategy for dealing with patients;
- inadequate monitoring of fluid balance and an apparent unawareness of the dangers of acute renal failure;
- delay in referral from smaller to the larger hospitals.

Haemorrhage

Sixteen of the women who died from postpartum haemorrhage delivered at home despite the fact that many of them were grand multiparae and should have been booked for hospital delivery. Of the 38 deaths directly due to haemorrhage, assessment of care was possible in 29 cases and in every case avoidable factors were considered to have been present. Factors identified within the hospital included delays in midwives appreciating the extent of blood loss and contacting a doctor; delays in doctors responding to midwives' requests for assistance; inadequate and delayed resuscitative procedures for blood loss; delays in manual removal of placentae when this was necessary; inadequate and/or inappropriate use of ergometrine.

Ectopic pregnancy

It was possible to assess the care given only in 14 of the deaths from ectopic pregnancy. Avoidable factors included misdiagnosis; delays in treating the patient when ectopic pregnancy was suspected; and inadequate resuscitation with blood before and during laparotomy.

Sepsis

Avoidable factors were present in 11 of the deaths due to non-abortion sepsis. The major factors included inadequate surveillance of temperature in women with prolonged first stage of labour and post-delivery; delays in ensuring delivery in women with prolongation of first stage of labour; failure to give antibiotics to women with prolonged rupture of the membranes; inadequate bacteriological investigations in women with puerperal pyrexia; and reluctance to treat women with puerperal pyrexia with broad spectrum antibiotics.

3.1.4 High risk groups

In all age groups para one women had higher risks of dying in pregnancy than para two and the risk thereafter increased with each additional birth. Women aged under 20 years had a higher risk of dying than those aged 20-24 years who had the lowest risk. The risk increased in each successive five-year age group, women over 40 years having almost an eight times higher risk than those aged 20-24 years.

MMR (per 100 000 live births*)

Age	| Parity 1	2	3	4	5-9	10+	Total
Under 20	88	64	–	–	–	–	79
20-24	77	44	45	18	155	–	71
25-29	142	70	37	28	66	–	93
30-34	–	95	242	156	116	211	182
35-39	–	583	657	317	83	144	241
40+	–	–	–	1 059	221	159	397
Total	86	63	78	75	102	157	108

*   Parity was known for all registered live births but maternal age was not stated for 0.5%. Of the 193 identified maternal deaths, age was known for all but 23%.

3.2   National, 1986-87 [2437, 2699]

The Jamaican Perinatal Mortality and Morbidity Study took place in 1986-87. A detailed study of deliveries included information on the mother's biological, environmental, social and medical background, the history of pregnancy, labour and delivery and events during the postpartum period. Additional information on maternal deaths was obtained from clinical records and post-mortem reports.

3.2.1   Rate

Live births	54 200
Maternal deaths	62
MMR (per 100 000 live births)	115

3.2.2 Causes of maternal deaths

	Number	%
Hypertensive disorders of pregnancy	19	31
Haemorrhage	15	24
Sepsis	11	18
Sickle cell disease	5	8
Embolisms	4	6
Other	6	10
Fortuitous	2	3
TOTAL	6	100

3.2.3 Avoidable factors

3.2.4 High risk groups

The most significant risk factors were age, parity and educational level of the mother. Date of attendance for prenatal care, marital status and living conditions were not found to be important risk factors. It should be noted, however, that the numbers of maternal deaths involved in each group are very small.

	Relative risk					
	Hypertensive disorders	Haemor-rhage	Sepsis	Other	Total	% of deaths
Age (20-24=1)						
<20 years	1	1	1	1	1	27
20-24	1	1	1	2	1	33
25-29	3	1	1	2	2	23
30-34	1	11	3	5	4	12
35+	4	12	–	5	4	7
Parity (parity 0=1)						
0-1	1	*	1	1	36	
1-2	1	3	*	1	1	40
3-4	2	7	*	1	2	15
5+	1	10	*	3	3	9
Distance from home to health centre (<2 miles=1)						
<2 miles	1	1	1	1	1	79
2+ miles	2	3	1	1	2	21
Gestation at first prenatal visit (<14 weeks=1)						
<14 weeks	1	1	1	1	1	26
14-27 weeks	1	2	1	1	1	52
28+ weeks	2	1	3	1	1	17
None	-	6	-	4	3	5
Marital status (common law=1)						
Married	1	2	*	2	1	15
Common law	1	1	*	1	1	37
Visiting	1	1	*	3	2	44

* Haemorrhage + sepsis.

	Relative risk					
	Hypertensive disorders	Haemor-rhage	Sepsis	Other	Total	% of deaths
Educational level of mother (secondary and above=1)						
Primary	4	5	2	10	4	32
Lower secondary	2	3	1	8	2	32
Secondary and higher	1	1	1	1	1	36
Occupation of household head (nonagricultural=1)						
Nonagri-cultural	1	1	*	1	1	81
Agricultural	2	3	*	2	2	19
Type of sanitary facilities (WC=1)						
WC	1	1	*	1	1	45
Other	1	6	*	2	2	55
Source of water supply (piped into dwelling=1)						
Piped into dwelling	1	1	*	1	1	41
Piped into yard	2	1	*	2	2	21
Public standpipe	2	6	*	3	3	21
Other	2	2	*	2	2	18

Logistic regression analysis showed that only maternal age and toilet facilities were independently associated with maternal mortality.

4. HOSPITAL STUDIES

4.1 Victoria Jubilee Hospital, Kingston, 1982 [0046]

4.1.1 Rate

Live births	13 410
Maternal deaths	8
MMR (per 100 000 live births)	60

5. CIVIL REGISTRATION DATA/GOVERNMENT ESTIMATES

5.1 National, 1960-84 (0825, 0826, 0827, 1625, 2713, 2827)

5.1.1 Rate

	Maternal deaths	MMR (per 100 000 live births)
1960	137	200
1965	123	176
1970	68	106
1982	22	36
1984	14	26

5.1.2 Causes of maternal deaths, 1984

	Number
Abortion	9
Hypertensive disorders of pregnancy	3
Haemorrhage	1
Other direct causes	1
TOTAL	14

6. OTHER SOURCES/ ESTIMATES

7. SELECTED ANNOTATED BIBLIOGRAPHY

Thomas, P. et al. *Pre-eclampsia, eclampsia and maternal mortality in Jamaica*. Report of a study for the World Health Organization, 1991. WHE 3154

Data were collected on over 10,000 singleton pregnancies through a combination of analysis of records and interviews on hypertensive disorders of pregnancy and outcome. It was found that over 10% of the women had raised blood pressure (diastolic over 90 mm Hg) and 4% had proteinuric pre-eclampsia. The overall incidence of eclampsia was 0.72%, distributed almost equally over the prenatal, intrapartum and postpartum periods. The most efficient predictor of eclampsia using combinations of blood pressure, proteinuria and oedema was the coexistence of two or more signs of a highest diastolic of 80 mm Hg or higher, proteinuria of 1+ or more and oedema. Women at high risk of developing hypertensive disorders were found to be all women with a pre-pregnancy weight of less than 175 lbs., all women with abnormal increases in body weight during pregnancy, all primigravidae aged 25 years or over, all multigravidae aged 35 or older and all multigravidae with a history of HDP.

8. FURTHER READING

Matadial, L. et al. Hypertensive diseases of pregnancy. *West Indian Journal of Medicine*, 1985; 34: 225-233.

Williams, L.L. Some observations on maternal mortality in Jamaica. *West Indian Medical Journal*, 1973; 22(1): 1-14. WHE 0783.

9. DATA SOURCES

WHE 0046   Ashley, D. *Study of perinatal deaths in Jamaica and the identification of the risk factors.* Unpublished research proposal presented at the Meeting of the STeering Committee of the Task Force on the Risk Approach and Programme Research in MCH/FP Care, Geneva, 1983.

WHE 0360   Jamaica, Ministry of Health. *A profile of maternal and child health and family planning in Jamaica*. Kingston, 1981.

WHE 0825   World Health Organization. Pan American Health Organization. *Health conditions in the Americas. 1969-72.* (PAHO scientific publication no. 306) PAHO, Washington, 1975.

WHE 0826   World Health Organization. Pan American Health Organization. *Health conditions in the Americas. 1973-1976.* (PAHO scientific publication no. 364) PAHO, Washington, 1982.

WHE 0827   World Health Organization. Pan American Health Organization. *Health conditions in the Americas. 1977-1980.* (PAHO scientific publication no. 427) PAHO, Washington, 1982.

WHE 0834   World Health Organization *World health statistics annual – vital statistics and causes of death.* Geneva, various years.

WHE 0991   Walker, G.J.A. et al. Maternal mortality in Jamaica. In: *Interregional meeting on the prevention of maternal mortality,* 11-15 November 1985 Geneva.

WHE 1343   Walker, G.J.A. et al. Maternal mortality in Jamaica. *Lancet,* 1986; 1(8479): 486-488.

WHE 1372   World Health Organization. Pan American Health Organization. *Documento de referencia sobre estudio y prevencion de la mortalidad materna.* Unpublished document HRM/HST, March 1986.

WHE 1534   World Health Organization, Pan American Health Organization. *Programa de salud materno infantil.* Documento de referencia sobre estudio y prevencion de la mortalidad materna, Fasciculo I. PAHO, Washington, 1986.

WHE 1625   World Health Organization, Pan American Health Organization. *Health conditions in the Americas.* 1981-84. Vol. I (PAHO Scientific Publication no. 500). PAHO, Washington, 1986.

WHE 1712   Mauldin W.P. and Segal, S.J., *Prevalence of contraceptive use in developing countries. A chart book.* Rockefeller Foundation, New York 1986.

WHE 1914   United Nations Children's Fund (UNICEF). *The state of the world's children,* Oxford, Oxford University Press, various years.

WHE 1915   United Nations. Department of International Economic and Social Affairs. *World population prospects: estimates and projections,* Population Studies, New York, various years.

WHE 2033   World Health Organization. *Global strategy for health for all by the year 2000. Second report on monitoring progress.* WHO document EB83/2 Add. 1, 1988.

WHE 2437   Jamaica, Department of Child Health. *The perinatal mortality and morbidity study,* University of the West Indies, Mona, Jamaica, 1989.

WHE 2699   Golding, J. et al. Maternal mortality in Jamaica. *Acta Obstetrica Gynecologica Scandinavia,* 1989; 68: 581-587.

WHE 2713   World Health Organization, Pan American Health Organization *Regional plan of action for the reduction of maternal mortality in the Americas,* Document No. CSP23/10, XXIII Pan American Sanitary Conference, Washington 1990.

WHE 2799   United Nations. Department of International Economic and Social Affairs. *Patterns of first marriage: timing and prevalence.* New York, 1990.

WHE 2827   World Health Organization. Pan American Health Organization. *Health conditions in the Americas,* Scientific Publication No. 524, Washington, 1990.

WHE 2934   Walker, G.J.A. et al. Identifying maternal deaths in developing countries: experience in Jamaica. *International Journal of Epidemiology,* 1990; 19(3): 599-605.

WHE 2977   Walker, G.J.A. et al. Maternal deaths in Jamaica. *World Health Forum,* 1987; 8: 75-79.

WHE 2996   Althaus, F. Three in four Jamaican pregnancies are either mistimed or unwanted. *International Family Planning Perspectives,* 1991; 17(1): 32-34.

MEXICO

		Year	Source

1. BASIC INDICATORS

1.1 Demographic

1.1.1 Population
Size (millions)	88.6	1990	(1915)
Rate of growth (%)	2.2	1985-90	(1915)

1.1.2 Life expectancy
Female	72	1985-90	(1915)
Male	66	1985-90	(1915)

1.1.3 Fertility
Crude Birth Rate	29	1985-90	(1915)
Total Fertility Rate	3.6	1985-90	(1915)

1.1.4 Mortality
Crude Death Rate	6	1985-90	(1915)
Infant Mortality Rate	43	1985-90	(1915)
Female	52	1977-87	(1964)
Male	60	1977-87	(1964)
1-4 years mortality rate			
Female	17	1977-87	(1964)
Male	15	1977-87	(1964)

1.2 Social and economic

1.2.1 Adult literacy rate (%)
Female	82	1985	(1914)
Male	88	1985	(1914)

1.2.2 Primary school enrolment rate (%)
Female	116	1986-88	(1914)
Male	119	1986-88	(1914)

1.2.3 Female mean age at first marriage
(years)	20.6	1980	(1918)

1.2.4 GNP/capita
(US $)	1 760	1987	(1914)

1.2.5 Daily per capita calorie supply
(as % of requirements)	135	1984-86	(1914)

2. HEALTH SERVICES

2.1 Health Expenditure

2.1.1 Expenditure on health
(as % of GNP)	3.8	1984	(2033)

2.1.2 Expenditure on PHC
(as % of total health expenditure)

2.2 Primary Health Care
(Percentage of population covered by):

2.2.1 Health services
National	91	1983-87	(2033)
Urban			
Rural			

2.2.2 Safe water
National	74	1983	(0834)
Urban	95	1985	(2033)
Rural	50	1985	(2033)

2.2.3 Adequate sanitary facilities
National	56	1983	(0834)
Urban	77	1985	(2033)
Rural	15	1985	(2033)

2.2.4 Contraceptive prevalence rate
(%)	41	1982	(1712)

2.3 Coverage of maternity care (%)

Area	Prenatal care	Trained attendant	Institutional deliveries	Postnatal care	Sample size	Year	Source
National			64			1981	(1534)
National	71	70				1982-87	(1964)
National	60	87				1983-87	(2033)

3. COMMUNITY STUDIES

4. HOSPITAL STUDIES

4.1 Hospital de la Mujer, Mexico City, 1969-73 [0711]

4.1.1 Rate

	Live births	Maternal deaths	MMR (per 100 000 live births)
1969	7 071	36	509
1970	7 324	32	437
1971	8 587	26	303
1972	7 902	31	389
1973	8 028	15	187
1969-73	38 972	140	357

4.1.2 Causes of maternal deaths

	Number	%
Hypertensive disorders of pregnancy	49	35
Sepsis	24	17
Haemorrhage	23	16
Abortion	10	7
Complications of anaesthesia	4	3
DIRECT CAUSES	110	79
INDIRECT CAUSES	10	7
Fortuitous	20	14
TOTAL	140	100

4.1.3 Avoidable factors

4.1.4 High risk groups

5. CIVIL REGISTRATION DATA/GOVERNMENT ESTIMATES

5.1 National, 1960-1984 [0825, 0826, 0827, 0834, 1625, 2713, 2827]

5.1.1 Rate

	Maternal deaths	MMR (per 100 000 live births)
1960	3 102	193
1965	3 109	165
1970	3 050	143
1975	2 558	113
1980	2 296	94
1981	2 199	87
1982	2 166	91
1983	2 133	82
1985	1 702	64
1986	1 681	65

5.1.2 Causes of maternal deaths, 1986

	Number	%
Haemorrhage	420	25
Hypertensive disorders of pregnancy	336	20
Abortion	151	9
Complications of the puerperium	152	9
Other direct causes	588	35
Indirect causes	34	2
TOTAL	1 681	100

5.2 National and by region, 1983 [2158]

	MMR (per 100 000 registered live births)
National	82
Aguascalientes	71
Baja California	31
Baja California Sur	35
Campeche	118
Coahuila	54
Colima	21
Chiapas	111
Chihuahua	93
Distrito Federal	50
Durango	55
Guanajuato	94
Guerrero	92
Hidalgo	119
Jalisco	38
Estado de México	107
Michoacan	94
Morelos	42
Nayarit	68
Nuevo Leon	13
Oaxaca	161
Puebla	152
Queretaro	91
Quintana Roo	46
San Luis Potosí	89
Sinaloa	43
Sonora	62
Tabasco	85
Tamaulipas	53
Tlaxcala	104
Veracruz	101
Yucatan	58
Zacatecas	61

5.2.3 Avoidable factors

5.2.4 High risk groups

Maternal mortality rates were lowest in the 15-29 age range and rose steadily for all ages over 30 years.

	Maternal deaths	MMR (per 100 000 registered live births)
<15	6	83
15-19	250	63
20-24	436	54
25-29	439	71
30-34	400	107
35-39	356	162
40-44	180	217
45-49	44	213
50+	6	–
Total	2 133	82

6. OTHER SOURCES/ ESTIMATES

6.1 National, 1986 [2713]

The maternal mortality rate was recalculated by PAHO using estimates for underreporting based on a study carried out in Brazil.

6.1.1 Rate

Births	2 569 000
Maternal deaths	5 138
MMR (per 100 000 births)	200

7. SELECTED ANNOTATED BIBLIOGRAPHY

World Health Organization. Pan American Health Organization. *Health conditions in the Americas*, Scientific Publication No. 524, Washington, 1990. WHE 2827

A report of the Pan American Health Organization quotes a hospital study in Mexico which found an institutional maternal mortality rate of 50 per 100 000 live births coupled with a rate of caesarean delivery of nearly 30%. It is noted that there is considerable variation in rates of caesarean delivery in different countries of the region. An epidemiological study of caesarean delivery, undertaken by the Centro Latino Americano de Perinatologia y Desarrollo Humano (CLAP) and PAHO in 1985 in 17 countries indicated that the frequency of caesarean delivery explains only 5% of the variations in perinatal mortality and that there is no correlation between frequency of operative delivery and reduction in maternal mortality. Indeed, caesarean delivery is associated with higher rates of mortality and morbidity than vaginal delivery and is a bigger strain on the human and financial resources of the health service.

8. FURTHER READING

Abdunis, R. et al. The use of focus groups in developing prenatal health education materials in Tijuana, Mexico. *Food and Nutrition Bulletin*, 1990; 12(2): 120-127. WHE 2764.

Browner, C.H. Women, household and health in Latin America. *Social Science and Medicine*, 1989; 28(5): 461-473. WHE 2120

Chackiel, J. *Medición indirecta de la mortalidad materna*. Unpublished document presented at the reunión regional sobre prevención de la mortalidad materna, Sao Paulo, 12-15 April 1988. WHE 2387

Diaz Saldana, J. et al. Hepatitis por virus durante el embarazo. *Ginecología y Obstetricia de México*, 1978; 43: 399-404. WHR 1453

Ruiz-Velasco, V. La operación cesarea en nuestro medio. *Ginecología y Obstetricia de México*, 1977; 42: 177-194. WHE 2684.

Urbina-Fuentes, M. and Echanove-Fernandez, El. Fecundidad y salud en México. *Salud Pública de México*, 1989, 31(2): 168-176. WHE 2306

Vargas López, E. et al. Epidemiología del alto riesgo materno. *Ginecología y obstetricia de México*, 1986; 54: 79-85. WHE 1736.

9. DATA SOURCES

WHE 0711   Trejo Ramírez, C.A. Maternal mortality in the Women's Hospital. *Ginecología y Obstetricia de México*, 1974; 36(217): 301-326.

WHE 0825   World Health Organization. Pan American Health Organization. *Health conditions in the Americas. 1969-72*. (PAHO scientific publication no. 306) PAHO, Washington, 1975.

WHE 0826   World Health Organization. Pan American Health Organization. *Health conditions in the Americas. 1973-1976*. (PAHO scientific publication no. 364) PAHO, Washington, 1982.

WHE 0827   World Health Organization. Pan American Health Organization. *Health conditions in the Americas. 1977-1980*. (PAHO scientific publication no. 427) PAHO, Washington, 1982.

WHE 0834   World Health Organization. *World health statistics annual – vital statistics and causes of death*. Geneva, various years.

WHE 1534   World Health Organization, Pan American Health Organization. *Programa de salud materno infantil*. Documento de referencia sobre estudio y prevención de la mortalidad materna, Fasciculo I. PAHO, Washington, 1986.

WHE 1625   World Health Organization, Pan American Health Organization. *Health conditions in the Americas*. 1981-84. Vol. I (PAHO Scientific Publication no. 500). PAHO, Washington, 1986.

WHE 1712   Mauldin W.P. and Segal, S.J., *Prevalence of contraceptive use in developing countries. A chart book*. Rockefeller Foundation, New York 1986.

WHE 1914   United Nations Children's Fund (UNICEF). *The state of the world's children*, Oxford, Oxford University Press, various years.

WHE 1915   United Nations. Department of International Economic and Social Affairs. *World population prospects: estimates and projections*, Population Studies, New York, various years.

WHE 1918   United Nations. Department of International Economic and Social Affairs. *First marriage: patterns and determinants*. New York 1988.

WHE 1964   Demographic and Health Surveys. *México: encuesta nacional sobre fecundidad y salud 1987*. Secretaría de Salud/Institute for Resource Development/Macro Systems Inc. 1989.

WHE 2033   World Health Organization. *Global strategy for health for all by the year 2000. Second report on monitoring progress*. WHO document EB83/2 Add. 1, 1988.

WHE 2158   del Carmen E. *La salud de la mujer en México. Cifras comentadas*. Programa Nacional Mujer y Salud, México, 1988.

WHE 2713   World Health Organization, Pan American Health Organization *Regional plan of action for the reduction of maternal mortality in the Americas,* Document No. CSP23/10, XXIII Pan American Sanitary Conference, Washington 1990.

WHE 2827   World Health Organization. Pan American Health Organization. *Health conditions in the Americas*, Scientific Publication No. 524, Washington, 1990.

NICARAGUA

		Year	Source

1. BASIC INDICATORS

1.1 Demographic

1.1.1 Population

		Year	Source
Size (millions)	3.9	1990	(1915)
Rate of growth (%)	3.4	1985-90	(1915)

1.1.2 Life expectancy

		Year	Source
Female	65	1985-90	(1915)
Male	62	1985-90	(1915)

1.1.3 Fertility

		Year	Source
Crude Birth Rate	42	1985-90	(1915)
Total Fertility Rate	5.5	1985-90	(1915)

1.1.4 Mortality

		Year	Source
Crude Death Rate	8	1985-90	(1915)
Infant Mortality Rate	62	1985-90	(1915)
Female	31	1980	(1444)
Male	39	1980	(1444)
1-4 years mortality rate			
Female	3	1980	(1444)
Male	4	1980	(1444)

1.2 Social and economic

1.2.1 Adult literacy rate (%)
Female
Male

1.2.2 Primary school enrolment rate (%)

		Year	Source
Female	104	1986-88	(1914)
Male	94	1986-88	(1914)

1.2.3 Female mean age at first marriage

		Year	Source
(years)	20.2	1971	(1918)

1.2.4 GNP/capita

		Year	Source
(US $)	830	1987	(1914)

1.2.5 Daily per capita calorie supply

		Year	Source
(as % of requirements)	110	1984-86	(1914)

2. HEALTH SERVICES

2.1 Health Expenditure

2.1.1 Expenditure on health

		Year	Source
(as % of GNP)	5.0	1984	(2033)

2.1.2 Expenditure on PHC
(as % of total health expenditure)

2.2 Primary Health Care
(Percentage of population covered by):

2.2.1 Health services
National
Urban
Rural

2.2.2 Safe water

		Year	Source
National	56	1983	(0834)
Urban	77	1985	(2033)
Rural	13	1985	(2033)

2.2.3 Adequate sanitary facilities

		Year	Source
National	28	1983	(0834)
Urban	35	1985	(2033)
Rural	16	1985	(2033)

2.2.4 Contraceptive prevalence rate

		Year	Source
(%)	9	1977	(1712)

2.3 Coverage of maternity care (%)

Area	Prenatal care	Trained attendant	Institutional deliveries	Postnatal care	Sample size	Year	Source
National			32			1976	(0826)
National			41			1984	(1534)
National: rural urban			5 40-50			(1987) (1987)	(1780) (1780)

3. COMMUNITY STUDIES

4. HOSPITAL STUDIES

4.1 IV Region, (1989) [2338]

A study was carried out in the context of a Mothers and Infants Programme. The women who died were campesinas of low socioeconomic status. Over 44% were illiterate. Only four of the women who died were high risk cases. It is thought that 64% of the deaths were avoidable and that in 40% of the cases the hospital treatment was inadequate.

4.1.1 Rate
Maternal deaths	34
MMR (per 100 000 live births)	219

5. CIVIL REGISTRATION DATA/GOVERNMENT ESTIMATES

5.1 National, 1960-84 [0825, 0826, 0827, 1625, 2827]

5.1.1 Rate

	Maternal deaths	MMR (per 100 000 live births)
1960	103	161
1975	87	94
1983	63	47
1984	50	47
1985	24	n.a.
1986	17	12

6. OTHER SOURCES/ ESTIMATES

6.1 National, 1987 [2713]

6.1.1 Rate
The rate was estimated by PAHO to be the same as that derived from a study in Peru.

Live births	149 000
Maternal deaths	447
MMR (per 100 000 live births)	300

7. SELECTED ANNOTATED BIBLIOGRAPHY

Bood, T. Experience with an active labour management protocol and reduction of caesarean section rate in Nicaragua. *Tropical Doctor*, 1989; 20: 115-118. WHE 2579

Prospective data were collected on the outcome of labour in 67 women with uncomplicated pregnancy, who attended a rural Nicaraguan hospital during 1987-88 and were managed actively in labour. No dystocia occurred and the rate of caesarean delivery was zero. Comparison with a similar hospital where active management was not practised found a caesarean delivery rate of nearly 13%. It is concluded that active management is safe and feasible in a rural setting and results in a low rate of caesarean delivery, and reduced maternal mortality and morbidity without compromising perinatal outcome.

8. FURTHER READING

Chackiel, J. *Medición indirecta de la mortalidad materna*. Unpublished document presented at the reunión regional sobre prevención de la mortalidad materna, Sao Paulo, 12-15 April 1988. WHE 2387

9. DATA SOURCES

WHE 0825   World Health Organization. Pan American Health Organization. *Health conditions in the Americas. 1969-72.* (PAHO scientific publication no. 306) PAHO, Washington, 1975.

WHE 0826   World Health Organization. Pan American Health Organization. *Health conditions in the Americas. 1973-1976.* (PAHO scientific publication no. 364) PAHO, Washington, 1982.

WHE 0827   World Health Organization. Pan American Health Organization. *Health conditions in the Americas. 1977-1980.* (PAHO scientific publication no. 427) PAHO, Washington, 1982.

WHE 0834   World Health Organization. *World health statistics annual – vital statistics and causes of death.* Geneva, various years.

WHE 1444   World Health Organization. Pan American Health Organization. *Health of women in the Americas.* Scientific publication no. 488. PAHO, Washington, 1985.

WHE 1534   World Health Organization. Pan American Health Organization. *Programa de salud materna infantil.* Documento de referencia sobre estudio y prevención de la mortalidad materna. Fasciculo I. PAHO, Washington, 1986.

WHE 1625   World Health Organization, Pan American Health Organization. *Health conditions in the Americas.* 1981-84. Vol. I (PAHO Scientific Publication no. 500). PAHO, Washington, 1986.

WHE 1712   Mauldin W.P. and Segal, S.J., *Prevalence of contraceptive use in developing countries. A chart book.* Rockefeller Foundation, New York 1986.

WHE 1780   Pascoe, M. and Stein, A. Midwifery work exchange project in Nicaragua. *Journal of Nurse Midwifery,* 1987; 32(2): 101-104.

WHE 1914   United Nations Children's Fund (UNICEF). *The state of the world's children*, Oxford, Oxford University Press, various years.

WHE 1915   United Nations. Department of International Economic and Social Affairs. *World population prospects: estimates and projections*, Population Studies, New York, various years.

WHE 1918   United Nations. Department of International Economic and Social Affairs. *First marriage: patterns and determinants.* New York 1988.

WHE 2033   World Health Organization. *Global Strategy for Health for All by the Year 2000. Second report on monitoring progress.* WHO document EB83/2 Add. 1, 1988.

WHE 2338   De la Fuente, M. Maternal mortality and morbidity: a call to women for action. *Women's Global Network for Reproductive Rights Newsletter* 30, July – September 1989.

WHE 2713   World Health Organization, Pan American Health Organization *Regional plan of action for the reduction of maternal mortality in the Americas,* Document No. CSP23/10, XXIII Pan American Sanitary Conference, Washington 1990.

WHE 2827   World Health Organization. Pan American Health Organization. *Health conditions in the Americas,* Scientific Publication No. 524, Washington, 1990.

NOTES

PANAMA

	Year	Source

1. BASIC INDICATORS

1.1 Demographic

1.1.1 Population

Size (millions)	2.4	1990	(1915)
Rate of growth (%)	2.1	1985-90	(1915)

1.1.2 Life expectancy

Female	74	1985-90	(1915)
Male	70	1985-90	(1915)

1.1.3 Fertility

Crude Birth Rate	27	1985-90	(1915)
Total Fertility Rate	3.1	1985-90	(1915)

1.1.4 Mortality

Crude Death Rate	5	1985-90	(1915)
Infant Mortality Rate	23	1985-90	(1915)
Female	17	1987	(2827)
Male	22	1987	(2827)
1-4 years mortality rate			
Female	2	1987	(2827)
Male	2	1987	(2827)

1.2 Social and economic

1.2.1 Adult literacy rate (%)

Female	86	1985	(1914)
Male	87	1985	(1914)

1.2.2 Primary school enrolment rate (%)

Female	104	1986-88	(1914)
Male	109	1986-88	(1914)

1.2.3 Female mean age at first marriage

(years)	21.2	1980	(1918)

	Year	Source

1.2.4 GNP/capita

(US $)	2 120	1987	(1914)

1.2.5 Daily per capita calorie supply

(as % of requirements)	107	1984-86	(1914)

2. HEALTH SERVICES

2.1 Health Expenditure

2.1.1 Expenditure on health

(as % of GNP)	10.1	1984	(2033)

2.1.2 Expenditure on PHC
(as % of total health expenditure)

2.2 Primary Health Care
(Percentage of population covered by):

2.2.1 Health services

National	82	1983-87	(2033)
Urban			
Rural			

2.2.2 Safe water

National			
Urban	100	1985	(2033)
Rural	64	1985	(2033)

2.2.3 Adequate sanitary facilities

National			
Urban	99	1985	(2033)
Rural	61	1985	(2033)

2.2.4 Contraceptive prevalence rate

(%)	61	1984	(1712)

2.3   Coverage of maternity care (%)

Area	Prenatal care	Trained attendant	Institutional deliveries	Postnatal care	Sample size	Year	Source
National:	89	89	88	81	8 240	1984	(1499):
urban	95	98	98	88	3 890	1984	(1499)
rural	84	80	80	75	4 350	1984	(1499)
Interior:							
Ladinos	89	91	85	79	1 537	1984-85	(1666)
Indians	56	73	46	53	341	1984-85	(1666)

3.   COMMUNITY STUDIES

4.   HOSPITAL STUDIES

5.   CIVIL REGISTRATION DATA/GOVERNMENT ESTIMATES

5.1   National, 1970-84 (0825, 0826, 0827, 1625, 2713, 2827)

5.1.1   Rate

	Maternal deaths	MMR (per 100 000 live births)
1970	72	135
1975	46	86
1980	38	72
1981	33	61
1982	49	90
1983	33	60
1984	28	49
1985	33	57
1986	36	62
1987	22	38

5.1.2   Causes of maternal deaths, 1987

	Number
Abortion	5
Hypertensive disorders of pregnancy	4
Haemorrhage	1
Other direct causes	11
Indirect causes	1
TOTAL	22

6.   OTHER SOURCES/ ESTIMATES

6.1   National, 1987 (2713)

The maternal mortality rate was adjusted to account for underreporting based on the estimated 39% under-registration observed in a study in the United States.

6.1.1   Rate

Births	68 000
Maternal deaths	40
MMR (per 100 000 births)	60

6.2   Provinces, 1983 (1626)

6.2.1   Rate

Province	MMR (per 100 000 live births)
Bocas del Toro	70
Cocle	50
Colon	40
Chiriqui	70
Darien	210
Los Santos	70
Panama	630
Veraguas	160
San Blas Region	390
Panama city	20
Colon city	50

7. SELECTED ANNOTATED BIBLIOGRAPHY

8. FURTHER READING

Chackiel, J. *Medición indirecta de la mortalidad materna*. Unpublished document presented at the reunión regional sobre prevención de la mortalidad materna, Sao Paulo, 12-15 April 1988. WHE 2387

9. DATA SOURCES

WHE 0753 United Nations, *Demographic Yearbook*. New York, various years.

WHE 0825 World Health Organization. Pan American Health Organization. *Health conditions in the Americas. 1969-72.* (PAHO scientific publication no. 306) PAHO, Washington, 1975.

WHE 0826 World Health Organization. Pan American Health Organization. *Health conditions in the Americas. 1973-1976.* (PAHO scientific publication no. 364) PAHO, Washington, 1982.

WHE 0827 World Health Organization. Pan American Health Organization. *Health conditions in the Americas. 1977-1980.* (PAHO scientific publication no. 427) PAHO, Washington, 1982.

WHE 1499 Guerra, L.F. *Maternal-child health/family planning survey.* Ministry of Health, Panama, 1984.

WHE 1625 World Health Organization, Pan American Health Organization. *Health conditions in the Americas.* 1981-84. Vol. I (PAHO Scientific Publication no. 500). PAHO, Washington, 1986.

WHE 1626 World Health Organization. Pan American Health Organization. *Health conditions in the Americas 1981-84.* Scientific publication no. 500, PAHO, Washington, 1986.

WHE 1666 Monteith, R.S. et al. Use of maternal and child health services and immunization coverage in Panama and Guatemala. *Bulletin of the Pan American Health Organization*, 1987; 21(1): 1-15.

WHE 1712 Mauldin W.P. and Segal, S.J., *Prevalence of contraceptive use in developing countries. A chart book.* Rockefeller Foundation, New York 1986.

WHE 1914 United Nations Children's Fund (UNICEF). *The state of the world's children*, Oxford, Oxford University Press, various years.

WHE 1915 United Nations. Department of International Economic and Social Affairs. *World population prospects: estimates and projections*, Population Studies, New York, various years.

WHE 1917 United Nations. Department of International Economic and Social Affairs. *Age structure of mortality in developing countries. A database for cross-sectional and time-series research.* New York 1986.

WHE 1918 United Nations. Department of International Economic and Social Affairs. *First marriage: patterns and determinants.* New York 1988.

WHE 2033 World Health Organization. *Global strategy for health for all by the year 2000. Second report on monitoring progress.* WHO document EB83/2 Add. 1, 1988.

WHE 2713 World Health Organization, Pan American Health Organization *Regional plan of action for the reduction of maternal mortality in the Americas,* Document No. CSP23/10, XXIII Pan American Sanitary Conference, Washington 1990.

WHE 2827 World Health Organization. Pan American Health Organization. *Health conditions in the Americas*, Scientific Publication No. 524, Washington, 1990.

NOTES

PARAGUAY

		Year	Source

1. BASIC INDICATORS

1.1 Demographic

1.1.1 Population

Size (millions	4.3	1990	(1915)
Rate of growth (%)	2.9	1985-90	(1915)

1.1.2 Life expectancy

Female	69	1985-90	(1915)
Male	65	1985-90	(1915)

1.1.3 Fertility

Crude Birth Rate	35	1985-90	(1915)
Total Fertility Rate	4.6	1985-90	(1915)

1.1.4 Mortality

Crude Death Rate	7	1985-90	(1915)
Infant Mortality Rate	42	1985-90	(1915)
Female	32	1985-90	(2761)
Male	38	1985-90	(2761)
1-4 years mortality rate			
Female	12	1985-90	(2761)
Male	10	1985-90	(2761)

1.2 Social and economic

1.2.1 Adult literacy rate (%)

Female	86	1985	(1914)
Male	91	1985	(1914)

1.2.2 Primary school enrolment rate (%)

Female	99	1986-88	(1914)
Male	104	1986-88	(1914)

1.2.3 Female mean age at first marriage

(years)	21.8	1982	(1918)

1.2.4 GNP/capita

(US $)	1 180	1987	(1914)

1.2.5 Daily per capita calorie supply

(as % of requirements)	123	1984-86	(1914)

2. HEALTH SERVICES

2.1 Health Expenditure

2.1.1 Expenditure on health

(as % of GNP)	1.7	1984	(2033)

2.1.2 Expenditure on PHC
(as % of total health expenditure)

2.2 Primary Health Care
(Percentage of population covered by):

2.2.1 Health services
National
Urban
Rural

2.2.2 Safe water

National	25	1983	(0834)
Urban	49	1985	(2033)
Rural	8	1985	(2033)

2.2.3 Adequate sanitary facilities

National	84	1983	(0834)
Urban	66	1985	(2033)
Rural	40	1985	(2033)

2.2.4 Contraceptive prevalence rate

(%)	48*	1990	(2761).

* Married or cohabiting women.

2.3 Coverage of maternity care (%)

Area	Prenatal care	Trained attendant	Institutional deliveries	Postnatal care	Sample size	Year	Source
National		22				1983	(0834)
National	65					1984	(0834)
National			22			1984	(1534)
National	57	30				1983-87	(2033)
National:	84				3 944w	1985-90	(2761)
urban	93				1 808w	1985-90	(2761)
rural	76				2 136w	1985-90	(2761)
Centro Sur	87				1 045w	1985-90	(2761)
Este	80				1 196w	1985-90	(2761)
Gran Asunción	94				1 117w	1985-90	(2761)
Norte	67				586	1985-90	(2761)

3. COMMUNITY STUDIES

4. HOSPITAL STUDIES

5. CIVIL REGISTRATION DATA/GOVERNMENT ESTIMATES

5.1 National (reporting areas only), 1980-1987 [(2827)]

	Maternal deaths	MMR (per 100 000 live births)
1980	164	365
1981	134	294
1982	149	297
1983	164	311
1984	155	275
1985	146	283
1986	140	261
1987	100*	194*

* Provisional

5.1.2 Causes of maternal deaths, 1986

	Number	%
Haemorrhage	43	31
Hypertensive disorders of pregnancy	25	18
Abortion	20	14
Complications of the puerperium	24	17
Other direct causes	22	16
Indirect causes	6	4
TOTAL	140	100

6. OTHER SOURCES/ ESTIMATES

6.1 National, 1986 [(2713)]

The rate was estimated by PAHO to be the same as that derived from a study in Peru.

6.1.1 Rate

Births	150 000
Maternal deaths	450
MMR (per 100 000 births)	300

7. SELECTED ANNOTATED BIBLIOGRAPHY

8. FURTHER READING

Chackiel, J. *Medición indirecta de la mortalidad materna*. Unpublished document presented at the reunión regional sobre prevención de la mortalidad materna, Sao Paulo, 12-15 April 1988. WHE 2387

9. DATA SOURCES

WHE 0834 World Health Organization. *World health statistics annual – vital statistics and causes of death*. Geneva, various years.

WHE 1534 World Health Organization, Pan American Health Organization. *Programa de salud materno infantil*. Documento de referencia sobre estudio y prevención de la mortalidad materna, Fasciculo I. PAHO, Washington, 1986.

WHE 1914 United Nations Children's Fund (UNICEF). *The state of the world's children*, Oxford, Oxford University Press, various years.

WHE 1915 United Nations. Department of International Economic and Social Affairs. *World population prospects: estimates and projections*, Population Studies, New York, various years.

WHE 1918 United Nations. Department of International Economic and Social Affairs. *First marriage: patterns and determinants*. New York 1988.

WHE 2033 World Health Organization. *Global strategy for health for all by the year 2000. Second report on monitoring progress*. WHO document EB83/2 Add. 1, 1988.

WHE 2713 World Health Organization, Pan American Health Organization *Regional plan of action for the reduction of maternal mortality in the Americas*, Document No. CSP23/10, XXIII Pan American Sanitary Conference, Washington 1990.

WHE 2761 Demographic and Health Surveys, *Paraguay encuesta nacional de demografía y salud 1990*. Centro Paraguayo de Estudios de Población/Institute for Resource Development/ Macro Systems Inc. 1991.

WHE 2827 World Health Organization. Pan American Health Organization. *Health conditions in the Americas*, Scientific Publication No. 524, Washington, 1990.

NOTES

PERU

	Year	Source

1. BASIC INDICATORS

1.1 Demographic

1.1.1 Population
Size (millions)	21.6	1990	(1915)
Rate of growth (%)	2.1	1985-90	(1915)

1.1.2 Life expectancy
Female	63	1985-90	(1915)
Male	60	1985-90	(1915)

1.1.3 Fertility
Crude Birth Rate	31	1985-90	(1915)
Total Fertility Rate	4.0	1985-90	(1915)

1.1.4 Mortality
Crude Death Rate	9	1985-90	(1915)
Infant Mortality Rate	88	1985-90	(1915)
Female	32	1983	(2827)
Male	36	1983	(2827)
1-4 years mortality rate			
Female	6	1983	(2827)
Male	6	1983	(2827)

1.2 Social and economic

1.2.1 Adult literacy rate (%)
Female	75	1985	(1914)
Male	90	1985	(1914)

1.2.2 Primary school enrolment rate (%)
Female	120	1986-88	(1914)
Male	125	1986-88	(1914)

1.2.3 Female mean age at first marriage
(years)	22.7	1981	(1918)

	Year	Source

1.2.4 GNP/capita
(US $)	1 300	1987	(1914)

1.2.5 Daily per capita calorie supply
(as % of requirements)	93	1984-86	(1914)

2. HEALTH SERVICES

2.1 Health Expenditure

2.1.1 Expenditure on health
(as % of GNP)	3.0	1984	(2033)

2.1.2 Expenditure on PHC
(as % of total health expenditure)

2.2 Primary Health Care
(Percentage of population covered by):

2.2.1 Health services
National
Urban
Rural

2.2.2 Safe water
National	52	1983	(0834)
Urban	73	1983	(0834)
Rural	18	1983	(0834)

2.2.3 Adequate sanitary facilities
National	35	1983	(0834)
Urban	67	1985	(2033)
Rural	13	1985	(2033)

2.2.4 Contraceptive prevalence rate
(%)	43	1981	(1712)

2.3 Coverage of maternity care (%)

Area	Prenatal care	Trained attendant	Institutional deliveries	Postnatal care	Sample size	Year	Source
National	46					1983	(0834)
National		44				1984	(0834)
National	65					1984	(2115)
National	60	78				1983-87	(2033)
National:	55	49			3 156	1981-86	(1662)
urban	79	80			1 641	1981-86	(1662)
rural	28	15			1 515	1981-86	(1662)
Area Metropolitana de Lima	88	94			651	1981-86	(1662)
Other coastal	65	62			795	1981-86	(1662)
Selva	40	34			463	1981-86	(1662)
Sierra	36	24			1 247	1981-86	(1662)

3. COMMUNITY STUDIES

3.1 Peri-urban areas of Lima, (1988) [2565]

A child mortality survey was carried out among a marginalised population in a poor peri-urban area of Lima where female life expectancy was estimated as 66 years and the total fertility rate was 3.6 children per woman. The "sisterhood method" was used to calculate maternal mortality rates. The lifetime risk of dying from pregnancy related causes was 1 in 98.

3.1.1 Rate
Maternal deaths	58
MMR (per 100 000 live births)	286

4. HOSPITAL STUDIES

4.1 Hospital San Bartolomé de Lima, 1962-65 [1820]

4.1.1 Rate
Deliveries	11 011
Maternal deaths	16
MMR (per 100 000 deliveries)	145

4.1.2 Causes of maternal deaths
Haemorrhage accounted for five maternal deaths, sepsis for four, hypertensive disorders of pregnancy for two, and vascular accidents for three maternal deaths.

4.1.3 Avoidable factors
Prenatal care

	MMR (per 100 000 live births)
Women with no prenatal care	109
Women with prenatal care	36

4.2 110 Ministry of Health hospitals and 19 Ministry of Social Security Hospitals, May-October 1985 [2115]

4.2.1 Rate
National

	Ministry of Health	Ministry of Social Security	TOTAL
Live births	84 540	17 060	101 603
Maternal deaths	163	5	168
MMR (per 100 000 live births)	193	29	165

By administrative region

	Live births	Maternal deaths	MMR (per 100 000 live births)
Amazonas	160	0	–
Ancash	2 663	9	338
Apurimac	893	1	112
Arequipa	6 012	7	116
Ayacucho	2 336	5	214
Cajamarca	1 368	2	146
Callao	3 603	5	139
Cusco	3 756	4	112
Huancavelica	223	1	448
Huanuco	2 262	4	177
Ica	5 445	3	55
Junin	3 754	9	240
La Libertad	5 245	12	229
Lambayeque	3 463	5	144
Lima	45 089	47	104
Loreto	3 193	8	251
Madre de Dios	289	0	–
Moquegua	660	1	151
Pasco	530	2	377
Piura	4 387	11	251
Puno	1 138	8	703
San Martin	1 550	14	903
Tacna	1 169	2	171
Tumbes	863	2	232
Ucayali	1 729	6	347

By geographic area

	Live births	Maternal deaths	MMR (per 100 000 live births)
Costa Baja (0-500 m)	65 761	87	132
Costa Alta (501-2000 m)	6 564	6	91
Sierra Baja (2001-3000 m)	17 159	37	216
Sierra Alta (>3000 m)	1 392	6	431
Selva Alta (501-2000 m)	6 462	25	387

4.2.2 Causes of maternal deaths

	Number	%
Abortion	37	22
Haemorrhage	32	19
Sepsis	30	18
Hypertensive disorders of pregnancy	29	17
Ruptured Uterus	6	4
Other direct causes	8	5
DIRECT CAUSES	142	85
INDIRECT CAUSES	26	15
TOTAL	168	100

Among women aged 35 years and older, haemorrhage was the most frequent cause of death accounting for 45% of the deaths in that age-group. Abortion was the most frequent cause of death among women aged 25-29 years.

4.2.3 Avoidable factors

Maternal deaths were more common among women who had not had prenatal care. 32% of the mothers who died had received prenatal care whereas 56% had not. By comparison, in a national community survey, 65% of the sample had received prenatal care and 35% had not.

5. CIVIL REGISTRATION DATA/GOVERNMENT ESTIMATES

5.1 National, 1970-83 [0825, 0826, 0827, 1625, 2827]

5.1.1 Rate

	Maternal deaths	MMR (per 100 000 live births)
1970	1 030	221
1975	802	189
1980	749	108
1981	648	92
1982	576	85
1983	611	89

5.1.2 Causes of maternal deaths, 1983 *(for 538 deaths)*

	Number	%
Abortion	59	11
Haemorrhage	178	33
Hypertensive disorders of pregnancy	43	8
Complications of the puerperium	75	14
Other direct causes	178	33
Indirect causes	5	1
TOTAL	538	100

6. OTHER SOURCES/ ESTIMATES

6.1 National (1984) [1354]

6.1.1 Rate

A report on the status of women in Peru, published in 1984, reports a maternal mortality rate of 314 per 100 000 live births.

6.2 National, 1983 [2713]

A Pan American Health Organization report estimated maternal deaths after adjusting for underreporting.

6.2.1

Births	759 000
Maternal deaths	2 277
MMR (per 100 000 births)	300

7. Selected Annotated Bibliography

8. Further Reading

Chackiel, J. *Medición indirecta de la mortalidad materna.* Unpublished document presented at the reunión regional sobre prevencion de la mortalidad materna, Sao Paulo, 12-15 April 1988. WHE 2387

Figueroa, M.L. et al. La situacion nutricional y de salud de la mujer Latinoamericana. *Archivos Latinoamericana de Nutricion,* 1988; 38(3): 705-722. WHE 3141

Singh S. and Wulf, D. Estimating abortion levels in Brazil, Colombia and Peru, using hospital admissions and fertility survey data. *International Family Planning Perspectives,* 1991; 17(1): 8-13. WHE 2994

9. Data Sources

WHE 0825   World Health Organization. Pan American Health Organization. *Health conditions in the Americas. 1969-72.* (PAHO scientific publication no. 306) PAHO, Washington, 1975.

WHE 0826   World Health Organization. Pan American Health Organization. *Health conditions in the Americas. 1973-1976.* (PAHO scientific publication no. 364) PAHO, Washington, 1982.

WHE 0827   World Health Organization. Pan American Health Organization. *Health conditions in the Americas. 1977-1980.* (PAHO scientific publication no. 427) PAHO, Washington, 1982.

WHE 0834   World Health Organization. *World health statistics annual – vital statistics and causes of death.* Geneva, various years.

WHE 1354   Jiménez La Rosa, R.E. *Participación de la mujer Peruana en la salud y el desarrollo.* Lima, 1984.

WHE 1625   World Health Organization, Pan American Health Organization. *Health conditions in the Americas.* 1981-84. Vol. I (PAHO Scientific Publication no. 500). PAHO, Washington, 1986.

WHE 1662   Demographic and Health Surveys. *Peru, encuesta demográfica y de salud familiar.* Instituto Nacional de Estadística/Institute for Resource Development/Westinghouse.

WHE 1712   Mauldin W.P. and Segal, S.J., *Prevalence of contraceptive use in developing countries. A chart book.* Rockefeller Foundation, New York 1986.

WHE 1820   Benavides, G. et al. Mortalidad materna. *Revista Ecuatoriana de Higiene y Medicina Tropical,* 1977; 30(1): 37-46.

WHE 1914   United Nations Children's Fund (UNICEF). *The state of the world's children,* Oxford, Oxford University Press, various years.

WHE 1915   United Nations. Department of International Economic and Social Affairs. *World population prospects: estimates and projections,* Population Studies, New York, various years.

WHE 1918   United Nations. Department of International Economic and Social Affairs. *First marriage: patterns and determinants.* New York 1988.

WHE 2033   World Health Organization. *Global strategy for health for all by the year 2000. Second report on monitoring progress.* WHO document EB83/2 Add. 1, 1988.

WHE 2115   Cervantes, R. et al. *Muerte materna y muerte perinatal en los hospitales del Peru.* Ministerio de Salud/Sociedad Peruana de Obstetricia y Ginecología, Lima, 1988.

WHE 2565   Maine, D. *Results of applications of the sisterhood method for estimating maternal mortality* London School of Hygiene and Tropical Medicine, 1990 (unpublished document).

WHE 2713   World Health Organization, Pan American Health Organization *Regional plan of action for the reduction of maternal mortality in the Americas,* Document No. CSP23/10, XXIII Pan American Sanitary Conference, Washington 1990.

WHE 2827   World Health Organization. Pan American Health Organization. *Health conditions in the Americas,* Scientific Publication No. 524, Washington, 1990.

PUERTO RICO

		Year	Source

1. BASIC INDICATORS

1.1 Demographic

1.1.1 Population

		Year	Source
Size (millions)	3.5	1990	(1915)
Rate of growth (%)	1.2	1985-90	(1915)

1.1.2 Life expectancy

Female	78	1985-90	(1915)
Male	72	1985-90	(1915)

1.1.3 Fertility

Crude Birth Rate	19	1985-90	(1915)
Total Fertility Rate	2.4	1985-90	(1915)

1.1.4 Mortality

Crude Death Rate	8	1985-90	(1915)
Infant Mortality Rate	15	1985-90	(1915)
Female	13	1987	(2827)
Male	16	1987	(2827)
1-4 years mortality rate			
Female			
Male			

1.2 Social and economic

1.2.1 Adult literacy rate (%)
Female
Male

1.2.2 Primary school enrolment rate (%)
Female
Male

1.2.3 Female mean age at first marriage

(years)	22.3	1980	(1918)

1.2.4 GNP/capita
(US $)

1.2.5 Daily per capita calorie supply
(as % of requirements)

2. HEALTH SERVICES

2.1 Health Expenditure

2.1.1 Expenditure on health
(as % of GNP)

2.1.2 Expenditure on PHC
(as % of total health expenditure)

2.2 Primary Health Care
(Percentage of population covered by):

2.2.1 Health services
National
Urban
Rural

2.2.2 Safe water
National
Urban
Rural

2.2.3 Adequate sanitary facilities.
National
Urban
Rural

2.2.4 Contraceptive prevalence rate

(%)	69	1982	(1712)

2.3 Coverage of maternity care (%)

Area	Prenatal care	Trained attendant	Institutional deliveries	Postnatal care	Sample size	Year	Source
National			99			1981	(0546)

3. COMMUNITY STUDIES

3.1 National Surveillance of all pregnancy related deaths, 1978-79 [1301, 1302]

An intensive survey of pregnancy-related deaths was conducted during 1978-79. By expanding surveillance through review of death certificates and selected medical records an additional 45 deaths were identified in addition to the 17 deaths registered through vital statistics. Thirteen of the additional deaths were identified by a review of death certificates and the remaining 32 by a review of selected medical records.

3.1.1 Rate

Live births	148 901
Maternal deaths*	62
MMR (per 100 000 live births)	42

* Deaths occurring within one year of termination of pregnancy.

3.1.2 Causes of maternal deaths*

	Number	%
Hypertensive disorders of pregnancy	22	35
Haemorrhage	16	26
Sepsis	12	19
Obstetric shock	10	16
Embolisms	4	6
Ectopic/molar pregnancy	3	5
Complications of anaesthesia	3	5
Cardiac diseases	3	5
Abortion	1	2
Others	1	2

* Causes not mutually exclusive.

3.1.3 Avoidable factors

3.1.4 High risk groups

Age

	Live births	Maternal deaths	MMR (per 100,000 live births)
<14	664	1	151
15-19	26 775	7	26
20-24	50 559	16	32
25-29	39 336	11	28
30-34	21 257	12	56
35-39	7 844	10	127
40-44	2 043	4	196
45+	260	1	485

3.1.5 Other findings

3.2 National, 1982 [3142]

Death certificates of women of childbearing age who died during 1982 were examined with a view to determining how many deaths has been misclassified and were, in fact, maternal deaths. Attempts were made to locate medical and autopsy records where the death had occurred in a health care facility. In 12% of these deaths the hospital failed to cooperate with the study. The review of death certificates yielded an additional three maternal deaths and the analysis of medical records a further 17 deaths. A total of 28 maternal deaths were identified, only eight of which had been classified as such by the Department of Health, an under-registration rate of over 70%. The maternal mortality rate was calculated to be 3.5 times higher than that indicated in the vital statistics.

3.2.1 Rate

Registered maternal deaths	8
MMR (per 100 000 live births)	12
Total maternal deaths	28
MMR (per 100 000 live births)	40

4. HOSPITAL STUDIES

5. CIVIL REGISTRATION DATA/GOVERNMENT ESTIMATES

5.1 National, 1960-83 [0825, 0826, 0827, 1625, 2713, 2827]

5.1.1 Rate

	Maternal deaths	MMR (per 100 000 live births)
1960	38	50
1965	37	46
1970	18	27
1975	11	16
1980	11	15
1981	12	17
1982	8	12
1983	4	6
1984	6	9
1985	8	13
1986	10	16
1987	11	17

5.1.2 Causes of maternal deaths

	Number
Hypertensive disorders of pregnancy	2
Haemorrhage	1
Complications of the puerperium	5
Other direct causes	3
TOTAL	11

6. OTHER SOURCES/ESTIMATES

6.1 National, (1990) [2713]

The maternal mortality rate was adjusted to account for underreporting based on the estimated 39% under-registration observed in a study in the United States.

6.1.1 Rate

Births	78 000
Maternal deaths	16
MMR (per 100 000 births)	21

7. SELECTED ANNOTATED BIBLIOGRAPHY

8. FURTHER READING

9. DATA SOURCES

WHE 0546   Puerto Rico, Departamento de Salud. *Informe anual de estadísticas vitales 1981.* 1982

WHE 0825   World Health Organization. Pan American Health Organization. *Health conditions in the Americas. 1969-72.* (PAHO scientific publication no. 306) PAHO, Washington, 1975.

WHE 0826   World Health Organization. Pan American Health Organization. *Health conditions in the Americas. 1973-1976.* (PAHO scientific publication no. 364) PAHO, Washington, 1982.

WHE 0827   World Health Organization. Pan American Health Organization. *Health conditions in the Americas. 1977-1980.* (PAHO scientific publication no. 427) PAHO, Washington, 1982.

WHE 1301   Speckhard, M.E. et al. Intensive surveillance of pregnancy-related deaths, Puerto Rico, 1978-1979. *Bulletin of the Association of Medicine of Puerto Rico,* 1985; 77(12).

WHE 1302   Speckhard, M.E. et al. Risk factors associated with pregnancy-related deaths in Puerto Rico. *Bulletin of the Association of Medicine of Puerto Rico,* 1986; 78(1).

WHE 1625   World Health Organization, Pan American Health Organization. *Health conditions in the Americas.* 1981-84. Vol. I (PAHO Scientific Publication no. 500). PAHO, Washington, 1986.

WHE 1712   Mauldin W.P. and Segal, S.J., *Prevalence of contraceptive use in developing countries. A chart book.* Rockefeller Foundation, New York 1986.

WHE 1915   United Nations. Department of International Economic and Social Affairs. *World population prospects: estimates and projections,* Population Studies, New York, various years.

WHE 1918   United Nations. Department of International Economic and Social Affairs. *First marriage: patterns and determinants.* New York 1988.

WHE 2713   World Health Organization, Pan American Health Organization *Regional plan of action for the reduction of maternal mortality in the Americas,* Document No. CSP23/10, XXIII Pan American Sanitary Conference, Washington 1990.

WHE 2827   World Health Organization. Pan American Health Organization. *Health conditions in the Americas,* Scientific Publication No. 524, Washington, 1990.

WHE 3142   Comas, A. et al. Misreporting of maternal mortality in Puerto Rico. *Bulletin of the Association of Medicine Puerto Rico,* 1990; 82(8): 343-346.

TRINIDAD AND TOBAGO

		Year	Source

1. BASIC INDICATORS

1.1 Demographic

1.1.1 Population

		Year	Source
Size (millions)	1.3	1990	(1915)
Rate of growth (%)	1.7	1985-90	(1915)

1.1.2 Life expectancy

Female	74	1985-90	(1915)
Male	69	1985-90	(1915)

1.1.3 Fertility

Crude Birth Rate	26	1985-90	(1915)
Total Fertility Rate	3.0	1985-90	(1915)

1.1.4 Mortality

Crude Death Rate	6	1985-90	(1915)
Infant Mortality Rate	16	1985-90	(1915)
Female	34	1977-87	(3140)
Male	29	1977-87	(3140)
1-4 years mortality rate			
Female	3	1977-87	(3140)
Male	3	1977-87	(3140)

1.2 Social and economic

1.2.1 Adult literacy rate (%)

Female	95	1985	(1914)
Male	97	1985	(1914)

1.2.2 Primary school enrolment rate (%)

Female	96	1983-86	(1914)
Male	93	1983-86	(1914)

1.2.3 Female mean age at first marriage

(years)	22.3*	1980	(1918)

* Includes legal, consensual and visiting unions.

1.2.4 GNP/capita

		Year	Source
(US $)	3 350	1987	(1914)

1.2.5 Daily per capita calorie supply

(as % of requirements)	126	1985	(1914)

2. HEALTH SERVICES

2.1 Health Expenditure

2.1.1 Expenditure on health

(as % of GNP)	2.8	1984	(2033)

2.1.2 Expenditure on PHC
(as % of total health expenditure)

2.2 Primary Health Care
(Percentage of population covered by):

2.2.1 Health services

National	99	1983-87	(2033)
Urban			
Rural			

2.2.2 Safe water

National	95	1985	(2033)
Urban	100	1985	(2033)
Rural	93	1985	(2033)

2.2.3 Adequate sanitary facilities

National	100	1985	(2033)
Urban	100	1985	(2033)
Rural	100	1985	(2033)

2.2.4 Contraceptive prevalence rate

(%)	53	1987	(3140)

2.3 Coverage of maternity care (%)

Area	Prenatal care	Trained attendant	Institutional deliveries	Postnatal care	Sample size	Year	Source
National	95	95				1983-87	(2033)
National:	98	98			1 929	1982-87	(3140)
urban	97	98			826	1982-87	(3140)
rural	98	97			1 103	1982-87	(3140)

3. COMMUNITY STUDIES

4. HOSPITAL STUDIES

4.1 Mount Hope Hospital, Port of Spain, 1981-86 [1589]

4.1.1 Rate

Deliveries	34 727
Maternal deaths	11
MMR (per 100 000 deliveries)	32

4.1.2 Causes of maternal deaths

Eight of the 11 deaths were attributable to hypertensive disorders of pregnancy.

5. CIVIL REGISTRATION DATA/GOVERNMENT ESTIMATES

5.1 National, 1950-87 [0712, 0825, 0826, 0827, 1625, 2713, 2827]

5.1.1 Rate

	Maternal deaths	MMR (per 100 000 live births)
1950	n.a.	380
1960	43	130
1970	34	130
1980	19	64
1981	19	59
1982	14	43
1983	18	54
1984	9	28
1986	18	56
1987	26	89

5.1.2 Causes of maternal deaths (1986)

	Number
Abortion	9
Hypertensive disorders of pregnancy	5
Haemorrhage	1
Complications of the puerperium	1
Other direct causes	1
Indirect causes	1
TOTAL	18

6. OTHER SOURCES/ESTIMATES

6.1 National, 1986 [2713]

The maternal mortality rate was adjusted to account for underreporting based on the estimated 39% underregistration observed in a study in the United States.

6.1.1 Rate

Births	31 000
Maternal deaths	34
MMR (per 100 000 births)	111

7. SELECTED ANNOTATED BIBLIOGRAPHY

8. FURTHER READING

9. DATA SOURCES

WHE 0712   Trinidad and Tobago, Ministry of Finance. *Population and vital statistics 1977*. Port of Spain, 1978.

WHE 0825   World Health Organization. Pan American Health Organization. *Health conditions in the Americas. 1969-72.* (PAHO scientific publication no. 306) PAHO, Washington, 1975.

WHE 0826   World Health Organization. Pan American Health Organization. *Health conditions in the Americas. 1973-1976.* (PAHO scientific publication no. 364) PAHO, Washington, 1982.

WHE 0827   World Health Organization. Pan American Health Organization. *Health conditions in the Americas. 1977-1980.* (PAHO scientific publication no. 427) PAHO, Washington, 1982.

WHE 1589   Roopnarinesingh, S. *Maternal mortality at the Mt. Hope Hospital.* (personal communication), 1987.

WHE 1625   World Health Organization, Pan American Health Organization. *Health conditions in the Americas.* 1981-84. Vol. I (PAHO Scientific Publication no. 500). PAHO, Washington, 1986.

WHE 1914   United Nations Children's Fund (UNICEF). *The state of the world's children*, Oxford, Oxford University Press, various years.

WHE 1915   United Nations. Department of International Economic and Social Affairs. *World population prospects: estimates and projections*, Population Studies, New York, various years.

WHE 1918   United Nations. Department of International Economic and Social Affairs. *First marriage: patterns and determinants.* New York 1988.

WHE 2033   World Health Organization. *Global strategy for health for all by the year 2000. Second report on monitoring progress.* WHO document EB83/2 Add. 1, 1988.

WHE 2713   World Health Organization, Pan American Health Organization *Regional plan of action for the reduction of maternal mortality in the Americas,* Document No. CSP23/10, XXIII Pan American Sanitary Conference, Washington 1990.

WHE 2827   World Health Organization. Pan American Health Organization. *Health conditions in the Americas*, Scientific Publication No. 524, Washington, 1990.

WHE 3140   Demographic and Health Surveys. *Trinidad and Tobago demographic and health survey 1987.* Family Planning Association/Institute for Resource Development/Westinghouse, 1988.

NOTES

URUGUAY

		Year	Source

1. BASIC INDICATORS

1.1 Demographic

1.1.1 Population
		Year	Source
Size (millions)	3.1	1990	(1915)
Rate of growth (%)	0.6	1985-90	(1915)

1.1.2 Life expectancy
		Year	Source
Female	75	1985-90	(1915)
Male	69	1985-90	(1915)

1.1.3 Fertility
		Year	Source
Crude Birth Rate	18	1985-90	(1915)
Total Fertility Rate	2.4	1985-90	(1915)

1.1.4 Mortality
		Year	Source
Crude Death Rate	10	1985-90	(1915)
Infant Mortality Rate	24	1985-90	(1915)
Female	21	1987	(2827)
Male	27	1987	(2827)
1-4 years mortality rate			
Female	1	1987	(2827)
Male	1	1987	(2827)

1.2 Social and economic

1.2.1 Adult literacy rate (%)
		Year	Source
Female	95	1985	(1914)
Male	96	1985	(1914)

1.2.2 Primary school enrolment rate (%)
		Year	Source
Female	109	1986-88	(1914)
Male	111	1986-88	(1914)

1.2.3 Female mean age at first marriage
		Year	Source
(years)	22.4	1975	(1918)

1.2.4 GNP/capita
		Year	Source
(US $)	2 470	1987	(1914)

1.2.5 Daily per capita calorie supply
		Year	Source
(as % of requirements)	100	1984-86	(1914)

2. HEALTH SERVICES

2.1 Health expenditure

2.1.1 Expenditure on health
		Year	Source
(as % of GNP)	8.0	1984	(2033)

2.1.2 Expenditure on PHC
(as % of total health expenditure)

2.2 Primary Health Care
(Percentage of population covered by):

2.2.1 Health services
National
Urban
Rural

2.2.2 Safe water
		Year	Source
National	83	1983	(0834)
Urban	95	1983	(0834)
Rural	27	1983	(0834)

2.2.3 Adequate sanitary facilities
		Year	Source
National	59	1983	(0834)
Urban	59	1983	(0834)
Rural	59	1983	(0834)

2.2.4 Contraceptive prevalence rate
(%)

2.3 Coverage of maternity care (%)

Area	Prenatal care	Trained attendant	Institutional deliveries	Postnatal care	Sample size	Year	Source
National	14		31			1972	(0825)
National		96	94			1977	(0827)
National			97			1983	(1534)

3. COMMUNITY STUDIES

4. HOSPITAL STUDIES

5. CIVIL REGISTRATION DATA/GOVERNMENT ESTIMATES

5.1 National, 1960-87 (0825, 0826, 0827, 1625, 2713, 2827)

5.1.1 Rate

	Maternal deaths	MMR (per 100 000 live births)
1960	71	117
1965	60	99
1970	50	77
1975	41	69
1980	27	50
1981	33	61
1982	20	37
1983	21	39
1984	20	38
1985	23	45
1986	14	26
1987	15	28

5.1.2 Causes of maternal deaths, 1986

	Number
Abortion	5
Hypertensive disorders of pregnancy	1
Haemorrhage	1
Complications of the puerperium	2
Other direct causes	5
TOTAL	14

6. OTHER SOURCES/ ESTIMATES

6.1 National, (1990) (2713)

A Pan American Health Organization report estimated maternal deaths after adjusting for underreporting. The correction factor was based on the 39% underreporting observed in a study in the United States.

6.1.1 Rate

Births	569 000
Maternal deaths	19
MMR (per 100 000 births)	36

7. SELECTED ANNOTATED BIBLIOGRAPHY

8. FURTHER READING

Chackiel, J. *Medición indirecta de la mortalidad materna*. Unpublished document presented at the reunión regional sobre prevención de la mortalidad materna, Sao Paulo, 12-15 April 1988. WHE 2387

9. DATA SOURCES

WHE 0825   World Health Organization. Pan American Health Organization. *Health conditions in the Americas. 1969-72.* (PAHO scientific publication no. 306) PAHO, Washington, 1975.

WHE 0826   World Health Organization. Pan American Health Organization. *Health conditions in the Americas. 1973-1976.* (PAHO scientific publication no. 364) PAHO, Washington, 1982.

WHE 0827   World Health Organization. Pan American Health Organization. *Health conditions in the Americas. 1977-1980.* (PAHO scientific publication no. 427) PAHO, Washington, 1982.

WHE 0834   World Health Organization *World health statistics annual – vital statistics and causes of death.* Geneva, various years.

WHE 1534   World Health Organization, Pan American Health Organization. *Programa de salud materno infantil.* Documento de referencia sobre estudio y prevención de la mortalidad materna, Fasciculo I. PAHO, Washington, 1986.

WHE 1625   World Health Organization, Pan American Health Organization. *Health conditions in the Americas.* 1981-84. Vol. I (PAHO Scientific Publication no. 500). PAHO, Washington, 1986.

WHE 1914   United Nations Children's Fund (UNICEF). *The state of the world's children*, Oxford, Oxford University Press, various years.

WHE 1915   United Nations. Department of International Economic and Social Affairs. *World population prospects: estimates and projections*, Population Studies, New York, various years.

WHE 1918   United Nations. Department of International Economic and Social Affairs. *First marriage: patterns and determinants.* New York 1988.

WHE 2033   World Health Organization. *Global strategy for health for all by the year 2000. Second report on monitoring progress.* WHO document EB83/2 Add. 1, 1988.

WHE 2713   World Health Organization, Pan American Health Organization *Regional plan of action for the reduction of maternal mortality in the Americas,* Document No. CSP23/10, XXIII Pan American Sanitary Conference, Washington 1990.

WHE 2827   World Health Organization. Pan American Health Organization. *Health conditions in the Americas*, Scientific Publication No. 524, Washington, 1990.

NOTES

VENEZUELA

		Year	Source

1. BASIC INDICATORS

1.1 Demographic

1.1.1 Population

		Year	Source
Size (millions)	19.7	1990	(1915)
Rate of growth (%)	2.6	1985-90	(1915)

1.1.2 Life expectancy

Female	73	1985-90	(1915)
Male	67	1985-90	(1915)

1.1.3 Fertility

Crude Birth Rate	31	1985-90	(1915)
Total Fertility Rate	3.8	1985-90	(1915)

1.1.4 Mortality

Crude Death Rate	5	1985-90	(1915)
Infant Mortality Rate	36	1985-90	(1915)
Female	22	1987	(2827)
Male	28	1987	(2827)
1-4 years mortality rate			
Female	1	1987	(2827)
Male	1	1987	(2827)

1.2 Social and economic

1.2.1 Adult literacy rate (%)

Female	88	1985	(1914)
Male	84	1985	(1914)

1.2.2 Primary school enrolment rate (%)

Female	107	1986-88	(1914)
Male	107	1986-88	(1914)

1.2.3 Female mean age at first marriage

(years)	21.2	1981	(1918)

		Year	Source

1.2.4 GNP/capita

(US $)	3 250	1987	(1914)

1.2.5 Daily per capita calorie supply

(as % of requirements)	102	1984-86	(1914)

2. HEALTH SERVICES

2.1 Health expenditure

2.1.1 Expenditure on health

(as % of GNP)	3.1	1984	(2033)

2.1.2 Expenditure on PHC
(as % of total health expenditure)

2.2 Primary Health Care
(Percentage of population covered by):

2.2.1 Health services
National
Urban
Rural

2.2.2 Safe water

National	83	1983	(0834)
Urban	88	1983	(0834)
Rural	65	1983	(0834)

2.2.3 Adequate sanitary facilities

National	45	1983	(0834)
Urban	57	1983	(0834)
Rural	6	1983	(0834)

2.2.4 Contraceptive prevalence rate

(%)	49	1977	(1712)

2.3   Coverage of maternity care (%)

Area	Prenatal care	Trained attendant	Institutional deliveries	Postnatal care	Sample size	Year	Source
National		82				1982	(0834)
National			98			1984	(1534)
National	74	69				1983-87	(2033)
National	32		16			1986-89	(3143)

3. COMMUNITY STUDIES

4. HOSPITAL STUDIES

4.1 "Doctor Armando Castillo Plaza" Maternity, Maracaibo University Hospital, Maracaibo, 1961-67 [1826]

4.1.1 Rate
Live births   67 252
Maternal deaths   84
MMR (per 100 000 live births)   125

4.1.2 Causes of maternal deaths

	Number	%
Abortion	28	34
Hypertensive disorders of pregnancy	16	21
Ruptured uterus	13	16
Haemorrhage	10	12
Sepsis	4	5
Embolisms	2	2
Ectopic pregnancy	1	1
Anaemia	1	1
Hepatitis	1	1
Hepatic failure	1	1
Tuberculosis	3	3
Others	4	3
Total	84	100

4.1.3 Avoidable factors

4.1.4 High risk groups
81% of the deaths were of multiparous women (3 or more previous deliveries), compared with 16% for primigravidas and 4% for women delivering their second child.

4.1.5 Other findings
42 of the 84 women who died arrived at the hospital moribund. 77% of the women who died were single.

4.2 Concepción Palacios Maternity Hospital, Caracas, 1939-74 [0019]

4.2.1 Rate

	Live births	Maternal deaths	MMR (per 100 000 live births)
1939-63	395 294	773	196
1964-72	374 146	469	125
1973-74	89 424	129	144
Total	858 864	1 371	160

4.2.2 Causes of maternal death

	Number	%
Sepsis	430	31
Haemorrhage	302	22
Hypertensive disorders of pregnancy	217	16
Complications of anaesthesia	37	3
Embolisms	12	1
Other direct causes	13	1
DIRECT CAUSES	1 011	74
Cardiac diseases	67	5
Hepatitis	3	0
Other indirect causes	26	2
INDIRECT CAUSES	96	7
Fortuitous	264	19
TOTAL	1 371	100

4.2.3 Avoidable factors

4.2.4 High risk groups

4.2.5 Other findings
The authors estimate that the official maternal mortality rate of 70 per 100,000 live births in 1974 is an underestimate. For example, officially there were 71 deaths from sepsis for the entire country in 1974, but in the Maternidad Concepcion Palacios alone there were 28 sepsis deaths.

4.3 Hospital Central "Dr.Manuel Nuñez Tovar" de Maturín, 1965-75 [0604]

4.3.1 Rate

	Live births	Maternal deaths	MMR (per 100 000 live births)
1965-67	8 657	11	127
1968-70	13 803	14	101
1971-73	15 022	19	126
1974-75	11 520	4	35
Total	49 002	48	98

4.3.2 Causes of maternal deaths

	Number	%
Haemorrhage	18	39
Hypertensive disorders of pregnancy	15	32
Sepsis	4	8
Ruptured uterus	2	4
Complications of anaesthesia	1	2
DIRECT CAUSES	40	83
Lung infections	3	7
Cardiac diseases	2	4
Liver infections	1	2
Kidney diseases	1	2
INDIRECT CAUSES	7	15
Fortuitous	1	2
TOTAL	48	100

5. CIVIL REGISTRATION DATA/GOVERNMENT ESTIMATES

5.1 National, 1960-87 [0825, 0826, 0827, 0834, 1625, 2722, 2827]

5.1.1 Rate

	Maternal deaths	MMR (per 100 000 live births)
1960	353	104
1965	409	108
1970	362	92
1975	305	68
1980	319	65
1981	265	52
1982	257	50
1983	303	59
1984	307	61
1985	291	58
1986	296	59
1987	284	55

5.1.2 Causes of maternal deaths, 1985

	Number	%
Abortion	67	23
Hypertensive disorders of pregnancy	67	23
Haemorrhage	44	15
Complications of the puerperium	43	15
Other direct obstetric causes	52	18
Indirect causes	18	6
TOTAL	291	100

5.2 City of Maracaibo, 1962-67 [1826]

5.2.1 Rate

Live births	110 382
Maternal deaths	138
MMR (per 100 000 live births)	125

6. OTHER SOURCES/ ESTIMATES

6.1 National, (1990) [2713]

The maternal mortality rate was recalculated by PAHO using estimates for underreporting based on a study carried out in Brazil.

6.1.1 Rate

Births	569 000
Maternal deaths	1 138
MMR (per 100 000 births)	200

7. SELECTED ANNOTATED BIBLIOGRAPHY

Lopez Gomez, J.R. et al. Operacion cesarean en el servicio de obstetricia del Hospital "Dr. Adolfo Prince Lara" Puerto Cabello – decenio 1974-1983. *Revista de Obstetricia y Ginecología de Venezuela*, 1985; 45(1): 37045. WHE 2842.

A retrospective analysis of caesarean deliveries over the period 1974-83 found that the proportion of births by caesarean increased from under 4% in 1974 to nearly 13% in 1983. Over 69% of the caesarean deliveries were performed on women aged between 19 and 32 years and 66% of the women had no previous deliveries. The most important indication for caesarean delivery was cephalo-pelvic disproportion (30%) followed by previous caesarean scar (28%). The maternal mortality rate for caesarean delivery was 379 per 100,000 births compared with 95 per 100,000 for vaginal deliveries. Sepsis was the major cause of death.

8. FURTHER READING

Chackiel, J. *Medicion indirecta de la mortalidad
   materna.* Unpublished document presented at the
   Reunion regional sobre prevencion de la
   mortalidad materna, Sao Paulo, 12-15 April 1988.
   WHE 2387

9. DATA SOURCES

WHE 0019   Aguero, O. et al. Mortalidad materna en
   la Maternidad Concepción Palacios, 1939-1974.
   Revista de Obstetricia y Ginecología de Venezuela,
   1977; 37(3): 361-366.

WHE 0604   Regardis Amaro, R. Mortalidad materna
   en el Hospital Central. *Revista de Obstetricia y
   Ginecología de Venezuela,* 1977; 37(1): 37-50.

WHE 0825   World Health Organization. Pan
   American Health Organization. *Health conditions
   in the Americas. 1969-72.* (PAHO scientific
   publication no. 306) PAHO, Washington, 1975.

WHE 0826   World Health Organization. Pan
   American Health Organization. *Health conditions
   in the Americas. 1973-1976.* (PAHO scientific
   publication no. 364) PAHO, Washington, 1982.

WHE 0827   World Health Organization. Pan
   American Health Organization. *Health conditions
   in the Americas. 1977-1980.* (PAHO scientific
   publication no. 427) PAHO, Washington, 1982.

WHE 0834   World Health Organization *World health
   statistics annual – vital statistics and causes of
   death.* Geneva, various years.

WHE 1534   World Health Organization, Pan
   American Health Organization. *Programa de salud
   materno infantil.* Documento de referencia sobre
   estudio y prevención de la mortalidad materna,
   Fasciculo I. PAHO, Washington, 1986.

WHE 1625   World Health Organization, Pan
   American Health Organization. *Health conditions
   in the Americas.* 1981-84. Vol. I (PAHO Scientific
   Publication no. 500). PAHO, Washington, 1986.

WHE 1712   Mauldin W.P. and Segal, S.J., *Prevalence
   of contraceptive use in developing countries. A chart
   book.* Rockefeller Foundation, New York 1986.

WHE 1826   Suarez Herrera, R. Maternal mortality in
   Maracaibo 1962-1967. *Revista de Obstetricia y
   Ginecología de Venezuela,* 1968; 28(4): 521-544.

WHE 1914   United Nations Children's Fund
   (UNICEF). *The state of the world's children,* Oxford,
   Oxford University Press, various years.

WHE 1915   United Nations. Department of
   International Economic and Social Affairs. *World
   population prospects: estimates and projections,*
   Population Studies, New York, various years.

WHE 1918   United Nations. Department of
   International Economic and Social Affairs. *First
   marriage: patterns and determinants.* New York
   1988.

WHE 2033   World Health Organization. *Global
   strategy for health for all by the year 2000. Second
   report on monitoring progress.* WHO document
   EB83/2 Add. 1, 1988.

WHE 2713   World Health Organization, Pan
   American Health Organization *Regional plan of
   action for the reduction of maternal mortality in the
   Americas,* Document No. CSP23/10, XXIII Pan
   American Sanitary Conference, Washington 1990.

WHE 2722   World Health Organization, *Maternal
   deaths and maternal mortality rates* (unpublished)
   1990.

WHE 2827   World Health Organization. Pan
   American Health Organization. *Health conditions
   in the Americas,* Scientific Publication No. 524,
   Washington, 1990.

WHE 3143   Expanded Programme on Immunization.
   Neonatal tetanus in Venezuela, 1986-1989. *EPI
   Newsletter,* 1990, 12(1): 5-6.

ASIA

AFGHANISTAN

		Year	Source

1. BASIC INDICATORS

1.1 Demographic

1.1.1 Population

		Year	Source
Size (millions)	16.6	1990	(1915)
Rate of growth (%)	2.6	1985-90	(1915)

1.1.2 Life expectancy

Female	42	1985-90	(1915)
Male	41	1985-90	(1915)

1.1.3 Fertility

Crude Birth Rate	49	1985-90	(1915)
Total Fertility Rate	6.9	1985-90	(1915)

1.1.4 Mortality

Crude Death Rate	23	1985-90	(1915)
Infant Mortality Rate	172	1985-90	(1915)
Female	191	1979	(0753)
Male	217	1979	(0753)
1-4 years mortality rate			
Female	26	1979	(0753)
Male	29	1979	(0753)

1.2 Social and economic

1.2.1 Adult literacy rate (%)

Female	8	1985	(1914)
Male	39	1985	(1914)

1.2.2 Primary school enrolment rate (%)

Female	14	1986-88	(1914)
Male	27	1986-88	(1914)

1.2.3 Female mean age at first marriage

(years)	17.8	1979	(1918)

1.2.4 GNP/capita
(US $)

1.2.5 Daily per capita calorie supply

		Year	Source
(as % of requirements)	94	1984-86	(1914)

2. HEALTH SERVICES

2.1 Health expenditure

2.1.1 Expenditure on health

(as % of GNP)	0.6	1984	(1888)

2.1.2 Expenditure on PHC

(as % of total health expenditure)	33	1987	(2033)

2.2 Primary Health Care
(Percentage of population covered by):

2.2.1 Health services

National	49	1984	(0834)
Urban			
Rural			

2.2.2 Safe water

National	19	1985	(2033)
Urban	38	1985	(2033)
Rural	17	1985	(2033)

2.2.3 Adequate sanitary facilities

National	2	1984	(0834)
Urban	5	1985	(2033)
Rural			

2.2.4 Contraceptive prevalence rate

(%)	2	1976	(1712)

2.3 Coverage of maternity care (%)

Area	Prenatal care	Trained attendant	Institutional deliveries	Postnatal care	Sample size	Year	Source
National	8	8				(1988)	(2033)
Greater Kabul	46	40	28		1 328	1973-74	(0011)

3. COMMUNITY STUDIES

3.1 Greater Kabul Area, 1973-74 [0011]

3.1.1 Rate
Deliveries 1 328
Maternal deaths 13
MMR (per 100 000 deliveries) 980

4. HOSPITAL STUDIES

4.1 Malalay Zejanton Hospital, 1980-81 [0244]

4.1.1 Rate
Births 16 723
Maternal deaths 31
MMR (per 100 000 births) 185

5. CIVIL REGISTRATION DATA/GOVERNMENT ESTIMATES

5.1 National, 1975 [0011]

5.1.1 Rate
According to the 1975 Afghan Demographic Survey, the maternal mortality rate for the country as a whole was 690 per 100 000 deliveries, and the rate in urban areas was 400 per 100 000 deliveries.

6. OTHER SOURCES/ ESTIMATES

6.1 National [0231]

6.1.1 Rate
A study published in 1978 quotes a maternal mortality rate of 640 per 100 000 deliveries.

6.2 National 1981 (2608)

6.2.1 Rate
MMR (per 100 000 live births) 600

7. SELECTED ANNOTATED BIBLIOGRAPHY

8. FURTHER READING

9. DATA SOURCES

WHE 0011   Afghanistan, Ministry of Health. *Infant and early childhood mortality in relation to fertility patterns: Report on an ad hoc survey in Greater Kabul, Afghanistan, 1973-74* Eastern Mediterranean Regional Office, 1976.

WHE 0231   Furnia, A.H. *Syncrisis: the dynamics of health: an analytic series on the interactions of health and social development,* US Department of Health, Education and Welfare, 1978.

WHE 0244   Grischenko, V.I. Personal communication, 1982.

WHE 0753 United Nations, *Demographic Yearbook.* New York, various years.

WHE 0834   World Health Organization *World health statistics annual – vital statistics and causes of death.* Geneva, various years.

WHE 1712   Mauldin W.P. and Segal, S.J., *Prevalence of contraceptive use in developing countries. A chart book.* Rockefeller Foundation, New York, 1986.

WHE 1888   World Health Organization, Eastern Mediterranean Regional Office, *Evaluation of the strategy for Health for All by the year 2000. Seventh report of the world health situation.* EMRO, Alexandria, 1987.

WHE 1914   United Nations Children's Fund (UNICEF). *The state of the world's children,* Oxford, Oxford University Press, various years.

WHE 1915   United Nations. Department of International Economic and Social Affairs. *World population prospects: estimates and projections,* Population Studies, New York, various years.

WHE 1918   United Nations. Department of International Economic and Social Affairs. *First marriage: patterns and determinants.* New York, 1988.

WHE 2033   World Health Organization. *Global strategy for health for all by the year 2000. Second report on monitoring progress.* WHO document EB83/2 Add. 1, 1988.

WHE 2608 United Nations Children's Fund, *1988 Asian and Pacific atlas of children in national development.* UNICEF/ESCAP, Bangkok, 1987.

NOTES

BAHRAIN

		Year	Source

1. BASIC INDICATORS

1.1 Demographic

1.1.1 Population

		Year	Source
Size (millions)	0.5	1990	(1915)
Rate of growth (%)	3.8	1985-90	(1915)

1.1.2 Life expectancy

Female	73	1985-90	(1915)
Male	67	1985-90	(1915)

1.1.3 Fertility

Crude Birth Rate	28	1985-90	(1915)
Total Fertility Rate	4.1	1985-90	(1915)

1.1.4 Mortality

Crude Death Rate	4	1985-90	(1915)
Infant Mortality Rate	26	1985-90	(1915)
Female			
Male			
1-4 years mortality rate			
Female			
Male			

1.2 Social and economic

1.2.1 Adult literacy rate (%)

Female	64	1985	(1914)
Male	79	1985	(1914)

1.2.2 Primary school enrolment rate (%)

Female	108	1986-88	(1914)
Male	111	1986-88	(1914)

1.2.3 Female mean age at first marriage
(years)

1.2.4 GNP/capita

(US $)	8 510	1987	(1914)

1.2.5 Daily per capita calorie supply
(as % of requirements)

2. HEALTH SERVICES

2.1 Health expenditure

2.1.1 Expenditure on health

(as % of GNP)	5.0	1986	(2033)

2.1.2 Expenditure on PHC
(as % of total health

expenditure)	22	1986	(2033)

2.2 Primary Health Care
(Percentage of population covered by):

2.2.1 Health services

National	100	1985	(0834)
Urban			
Rural			

2.2.2 Safe water

National	100	1985	(0834)
Urban	100	1985	(0834)
Rural	100	1985	(0834)

2.2.3 Adequate sanitary facilities

National	100	1985	(0834)
Urban	100	1985	(0834)
Rural	100	1985	(0834)

2.2.4 Contraceptive prevalence rate (%)

2.3 Coverage of maternity care (%)

Area	Prenatal care	Trained attendant	Institutional deliveries	Postnatal care	Sample size	Year	Source
National	80	100	85			1981	(0800)
National	85	98				1984	(0834)

3. COMMUNITY STUDIES

4. HOSPITAL STUDIES

5. CIVIL REGISTRATION DATA/GOVERNMENT ESTIMATES

5.1 National, 1981 (0055)

5.1.1 Rate
Live births 10 300
Maternal deaths 2
MMR (per 100 000 live births) 19

5.2 National, 1977-86 (2258)

5.2.1 Rate
Live births 10 921
Maternal deaths 37
MMR (per 100 000 live births) 34

5.2.2 Causes of maternal deaths

	Number	%
Haemorrhage	7	19
Hypertensive disorders of pregnancy	5	14
Embolisms	3	8
Abortion	2	5
Complication of Caesarean section	1	3
DIRECT CAUSES	18	49
Infections	7	19
Pulmonary embolism	5	14
Cardiac failure	2	5
Cerebrovascular accident	2	5
Other indirect causes	3	8
INDIRECT CAUSES	19	51
TOTAL	37	100

5.2.3 Avoidable factors
Avoidable factors were present in 14 (38%) of the 37 cases, the majority (ten cases) being due to the failure of the patients to seek medical care or follow medical advice. In four cases avoidable factors were associated with inappropriate clinical management or inadequate medical facilities.

5.2.4 High risk groups

5.2.5 Other findings
Sickle cell disease was found to be an underlying cause in about one third of the maternal deaths.

6. OTHER SOURCES/ ESTIMATES

7. SELECTED ANNOTATED BIBLIOGRAPHY

8. FURTHER READING

9. DATA SOURCES

WHE 0055   Bahrain, Ministry of Health. *Annual report 1981,* Bahrain, 1981.

WHE 0800   World Health Organization. *Country reports to regional offices of the progress in implementing Health for All by the Year 2000.* (Unpublished documents) 1983

WHE 0834   World Health Organization. *World health statistics annual – vital statistics and causes of death.* Geneva, various years.

WHE 1914   United Nations Children's Fund (UNICEF). *The state of the world's children,* Oxford, Oxford University Press, various years.

WHE 1915   United Nations. Department of International Economic and Social Affairs. *World population prospects: estimates and projections,* Population Studies, New York, various years.

WHE 2033   World Health Organization. *Global strategy for health for all by the year 2000. Second report on monitoring progress.* WHO document EB83/2 Add. 1, 1988.

WHE 2258   El-Shafei, A.M. et al., Maternal mortality in Bahrain with special reference to sickle cell disease. *Australia and New Zealand Journal of Obstetrics and Gynaecology,* 1988; 28(1): 36-40.

NOTES

BANGLADESH

		Year	Source

1. BASIC INDICATORS

1.1 Demographic

1.1.1 Population

		Year	Source
Size (millions)	117.7	1990	(1915)
Rate of growth (%)	3.0	1985-90	(1915)

1.1.2 Life expectancy

Female	50	1985-90	(1915)
Male	51	1985-90	(1915)

1.1.3 Fertility

Crude Birth Rate	42	1985-90	(1915)
Total Fertility Rate	5.5	1985-90	(1915)

1.1.4 Mortality

Crude Death Rate	16	1985-90	(1915)
Infant Mortality Rate	119	1985-90	(1915)
Female	140	1981	(1917)
Male	145	1981	(1917)
1-4 years mortality rate			
Female	25	1981	(1917)
Male	22	1981	(1917)

1.2 Social and economic

1.2.1 Adult literacy rate (%)

Female	22	1985	(1914)
Male	43	1985	(1914)

1.2.2 Primary school enrolment rate (%)

Female	64	1986-88	(1914)
Male	76	1986-88	(1914)

1.2.3 Female mean age at first marriage

(years)	16.7	1981	(1918)

1.2.4 GNP/capita

(US $)	160	1987	(1914)

1.2.5 Daily per capita calorie supply

(as % of requirements)	83	1984-86	(1914)

2. HEALTH SERVICES

2.1 Health expenditure

2.1.1 Expenditure on health

(as % of GNP)	1.1	1987-88	(2033)

2.1.2 Expenditure on PHC

(as % of total health expenditure)	65	1987-88	(2033)

2.2 Primary Health Care
(Percentage of population covered by):

2.2.1 Health services

National	38	1987	(2033)
Urban			
Rural			

2.2.2 Safe water

National	40	1983	(0834)
Urban	25	1987	(2033)
Rural	66	1987	(2033)

2.2.3 Adequate sanitary facilities

National	4	1983	(0834)
Urban	20	1987	(2033)
Rural	6	1987	(2033)

2.2.4 Contraceptive prevalence rate

(%)	25	1985	(1712)

2.3   Coverage of maternity care (%)

Area	Prenatal care	Trained attendant	Institutional deliveries	Postnatal care	Sample size	Year	Source
National			1			1984	(0917)
National			5			(1984)	(0298)
National		5				1985	(1087)
National	12	5				1988	(2033)

3.   COMMUNITY STUDIES

3.1   Matlab Thana, 1967-70 and 1976-85 (0131, 0597, 1576, 1579, 2242)

Two studies were carried out over the period 1967-70. The first, covering 132 villages took place between December 1967 and November 1968 and the second, covering an additional 101 villages, took place between May 1968 and April 1970. During the period 1976-85 studies were carried out in 70 villages where a special family planning programme was set up and, for comparison, in another 79 villages where no such programme existed.

3.1.1   Rate

	1967-68	1968-70	1976-85
Live births	5 329	20 816	70 286
Maternal deaths	41	119	387
MMR (per 100 000 live births)	769	572	550
MMR (per 100 000 women aged 15-44 years)	–	–	101

3.1.2   Causes of maternal deaths (%)

	1967-68	1976-85 MCH-FP*	COMP**	Total
Haemorrhage	12	20	19	20
Abortion	7	21	16	18
Hypertensive disorders of pregnancy	25	12	12	12
Sepsis	7	5	8	7
Ruptured uterus / Obstructed labour	12	7	6	7
Ectopic pregnancy	2	0	0	0
Other obstetric causes	15	14	14	14
Medical diseases	10	7	11	9
Injuries, violence	–	9	9	9
Other	10	5	5	4
Total	100	100	100	100
(N)	41	168	219	387

*   MCH-FP – Area where a maternal and child health and family planning programme was in action.
**   COMP – Area (from the same thana) comparable to the project area, but where no programme was in action.

Causes of maternal deaths by age and parity, 1976-85 (%)

	Maternal age 15-19	20-34	35-44	Prior parity 0	1-5	6+
Haemorrhage	15	20	24	14	20	29
Abortion	16	15	29	16	16	25
Hypertensive disorders of pregnancy	18	13	0	20	11	0
Sepsis	5	8	6	9	6	5
Obstructed labour	6	6	7	7	5	8
Other obstetric causes	12	17	9	14	14	14
Injuries, violence	17	7	5	13	8	4
Medical diseases	6	8	16	5	13	9
Other and unspecified	5	6	3	2	7	6
Total	100	100	100	100	100	100
(N)	94	209	84	141	167	79

3.1.3 Avoidable factors

3.1.4 High risk groups

Age

	MMR (per 100 000 live births)	
	1968-70	1976-85
10-14	1 770	n.a.
15-19	740	743
20-24	380	412
25-29	520	447
30-34	620	460
35-39	480	988
40-44	810	791
45-49	0	n.a.

Parity

	MMR (per 100 000 live births)	
	1968-70	1976-85
0	1 270	971
1	240	407
2	1260	310
3	240	315
4	470	488
5	600	343
6	680	590
7	740	693
8	650	830*
9 or more	660	

*   for gravidity 8+.

Age and parity, 1976-85

	MMR (per 100 000 live births)						
	Parity						
Age	0	1-2	3-4	5-6	7-8	9+	Total
15-19	900	330	*	*	*	*	740
20-24	900	270	250	0	*	*	410
25-29	3 160	500	320	350	0	*	450
30-34	*	730	550	340	450	400	460
35-44	*	1 780	1 230	640	1 070	980	940
Total	960	350	420	430	840	890	550

*   N < 100 live births

With few exceptions, at each parity level maternal mortality risks increased with age. For all maternal age categories nulliparous women faced substantially higher maternal mortality risks.

3.1.5 Other findings

Time of death

During 1976-85, the majority of maternal deaths occurred postpartum.

	% of maternal deaths
During pregnancy	17
During labour	15
Post abortion	18
Postpartum	50
0-1 day	21
2-7 days	11
8-22 days	9
23-42 days	5
43-90 days	5
	100

The impact of family planning programmes

An important finding of the 1976-85 study concerned the impact of family planning on maternal mortality rates and ratios. In 1977 a family planning programme was introduced in the Matlab treatment area. At the start of the programme contraceptive prevalence had been low but it rose to nearly 44% by 1985. In the control area, by contrast, which received only the less intensive services provided by the Government programme, contraceptive prevalence remained low, at around 16%.

Prior to the introduction of the FP programme, maternal mortality rates (deaths per 100 000 women of reproductive age) were similar in both areas. Beginning in 1978, when the effects of the FP programme began to become apparent, consistently lower maternal mortality rates were evident in the treatment area. By 1985 the maternal mortality rate in the comparison area was twice that in the treatment area (121 per 100 000 women compared with 66 per 100 000.)

A substantially different picture is observed when trends in maternal mortality ratios (deaths per 100 000 live births) are examined. Overall maternal mortality ratios were not consistently different in treatment and comparison areas.

In the treatment area, total fertility rates are estimated to have declined by 25% in the initial years of the programme while remaining stable in the comparison area. The family planning programme, by reducing the number of pregnancies and births, reduced the number of women who died from maternity-related causes - hence the low maternal mortality rate in the treatment areas. The FP programme did not, however, substantially alter the mortality risks associated with pregnancy and childbirth and had, therefore, little impact on maternal mortality ratios.

Birth spacing

Another important finding was the relationship between birth-spacing and maternal deaths. Higher parity-for-age, or lower age-for-parity both imply shorter average intervals between births. If shorter intervals between births were an important determinant of maternal mortality, then at a given age, mortality risks should increase with higher parity, and conversely, at a given parity level, mortality rates should increase with decreasing age. There was no evidence to support this hypothesis from the results of the study.

3.2   Tangail district, 1982-83 [1279]

This was a prospective study carried out between September 1982 and August 1983 in two upazillas of Tangail district. Twelve field workers, each responsible for around 27 villages, collected data. They were assisted by one or more contact persons in each village who provided information about any reproductive event or any death in the village. The investigator then interviewed a member of the household where the event had occurred.

3.2.1   Rate

Live births	8 485
Maternal deaths	48
MMR (per 100 000 live births)	566

3.2.2   Causes of maternal deaths

A careful review of the symptoms associated with maternal death in this study revealed that anaemia was a common factor in nearly all the maternal deaths. This explains the high death rate from haemorrhage. All abortions except one were induced, and all the women died of sepsis. In the case of the one suicide death the predisposing factor was pregnancy in an unmarried woman.

	Number	%
Haemorrhage	18	38
Abortion	8	17
Hypertensive disorders of pregnancy	7	15
Prolonged labour	6	12
Sepsis	5	10
Anaemia	2	4
Gastroenteritis	1	2
Suicide	1	2
Total	48	100

3.2.3   Avoidable factors

3.2.4.   High risk groups

Age	MMR (per 100 000 live births)			
	Parity 0-2	Parity 3-4	Parity >4	All parities
<20	861	*	*	860
20-29	290	411	1 465	357
30+	476	372	1 242	835
All ages	404	392	1 280	566

*   None of the women aged 20 and below exceeded parity 2.

Analysis of maternal mortality simultaneously by age and parity shows that mothers who were under 20 years of age and mothers, regardless of age, at parity higher than four were at greatest risk of death. The effect of higher parity in the 20-29 age group may reflect the consequences of short birth spacing, while the effect in the 30+ age group may reflect both high parity and older age.

3.2.5   Other findings

Time of death

Of the 48 maternal deaths, thirteen occurred during pregnancy but prior to delivery, eight during labour and childbirth and 27 (56%) postpartum.

Place of death

With the exception of one woman who died in a hospital, all the maternal deaths occurred at home. Of the 35 postpartum deaths only five were attended by a medical practitioner. The remaining 30 mothers were attended either by relatives or TBAs. All thirteen mothers who died during pregnancy but before childbirth had received some medical care except one who committed suicide.

Selected demographic characteristics

The women who died were, on average, 28 years old at the time of death and had been married since the age of 16 years. They averaged five previous pregnancies and had an average of 3.3 living children. They were either illiterate or could read very little and were mainly wives of agricultural workers. Thirty of the women who died were from households where income and/or harvest was lower than required to meet basic needs.

Data collection

The method of data collection, which relied heavily on informers, probably led to an underestimation of both live births and maternal deaths, especially those occurring early in pregnancy such as those associated with ectopic pregnancy and abortion.

3.3 Jamalpur district, 1982-83 [1254, 1357]

This was a prospective study carried out between 1982 and 1983 along similar lines to that carried out in Tangail district (3.2 above).

3.3.1 Rate

Live births	9 317
Maternal deaths	58
MMR (per 100 000 live births)	623

3.3.2 Causes of maternal deaths

	Number	%
Abortion	12	21
Hypertensive disorders of pregnancy	12	21
Sepsis/tetanus	10	17
Haemorrhage	10	17
Obstructed labour	6	10
Anaemia	5	9
Suicide	1	2
Other	2	3
Total	58	100

3.3.3 Avoidable factors

3.3.4 High risk groups

Age

	Live Births	Maternal deaths	MMR (per 100 000 births)
<20	1 744	10	573
20-24	3 006	8	266
25-29	2 337	11	471
30-34	1 221	9	737
35-39	729	13	1 783
>40	280	7	2 500
Total	9 317	58	623

Age and parity

	MMR (per 100 000 live births)				
		Parity			All
Age in years	0	1-2	3-4	5+	parities
<25	406	379	0	0	379
25-35	0	366	663	914	562
35	0	3 571	2 222	1 813	1 982
All ages	383	421	764	1 424	623

3.4.5 Other findings

Time and place of death

53 of the 58 deaths took place at home. All the cases admitted to hospital before death were cases of toxaemia. Half of the maternal deaths occurred before delivery.

Time of death	% of deaths
Before delivery	50
Within one day of delivery	10
1-7 days postpartum	12
1-2 weeks postpartum	10
2-4 weeks postpartum	12
4-6 weeks postpartum	5
Total	100

Medical care

Only 13 of the mothers who died received medical attention from a qualified physician prior to death. Unqualified local practitioners were the sole attendants for 21 mothers and the remaining 24 mothers did not receive any medical attention at all before death. Proportionately more women who died as a result of toxaemia received medical care from qualified physicians than women who died from other causes. This is consistent with the fact that three of these women were hospitalized before death. A relatively high proportion of women who experienced difficult labour prior to death received no medical care whatsoever.

Abortion [1357]

There were 412 cases of induced abortion, carried out by indigenous health practitioners, which resulted in ten maternal deaths, or 17% of total maternal deaths. The death rate was higher for women aged 35 years or older and for higher parity women.

	Induced abortions	Abortion deaths	Deaths to case rate *	Abortion mortality rate **
Age				
<25	150	2	1.3	42
25-34	179	3	1.7	84
35+	83	5	6.0	496
Parity				
0	75	1	1.3	43
1-4	209	5	2.4	89
5+	128	4	3.1	300
Total	412	10	2.4	107

* Abortion deaths as % of induced abortions.
** Deaths due to induced abortions per 100 000 live births.

3.4 Gopalpur, Raipura, Singra and Godagari Upazillas, 1985 [1505, 2690]

The study consisted of two phases: a baseline survey and a longitudinal surveillance study. For the latter, women at the beginning of a pregnancy were registered and followed up for pregnancy management, food and work habits, health care, delivery management and birth outcome. The investigators noted that ectopic pregnancies and early abortions, particularly if induced, would probably have been missed by the method of data collection as would women who returned to their mother's home for delivery.

3.4.1 Rate

	Live births	Maternal deaths	MMR (per 100 000 live births)
Gopalpur	1 892	9	476
Raipura	892	8	897
Singra	1 708	7	410
Godagari	1 629	5	307
All areas	6 121	29	474

3.4.2 Causes of maternal deaths

	Number	%
Hypertensive disorders of pregnancy	11	38
Haemorrhage	9	32
Abortion	5	17
Sepsis	2	7
Obstructed labour	1	3
Others	1	3
Total	29	100

3.4.3 Avoidable factors.

3.4.4 High risk groups

Age

	Live births	Maternal deaths	MMR (per 100 000 live births)
<15	22	0	–
15-19	1 002	3	290
20-24	1 789	10	560
25-29	1 523	5	330
30-34	813	4	490
35-39	593	4	670
40-44	266	2	750
45-49	113	1	880

3.4.5 Other findings

Nearly 5% of pregnancies ended in abortion, of which 30% were induced.

Postpartum infection and postpartum haemorrhage [2690]

During the follow-up study women were interviewed to ascertain the extent of postpartum infection and postpartum haemorrhage. Postpartum infection was defined as reported fever and foul smelling lochial discharge for more than two days. Postpartum haemorrhage was defined as reported excessive bleeding after the expulsion of the placenta and any excessive bleeding thereafter. Symptoms were reported by the study subjects themselves to the interviewers who made postpartum visits every two weeks until six weeks after termination of the pregnancy.

Of the 6 513 women who participated in the study, 14.5% reported postpartum infection and 17.9% reported postpartum haemorrhage. Risk factors for both infection and haemorrhage were length of labour more than 48 hours, abnormal delivery or malpresentation.

Trained attendant during delivery

Only 4% of the women delivered with the assistance of a health/family planning worker or doctor. A further 12% were assisted by a trained birth attendant. Over a third of the women were assisted by relatives, 22% by an untrained traditional birth attendant, 18% by friends or neighbours and 10% of the women delivered alone.

3.5 Monirampur and Cox's Bazar, Jessore District, 1986 [2617]

Household listings were used to identify women aged 23 years or less who were interviewed using a structured questionnaire. Pregnant women were identified and women with 6 weeks amenorrhoea were followed for possible pregnancy. Female paramedics visited each identified pregnant woman twice during the pregnancy and twice postpartum. All deliveries were conducted at home. Additional supervision was carried out by medical doctors. All cases of maternal and neonatal death, abnormal pregnancy and abnormal outcome were analyzed. A total of 6 588 married women aged 23 years or less were identified of which 95% were followed completely. The mean age at first marriage was 14.4 years. The women were divided into two age groups, 13-17 years (556 women) and 18-23 years (1 209 women). The relatively low maternal mortality rate compared with those found in other studies is thought to be related to the small sample size.

3.5.1 Rate

	Maternal deaths	MMR (per 100 000 births)
Women aged 13-17 years	3	580
Women aged 18-23 years	2	180
Total	5	300

3.5.2 Causes of maternal deaths

There were two deaths from postpartum haemorrhage and one each from tetanus and toxaemia.

3.5.3 Avoidable factors

Most of the women received no prenatal care and 89% of the deliveries were attended by untrained persons.

4. HOSPITAL STUDIES

5. CIVIL REGISTRATION DATA/GOVERNMENT ESTIMATES

5.1 National, 1968 [0063]

5.1.1 Rate

A government report quotes a maternal mortality rate of 2 540 per 100 000 live births in Bangladesh in 1968.

5.2 National, 1985 [1087, 2629]

5.2.1 Rate

A report published by the Ministry of Health and Population Control in 1985 estimated the maternal mortality rate to be 600 per 100 000 live births.

5.2.2 Causes of maternal deaths

	%
Abortion	21
Hypertensive disorders of pregnancy	21
Obstructed labour	17
Sepsis	10
Haemorrhage	10
Tetanus	7
Indirect causes	14
Total	100

6. OTHER SOURCES/ ESTIMATES

6.1 National, 1965, 1970, 1975, 1980 [0829, 1522]

6.1.1 Rate

According to the WHO Regional Health Information Bulletin, the maternal mortality rates in Bangladesh were as follows:

	MMR (per 100 000 live births)
1965	3 000
1970	2 500
1975	3 000
1980	3 000

6.2 National, 1978 [0688]

6.2.1 Rate

A report by a UNICEF consultant to Bangladesh estimated the maternal mortality rate in Bangladesh to be around 1 500 per 100 000 live births in 1978.

6.3 National, 1978 [0726]

6.3.1 Rate

The UNFPA Mission for Needs Assessment for Population Assistance published in 1978 estimated the maternal mortality rate to be 700 per 100 000 live births.

6.4 Chandina, Gabtali and Tongi, 1982-83 [1386]

6.4.1 Rate

A study by the Bangladesh Association for Maternal and Neonatal Health in the Chandina, Gabtali and Tongi areas in 1982-83 estimated the maternal mortality rate to be 480 per 100 000 live births.

7. SELECTED ANNOTATED BIBLIOGRAPHY

Abdullah, M., and Wheeler, F. Seasonal variations, and the intra-household distribution of food in a Bangladeshi village *American Journal of Clinical Nutrition,* 1985; 41: 1305-1313. WHE 1007

Individual food intakes and body weights were measured in 53 rural Bangladeshi households at four seasons. Women's and older children's proportional energy intakes remained constant throughout the year, and were in line with expected values. Young children's proportional intakes were low, especially for girls.

Ali, S.E. *Repair of vesicovaginal fistula.* Dhaka. 1989. 6p. (Unpublished). WHE 2173

A review of 64 cases of vesico-vaginal fistula treated at Chittagong Medical College Hospital and Sir Salimullah Medical College Hospital, Bangladesh, from 1973-1978, is presented. VVF comprised 2% of all major gynaecological conditions during that period. Pre-operative and operative management are described. Thirty-two (50%) operations were performed vaginally, and 15 cases (23%) were given urinary diversions. Fifty-two operations were successful, giving a success rate of 81%.

Amin, R. and Khan, A.H. Characteristics of traditional midwives and their beliefs and practices in rural Bangladesh. *International Journal of Gynecology and Obstetrics,* 1989; 28: 119-125. WHE 2689

A study analyzed the characteristics, beliefs and practices of rural midwives. They were mainly older than 30, married or widowed and illiterate. Most had learned their midwifery from informal sources such as female relatives or neighbours. They frequently imposed dietary restrictions on mothers during pregnancy, childbirth and post-partum. Devices used in the cutting of the umbilical cord were not properly sterilized and potentially dangerous substances were applied at the navel. There was a practice of withholding breastfeeding up to three days after the delivery.

Begum, A. Vesico-vaginal fistula: surgical management of 100 cases. *Journal of Bangladesh College of Physicians and Surgeons,* 1989: 6(2); 29-32. WHE 2194

One hundred women with vesicovaginal fistula were admitted to Dhaka Medical College Hospital and Mymensingh Medical College Hospital, Dhaka, Bangladesh from January 1987 to December 1988. All the fistulae were of obstetric origin. 48% of the women were 20 years of age and under, and all but four were under 31. Primiparous women accounted for 73% of cases. Most (73%) had had no formal education, and 98% had had no prenatal care. 86% were from very poor families.

Blanchet, T. *Maternal mortality in Bangladesh: anthropological assessment report.* (unpublished) Report prepared for NORAD, 1988. WHE 2032

An anthropological study undertaken in an area with high maternal mortality rates found a combination of inadequate health services coupled with lack of community awareness about women's health needs, especially during pregnancy and childbirth. Constraints such as limited mobility of village women, preference for home deliveries, low priority given to a wife's health, fear of hospitals and extreme shortage of female doctors result in a weak demand for services and acceptance of ill-health and death related to childbearing.

Brown, K. et al. Consumption of food and nutrients by weanlings in rural Bangladesh *American Journal of Clinical Nutrition,* 1982; 36: 878-889. WHE 1084

Longitudinal studies of the consumption of food and nutrients by 70 children between 5 and 30 months of age were carried out. There was little difference in the feeding of boys and girls less than 18 months old except that the boys received more dairy products. In the older age groups, however, boys received more breast milk, cereals and dairy products.

Carloni, A.S. Sex disparities in the distribution of food within rural households. *Food and Nutrition,* 1981; 7(1): 3-12. WHE 1306

A survey of nutritional habits in rural Bangladesh found that food was inequitably divided among household members in relation to their nutritional requirements. Women and girls were disadvantaged in comparison to men and boys, resulting in a higher incidence of severe malnutrition among females and excess female mortality.

Chen, L.C. et al. Epidemiology and causes of death among children in a rural area of Bangladesh. *International Journal of Epidemiology,* 1980; 9(1): 25-33. WHE 1085

An analysis of the causes of childhood deaths was undertaken based on the study of 260,000 people living in 228 rural villages. A substantial proportion (44%) of infant deaths could not be categorized, suggesting that the causes may have been low birth weight, obstetrical-related bleeding and infection problems, prematurity, birth injuries, congenital anomalies, asphyxia and atelectasis. Many of these conditions arise from the inadequate care of the mother during pregnancy and delivery.

A marked sex differential was also observed. While there were more male than female deaths among neonates, this situation was reversed thereafter, with the greatest excess female mortality occurring among 1-year olds for all causes except drowning and tetanus. The researchers surmise that these differences may reflect socio-cultural forces operating in the traditional society. Thus, a strong preference for male children and an inferior status for women may have resulted in reduced care, poorer nutrition and other health practices inimical to girls.

Fauveau, V. and Blanchet, T. Deaths from injuries and induced abortion among rural Bangladeshi women. *Social Science and Medicine,* 1989: 29(9); 1121-1127. WHE 2448

Detailed information on 1,139 women aged 15-44 years who died between 1976 and 1986 was analyzed. Injuries and violence accounted for 31% of all deaths among women aged 15-19 years. The proportion was particularly high among unmarried women. 7% of all women of reproductive age died as a result of either suicide or homicide and of these, 32% were pregnant at the time of death. A further 5% of all the deaths resulted from complications of induced abortion. The authors conclude that special attention should be given to violent deaths during pregnancy, especially among young unmarried women. In a male-dominated society such as the one under study, suicide and homicide are two frequent consequences of illegitimate pregnancy.

Fauveau, V. et al. The effect of maternal and child health and family planning services on mortality: Is prevention enough? *British Medical Journal,* 1990; 301: 103-108. WHE 2571

A study was undertaken to examine the impact on mortality of a child survival strategy, mostly based on preventive interventions, in Matlab, Bangladesh. The interventions consisted of advice on contra-ception; information on feeding and weaning babies; the distribution of oral rehydration solution; vitamin supplementation for children; provision of iron and folic acid during pregnancy; immunization of children; trained birth attendants during delivery; and referral of the seriously ill to a central clinic. The study found that the programme was effective in preventing some deaths both among children and women. The main factor resulting in the reduction in the numbers of deaths among women was the decrease in the number of unsafe abortions.

Hossain, M., and Glass, R.I. Parental son preference in seeking medical care for children less than five years of age in a rural community in Bangladesh. *American Journal of Public Health,* 1988; 78(10): 1349-1350. WHE 2028

Examination of drug purchases from privately owned pharmacies in Matlab for children under 5 confirmed previous observations in this community of parental son preference in caring for children. The male to female incidence rate ratio for overall drug purchases was 1.71, and this despite the absence of any significant differences in sex specific incidence rates of common illnesses in the children.

Hussain, M.A. Vesico-vaginal fistula: a review. *Bangladesh Journal of Obstetrics and Gynaecology,* 1986; 1(1): 21-32. WHE 2182

During the year 1984-85 at Dhaka Medical College Hospital, Bangladesh, a total of 80 women with VVF were admitted. Of these fistulae, 96% were of obstetrical origin.

Koenig, M.A. and D'Souza, S., Sex differences in childhood mortality in rural Bangladesh. *Social Science and Medicine,* 1986; 22(1): 15-22. WHE 1328

An analysis of longitudinal data from children in rural Bangladesh found evidence of higher female than male mortality during childhood. The analysis showed that female mortality began systematically to exceed male mortality during the second half of the first year of life and that thereafter this differential became increasingly pronounced. The authors suggest that an explanation of sex differences in mortality which emphasizes solely the role of culture is inadequate, and oversimplifies a complex area of behaviour. They postulate that economic pressures force parents to selectively distribute limited resources such as food, clothing and medical care to their offspring. Faced with the necessity of allocating resources parents may be forced to prioritize their children in terms of levels of investments.

Miller, B.D. Son preference, daughter neglect, and juvenile sex ratios: Pakistan and Bangladesh compared. *Michigan State University Working Paper No. 30,* 1983. WHE 1134

A longitudinal study of over 2000 married women was carried out during 1975-77. Weight fluctuated throughout the study period corresponding to seasonal food shortages. Maternal weight (controlling for height) was consistently lower for older, higher parity women, illustrating the negative impact of increasing numbers of births on the mother's nutrient stores.

Shah, K.P. *Enquiry on the epidemiology and surgical repair of obstetric related fistula in South-East Asia.* Paper prepared for a Technical Working Group. WHO, Geneva, 1989. 11p. (Unpublished). WHE 2122

Based on a postal enquiry and a review of published and unpublished material this report summarizes some overall findings on fistula in this region. In Bangladesh the condition was most common in areas where the obstetric services are poor. The overwhelming majority of fistulae admitted to the hospitals were of obstetric origin. Most of the women suffering from fistulae were young, primiparous and from the lowest socio-economic group, with a literacy rate of 27% in Dhaka. Most women had received no prenatal care, and many travelled very long distances to reach a hospital. Most of the women who developed vesico-vaginal fistula had been abandoned by their husbands, and rendered social rejects.

Wasserheit, J. et al. Reproductive tract infections in a family planning population in rural Bangladesh. *Studies in Family Planning,* 1989; 20(2): 1989. WHE 2656

A study to determine the magnitude and nature of reproductive tract infections was carried out among currently married women of reproductive age women living in the Comilla district villages and receiving maternal and child health care and family planning services from the Matlab field station. Overall, 22% of the 2,929 women surveyed reported symptoms of reproductive tract infections. Of the 472 symptomatic women examined, 68% had clinical or laboratory evidence of infection. Users of intrauterine devices and tubectomy were each approximately four times and seven times as likely to have examination-confirmed infection as non-users.

8. FURTHER READING

Amin, R. et al. Community health services and health care utilization in rural Bangladesh. *Social Science and Medicine,* 1989; 29(12): 1343-1349. WHE 2631

Amin R. and Mariam, A.G. Son preference in Bangladesh: an emerging barrier to fertility regulation. *Journal of Biosocial Science,* 1987; 19: 221-228. WHE 2042

Bhatia, S. Traditional childbirth practices: implications for a rural maternal and child health programme. *Studies in Family Planning,* 1981; 12(2): 66-75. WHE 0090

Bhatia, S. et al. Assessing menstrual regulation performed by paramedics in rural Bangladesh. *Studies in Family Planning,* 1980; 11(6): 213-218. WHE 0091

Bhiuyan, S.N., and Burkhart, M.C. Maternal and public health benefits of menstrual regulation in Chittagong *International Journal of Gynaecology and Obstetrics,* 1982; 20(20): 105-109. WHE 0094

Bhuiya, A. et al., Socioeconomic determinants of child nutritional status: boys versus girls. *Food and Nutrition Bulletin,* 1985; 8(3): 3-7. WHE 1646

Blanchet, T. Meanings and rituals of birth in rural Bangladesh. University Press Limited, Dhaka, 1984. WHE 1653

Chen, L.C. Where have all the women gone? *Economic and Political Weekly,* 1982; March 6: 364-372. WHE 0130

Chen, L.C. Sex bias in the family allocation of food and health care in rural Bangladesh *Population and Development Review,* 1981; 7(1): 55-70. WHE 0132

Fauveau, V. et al. Epidemiology and cause of deaths among women in rural Bangladesh. *International Journal of Epidemiology,* 1989; 19(1): 139-145. WHE 2243

Feldman, S. The use of private health care providers in rural Bangladesh: a response to Claquin *Social Science and Medicine,* 1983; 17(23): 1887-1896. WHE 0218

Islam, M. Child wives of Bangladesh. *People,* 1985; 12(3): 8-9. WHE 1427

Kabir, S. Women in the dark ages. *People,* 1988; 15(4): 7-8. WHE 2046

Lindenbaum, S. Implications for women of changing marriage transactions in Bangladesh *Studies in Family Planning,* 1981; 12(11): 394-401. WHE 0439

Measham, A.R. et al. Complications from induced abortion in Bangladesh related to types of practitioner and methods, and impact on mortality *Lancet,* 1981; 1(8213): 199-202. WHE 0448

Miller, B.D. Daughter neglect, women's work and marriage: Pakistan and Bangladesh compared. *Medical Anthropology,* 1984; 8(2): 109-126. WHE 1364

Mohan, A. et al. *Health problems and awareness in Sreepur and Kalihati Bangladesh.* National Institute of Preventive and Social Medicine, 1988. WHE 2284

Obaidullah, M. et al. Induced abortion in rural Bangladesh. *Rural Demography,* 1981; 8(1): 89-120. WHE 0501

Rahman, S. *Determinants of the utilization of maternal and child health services.* National Institute of Population, Research and Training, 1981. WHE 1751

Rochat, P.W. et al. Maternal and abortion related deaths in Bangladesh, 1978-79 *International Journal of Gynaecology and Obstetrics,* 1981; 19: 155-164. WHE 0610

9. DATA SOURCES

WHE 0063 Bangladesh, Ministry of Health and Population, *Bangladesh health profile 1977* Dacca, 1981.

WHE 0131 Chen, L.C. et al. Maternal mortality in rural Bangladesh. *Studies in Family Planning,* 1974: 5(11); 334-341.

WHE 0298 Begum, S.F. *Role of TBAs in controlling maternal and neonatal health in Bangladesh: a long term programme need,* (unpublished paper). 1984

WHE 0597 Lindpainter, L.S. et al. *Maternal mortality in Matlab Thana, Bangladesh 1982:* final report for research protocol 83-021(P) of the Community Service Research Working Group, International Centre for Diarrhoeal Disease Research (unpublished paper), 1984.

WHE 0688 Tatochenko, V. *Report of a visit to Bangladesh* (unpublished paper) 1978.

WHE 0726 United Nations Fund for Population Activities. *Report of a mission on needs assessment of population assistance – Bangladesh,* UNFPA, New York, 1978.

WHE 0829 World Health Organization. Southeast Asia Regional Office. *Bulletin of regional health information,* (unpublished document no. SEA/VHS/165 Rev.1), New Delhi, 1981.

WHE 0834 World Health Organization *World health statistics annual – vital statistics and causes of death.* Geneva, various years.

WHE 0917 United Nations Economic and Scoail Commission for Asia and the Pacific. *The Asian and Pacific atlas of children in national development 1984,* UNICEF, Bangkok, 1984.

WHE 1087 Bangladesh, Ministry of Health and Population Control, MCH Task Force *National strategy for a comprehensive MCH programme,* Dhaka, 1985.

WHE 1254 Khan, A.R. et al. Maternal mortality in rural Bangladesh. The Jamalpur district. *Studies in Family Planning,* 1986: 17(1); 7-12.

WHE 1279 Alauddin, M. Maternal mortality in rural Bangladesh. The Tangail District. *Studies in Family Planning,* 1986: 17(1); 13-21.

WHE 1357 Khan, A.R. et al. Induced abortion in a rural area of Bangladesh. *Studies in Family Planning,* 1986: 17(2); 95-99.

WHE 1386 Ahmed, A.U. *Mortality, health and nutrition.* Perspectives in Bangladesh in ESCAP. Interim meeting. Analysis of trends and patterns of mortality in the ESCAP region. Changmai, Thailand, 4-5 November 1985.

WHE 1505 Alauddin, F. *Pregnancy outcome and neonatal mortality in four upazilas of Bangladesh,* BAMANEH, Dhaka, 1987.

WHE 1522 World Health Organization. Southeast Asia Regional Office. *Bulletin of regional health information,* New Delhi, 1986.

WHE 1576 Koenig, M.A. et al. Maternal mortality in Matlab, Bangladesh. *Studies in Family Planning,* 1988; 19(2): 69-80.

WHE 1579 Faveau, V. et al. *Causes of maternal mortality in rural Bangladesh,* 1987 (Unpublished) see WHE 1576 above.

WHE 1712 Mauldin W.P. and Segal, S.J., *Prevalence of contraceptive use in developing countries. A chart book.* Rockefeller Foundation, New York, 1986.

WHE 1914 United Nations Children's Fund (UNICEF). *The state of the world's children,* Oxford, Oxford University Press, various years.

WHE 1915 United Nations. Department of International Economic and Social Affairs. *World population prospects: estimates and projections,* Population Studies, New York, various years.

WHE 1917 United Nations. Department of International Economic and Social Affairs. *Age structure of mortality in developing countries. A database for cross-sectional and time-series research.* New York, 1986.

WHE 1918 United Nations. Department of International Economic and Social Affairs. *First marriage: patterns and determinants.* New York, 1988.

WHE 2033 World Health Organization. *Global strategy for health for all by the year 2000. Second report on monitoring progress.* WHO document EB83/2 Add. 1, 1988.

WHE 2242 Fauveau, V. et al. Causes of maternal mortality in rural Bangladesh. *Bulletin of the World Health Organization,* 1988; 66(5): 642-651.

WHE 2617 Rahman, S. et al. Reproductive health of adolescents in Bangladesh. *International Journal of Gynecology and Obstetrics,* 1989: 29; 329-335.

WHE 2629 Begum, A.I. *Towards development of safe motherhood in Bangladesh* (unpublished) Directorate-General of Health Services/ Ministry of Health and Family Planning, 1990.

WHE 2690 Faisel, A.J. *Postpartum infection and hemorrhage in rural Bangladesh, 1985-86.* Thesis submitted to Emory University. (unpublished), 1989.

BHUTAN

		Year	Source

1. BASIC INDICATORS

1.1 Demographic

1.1.1 Population
		Year	Source
Size (millions)	1.5	1985-90	(1915)
Rate of growth (%)	2.1	1985-90	(1915)

1.1.2 Life expectancy
Female	47	1985-90	(1915)
Male	49	1985-90	(1915)

1.1.3 Fertility
Crude Birth Rate	38	1985-90	(1915)
Total Fertility Rate	5.5	1985-90	(1915)

1.1.4 Mortality
Crude Death Rate	17	1985-90	(1915)
Infant Mortality Rate	127	1988	(1914)
Female			
Male			
1-4 years mortality rate			
Female			
Male			

1.2 Social and economic

1.2.1 Adult literacy rate (%)
Female			
Male			

1.2.2 Primary school enrolment rate (%)
Female	20	1986-88	(1914)
Male	32	1986-86	(1914)

1.2.3 Female mean age at first marriage
(years)

1.2.4 GNP/capita
(US $)	150	1987	(1914)

1.2.5 Daily per capita calorie supply
(as % of requirements)

2. HEALTH SERVICES

2.1 Health Expenditure

2.1.1 Expenditure on health
(as % of GNP)	4.9	1982	(1489)

2.1.2 Expenditure on PHC
(as % of total health expenditure)	60	(1988)	(2033)

2.2 Primary Health Care
(Percentage of population covered by):

2.2.1 Health services
National	65	1986	(2033)
Urban			
Rural			

2.2.2 Safe water
National			
Urban	50	1987	(2727)
Rural	26	1987	(2727)

2.2.3 Adequate sanitary facilities
National			
Urban	60	1987	(2727)
Rural	7	1987	(2033)

2.4 Contraceptive prevalence rate
(%)

2.3   Coverage of maternity care (%)

Area	Prenatal care	Trained attendant	Institutional deliveries	Postnatal care	Sample size	Year	Source
National	3	3				1984	(0834)
National	16	7				1988	(2033)
National	22		5			(1989)	(2373)
Chirang	20	3	2			1985	(1293)

3. COMMUNITY STUDIES

4. HOSPITAL STUDIES

4.1   Eighteen districts, 1990 [2600]

A pilot project on maternal mortality and morbidity was carried out among District Health Supervisory Officers in eighteen districts who were asked to complete monthly hospital death registration forms.

4.1.1   Rate
Deliveries	843
Maternal deaths	11
MMR (per 100 000 deliveries)	1 305

4.1.2   Causes of maternal deaths

	Number
Retained placenta	5
Haemorrhage	3
Other	3
Total	11

4.1.3   Avoidable factors

4.1.4   High risk groups

4.1.5   Other findings

A further 30 deaths were registered as having occurred either at home or during transfer to the hospital. Of the home deaths, 12 were due to haemorrhage, four to sepsis and three were due to eclampsia.

4.2   Thimphu General Hospital, 1977-87 [2724]

4.2.1   Rate
Deliveries	5 440
Maternal deaths	44
MMR (per 100 000 deliveries)	809

4.2.2   Causes of maternal deaths

	Number	%
Haemorrhage	11	25
Hypertensive disorders of pregnancy	6	14
Sepsis	4	9
Ruptured uterus	3	7
Obstructed labour	3	7
Abortion	3	7
Complications of anaesthesia	1	2
Complications of caesarean section	1	2
Embolisms	1	2
Anaemia	3	7
Hepatitis	5	11
Cardiac failure	1	2
Infections	2	4
TOTAL	44	100

In 1984-85 there was an outbreak of infective hepatitis which resulted in several maternal deaths.

4.2.3   High risk groups

4.2.4   Avoidable factors

The majority of women in the area expect to deliver at home and few attend for regular prenatal checks. There were delays in seeking treatment when complications arose. Cases of eclampsia, which is thought to be caused by evil spirits, were treated unsuccessfully by monks or traditional healers for several days before being brought to the hospital.

The vast majority of the deaths occurred on the day of admission. Most of the women were admitted moribund following transfer to the hospital from local health centres. In several cases of retained placenta, the women had delivered at home but waited several days before seeking help when the placenta was not spontaneously expelled. Several women were found to be severely anaemic at the local health clinic but went into labour before the condition could be corrected and died immediately postpartum. Several women who were admitted with obstructed labour had been in labour at home for several days prior to admission.

There is no blood bank available at the hospital and blood is taken directly from matching available donors. More often than not it was impossible to find matching blood quickly enough.

4.2.5   Other findings

5.   CIVIL REGISTRATION DATA/GOVERNMENT ESTIMATES

6.   OTHER SOURCES/ ESTIMATES

6.1   National, 1983 [1949, 2373]

6.1.1   Rate

MMR (per 100 000 live births)	773

7.   SELECTED ANNOTATED BIBLIOGRAPHY

Giri, K. *Notes on a visit to Bhutan* (unpublished document), 1989. WHE 2210

A study on unmet needs in maternal and child health and family planning was carried out from 1987-89. A total of 2,097 women of reproductive age were interviewed. Of the pregnant women only 69% were attending prenatal clinics and over half of them had to travel around 2 hours to reach the health centre. Nonattendance was related to a variety of factors including distance, pressure of household and other tasks and shyness. Only 8% of deliveries were attended by a trained person.

8.   FURTHER READING

9.   DATA SOURCES

WHE 0834   World Health Organization *World health statistics annual – vital statistics and causes of death.* Geneva, various years.

WHE 1293   World Health Organization, EPI Programme Review. Bhutan. *Weekly Epdiemiological Record,* 1986; 61 (4): 21-28.

WHE 1489   World Health Organization. Regional Office for Southeast Asia. *Evaluation of the strategy of Health for All by the year 2000.* Seventh Report on the World Health Situation. New Delhi, 1986.

WHE 1914   United Nations Children's Fund (UNICEF). *The state of the world's children ,* Oxford, Oxford University Press, various years.

WHE 1915   United Nations. Department of International Economic and Social Affairs. *World population prospects: estimates and projections,* Population Studies, New York, various years.

WHE 1949   Gupta, J.P. *Health manpower policy and planning in Bhutan.* Assignment report: 9 November - 8 December 1987.

WHE 2033   World Health Organization. *Global strategy for Health for All by the year 2000. Second report on monitoring progress.* WHO document EB83/2 Add. 1, 1988.

WHE 2373   Singay, J. *Maternal mortality and morbidity surveillance within the national health information system.* (unpublished paper) 1989.

WHE 2600   World Health Organization. Southeast Asia Regional Office. *Report on pilot studies of maternal mortality and morbidity,* (unpublished document), 1990.

WHE 2724   Norbhu, H. *A retrosprctive study of maternal mortality at General Hospital Thimphu between 1976 and 1987.* (unpublished), 1988.

WHE 2727   Bhutan, Ministry of Social Affairs. *Basic health indicators.* 1987.

NOTES

BRUNEI DARUSSALAM

		Year	Source

1. BASIC INDICATORS

1.1 Demographic

1.1.1 Population

Size (millions)	0.2	1988	(0753)
Rate of growth (%)	2.8	1985-88	(0753)

1.1.2 Life expectancy

Female	73	1981	(0753)
Male	70	1981	(0753)

1.1.3 Fertility

Crude Birth Rate	31	1986	(0753)
Total Fertility Rate	3.5	1986	(0753)

1.1.4 Mortality

Crude Death Rate	3	1986	(0753)
Infant Mortality Rate	12	1989	(1914)
Female			
Male			
1-4 years mortality rate			
Female			
Male			

1.2 Social and economic

1.2.1 Adult literacy rate (%)

Female	69	1985	(0753)
Male	85	1985	(0753)

1.2.2 Primary school enrolment rate (%)

Female	
Male	

1.2.3 Female mean age at first marriage

(years)	25.0	1986	(2799)

		Year	Source

1.2.4 GNP/capita

(US $)	20 760	1988	(1914)

1.2.5 Daily per capita calorie supply
(as % of requirements)

2. HEALTH SERVICES

2.1 Health Expenditure

2.1.1 Expenditure on health

(as % of GNP)	8.0	1984	(2033)

2.1.2 Expenditure on PHC
(as % of total health expenditure)

2.2 Primary Health Care
(Percentage of population covered by):

2.2.1 Health services

National	96	1984	(2033)
Urban			
Rural			

2.2.2 Safe Water

National
Urban
Rural

2.2.3 Adequate sanitary facilities

National
Urban
Rural

2.2.4 Contraceptive prevalence rate
(%)

2.3 Coverage of maternity care (%)

Area	Prenatal care	Trained attendant	Institutional deliveries	Postnatal care	Sample size	Year	Source
	–	–	–	–	–	–	–

3. COMMUNITY STUDIES

4. HOSPITAL STUDIES

5. CIVIL REGISTRATION DATA/GOVERNMENT ESTIMATES

6. OTHER SOURCES/ ESTIMATES

7. SELECTED ANNOTATED BIBLIOGRAPHY

8. FURTHER READING

9. DATA SOURCES

WHE 0753   United Nations, *Demographic Yearbook.* New York, various years.

WHE 1914   United Nations Children's Fund (UNICEF). *The state of the world's children*, Oxford, Oxford University Press, various years.

WHE 2033   World Health Organization. *Global strategy for health for all by the year 2000. Second report on monitoring progress.* WHO document EB83/2 Add. 1, 1988.

WHE 2799   United Nations. Department of International Economic and Social Affairs. *Patterns of first marriage: timing and prevalence.* New York, 1990.

CAMBODIA

		Year	Source

1. BASIC INDICATORS

1.1 Demographic

1.1.1 Population

		Year	Source
Size (millions)	8.2	1990	(1915)
Rate of growth (%)	2.5	1985-90	(1915)

1.1.2 Life expectancy

		Year	Source
Female	50	1985-90	(1915)
Male	47	1985-90	(1915)

1.1.3 Fertility

		Year	Source
Crude Birth Rate	41	1985-90	(1915)
Total Fertility Rate	4.7	1985-90	(1915)

1.1.4 Mortality

		Year	Source
Crude Death Rate	17	1985-90	(1915)
Infant Mortality Rate	130	1985-90	(1915)
Female			
Male			
1-4 years mortality rate			
Female			
Male			

1.2 Social and economic

1.2.1 Adult literacy rate (%)

		Year	Source
Female	17	1985	(1914)
Male	41	1985	(1914)

1.2.2 Primary school enrolment rate (%)

		Year	Source
Female			
Male			

1.2.3 Female mean age at first marriage

		Year	Source
(years)	21.3	1962	(2799)

1.2.4 GNP/capita
(US $)

1.2.5 Daily per capita calorie supply

		Year	Source
(as % of requirements)	98	1984-86	(1914)

2. HEALTH SERVICES

2.1 Health Expenditure

2.1.1 Expenditure on health
(as % of GNP)

2.1.2 Expenditure on PHC
(as % of total health expenditure)

2.2 Primary Health Care
(Percentage of population covered by):

2.2.1 Health services

		Year	Source
National	53	1985-88	(1914)
Urban	80	1985-88	(1914)
Rural	50	1985-88	(1914)

2.2.2 Safe Water

		Year	Source
National	3	1985-88	(1914)
Urban	10	1985-88	(1914)
Rural	2	1985-88	(1914)

2.2.3 Adequate sanitary facilities
National
Urban
Rural

2.2.4 Contraceptive prevalence rate
(%)

2.3   Coverage of maternity care (%)

Area	Prenatal care	Trained attendant	Institutional deliveries	Postnatal care	Sample size	Year	Source
	–	–	–	–	–	–	–

3. COMMUNITY STUDIES

4. HOSPITAL STUDIES

5. CIVIL REGISTRATION DATA/GOVERNMENT ESTIMATES

6. OTHER SOURCES/ ESTIMATES

6.1   National, 1981 [2608]

6.1.1   Rate

MMR (per 100 000 live births)   500

7. SELECTED ANNOTATED BIBLIOGRAPHY

8. FURTHER READING

9. DATA SOURCES

WHE 1914   United Nations Children's Fund (UNICEF). *The state of the world's children*, Oxford, Oxford University Press, various years.

WHE 1915   United Nations. Department of International Economic and Social Affairs. *World population prospects: estimates and projections*, Population Studies, New York, various years.

WHE 2608   United Nations Children's Fund, *1988 Asian and Pacific atlas of children in national development*. UNICEF/ESCAP, Bangkok, 1987.

WHE 2799   United Nations. Department of International Economic and Social Affairs. *Patterns of first marriage: timing and prevalence*. New York, 1990.

CHINA

	Year	Source

1. BASIC INDICATORS

1.1 Demographic

1.1.1 Population

		Year	Source
Size (millions)	1,355	1990	(1915)
Rate of growth (%)	1.4	1985-90	(1915)

1.1.2 Life expectancy

		Year	Source
Female	71	1985-90	(1915)
Male	68	1985-90	(1915)

1.1.3 Fertility

		Year	Source
Crude Birth Rate	21	1985-90	(1915)
Total Fertility Rate	2.4	1985-90	(1915)

1.1.4 Mortality

		Year	Source
Crude Death Rate	6.7	1985-90	(1915)
Infant Mortality Rate	32	1985-90	(1915)
Female			
Male			
1-4 years mortality rate			
Female			
Male			

1.2 Social and economic

1.2.1 Adult literacy rate (%)

		Year	Source
Female	56	1985	(1914)
Male	82	1985	(1914)

1.2.2 Primary school enrolment rate (%)

		Year	Source
Female	124	1986-88	(1914)
Male	140	1986-88	(1914)

1.2.3 Female mean age at first marriage

		Year	Source
(years)	22.4	1982	(1918)

1.2.4 GNP/capita

		Year	Source
(US $)	290	1987	(1914)

1.2.5 Daily per capita calorie supply

		Year	Source
(as % of requirements)	111	1984-86	(1914)

2. HEALTH SERVICES

2.1 Health expenditure

2.1.1 Expenditure on health

		Year	Source
(as % of GNP)	3.1	1988	(3153)

2.1.2 Expenditure on PHC

		Year	Source
(as % of total health expenditure)	40	1985	(2033)

2.2 Primary Health Care
(Percentage of population covered by):

2.2.1 Health services

National
Urban
Rural

2.2.2 Safe water

		Year	Source
National			
Urban	85	1980-87	(1914)
Rural			

2.2.3 Adequate sanitary facilities

National
Urban
Rural

2.2.4 Contraceptive prevalence rate

		Year	Source
(%)	74	1985	(1913)

2.3   Coverage of maternity care (%)

Area	Prenatal care	Trained attendant	Institutional deliveries	Postnatal care	Sample size	Year	Source
National		94				1986	(2033)
Hebei		30				1980-84	(2000)
Shaanxi		38				1980-84	(2000)
Shandong Province	95		40			1980	(0526)
Shanghai	98		100			1980	(0526)
Shanghai County	97		98			1980	(1829)
Shanghai		98				1980	(2000)

3.   COMMUNITY STUDIES

3.1   Twenty-one provinces, cities and autonomous regions, 1984-1988 (2632, 2642)

This cross-sectional study covered 21 of the total 30 provinces, cities and autonomous regions with a total population of over 177 million, constituting 19.5% of the total population of China.

3.1.1   Rate

	National	Urban	Rural
Live births	15 466 368	–	–
Maternal deaths	7 485	882	6 603
MMR (per 100 000 live births)	48	19	61

By Region

MMR (per 100 000 live births)		MMR (per 100 000 live births)	
Gansu	101	Fujian	49
Shanxi	93	Jiangxi	43
Henan	86	Zhejiang	41
Ningxia	85	Heilongjiang	41
Sichuan	84	Liaoning	39
Hunan	82	Guangdong	36
Yunnan	77	Beijing	35
Shaanxi	73	Jiangsu	32
Hebei	65	Tianjin	32
Hubei	58	Shanghai	24
Neimenggu	52		

3.1.2   Causes of maternal deaths (%)

	National	Urban	Rural
Haemorrhage	47	16	51
Hypertensive disorders of pregnancy	10	15	9
Sepsis	5	3	5
Embolisms	5	11	5
Ectopic pregnancy	1	4	2
Abortion	1	0	1
Other direct obstetrical causes	2	1	2
DIRECT CAUSES	71	52	75
Heart disease	10	15	10
Hepatic diseases	4	11	4
Kidney diseases	1	1	2
Cerebrovascular diseases	1	3	1
Anaemia	1	1	2
Other INDIRECT CAUSES	12	17	6
TOTAL	100	100	100

The ranking of causes of death by order of importance for rural and urban areas was as follows:

	Ranking	
	Urban	Rural
Haemorrhage	1	1
Heart disease	3	2
Hypertensive disorders of pregnancy	2	3
Sepsis	–	4
Amniotic fluid embolism	5	5
Hepatitis	4	6

3.2 30 provinces, 1989 [2780, 3014]

The study described in section 3.1 above, was extended in 1989 to cover all 30 provinces, municipalities and autonomous regions, covering a total population of 100,000,000. The survey found serious underreporting of maternal deaths (34%) and of births (15%).

3.2.1 Rate

	National	Urban	Rural
MMR (per 100 000 live births)	95	50	115

3.2.2 Causes of maternal deaths

	%	MMR (per 100 000 live births)
Haemorrhage	49	36
Hypertensive disorders of pregnancy	10	8
Cardiac diseases	9	7
Sepsis	6	4
Embolisms	5	4
Hepatitis	4	3
Other	17	–

3.2.3 Avoidable factors

Mortality rates were highest among women who had received little or no prenatal care and among those whose first prenatal visit took place later than 28 week's gestation. Women who delivered at home had a threefold risk of death compared with those who delivered at hospital.

	MMR (per 100 000 live births)	Relative risk
Number of prenatal visits		
None	778	35
1-2	199	9
3-4	71	3
5-6	32	1
6+ (6+ = 1)	23	1
Gestation time of first visits		
< 12 weeks (<12 = 1)	27	1
12-27 weeks	54	2
27+ weeks	71	3
Place of delivery		
Provincial hospital (=1)	23	1
County hospital	46	2
Village hospital	47	2
At home	113	5

3.2.4 High risk groups

	MMR (per 100 000 live births)	Relative risk
Age		
15-19	196	4
20-24	64	1
25-29 (= 1)	50	1
30-34	125	3
35-39	360	7
40+	1 028	20
Parity		
Primiparous (= 1)	42	1
Parity 2	82	2
Parity 3	217	5
Parity 4+	634	15
Literacy and educational level		
Illiterate	359	67
Primary level education	124	23
Junior middle school	44	8
Higher middle school	21	4
University (= 1)	5	1
Family monthly income		
<20 yuan	211	5
20-49 yuan	98	3
50-99 yuan	31	1
100+ yuan (= 1)	36	1
Geographic residence		
Mountains	181	4
Plains (= 1)	46	1
Other	61	1

3.3 Meiyun County, 1985-88 [2449, 2640]

A retrospective analysis of maternal deaths was carried out in a rural area. All deaths of women of reproductive age were investigated. Of the total 521 deaths, 33 were found to be maternal deaths, of which 9 had not been reported as such.

3.3.1 Rate

Maternal deaths	33
MMR (per 100 000 live births)	114

3.3.2 Causes of maternal deaths

	Number	%
Haemorrhage	7	21
Sepsis	5	15
Hypertensive disorders of pregnancy	3	9
Ectopic pregnancy	3	9
Cardiac diseases	3	9
Hepatic disease	3	9
Embolism	2	6
Others/unknown	7	21
TOTAL	33	100

3.3.3 Avoidable factors

Avoidable factors were present in 13 cases and a further three cases might have been avoided given improvements in technology and facilities. None of the women who died had had a prenatal examination early in the pregnancy with the result that several anaemic women and some with cardiac diseases remained untreated. The village birth attendants were largely illiterate and untrained. Four women died following sepsis caused by examination or delivery in unsterile conditions; three women died following postpartum haemorrhage as a result of mismanagement of the third stage of labour.

3.4 Jiangsu and Henan provinces, 1988-89 [2641, 2704]

The study was carried out in 25 counties in Jiangsu province and seven counties in Henan province. All maternal deaths were registered and family members interviewed to determine the circumstances of the death. For each maternal death two surviving mothers, in the same locality, of the same parity and similar age group, and with the same obstetrical condition were interviewed. By the end of the study a total of 195 maternal deaths had been registered and another 585 case records were available for comparative analysis.

3.4.1 Rate

	MMR (per 100 000 live births)
Jiangsu	45
Henan	147

3.4.2 Causes of maternal deaths

	Henan No.	Henan %	Jiangsu No.	Jiangsu %
Haemorrhage	66	60	39	46
Sepsis	12	11	3	4
Hypertensive disorders of pregnancy	11	10	9	11
Rupture of the uterus	3	3	0	–
Embolism	1	1	1	1
Ectopic pregnancy	0	–	6	7
DIRECT CAUSES	93	85	58	68
INDIRECT CAUSES	17	15	27	32
TOTAL	110	100	85	100

The comparatively low maternal mortality rate in Jiangsu, together with the higher proportion of deaths due to indirect causes, are indicative of the better quality and availability of obstetric services in the province compared with Henan. Per capita incomes were, on average, higher in Jiangsu.

3.4.3 Avoidable factors

Inadequate facilities at township clinics, village health stations and private doctors resulted in many of the deaths. Few local health care posts had facilities for blood transfusions. Staff were not sufficiently trained to deal with emergencies. Women with complications reporting to the local clinic or health post often faced inordinate delays in being transferred to the hospital, mainly because the staff did not realize the gravity of the situation and take immediate action.

3.4.4 High risk groups

Income

Income below 500 yuan was found to be positively correlated with maternal mortality in both provinces. Income affects both the socioeconomic situation of the families and also the nutritional status of the mother. Controlling for income levels, there was no statistically significant difference in the mortality rates for the two provinces. The authors suggest that women from low income families should be classified prenatally as high risk cases and treated accordingly.

Educational level

In both provinces, illiterate women were at greater risk of maternal death but there was evidence that widespread dissemination of health messages could offset lack of education to some extent. Knowledge of a minimum of three health messages on the part of either husband or wife, but particularly husband, was found to be positively correlated with use of prenatal care services and delivery in county hospitals.

History of previous abortion

Women with an unplanned pregnancy and/or a history of abortion were at greater risk of death.

Prenatal care

Women who had prenatal care at the county hospitals were at lower risk than those who received it from private doctors. Women from families which had some information about the importance of prenatal care were less likely to die than those who knew little or nothing. This was true even when controlling for illiteracy. It is suggested that efforts be directed to disseminating health messages through the media, in particular, radio and television.

Institutional delivery

The highest risk of maternal death was for delivery at home with untrained birth attendants. Delivery in county hospitals carried the lowest risk of maternal death whereas women who delivered at private clinics were more likely to succumb to serious complications. It was found that private doctors were sometimes unable to treat life threatening emergencies such as retained placenta and were liable to make incorrect diagnoses of a variety of obstetric complications. Township and private clinics had no blood transfusion facilities and the staff were frequently inadequately trained. In particular it was noted that they lacked the skills to prevent and manage postpartum haemorrhage, to check blood types and to organize local "walking blood banks".

3.4.5 Other findings

In both provinces, although around 70% of the villages had telephones in working order, only approximately 12% of both maternal death cases and controls availed themselves of the telephone in an emergency. The main reasons given were that the room containing the telephone was locked and that people were unable or unwilling to use the system due to lack of familiarity.

4. HOSPITAL STUDIES

4.1 Beijing urban districts, institutional deliveries, 1959-83 [1675, 2632]

4.1.1 Rate

	Live Births	Maternal deaths	MMR (per 100 000 births)
1959-63	347 687	68	20
1964-68	163 175	35	21
1969-73*	127 605	46	36
1974-78*	80 323	38	47
1979-83	217 884	46	21

* During the "cultural revolution" (1969-78) many midwifery schools were closed, the health services network was severely disrupted, fewer deliveries occurred in institutional settings and there was an increase in maternal deaths.

4.1.2 Causes of maternal deaths

	1959-63		1979-83	
	No.	%	No.	%
Cardiac diseases	10	15	12	26
Embolisms	3	4	8	17
Hypertensive disorders of pregnancy	8	12	7	15
Hepatitis	2	3	6	13
Sepsis	0	0	2	4
Ectopic pregnancy	0	0	1	2
Abortion	1	2	0	0
Haemorrhage	23	34	0	0
Ruptured uterus	8	12	0	0
Operative injury	0	0	0	0
Anaemia	2	3	0	0
Others	11	16	10	22
Total	68	100	46	100

Ranking of different causes, 1959-63 and 1979-83

	Rank	
	1959-63	1979-83
Haemorrhage	1	–
Cardiac diseases	2	1
Hypertensive disorders of pregnancy	3	3
Embolisms	4	2
Hepatitis	5	4
Abortion	6	–
Sepsis	–	5

4.2 Shanghai International Peace Hospital, 1962-71 [0835]

4.2.1 Rate

Deliveries	46 000
Maternal deaths	5
MMR (per 100 000 deliveries)	11

5. CIVIL REGISTRATION DATA/GOVERNMENT ESTIMATES

5.1 National, 1982 [0837]

5.1.1 Rate

According to a communication from the Ministry of Public Health, the maternal mortality rate for China was 50 per 100 000 live births in 1982.

5.2 Selected urban areas, 1975, 1980, 1982 [1361]

5.2.1 Rate

Area	MMR (per 100 000 live births)		
URBAN	1975	1980	1982
Beijing	28	13	22
Shanghai	8	11	10
Tienjin	26	13	18

5.3 Shanghai, 1978-87 [1094, 2005]

5.3.1 Rate

	Live births	Maternal deaths	MMR (per 100 000 live births)		
			Urban	Rural	Total
1978	138 586	37	30	23	27
1979	151 292	43	30	27	28
1980	142 402	43	26	35	30
1981	190 791	43	25	20	23
1982	221 117	58	26	26	26
1983	190 403	47	28	19	25
1984	167 051	30	13	22	18
1985	156 551	46	28	33	29
1986	184 211	38	22	18	21
1987	189 828	53	27	29	27

5.3.2 Causes of maternal deaths, 1975-84 and 1985-87

	1975-84		1985-87	
	Number	%	Number	%
Haemorrhage	96	25	16	12
Ectopic pregnancy	11	3	12	9
Sepsis	15	4	9	7
Embolisms	46	12	10	7
Hypertensive disorders of pregnancy	50	13	6	4
Uterine rupture	8	2	1	1
DIRECT CAUSES	226	58	54	39
Cardiac diseases	47	12	18	13
Hepatitis	43	11	12	9
Anaemia	5	1	2	1
Other infections	13	3	4	3
Other	56	14	47	34
INDIRECT CAUSES	164	42	83	61
TOTAL	390	100	137	100

5.4 Province of Taiwan, 1970-80 [0144]

5.4.1 Rate

	MMR (per 100 000 live births)
1970	40
1971	40
1972	35
1973	40
1974	32
1975	25
1976	30
1977	30
1978	23
1979	17
1980	19

5.5 Province of Taiwan, 1981-84 [1473]

5.5.1 Rate

Live births	1 569 697
Maternal deaths	259
MMR (per 100 000 live births)	17

5.5.2 Causes of maternal deaths

	Number	%
Haemorrhage	102	39
Hypertensive disorders of pregnancy	51	20
Embolisms	35	14
Ectopic pregnancy	16	6
Abortions	13	6
Obstetrical trauma	9	3
Sepsis	6	2
Obstructed labour	6	2
Complications of anaesthesia	2	1
Others	20	8
Total	259	100

6. OTHER SOURCES/ ESTIMATES

6.1 Selected rural areas, 1975, 1980, and 1982 [1361]

6.1.1 Rate

Data were obtained from counties participating in the first World Bank health project.

	MMR (per 100 000 live births)		
	1975	1980	1982
Heilongjiang (10 counties)	45	42	25
Shangdong (15 counties)	41	37	28
Sichuan (16 counties)	51	64	39
Ningxia (5 counties)	117	92	86

7. SELECTED ANNOTATED BIBLIOGRAPHY

Hua Jiazhen, *Epidemiology of pregnancy induced hypertension in China.* (unpublished reports). PIH Research Cooperation Groups, 1988 and 1990. WHE 2801 and WHE 2705

Over the period 1984-1986 a prospective study was undertaken in 21 provinces and cities with a total population of over 2 million women. The incidence of pregnancy-induced hypertension (PIH), its causes and maternal and fetal outcomes were examined in 48,472 pregnant women. The incidence of PIH was 10.4%, of preeclampsia 1.8% and of eclampsia 0.2%. Regional differences were pronounced. In general, the incidence was higher in urban areas (11.3%) than in rural areas (4.5%). There were five maternal deaths of which three were due to hypertensive disorders of pregnancy. Among women with PIH the rates of caesarean and operative delivery were higher than among women with no PIH.

In 1988 the study was expanded to cover all provinces except Tibet and Province of Taiwan There were 67,813 pregnant women and the incidence of pregnancy induced hypertension (PIH) was 9.4%. The incidence of preeclampsia and of eclampsia was the same as in the earlier survey. There were three deaths, one from preeclampsia and two from eclampsia. The mortality rate in rural areas was 179 per 100,000 live births compared with 26 per 100,000 in urban areas. Among the women with PIH there was a statistically significant higher rate of caesarean delivery, operative vaginal delivery, postpartum hypertension and premature placental separation. The incidence of PIH was found to be higher in hot, humid zones as well as in cold areas where household heating was inadequate.

World Health Organization. International Collaborative Study of Hypertensive Disorders of Pregnancy. Geographic variation in the incidence of hypertension in pregnancy *American Journal of Obstetrics and Gynecology,* 1988; 158(1): 80-83. WHE 2552.

Prospectively collected information on blood pressure and proteinuria was available for 4 723 primigravidas in part of the city of Shanghai. Clinical diagnosis of hypertensive disorders of pregnancy was made in 31% of the women and proteinuric preeclampsia occurred in 8.3% but only 0.17% developed eclampsia. There were marked differences in the incidence of hypertensive disorders and eclampsia in the different countries participating in the study, Burma, China, Thailand and Viet Nam but there is no satisfactory explanation for these variations (see relevant country profiles).

8. FURTHER READING

Arnold, F. and Liu Zhaoxiang. Son preference, fertility and family planning in China. *Population and Development Review,* 1986; 12(2): 221-246. WHE 1470

Chinese Medical Association. Medical progress in China. *Chinese Medical Journal,* 1989; 102(6): 407-410. WHE 2596

Hull, T.H. Recent trends in sex ratios at birth in China. *Population and Development Review,* 1990; 16(1): 63-83. WHE 2683

Li Bo-Ying et al. Outcomes of pregnancy in Hong-qiao and Qi-yi communes. *American Journal of Public Health,* 1982; 72(suppl.): 30-32. WHE 1846

Sun, T.H. et al. Trends in fertility, family size preference and family planning practice: Taiwan, 1961-76. *Studies in Family Planning,* 1978; 9(4): 54-70. WHE 1740

Yan, R.Y. How Chinese clinicians contribute to the improvement of maternity care. *International Journal of Gynecology and Obstetrics,* 1989; 30: 23-26. WHE 2703

Zhang, N. Maternity care in China. *Midwives' Chronicle and Nursing Notes,* 1988, 100-101. WHE 2066

Zhang, L. and Ding, H. Analysis of the causes of maternal death in China. *Bulletin of the World Health Organization,* 1988; 66(3): 387-389. WHE 1419

9. DATA SOURCES

WHE 0144   China, Directorate General of Budget, Accounting and Statistics. *Social indicators of the Republic of China, 1981.* 1982.

WHE 0526   Perera, T. *Maternal and child health and family planning in the People's Republic of China.* World Health Organization, New Delhi, 1981.

WHE 0835   Wray, J.D. Child care in the People's Republic of China – 1973. Part II. *Pediatrics,* 1975; 55(5): 723-734.

WHE 0837   Xu, S. *Personal communication,* 1983.

WHE 1094   Chen, Ru-Jun. *Maternal mortality in Shanghai.* Paper presented to the Interregional Meeting on Prevention of Maternal Mortality, WHO doc. no. FHE/PMM/85.9.2, Geneva, 15-20 November 1985.

WHE 1361   Young, M.E. and Prost, A. Child health in China. *World Bank Staff Working Papers,* No. 767, Washington, 1985.

WHE 1473   China, Department of Health. Maternal mortality in the Taiwan area. *Epidemiology Bulletin,* 1986; 2(9): 73-76.

WHE 1675   Woman's Care Institution, The analysis of the maternal mortality in Beijing Urban Districts from 1959 to 1983. *Beijing Medicine,* 1985; 8(2).

WHE 1829   Xing-Juan, H. and Bao-Juan, Z. Women's health care. *American Journal of Public Health,* 1982; 72(suppl.): 33-35.

WHE 1913   United Nations. Department of International Economic and Social Affairs. *World Population Policies.* New York, 1987.

WHE 1914   United Nations Children's Fund (UNICEF). *The state of the world's children,* Oxford, Oxford University Press, various years.

WHE 1915   United Nations. Department of International Economic and Social Affairs. *World population prospects: estimates and projections,* Population Studies, New York, various years.

WHE 1918   United Nations. Department of International Economic and Social Affairs. *First marriage: patterns and determinants.* New York, 1988.

WHE 2000   Yimin, S. Selected findings from recent fertility surveys in three regions of China. *International Family Planning Perspectives,* 1987; 13(3): 80-85.

WHE 2005   Chen, Ru-Jun. *Maternal mortality in Shanghai, China – 1975-87.* (unpublished), 1988.

WHE 2033   World Health Organization. *Global strategy for health for all by the year 2000. Second report on monitoring progress.* WHO document EB83/2 Add. 1, 1988.

WHE 2449   Zhengxuan, X. *Work report of the first period of investigation and reduction of maternal mortality to ensure safe motherhood in Meiyun County of Beijing.* (unpublished), 1989.

WHE 2632   Yan, Ren-Ying. Maternal mortality in China. *World Health Forum,* 1989; 10: 327-330.

WHE 2640   Zhengxuan, X. *Analysis of maternal mortality of 1985 to 1988 in Meiyun County after case audit.* (unpublished), 1990.

WHE 2641   Yan, Ren-Ying *An analysis of social factors which may influence maternal mortality in rural areas of China – a case-control study of maternal mortality in Henan and Jiangsu provinces.* (unpublished), 1990.

WHE 2642   Zhang, Lin Mei, *Analysis of cause and rate of maternal death in pilot areas of 21 provinces, municipalities and autonomous regions of China.* (unpublished), 1989.

WHE 2704   Yan, Ren-Ying *Study on the social risk factors influencing maternal mortality in rural China,* (personal communication), 1989.

WHE 2780   Wenzhen, Chen, *WHO Collaborating Center for Research and Training on Perinatal Care. Annual report 1990.* (unpublished) Beijing, 1990.

WHE 3014   Zhang Lingmei, *Analysis of surveillance results on maternal death in 30 provinces, municipalities and autonomous regions of China,* (unpublished) Beijing Municipal Health Institute, Beijing, 1991.

WHE 3153   World Health Organization. Western Pacific Regional Office. *Country data sheets.* (unpublished), 1991.

DEMOCRATIC PEOPLE'S REPUBLIC OF KOREA

		Year	Source
1. BASIC INDICATORS			

1.1 Demographic

1.1.1 Population

		Year	Source
Size (millions)	22.9	1990	(1915)
Rate of growth (%)	2.4	1985-90	(1915)

1.1.2 Life expectancy

Females	73	1985-90	(1915)
Males	66	1985-90	(1915)

1.1.3 Fertility

Crude Birth Rate	29	1985-90	(1915)
Total Fertility Rate	3.6	1985-90	(1915)

1.1.4 Mortality

Crude Death Rate	5	1985-90	(1915)
Infant Mortality Rate	24	1985-90	(1915)
Female			
Male			
1-4 years mortality rate			
Female			
Male			

1.2 Social and economic

1.2.1 Adult literacy rate (%)
Female
Male

1.2.2 Primary school enrolment rate (%)
Female
Male

1.2.3 Female mean age at first marriage
(years)

		Year	Source

1.2.4 GNP/capita
(US $)

1.2.5 Daily per capita calorie supply

(as % of requirements)	135	1984-86	(1914)

2. HEALTH SERVICES

2.1 Health Expenditure

2.1 Expenditure on health
(as % of GNP)

2.1.2 Expenditure on PHC
(as % of total health expenditure)

2.2 Primary Health Care
(Percentage of population covered by):

2.2.1 Health services

National	100	1987	(2033)
Urban			
Rural			

2.2.2 Safe Water

National	100	1987	(2033)
Urban	100	1987	(2033)
Rural	100	1987	(2033)

2.2.3 Adequate sanitary facilities

National	100	1987	(2033)
Urban	100	1987	(2033)
Rural	100	1987	(2033)

2.2.4 Contraceptive prevalence rate
(%)

2.3   Coverage of maternity care (%)

Area	Prenatal care	Trained attendant	Institutional deliveries	Postnatal care	Sample size	Year	Source
National	78	65				1983	(1488)
National	100	100				1987	(2033)

3. COMMUNITY STUDIES

4. HOSPITAL STUDIES

5. CIVIL REGISTRATION DATA/GOVERNMENT ESTIMATES

6. OTHER SOURCES/ ESTIMATES

7. SELECTED ANNOTATED BIBLIOGRAPHY

8. FURTHER READING

9. DATA SOURCES

WHE 1488   World Health Organization. Regional Office for the Western Pacific. *Evaluation of the strategy for health for all by the year 2000*, Seventh report on the world health situation. Manila, 1980.

WHE 1914   United Nations Children's Fund (UNICEF). *The state of the world's children*, Oxford, Oxford University Press, various years.

WHE 1915   United Nations. Department of International Economic and Social Affairs. *World population prospects: estimates and projections*, Population Studies, New York, various years.

WHE 2033   World Health Organization. *Global strategy for health for all by the year 2000. Second report on monitoring progress.* WHO document EB83/2 Add. 1, 1988.

EAST TIMOR

		Year	Source

1. BASIC INDICATORS

1.1 Demographic

1.1.1 Population

		Year	Source
Size (millions)	0.7	1990	(1915)
Rate of growth (%)	2.2	1985-90	(1915)

1.1.2 Life expectancy

		Year	Source
Female	43	1985-90	(1915)
Male	42	1985-90	(1915)

1.1.3 Fertility

		Year	Source
Crude Birth Rate	44	1985-90	(1915)
Total Fertility Rate	5.4	1985-90	(1915)

1.1.4 Mortality

		Year	Source
Crude Death Rate	22	1985-90	(1915)
Infant Mortality Rate	166	1985-90	(1915)
Female			
Male			
1-4 years mortality rate			
Female			
Male			

1.2 Social and economic

1.2.1 Adult literacy rate (%)
Female
Male

1.2.2 Primary school enrolment rate (%)
Female
Male

1.2.3 Female mean age at first marriage
(years)

1.2.4 GNP/capita
(US $)

1.2.5 Daily per capita calorie supply
(as % of requirements)

2. HEALTH SERVICES

2.1 Health Expenditure

2.1.1 Expenditure on health
(as % of GNP)

2.1.2 Expenditure on PHC
(as % of total health expenditure)

2.2 Primary Health Care
(Percentage of population covered by):

2.2.1 Health services
National
Urban
Rural

2.2.2 Safe Water
National
Urban
Rural

2.2.3 Adequate sanitary facilities
National
Urban
Rural

2.2.4 Contraceptive prevalence rate
(%)

2.3   Coverage of maternity care (%)

Area	Prenatal care	Trained attendant	Institutional deliveries	Postnatal care	Sample size	Year	Source
	–	–	–	–	–	–	–

3. COMMUNITY STUDIES

4. HOSPITAL STUDIES

5. CIVIL REGISTRATION DATA/GOVERNMENT ESTIMATES

6. OTHER SOURCES/ ESTIMATES

7. SELECTED ANNOTATED BIBLIOGRAPHY

8. FURTHER READING

9. DATA SOURCES

WHE 1915 United Nations. Department of International Economic and Social Affairs. *World population prospects: estimates and projections*, Population Studies, New York, various years.

HONG KONG

		Year	Source

1. BASIC INDICATORS

1.1 Demographic

1.1.1 Population

		Year	Source
Size (millions)	5.8	1990	(1915)
Rate of growth (%)	1.4	1985-90	(1915)

1.1.2 Life expectancy

Female	79	195-905	(1915)
Male	73	1985-90	(1915)

1.1.3 Fertility

Crude Birth Rate	16	1985-90	(1915)
Total Fertility Rate	1.7	1985-90	(1915)

1.1.4 Mortality

Crude Death Rate	5.8	1985-90	(1915)
Infant Mortality Rate	8	1985-90	(1915)
Female	9	1981	(1917)
Male	11	1981	(1917)
1-4 years mortality rate			
Female	0.6	1981	(1917)
Male	0.6	1981	(1917)

1.2 Social and economic

1.2.1 Adult literacy rate (%)

Female	81	1985	(1914)
Male	95	1985	(1914)

1.2.2 Primary school enrolment rate (%)

Female	105	1986-88	(1914)
Male	106	1986-88	(1914)

1.2.3 Female mean age at first marriage

(years)	25.3	1981	(1918)

		Year	Source

1.2.4 GNP/capita

(US $)	8 070	1987	(1914)

1.2.5 Daily per capita calorie supply

(as % of requirements)	121	1984-86	(1914)

2. HEALTH SERVICES

2.1 Health expenditure

2.1.1 Expenditure on health

(as % of GNP)	3.7	1983	(1488)

2.1.2 Expenditure on PHC

(as % of total health expenditure)	7.2	1983	(1488)

2.2 Primary Health Care
(Percentage of population covered by):

2.2.1 Health services
National
Urban
Rural

2.2.2 Safe water
National
Urban
Rural

2.2.3 Adequate sanitary facilities
National
Urban
Rural

2.2.4 Contraceptive prevalence rate

(%)	73	1984	(1712)

2.3   Coverage of maternity care (%)

Area	Prenatal care	Trained attendant	Institutional deliveries	Postnatal care	Sample size	Year	Source
National	99	99				1976-83	(1488)
National		89				1980	(1350)
National		92				1984	(1350)

3.   COMMUNITY STUDIES

4.   HOSPITAL STUDIES

4.1   Tsan Yuk Hospital, 1945-83 [1481]

4.1.1   Rate

	Births	Maternal deaths	MMR (per 100 000 deliveries)
1945-83	235 319	118	50
1945-54	–	–	89
1975-83	–	–	10

4.1.2   Causes of maternal deaths.

	No.	%
Hypertensive disorders of pregnancy	34	28
Haemorrhage	23	19
Sepsis	9	8
Embolisms	6	5
Complications of anaesthesia	2	2
DIRECT CAUSES	74	63
Cardiac diseases	17	14
Hepatitis	6	5
Anaemia	2	2
Malaria	1	1
Other infections	2	2
Others	16	14
INDIRECT CAUSES	44	37
TOTAL	118	100

Hypertensive disorders of pregnancy, haemorrhage and infection were the most important causes of death between 1945 and 1964. There were no deaths from these causes after 1975. Of the three direct obstetric deaths which occurred after 1975, two were from amniotic fluid embolism and one from mismatched blood transfusion.

4.1.3   Avoidable factors

4.1.4   High risk groups

	Maternal deaths	MMR (per 100 000 births)
Age		
<20	1	11
20-29	12	14
30-39	18	52
>40	7	173
Parity		
0	38	41
1-4	53	37
5+	27	82

5.   CIVIL REGISTRATION DATA/GOVERNMENT ESTIMATES

5.1   National, 1975-87 [0753, 0834, 1350, 2722]

5.1.1   Rate

Year	Live births	Maternal deaths	MMR (per 100 000 live births)
1975	78 200	2	3
1976	76 342	14	18
1977	78 807	13	16
1978	79 173	5	6
1979	82 157	7	8
1980	85 406	4	5
1981	87 104	7	8
1982	86 036	1	1
1983	82 015	6	7
1984	77 635	5	6
1985	–	–	5
1986	–	–	3
1987	–	–	4

5.2 National, 1961-85 [2099]

5.2.1 Rate

	Total births	Maternal deaths	MMR (per 100 000 live births)
1961-65	546 672	214	39
1981-85	409 508	23	6

5.2.2 Causes of maternal deaths

	1961-65 No.	1961-65 %	1981-85 No.	1981-85 %
Haemorrhage	77	36	8	35
Hypertensive disorders of pregnancy	49	23	5	22
Ectopic pregnancy	20	9	4	17
Sepsis	9	4	0	–
Other	59	28	6	26
Total	214	100	23	100

6. OTHER SOURCES/ ESTIMATES

7. SELECTED ANNOTATED BIBLIOGRAPHY

8. FURTHER READING

9. DATA SOURCES

WHE 0753   United Nations, *Demographic Yearbook.* New York, various years.

WHE 0834   World Health Organization *World Health Statistics annual – vital statistics and causes of death.* Geneva, various years.

WHE 1350   Hong Kong, Ministry of Health. Statistical data, (unpublished), 1984.

WHE 1481   Yam, A. et al. Maternal mortality yet to be minimized. *Asia-Oceania Journal of Obstetrics and Gynaecology,* 1986; 12(1): 79-87.

WHE 1488   World Health Organization. Western Pacific Regional Office. *Evaluation of the strategy for health for all by the year 2000.* Seventh report of the world health situation, 1980.

WHE 1712   Mauldin W.P. and Segal, S.J., *Prevalence of contraceptive use in developing countries. A chart book.* Rockefeller Foundation, New York, 1986.

WHE 1914   United Nations Children's Fund (UNICEF). *The state of the world's children,* Oxford, Oxford University Press, various years.

WHE 1915   United Nations. Department of International Economic and Social Affairs. *World population prospects: estimates and projections,* Population Studies, various years, New York, 1986.

WHE 1917   United Nations. Department of International Economic and Social Affairs. *Age structure of mortality in developing countries. A database for cross-sectional and time-series research.* New York, 1986.

WHE 1918   United Nations. Department of International Economic and Social Affairs. *First marriage: patterns and determinants.* New York, 1988.

WHE 2099   Duthie, S.J. and Ghosh, H.K. Maternal mortality in Hong Kong 1961-85. *British Journal of Obstetrics and Gynaecology,* 1989; 96: 4-8.

WHE 2722   World Health Organization, Maternal deaths and mortality rates (unpublished) 1990.

NOTES

INDIA

		Year	Source

1. BASIC INDICATORS

1.1 Demographic

1.1.1 Population

Size (millions)	853.3	1990	(1915)
Rate of growth (%)	2.1	1985-90	(1915)

1.1.2 Life expectancy

Female	58	1985-90	(1915)
Male	58	1985-90	(1915)

1.1.3 Fertility

Crude Birth Rate	32	1985-90	(1915)
Total Fertility Rate	4.3	1985-90	(1915)

1.1.4 Mortality

Crude Death Rate	11	1985-90	(1915)
Infant Mortality Rate	99	1985-90	(1915)
Female	97	1986	(2430)
Male	96	1986	(2430)
1-4 years mortality rate			
Female	29	1971-76	(1917)
Male	25	1971-76	(1917)

1.2 Social and economic

1.2.1 Adult literacy rate (%)

Female	29	1985	(1914)
Male	57	1985	(1914)

1.2.2 Primary school enrolment rate (%)

Female	81	1986-88	(1914)
Male	113	1986-88	(1914)

1.2.3 Female mean age at first marriage

(years)	18.7	1981	(1918)

1.2.4 GNP/capita

(US $)	300	1987	(1914)

1.2.5 Daily per capita calorie supply

(as % of requirements)	100	1984-86	(1914)

2. HEALTH SERVICES

2.1 Health expenditure

2.1.1 Expenditure on health

(as % of GNP)	3.1	1986-87	(2033)

2.1.2 Expenditure on PHC

(as % of total health expenditure)	30	1985-86	(2033)

2.2 Primary Health Care
(Percentage of population covered by):

2.2.1 Health services

National	100	1987	(2033)
Urban			
Rural			

2.2.2 Safe water

National	81	1987	(2033)
Urban	79	1987	(2033)
Rural	85	1987	(2033)

2.2.3 Adequate sanitary facilities

National	8	1983	(0834)
Urban	40	1987	(2033)
Rural	4	1987	(2033)

2.2.4 Contraceptive prevalence rate

(%)	34	1982	(1712)

2.3   Coverage of maternity care (%)

Area	Prenatal care	Trained attendant	Institutional deliveries	Postnatal care	Sample size	Year	Source
National			10-15			1981	(0917)
National	45	33				1983	(0834)
National	40-50	30-35				1985	(0486)
National:							
rural			13			(1988)	(2430)
urban			45			(1988)	(2430)
3 rural areas	12		2		4 389	1981-85	(1375)
3 urban areas		80		15	3 197	1981-85	(1375)
Gujarat:							
rural		39			2 056	(1982)	(0813)
Maharashtra:							
rural		43			2 141	(1982)	(0813)
Orissa:							
rural		25			2 090	(1982)	(0813)
Pachod:							
rural	78					1987-88	(2732)
Uttar Pradesh:							
rural		13			2 279	(1982)	(0813)
West Bengal:							
rural		24			2 101	(1982)	(0813)

3.   COMMUNITY STUDIES

3.1   Baskripalnagar village, Alwar, Rajasthan, 1974-79 [(0256)]

3.1.1   Rate

A longitudinal morbidity survey was carried out in the village of Baskripalnagar (population about 3 000). A total of 281 women had 349 pregnancies which were followed up. There were two maternal deaths, both from postpartum haemorrhage.

Live births	338
Maternal deaths	2
MMR (per 100 000 pregnancies)	592

3.2   Sirur, Maharashtra, 1981-84 [(1981)]

A study on the risk approach in MCH care was carried out in a rural area, total population around 48 000. Community health workers were trained to register pregnant women, make regular home visits during the pregnancy, identify pregnancies at high risk of complications and carry out preliminary examinations of the newborns. In order to foster community participation, local leaders, traditional birth attendants and general practitioners were also involved and the principles of child care were discussed with women's groups throughout the area.

3.2.1 Rate

Births	5 919
Maternal deaths	15
MMR (per 100 000 live births)	253

Of the 15 deaths, eleven occurred in the 1 107 women who had been classified as high risk, a mortality rate of 994 per 100 000 deliveries. Among the 4 887 women who were described as low risk there were 4 maternal deaths, a mortality rate of 82 per 100 000.

3.2.2 Causes of maternal deaths

	Number
Sepsis	3
Haemorrhage	3
Hypertensive disorders of pregnancy	2
Other direct causes	1
Hepatitis	3
Thrombosis	2
Unknown	1
TOTAL	15

3.2.3 Avoidable factors

3.2.4 High risk groups

	Deliveries	Maternal deaths	MMR (per 100 000 deliveries)
Age			
<20 years	598	2	334
20-29	4 382	9	205
30+	1 014	4	395
Parity			
0	1 727	5	290
1-4	3 990	9	226
5+	277	1	361

3.2.5 Other findings

Fate of the child

Of the pregnancies that resulted in a maternal death, there were six perinatal deaths, five neonatal deaths and one infant death during the post neonatal period. Only six children survived following the death of the mother. The perinatal and neonatal death rates were 10 times higher than the rates observed among children of mothers who survived.

3.3 Urban slums in Madras, Delhi and Calcutta and rural areas near Chandigarh, Varanasi and Hyderabad, 1981-85 [1375]

This was a community based study carried out between 1981 and 1985 under the auspices of the Indian Council for Medical Research. Each area comprised a population of around 30 000. (No maternal deaths were reported from Hyderabad).

3.3.1 Rate

	Deliveries	Maternal deaths	MMR (per 100 000 deliveries)
Urban			
Calcutta	886	1	120
Delhi	1 082	5	460
Madras	881	4	450
Rural			
Chandigarh	1 338	2	150
Varanasi	1 306	7	530

3.4 Anantapur district, Andhra Pradesh, 1984-85 [1259]

This was a case-control study carried out with the objective of identifying maternal deaths, investigating their causes and determining the characteristics of cases of maternal mortality (i.e. how women who died differed from those who survived). The study covered both the rural and urban areas of the district.

Information on maternal deaths was collected from the fifteen hospitals in the district, and from death certificates obtained from civil registration authorities. For information from the rural areas, the study team visited each of the 22 Primary Health Centres (PHCs) in the district and interviewed the staff. A sample of 50% of the sub-centres under each PHC was visited by the study team which examined the records maintained and interviewed the staff in order to identify additional deaths. All the villages and hamlets covered by the sub-centres were also visited, and information on deaths to women in the reproductive age-group was obtained through interviews with key informants. The field interviewers visited the village school and made enquiries of the children, and this proved to be a very useful source of information. All cases of death identified were followed up, and data collected in detail. The control cases were randomly selected from among women who gave birth during the reference period and survived.

3.4.1 Rate

Location	Live births *	Maternal deaths *	MMR (per 100 000 live births)	MMR (per 100 000 women aged 15-49 years)
Urban	10 650	58	545	41
Rural	84 924	705	830	142
Both	95 574	763	798	120

* Estimates for the district projected from area sample survey results

3.4.2 Causes of maternal deaths *(data for area surveys, 284 deaths)*

Urban/rural

	Rural No.	Rural %	Urban No.	Urban %	Total No.	Total %
Sepsis	65	25	6	27	71	25
Haemorrhage/retained placenta	40	15	3	14	43	15
Abortion	27	10	4	18	31	11
Hypertensive disorders of pregnancy	21	8	5	23	26	9
Ruptured uterus	13	6	2	9	15	5
Other direct causes	4	2	–	0	4	2
DIRECT CAUSES	170	65	20	91	190	67
Anaemia	24	9	2	9	26	9
Hepatitis	28	11	0	0	28	10
Other infections	31	12	0	0	31	11
Others	9	3	0	0	7	3
INDIRECT CAUSES	92	34	2	9	92	32
TOTAL	262	100	22	100	284	100

Age

	15-19	20-24	25-29	30-34	35-39	40-44	Total
Sepsis	11	28	21	4	7	–	71
Abortion	7	5	6	7	5	1	31
Hypertensive disorders	5	13	3	1	4	–	26
Haemorrhage	4	5	6	4	2	–	21
Other direct causes	8	13	17	2	1	–	41
Infective hepatitis	4	11	7	4	2	–	28
Anaemia	2	7	4	4	6	3	26
Other indirect causes	11	9	8	7	5	–	40
Total	52	91	72	33	32	4	284

Parity

	0	1	2	3	4+	Total
Sepsis	4	27	10	13	17	71
Abortion	8	4	3	5	11	31
Hypertensive disorders	6	9	6	2	3	26
Haemorrhage	4	6	3	2	6	21
Other direct causes	2	19	5	3	12	41
Infective hepatitis	4	10	7	5	2	28
Anaemia	2	7	4	3	10	26
Other indirect causes	2	4	10	5	19	40
Total	32	86	48	38	80	284

3.4.3 Avoidable factors

41% of deaths were considered definitely preventable, 37% possibly preventable and the remaining unavoidable. Control of infection and early transfer of patients to hospital for skilled care were the most important actions which could have prevented maternal deaths.

Action required	Preventable deaths Number	Preventable deaths %
Antibiotic therapy for infection control	44	20
Early transfer to hospital and adequate treatment	42	19
Treatment of anaemia during pregnancy	26	12
Early and adequate prenatal care	18	8
Institutional delivery	18	8
Blood transfusion	18	8
Medical termination of pregnancy	18	8
Control of dehydration	10	3
Treatment of hepatitis	7	3
Early caesarean section	7	3
Tetanus toxoid immunization	6	3
Other	7	3
Total	221	100

3.4.4 High risk groups

Age

	MMR (per 100 000 live births) Rural	Urban	Both
15-19	796	131	539
20-24	826	532	793
25-29	702	222	602
30-34	1 162	696	1 090
35-39	1 327	857	1 285
40-44	361	1 786	436
45-49	271	–	221
Total	830	545	798

	MMR (per 100 000 women aged 15-49 years) Rural	Urban	Both
15-19	104	29	84
20-24	232	75	195
25-29	179	33	150
30-34	163	72	145
35-39	128	30	106
40-44	30	28	30
45-49	7	–	5
Total	142	41	120

3.4.5   Other findings

Comparison of characteristics of maternal deaths and controls in rural areas (262 deaths)

Development status of the village

	Number of villages	Population as % of total	MMR (per 100 000 live births)
Poorly developed	60	1	2 166
Somewhat developed	465	17	1 523
Adequately developed	604	43	803
Highly developed	266	39	516
Total	1 395	100	830

*   Villages were classified according to development status based on the following variables: location of the village; condition of the road to subcentre; condition of the road to PHC; condition of road to nearest town; distance to nearest town; distance to nearest railway station; distance to nearest bus station; existence of educational institutions in the village; electricity in the village; existence of post office in the village.

Socio-economic group

	Maternal deaths		Control cases	
	Number	%	Number	%
Poor	181	69	97	37
Middle	67	26	123	47
High	14	5	42	16
Total	262	100	262	100

Caste

	Maternal deaths		Control cases	
	Number	%	Number	%
Scheduled castes/tribes	63	24	39	15
Non-scheduled castes/tribes	199	76	223	85
Total	262	100	262	100

Literacy

There were twice as many literate women in the control group as among the women who died. The husbands of women who survived also had a higher educational status than husbands of women who died. The differences in both cases were statistically significant.

Prenatal care

Less than one half (46%) of the women who died of maternal causes were registered for prenatal care, and they made on average only 0.33 visits to the health facility for prenatal care. The comparable figures for the control group were 66% and 0.63 visits. The differences are statistically significant.

Special circumstances in rural areas

Place of death

About two-fifths of the deaths (41%) occurred at home and 9% on the way to hospital. The belief that in an emergency pregnant women are able to reach hospitals, even if in a morbid condition, is not supported by this study.

Awareness of seriousness of condition

When family members of the women who died were asked if they were aware of the seriousness of the patient's condition, 22% of the respondents indicated that they were not. Of those who were aware of it the great majority took steps to call a health worker/doctor, or move the patient to a hospital.

Transport

Availability of transportation was an important factor in averting maternal deaths. Of 140 women who were taken to hospital in a serious condition, 96 (69%) were transported by public bus, 27 (19%) by bullock carts, 5 (3%) by manually drawn rickshaws and only 12 were taken to the hospital in a motor driven vehicle or by ambulance. 24 women died on the way to hospital, and another 54 died immediately upon arrival.

Predisposing adverse health conditions

About half (49%) of the women who died had predisposing health conditions such as anaemia or hypertension which complicated the pregnancy, and 58% had had danger signals such as excessive bleeding, high fever and eclamptic fits during pregnancy. The comparable figures for women who survived childbirth were 11% and 8% respectively.

Abortion

27 of the 262 maternal deaths were due to abortions carried out by unqualified persons to terminate unwanted pregnancies. Although abortion has been legalized in India, most rural women were unaware of the fact or else did not know which facilities provided medical termination of pregnancy.

Number of living sons

In India the desire for a male child is well documented. The prestige of a woman depends to a great extent on the number of male children she bears. Couples are reluctant to use family planning methods unless they have at least one living son. It can be assumed that in rural areas, couples who do not have at least one son will not be using contraception. The number of male children can, therefore, be used as a proxy for contraceptive use. Analysis reveals that 55% of the women who died had no living sons compared with 25% of the women who survived childbirth.

No. of living male children	Maternal deaths		Control cases	
	Number	%	Number	%
none	143	55	65	25
1	68	26	118	45
2	36	14	56	21
3	6	2	15	6
4 or more	9	3	8	3
Total	262	100	262	100

3.5 Ambala, North India, 1985-86 [2630]

A community study was carried out in a rural area comprising 774 villages and a total population of around 716,000. Indigenous medical practitioners and traditional birth attendants are available in every village. Peripheral health posts provided by the State Government have auxiliary nurse midwives, in a ratio of one to every 5 000 population. There are five Primary Health Centres and 15 Rural Dispensaries with qualified doctors. Referral services are provided by four Government and two Mission Hospitals situated in towns. There are also a number of private maternity hospitals in the towns.

Fifteen field assistants were trained to assemble data by contacting village leaders, TBAs, health workers and volunteers, village "Chowkidar" (persons responsible for registering births and deaths) and a number of women in each village. Information was sought about the deaths of all women of reproductive age during the previous year. Surviving family members of the deceased were interviewed to determine whether the death occurred during or shortly after a pregnancy. A team of doctors trained in community medicine evaluated the completed questionnaires and identified maternal deaths.

3.5.1 Rate

Live births*	23 910
Maternal deaths	55
MMR (per 100 000 live births)	230

* Estimated on the basis of a birth rate of 33.4 per 1000 population.

The authors suggest that the relatively low mortality rate compared with national figures (400-500 per 100 000 live births) may be due to improvments in socioeconomic conditions, health care infrastructure and maternal and child health care made since 1984.

3.5.2 Causes of maternal deaths

	Number	%
Haemorrhage	10	18
Sepsis	9	16
Abortion	5	9
Obstructed labour	4	7
Hypertensive disorders of pregnancy	3	6
Retained placenta	2	4
Complications of anaesthesia	1	2
INDIRECT CAUSES	34	62
Anaemia	9	16
Stroke	2	4
Tuberculosis	2	4
Gastroenteritis	1	2
Suicide	1	2
Others/unknown	6	11
TOTAL	55	100

3.6 Pachod, Maharashtra, 1977-88 [2732]

A Comprehensive Health and Development Project was started in Pachod in 1977 following a needs assessment study which revealed that maternal health services were the highest priority for the community. The programme provided maternal and neonatal health services through village Dais. The Pachod project currently covers 50 villages with a total population of 50,976 in Paithan Taluka of Aurangabad District in Maharashtra. The health delivery system is based on the interaction of village Health Posts with Dais, Community Health Volunteers and Female Multipurpose Workers who all contact and follow up pregnant women in their areas.

Programme indicators were evaluated in 1987. The authors point out that in view of the difficulties in obtaining information on pregnancies in a rural area, it is likely that many pregnancies were not detected until after the fifth month of gestation and that maternal deaths occurring early in the pregnancy due to abortion, ectopic pregnancy, trophoblastic disease etc. were missed. Moreover, because the numbers are relatively small the decline in maternal mortality rates may not be significant. However, it was felt that the programme had succeeded in ensuring that more women received prenatal care during the latter part of the pregnancy and that there were some real improvements in women's and children's health over the period. The proportion of deliveries by trained Dais increased from 51% to 74% and prenatal care coverage from 58% to 78%.

3.6.1 Rate

	MMR (per 100 000 live births)
1977-78	1 200
1981-82	440
1987-88	210

4. HOSPITAL STUDIES

4.1 41 teaching institutions, 1978-81 [0284, 1098]

4.1.1 Rate

Deliveries	652 859
Maternal deaths	4 707
MMR (per 100 000 live births)	721

The MMR ranged from as low as 55 to as high as 3 245 per 100 000 live births. The high rates were mainly due to the fact that the institutions were referral centres receiving unbooked and emergency obstetric cases, often late in labour. Of 4 703 maternal deaths analysed, only 5% were booked cases; 85% were emergencies of which 15% were admitted in a state of shock.

4.1.2 Causes of maternal deaths *(available for 4 703 cases)*

Abortion accounted for 15% of the total deaths, 80% of the abortion deaths were due to septic illegal abortions and 13% followed legally induced abortions. Despite the availability of broad-spectrum antibiotics, sepsis was still an important cause of maternal deaths, closely followed by haemorrhage. Jaundice, which accounted for between 0.5% and 3% of maternal deaths in Madras and Bombay 50 years earlier, assumed alarming proportions, accounting for many maternal deaths in this series.

	Number	%
Abortion	710	15
Haemorrhage	684	15
Sepsis	658	14
Hypertensive disorders of pregnancy	505	11
Embolisms	275	6
Ruptured uterus	233	5
Ectopic and molar pregnancy	83	2
Complications of anaesthesia	54	1
Obstetric shock	27	1
Obstructed labour	3	0
DIRECT CAUSES	3 232	69
Hepatitis	535	11
Anaemia	347	7
Cardiac diseases	189	4
Malaria, tuberculosis and other infections	183	4
Other indirect causes	217	5
INDIRECT CAUSES	1 471	31
TOTAL	4 703	100

4.1.3 Avoidable factors

Avoidable factors were present in 69% of the deaths.*

	% of deaths
Delay by patients or relatives in seeking medical care	65
Defective obstetric care	47
Poor transportation	12
Inadequate blood transfusion and other facilities	6

*   factors not mutually exclusive

4.2 Eight teaching hospitals, 1978-81 [1098]

4.2.1 Rate

Hospital	MMR (per 100 000 live births)
AFMC, Pune	55
J.J. Hospital, Bombay	366
Women's Hospital, Madras	418
Eden Hospital, Calcutta	969
V.V. Hospital, Bangalore	1 249
AIIMS, New Delhi	1 387
Medical College Hospital, Jaipur	2 308
Medical College Hospital, Tirunelveli	3 245

4.3 Nowrosjee Wadia Maternity Hospital, Bombay, 1929-1983 [2007]

4.3.1 Rate

	Deliveries	Maternal deaths	MMR (per 100 000 live births)
1929-39	47 310	909	1 920
1940-49	90 783	857	940
1950-59	122 135	476	390
1960-69	120 348	355	290
1970-79	72 202	135	190
1980-83	34 912	28	80

4.3.2 Causes of maternal deaths, 1929-69

During the 1970-83 period there were considerable reductions in mortality in cases of placenta praevia, accidental haemorrhage and postpartum haemorrhage as well as in cases of ectopic or molar pregnancy and ruptured uterus. The author asserts that this is due to prompt obstetric intervention and availability of an adequate supply of blood. However, during the period 1970-83 eleven patients succumbed to disseminated intravascular coagulation and hypofibrinogenemia. The majority of these patients were admitted very late and in extremis and died despite administration of fibrinogen, plasma and blood transfusion.

Puerperal sepsis accounted for only 14 deaths during 1970-83, compared with 89 deaths during 1929-39 – a reduction largely accounted for by the use of chemo-therapeutic drugs and powerful antibiotics. However, the injudicious use of such drugs has resulted in drug resistant organisms which may be a factor in some of the cases of mortality in this group. Septic abortion due to induction outside the hospital is also a contributory factor in sepsis deaths.

Deaths due to hypertensive disorders of pregnancy fell from 85 during 1929-39 to 12 during 1970-79 and four during 1980-83. The author estimates that continuing education of women and their relatives in the importance of prenatal care could reduce still further the mortality from hypertensive disorders.

Mortality from indirect obstetric causes has also fallen appreciably since the 1920s. There were 23 maternal deaths due to cardiovascular complications during 1929-39 compared with only two during 1980-83. Deaths due to anaemia fell from 235 during 1929-39 to two during 1980-83. These striking reductions in maternal mortality are due to adequate prenatal supervision, early detection of medical and surgical disorders and regular prenatal checks.

	Number
Haemorrhage	4
Hypertensive disorders of pregnancy	4
Embolisms	4
Associated with caesarean section	4
Complications of anaesthesia	3
Ruptured uterus	3
Sepsis	1
Obstetric shock	1
Ectopic/molar pregnancy	0
DIRECT CAUSES	24
Anaemia	2
Cardiovascular diseases	2
Other indirect causes	1
INDIRECT CAUSES	5
Fortuitous	0
TOTAL	29

4.4 N.R.S. Medical College Hospital, Calcutta, West Bengal, 1956-58 and 1966-68 [0172]

4.4.1 Rate

	1956-58	1966-68
Births	12 857	13 559
Maternal deaths	108	80
MMR (per 100 000 live births)	840	590

4.4.2 Causes of maternal deaths

Haemorrhage, hypertensive disorders of pregnancy, rupture of the uterus and abortion accounted for 83% of all direct obstetric causes in both series. By 1966-68 there had been a significant fall in number and percentage of deaths from hypertensive disorders of pregnancy. However, there was a steep rise in deaths from infective hepatitis. Of the ten eclamptic deaths in 1966-68, seven occurred in women aged below 20 years.

	1956-58		1966-68	
	Number	%	Number	%
Haemorrhage	17	16	22	28
Hypertensive disorders of pregnancy	30	28	10	13
Ruptured uterus	5	5	9	11
Abortions	10	9	7	9
Ectopic/molar pregnancy	0	0	4	5
Sepsis	9	8	3	4
Associated with operative delivery	3	3	3	4
DIRECT CAUSES	74	69	58	73
Anaemia	26	24	10	13
Hepatitis	2	2	8	10
Cardiac diseases	4	4	1	1
Others	2	2	3	4
INDIRECT CAUSES	34	31	22	28
TOTAL	108	100	80	100

4.4.3 Avoidable factors

Avoidable factors were found in 92% of all deaths due to obstetric causes. In half the cases the patient and/or relatives were responsible. Inadequate care by medical staff was responsible in 43% of the cases and lack of hospital facilities in the remaining 7%.

Of the 22 *haemorrhage deaths* 19 were considered avoidable. Except in four cases, all the deaths resulted from deficiencies in the health services. Twelve deaths resulted from failures on the part of medical staff to provide appropriate care: these included refusal of prenatal admission to an anaemic woman (Hb. 46%); allowing prolonged labour; internal podalic version by inexperienced doctors; death as a result of the administration of anaesthesia by a non-anaesthetist; delayed manual removal of placentae; and treatment of retained placenta and placenta praevia in ill-equipped maternity centres. Three deaths were due to inadequate blood supply.

All nine deaths due to *ruptured uterus* were avoidable. Eight women had received no prenatal care. In one case death resulted from a caesarean scar rupture which remained undetected following a forceps delivery.

Delay in seeking medical help and lack of adequate facilities in the hospital contributed to deaths from *abortion*. Seven women died of abortion due to delays in evacuation to a treatment facility and inadequate arrangement for blood transfusion.

Lack of prenatal care contributed to several deaths from *hypertensive disorders of pregnancy* and *anaemia*.

4.5 Eden Hospital, Calcutta, West Bengal, 1962-71 and 1972-74 [0395, 0403, 0615]

4.5.1 Rate

	Deliveries	Maternal deaths	MMR (per 100 000 deliveries)
1962-71	121 056	596	492
1972-74	8 938	76	850

4.5.2 Causes of maternal deaths

During both periods, 21% of all maternal deaths were due to abortion. The causes of death for the 76 maternal deaths in 1972-74 are given below:

	Number	%
Haemorrhage	21	28
Abortion	16	21
Hypertensive disorders of pregnancy	10	13
Associated with caesarean section	9	12
Obstetric shock	4	5
Ectopic /molar pregnancy	2	3
Ruptured uterus	1	1
DIRECT CAUSES	51	67
Anaemia	6	8
Hepatitis	4	5
Other infections	3	4
INDIRECT CAUSES	13	17
TOTAL	76	100

4.5.4 Avoidable factors

4.5.4 High risk groups

4.5.5 Other findings

A study covering the period 1962-71 [0395] surveys abortion mortality and provides a detailed analysis of deaths due to abortion for the years 1969-71. Over the whole period 1962-71, there were 125 abortion deaths in a total of 12 683 abortion cases admitted and treated, a fatality rate of 9.8 per 1 000. The more detailed analysis for 1969-71 shows that most of the abortion deaths (53%) were among women aged 21-30 years and that the majority of the women (56%) were of parity five or higher.

In more than four-fifths of the abortion deaths there was evidence of interference. Sepsis continued to be the major factor in abortion deaths. Of the 45 abortion deaths between 1969-71, 31 were caused by sepsis.

A study on abortions covering the years 1969-73 [0403] found a total of 8 029 abortion admissions and 81 deaths, a fatality rate of 10 per 1 000.

During 1972-74, there were 1 515 medical terminations of pregnancy in Eden Hospital, of which only one resulted in death [0403]. Over the same period, there were 3 319 abortion admissions and 26 deaths. Even assuming that only 50% of these were induced, the great margin of safety in medical terminations is evident.

An analysis of maternal deaths due to haemorrhage in Eden Hospital between 1972 and 1974 [0615] shows a steady increase in both numbers and proportion of deaths due to postpartum haemorrhage and a decline in deaths due to placenta praevia. The latter is thought to be a result of judicious and liberalised use of caesarean section. Three quarters of the deaths due to haemorrhage were in unbooked patients and 40% of the deaths occurred within 24 hours of admission.

4.6 Lady Dufferin Victoria Hospital, Calcutta, 1968-70 [0247]

4.6.1 Rate

Births	17 798
Maternal deaths	59
MMR (per 100 000 live births)	331

4.6.2 Causes of maternal deaths

Anaemia was the major cause of death; in eleven of the twelve deaths the patients had a haemoglobin level below 40% of normal on admission.

	Number	%
Haemorrhage	14	24
Abortion	7	12
Hypertensive disorders of pregnancy	4	7
Ruptured uterus	3	5
Sepsis	2	3
Obstetric shock	2	3
Embolisms	2	3
DIRECT CAUSES	34	58
Anaemia	12	20
Cardiac diseases	5	8
Hepatitis	4	7
Other infections	2	3
Other indirect causes	2	3
INDIRECT CAUSES	25	42
TOTAL	59	100

4.6.3 Avoidable factors

4.6.4 High risk groups

Parity	Deliveries	Maternal deaths	MMR (per 100 000 deliveries)
Primipara	5 235	18	344
2	4 361	8	183
3	3 400	6	176
4	2 395	4	167
5	1 418	5	353
6	989	5	506

Maternal mortality was high in patients from low socioeconomic groups, who had a higher incidence of anaemia mainly caused by parasitic diseases.

4.7 Baroda Medical College, Gujarat, 1967-68 and 1983-84 [2482]

Baroda Medical College and the affiliated Shree Sayajee General Hospital, treat difficult obstetric cases from a catchment area of some 40-60 km. Maternal mortality rates were very high and were accepted as inevitable; as a result few hospital records were kept. In 1965, Baroda Medical College initiated a process of medical audit of maternal and perinatal deaths. The following factors were found to lead to high maternal mortality: failure to supervise junior staff and in particular allowing them to perform obstetric procedures in high risk cases without supervision; failure of consultants to examine patients before prescribing treatment; and neglect of responsibilities during weekends and holidays. The impact of the detailed investigation of each maternal death, regular departmental meetings and discussions, was rapidly reflected in improvements in the quality of care. In 1983-84 it was estimated that errors of judgement by members of the obstetrics department were responsible for 1.5% of the maternal deaths compared with 10% during 1967-68.

4.7.1 Rate

	Deliveries	Maternal deaths	MMR (per 100 000 deliveries)
1967-68	2 968	43	1 449
1983-84	3 125	36	1 152

4.8 R.M.C. Hospital, Imphal, Manipur, 1976-85 [1812]

4.8.1 Rate

Deliveries and abortions	42 614
Maternal deaths	128
MMR (per 100 000 pregnancies)	300

4.8.2 Causes of maternal deaths

	Number	%
Haemorrhage	45	35
Abortions	32	25
Hypertensive disorders of pregnancy	11	9
Sepsis	9	7
Ruptured uterus	9	7
Associated with caesarean section	8	6
Obstetric shock	4	3
Embolisms	3	2
Ectopic pregnancy	1	1
DIRECT CAUSES	122	95
Hepatitis	1	1
Other infections	1	1
Others	4	3
INDIRECT CAUSES	6	5
TOTAL	128	100

4.8.3 Avoidable factors

More than 60% of the deaths were considered to have been avoidable through a combination of improvements in blood bank facilities, use of antibiotic therapy and more adequate supply of emergency medicines. A critical review of all first hour deaths suggested the need for more active and prompt intensive care by experienced obstetricians. In five cases, immediate surgical intervention could have prevented death.

4.8.4 High risk groups

4.8.5 Other findings

4.9 Queen Mary's Hospital, Lucknow, Uttar Pradesh, 1970-73 [0208]

4.9.1 Rate

	Total
Deliveries	12 838
Maternal deaths	150
MMR (per 100 000 deliveries)	1 168

4.9.2 Causes of maternal deaths

Sepsis, both postabortal and postpartum, was the major cause of death. All 17 abortion deaths were from sepsis, the abortions having been illegally induced in all cases. In the postnatal sepsis deaths, twelve cases were unbooked patients who had delivered at home. Anaemia was the second most frequent cause of death. Sixteen of the 24 women who died had been admitted as postnatal cases, with severe anaemia (haemoglobin range of 2 to 4 gms.)

	Number	%
Abortion	17	11
Ruptured uterus	14	9
Embolisms	14	9
Sepsis	13	9
Haemorrhage	13	9
Hypertensive disorders of pregnancy	13	10
Obstetric shock	3	2
Other direct causes	9	6
DIRECT CAUSES	96	64
Anaemia	24	16
Cardiac diseases	10	7
Hepatitis	7	5
Other indirect causes	13	9
INDIRECT CAUSES	54	36
TOTAL	150	100

4.9.3 Avoidable factors

Booking status

	MMR (per 100 000 deliveries)	
	Booked	Unbooked
Deliveries	9 467	3 371
Maternal deaths	3	147
MMR (per 100 000 deliveries)	31	4 360

4.10 Four City Hospitals, Madras, Tamil Nadu, 1974-75 (0605)

4.10.1 Rate

Deliveries	87 438
Maternal deaths	393
MMR (per 100 000 deliveries)	449

The author estimates that over 95% of all deliveries in Madras City are institutional or are carried out under skilled supervision and supported by a good transport and communications system. There were 192 642 births in the city during 1974-75, of which 87 438 (46%) delivered in these four institutions. On the basis of total births the maternal mortality rate was 204 per 100 000 for Madras City as a whole.

4.10.2 Causes of maternal deaths

An epidemic of infective hepatitis was responsible for an appreciable rise in the maternal mortality rate in 1975. Abortion was the third most frequent cause of death after infective hepatitis and haemorrhage. Despite the availability of medical terminations of pregnancy, all 50 abortion deaths in this series were from septic illegally induced abortions.

	Number	%
Haemorrhage	54	14
Abortion	50	13
Ruptured uterus	27	7
Sepsis	26	7
Hypertensive disorders of pregnancy	18	4
Obstructed labour	6	1
Other direct causes	19	5
DIRECT CAUSES	200	51
Hepatitis	66	17
Anaemia	38	10
Cardiac diseases	25	6
Cerebrovascular accidents	22	6
TB and pneumonia	12	3
Other infections	30	8
INDIRECT CAUSES	193	49
TOTAL	393	100

4.10.3 Avoidable factors

Avoidable factors were present in 238 deaths (61%). The patient or her relatives were responsible in almost one third of cases and in about 20%, the physician, midwife or institution was at fault. In 8% of the deaths multiple factors were contributory and in about 10% there was a lack of prompt transport facilities. Most of the deaths occurred among unbooked cases and emergency admissions.

4.11 Government Erskine Hospital, Madurai, Tamil Nadu, 1960-72 (0089, 0577)

4.11.1 Rate

Deliveries	74 384
Maternal deaths	1 245
MMR (per 100 000 deliveries)	1 674

Over the 13-year period it was estimated that there were 321 351 deliveries in the city as a whole. Taking this figure as the denominator gives a maternal mortality rate of 387 per 100 000 live births.

4.11.2 Causes of maternal deaths

The leading cause of death over the period was obstetric haemorrhage (231 cases), followed by rupture of the uterus and hypertensive disorders of pregnancy. The percentage of deaths from hypertensive disorders of pregnancy fell from 21% in 1960-64 to 11% in 1970-72. The proportion of deaths resulting from septic abortions rose from 6% at the beginning of the period to 22% in 1970-72. There was a significant decrease in the number of deaths from haemorrhage over the 13 years but deaths from uterine rupture remained unchanged. A strikingly large number of deaths were from anaemia (108 cases). An epidemic of infectious hepatitis in 1969-70 accounted for 40 of the 60 hepatitis deaths over the entire period.

	Number	%
Haemorrhage	231	19
Ruptured uterus	193	16
Hypertensive disorders of pregnancy	133	10
Abortion	101	8
Obstructed labour	69	6
Sepsis	65	5
Embolisms, complications of anaesthesia, etc.	62	5
DIRECT CAUSES	854	69
Anaemia	108	9
Cerebrovascular accidents	96	8
Hepatitis	60	5
Cardiac diseases	52	4
Tuberculosis, typhoid and pneumonia	28	2
Other infections	28	2
Others	19	1
INDIRECT CAUSES	391	31
TOTAL	1 245	100

4.11.3 Avoidable factors

Avoidable factors were discerned in 83% of maternal deaths. The patients or their relatives were responsible for about half of these, the institution or its staff for about 20%. In one fifth of the deaths poor transport facilities contributed to dangerous delays in starting therapy. The majority of the 204 women who were admitted moribund were cases of uterine rupture or of obstetric haemorrhage and many of these could have been saved if communication and transport facilities had been better. During the last five years of the study avoidable factors occurred principally among parturients brought to the hospital from outside the city. The author suggests that such factors could be eliminated by a concerted effort by the health authorities of the district, by better health education of patients and by the use of mobile obstetric services.

4.11.4 High risk groups

4.11.5 Other findings

A study of cases of septic abortion admitted to the hospital between 1971 and 1973 [0577] found 79 deaths out of 393 cases of septic abortion but only four deaths among the 1 479 medical terminations of pregnancy carried out in the hospital. It was usually the grand multiparae who resorted to illegal abortion to terminate an unwanted pregnancy. 87% of the patients came from families with monthly incomes of 100 rupees or less, which is far below the subsistence level. 62% of them were rural women.

4.12 Cheluvamba Hospital, Mysore, Karnataka, 1967-71 [0522]

4.12.1 Rate

Births	22 887
Maternal deaths	310
MMR (per 100 000 live births)	1 354

4.12.2 Causes of maternal deaths *(available for 307 deaths)*

Anaemia was the most frequent cause of death, claiming 67 lives. In 60% of the women who died, the haemoglobin level ranged from 10-30%, and in the rest, between 30 and 50%.

	Number	%
Abortion	44	14
Obstetric shock	40	13
Hypertensive disorders of pregnancy	30	10
Haemorrhage	26	8
Embolisms	11	4
Ruptured uterus	10	3
Sepsis	9	3
Transfusion reaction	4	1
Complications of anaesthesia	2	1
Other direct causes	3	1
DIRECT CAUSES	179	58
Anaemia	67	22
Hepatitis	8	3
Other infections	6	2
Cardiac diseases	3	1
Central nervous system involvement*	30	10
Others	14	5
INDIRECT CAUSES	128	42
TOTAL	307	100

*   Meningitis, encephalitis, cerebral thrombosis etc.

4.12.3 Avoidable factors

Many patients were admitted moribund and too late to be helped. 32% of the deaths took place within 12 hours of admission and a further 9% between 12 hours and 24 hours of admission. Transportation facilities were inadequate and many patients were brought exsanguinated, dehydrated and highly infected.

4.12.4 High risk groups

4.12.5 Other findings

Anaemia was a contributory factor in many women who died from haemorrhage and sepsis. Parasitic infestation was very common and was an important cause of anaemia alongside poor nutrition.

4.13 JIPMER Rural Health Centre, Pondicherry, 1967 and 1971 [0169]

4.13.1 Rate

	1967	1971
MMR (per 100 000 deliveries)	680	280

4.13.2 Causes of maternal deaths

Abortion [1844]

A study of septic abortion cases at the hospital between 1971 and 1979 found 1,958 cases of septic abortion, constituting 22% of all abortion admissions. There was a case fatality rate of 14.3%. Medical termination of pregnancy became available in 1973; thereafter there were no deaths resulting from this procedure.

5. CIVIL REGISTRATION DATA/GOVERNMENT ESTIMATES

5.1 National, 1976-80 [0175, 0339, 0486, 0914, 0918, 1098, 1109]

5.1.1 Rate

	MMR (per 100 000 live births)
1974-78	500
1976	400-500
1979	700
1980	480
1984	460

For towns with populations of 30 000 and over, the maternal mortality rate in 1976 was 157 per 100 000 live births.

5.1.2 Causes of maternal deaths in several rural areas*

As percentage of all maternal deaths

	1975	1976	1977	1978	1979	1980
Haemorrhage	19	17	21	18	20	16
Abortion	8	12	8	11	12	13
Obstructed labour	9	9	9	10	10	13
Sepsis	20	14	19	12	12	12
Hypertensive disorders of pregnancy	7	10	11	21	16	12
Anaemia	21	22	16	15	15	16
Others	16	16	16	14	15	18
Total	100	100	100	100	100	100
Deaths in sample	164	163	170	137	180	209

* Based on a rural sample, in a survey conducted as part of the Model Registration Scheme.

Distribution by cause and age group, 1980

	Age (years)		
	15-24	25-34	35-44
Sepsis	16	8	15
Abortion	14	8	21
Haemorrhage	14	23	3
Obstructed labour	13	12	21
Hypertensive disorders of pregnancy	13	12	15
Anaemia	14	18	12
Others	18	20	12
Total	100	100	100
Number of deaths in sample	88	86	33

5.2 Greater Bombay City, 1969-80 [0680]

5.2.1 Rate

	MMR (per 100 000 live births)			
	1969	1974	1979	1980
City	600	400	800	500
Suburbs	700	300	600	500
Extended suburbs	600	300	600	300
Greater Bombay	–	–	700	500

6. OTHER SOURCES/ESTIMATES

6.1 National, 1978-80 [0829, 1522]

6.1.1 Rate

A WHO Regional Health Information Bulletin quoted a maternal mortality rate of between 700 per 100 000 live births in urban areas and 1 360 per 100 000 in rural areas, an average of 1 250 per 100 000 for the country as a whole over the period 1978-80.

7. SELECTED ANNOTATED BIBLIOGRAPHY

Bang R. et al. High prevalence of gynaecological diseases in rural Indian women. *Lancet,* January 14 1989; 85-89. WHE 2097

In a community based, cross-sectional study, carried out in two rural villages, 55% of the women had gynaecological complaints and 45% were symptom free. However, 92% of the women were found on examination to have one or more gynaecological or sexually transmitted diseases and the average was 3.6 diseases per woman. Only 8% of the women had undergone gynaecological examination or treatment in the past. Infections constituted half of the morbidities, mainly, vaginitis, cervicitis and pelvic inflammatory disease. Menstrual disorders were also common with genital tract infection a likely contributory cause.

There was a very high prevalence of iron deficiency anaemia (83%) and vitamin A deficiency (58%) due to the poor economic status of the region and of the women in particular. Even symptomless women were very likely to have reproductive tract disease. There was a statistically significant association between certain gynaecological diseases and past or present female contraception but this explains only a small fraction of overall morbidity since 78% of the ever married women had never used such contraception yet had a high prevalence of disease.

Bang A. et al. Commentary on a community based approach to reproductive health care. *International Journal of Gynecology and Obstetrics,* 1989, Suppl. 3: 125-129. WHE 2635

The authors describe a community based approach to comprehensive reproductive care by undertaking participatory research, fostering mass education with the people's involvement, and by making care available through village based female workers and improved referral services. Their approach is based on the findings from their epidemiological study of rural women cited above.

Basu, A.M. Is discrimination in food really necessary for explaining sex differentials in childhood mortality? *Population Studies,* 1989; 43: 193-210. WHE 2315

The author suggests that sex differences in nutrition are not responsible for significant observed differences in childhood mortality and that differential use of health care by the two sexes is probably a more important explanatory factor.

Das B. et al. Caesarian section – present and past. *Journal of the Indian Medical Association,* 1984; 82(8): 276-278. WHE 1819

913 cases of caesarian section (CS) performed in a Calcutta hospital between 1980 and 1981 were analysed. The incidence of CS was 5.4% of all confinements. The most common indications for caesarean section were previous CS (25%), and cephalopelvic disproportion or contracted pelvis (15%). There was one maternal death in 1980 due to intractable haemorrhage.

Deodar, N.S. et al. Maternal health. In: *Health conditions of mothers and children in Sikkim,* All India Institute of Hygiene and Public Health/UNICEF, 1982. WHE 0176

This review of the health conditions of pregnant and nursing mothers examines socioeconomic background, physical growth, haemoglobin levels, leading causes and extent of morbidity, prenatal and maternity care, family planning and utilization of services. 90% of the women were illiterate; 36% had haemoglobin levels of less than 80%; intestinal infections, anaemias, upper respiratory infections, dysentery and diarrhoea, and skin diseases were the commonest conditions. Only 12.7% of women received prenatal care and 95% of deliveries took place at home with the assistance of untrained persons.

Ghose N. and Das B. Treatment of eclampsia. *Journal of the Indian Medical Association,* 1985; 83(9): 299-302. WHE 1815

152 consecutive cases of eclampsia were admitted to a Calcutta hospital between 1976 and 1983 and were treated with intravenous diazepam instead of chlorpromazine hydrochloride and promethazine hydrochloride, the previous hospital regime. There were nine maternal deaths, a case fatality rate of 5.9%. Late admission was the commonest finding in all the fatal cases. Patients for whom treatment could be started early after the onset of convulsions, mostly survived.

Goswami B. et al. A study on caesarian section in a rural hospital. *Journal of the Indian Medical Association,* 1985; 83(12): 404-406. WHE 1816

The incidence of caesarian section in this rural area was low (4.8%) and the indications mainly maternal. About 77% of the patients had no prenatal care and 85% were admitted as emergencies. Obstructed labour was the commonest indication (19.6%) and the perinatal loss was high (17.32%). There were five maternal deaths (1.4%).

Khan M.E. at al. Health practices in Uttar Pradesh: a study of discrimination against women. Working paper No 45. *Studies in Population, Health and Family Planning,* Baroda, 1985. WHE 1126

Daily food intake of pregnant village women in the study was grossly inadequate and they were frequently required to perform strenuous work 13-14 hours a day until labour started. During pregnancy they had almost no medical care. The majority of the women were unaware of preventive measures to be observed during pregnancy or of MCH services provided at the Primary Health Care Centre. The auxiliary nurse-midwife's services were not generally available to the women, she rarely visited the villages and did not see patients with complications. The MCH centre in the study village was closed most of the time.

Jain M. et al. Rupture Uterus. *Journal of the Indian Medical Association,* 1988; 86(11): 297-298. WHE2619

A retrospective study was carried out in the Institute of Medical Sciences, Banares Hindu University, Varansi between 1974 and 1985. There were 188 cases of ruptured uterus, an incidence of 1 in 99 deliveries. Most of the cases were from rural areas, were of low socioeconomic status and were unbooked. There were 18 maternal deaths, a case fatality rate of 9.5%. Four patients developed vesico-vaginal fistulae and 133 women (71%) suffered other morbidities. Only four babies were born alive, two of which died after delivery.

Jejeebhoy, S.J. and Kulkarni, S. Reproductive motivation: a comparison of wives and husbands in Maharashtra, India. *Studies in Family Planning,* 1989; 20(5): 264-272. WHE 2368

Family size preferences, ideal sex compositions and the motivation underlying these preferences between currently married women and their husbands in a transitional rural society are compared. Women's family size preferences are largely shaped by their dependence on sons for old age and other support. Husbands are affected by this consideration but are also influenced by a desire to continue the family line and perform ritual obligations. However, it is primarily the women who feel the constraints imposed on their time, resources, and other opportunities by large numbers of children, which affect their family size preferences negatively. Both spouses are similarly concerned about the health risks to the mother imposed by frequent childbearing.

Mani S.B. A review of midwife training programmes in Tamil Nadu. *Studies in Family Planning,* 1980; 11(12): 395-400. WHE 0434

More than two-thirds of all deliveries in Tamil Nadu are attended by untrained persons, including relatives, friends and traditional birth attendants. Realizing that village TBAs might serve as a key link in the chain of delivery of maternal health services to remote rural populations, a TBA training programme was launched. This report reveals that the training and follow up programmes failed to attract a large number of TBAs for training and active involvement in the promotion of family planning. The reasons cited for this failure include: administrative and communication problems, inadequate supply of materials, poor supervision and follow-up, urban and elite-oriented training syllabus, and inadequate assessment of community needs and of the socio-cultural characteristics of the practicing TBAs and their clients. The author points out that trained TBAs were simply supplied to the communities without educating them about the value of such improved services. The author and medical officers concerned feel that TBAs have an important role to play in MCH/FP activities in rural areas but that their potential has not been properly tapped.

Mehta S. *Study of induced abortion in India.* Doctoral Thesis in Public Health submitted to the School of Hygiene and Public Health of the Johns Hopkins University, Baltimore, 1986. WHE 2546

Abortion has been legally available in certain circumstances since 1972. The study analysed hospital data on 32,227 abortions carried out over a 16 month period in 107 teaching hospitals in four distinct geographic areas. The majority of abortion seekers were married, aged 20-34 and had 2-3 children. Women with no living sons were less likely to seek an abortion. Women under 20, unmarried and socioeconomically disadvantaged, were more likely to delay seeking an abortion until the second trimester of pregnancy. Younger women (under 20) and those pregnant for the first time were at maximum risk of suffering from excessive bleeding and visceral injuries. The risk of developing sepsis was associated with anaemia and with low educational status.

Mitra R. Rupture of uterus. *Journal of Obstetrics and Gynaecology of India,* 1973; 23: 474-79. WHE 1843

106 cases of ruptured uterus were studied between 1961 and 1970. The incidence was 1:319. There were 24 maternal deaths, a case fatality rate of 22.6%. 95% of the cases were emergencies, only 5% were booked. The common aetiological factor was contracted pelvis which was found in 48 (45%) cases. 23 cases were moribund on admission.

Murthy N. Reluctant patients – the women of India. *World Health Forum,* 1982; 3(3): 315-316. WHE 0474

A study conducted by the Indian Institute of Management found that the ratio of men to women seeking medical treatment at a primary health care centre was 5 to 1. The author concludes that women fail to seek medical care for themselves for a variety of behavioural reasons rather than because of faults in the health system. Because of their household responsibilities, and out of ignorance, women tend to neglect their illnesses until they become too sick either to lead their normal lives or to seek medical help. The implications are that Indian women need health care literally on their doorstep. Health workers must identify patients in need, women must be encouraged to seek early help and the health system must be able to handle emergencies in the field.

Sarkar B. Eclampsia in a remote district hospital of Bengal. *Journal of the Indian Medical Association,* 1986; 84(11): 338-340. WHE 1727

255 cases of eclampsia out of 9932 deliveries (an incidence of 2.6%), were studied. The incidence of eclampsia increased in winter. Patients were treated with chlorpromazine, promethazine and pethidine injections supplemented by diazepam drip to control recurrence of fits, and caesarean section in 2.9% of cases. Rates of maternal mortality (19.6%) and perinatal mortality (65.7%) were high. Rural women need to be made aware of the importance of prenatal care and encouraged to use available services. Medical personnel need more training and modern anaesthetic techniques need to be made available in district hospitals.

Shah, K.P. *Enquiry on the epidemiology and surgical repair of obstetric related fistula in South-East Asia.* Paper prepared for a WHO Technical Working Group, (unpublished) Geneva, 1989. WHE 2122

Based on a postal enquiry and a review of published and unpublished material from Bangladesh, India, Nepal, Pakistan, Sri Lanka and Thailand, this report summarizes some overall findings on fistula in this region. Trends in some parts of India seemed to show that the incidence of fistula as a result of obstructed labour was declining, but that there was an increase in fistulae caused by surgical trauma.

Shroff, C.P. and Roy, S. Autopsy study in obstetric deaths – a clinicopathologic evaluation. *The Indian Practitioner,* 1987: 687-694. WHE 1813

Over a period of four years at the LTMM College Hospital, Sion, Bombay, Maharashtra there were 855 admissions with antepartum and postpartum complications. Of these 150 died in the hospital. Autopsies performed on 69 cases found the main causes of death to be haemorrhage and hypertensive disorders of pregnancy.

United Nations Children's Fund. *The lesser child,* UNICEF, 1990. WHE 2645

The report documents the treatment of girl children in many parts of India. Girls are likely to be breast fed less often and for shorter periods than boys and the resulting undernutrition continues throughout adolescence and adulthood. Girls are subject to a heavy workload and are less likely to receive medical attention than boys when they are ill. In Bihar, Haryana, Madhya Pradesh, Manipur, Punjab, Rajasthan, Tamil Nadu and Uttar Pradesh female mortality by the age of 5 years exceeds that of males by 20% or more. Girls are less likely to attend school than boys at primary as well as secondary levels. The report stresses the urgent need to address the problems facing India's 130 million girls aged under 20.

Walia I. Intranatal care in a rural community in Haryana, North India. *Midwifery,* 1986; 2: 119-125. WHE 1492

Of 1000 consecutive live births in a rural community in North India one third of the mothers were randomly selected and interviewed to ascertain practices relating to their intranatal care. 98% of the women delivered at home on locally made cots and dirty, unwashed bedding. Traditional birth attendants conducted 98% of the deliveries. Problems were perceived for 7% of the women and about 9% of the babies. A number of serious deficiencies or harmful practices were identified including poor hygiene, administration of injections or tablets by untrained persons, and lack of understanding of the importance of keeping newborns warm.

8. FURTHER READING

Bhaskara Rao, K. Tragedy of maternal deaths. *The Hindu,* March 27 1988. WHE 1959

Caldwell, J.C. et al. The causes of marriage change in South India. *Population Studies,* 1983; 37: 343-361. WHE 0119

Das Gupta, M. Selective discrimination against female children in rural Punjab, India. *Population and Development Review,* 1987; 13(1): 77-100. WHE 1641

Das Gupta, M. Death clustering, mothers' education and the determinants of child mortality in rural Punjab, India. *Population Studies,* 1990; 44: 489-505. WHE 2733

Deodhar, N.S. Primary health care in India. *Journal of Public Health Policy,* 1982, 3(1): 76-99. WHE 0175

Dyson, T. and Moore, M. On kinship structure, female autonomy, and demographic behaviour in India. *Population and Development Review,* 1983; 9(1): 35-60. WHE 0185

Ghosh, S. Discrimination begins at birth. *Indian Pediatrics,* 1986; 23: 9-15. WHE 1940

Jeffrey, R. et al. Female infanticide and amniocentesis. *Social Science and Medicine,* 1984; 19(11): 1207-1212. WHE 1145

Kadi, A.S. Age at marriage in India. *Asia-Pacific Population Journal,* 1987; 2(1): 41-56. WHE 1521

Karan, S. et al. Customs and beliefs relating to the mother and infant in an area of rural Andhra Pradesh. *Journal of Tropical Pediatrics,* 1983; 23: 81-84. WHE 0377

Key, P. Women, health and development, with special reference to Indian Women. *Health Policy and Planning,* 1987; 2(1): 58-69. WHE 1722

Khosla, T. The plight of female infants in India. *Journal of Epidemiology and Community Health,* 1980; 34: 143-146. WHE 1204

Lahiri D. et al. Jaundice in pregnancy. *Journal of the Indian Medical Association,* 1983; 80(7 & 8): 85-90. WHE 1818

Mandal D.and Roy Chowdhury N.N. Viral hepatitis in pregnancy. *Journal of the Indian Medical Association,* 1982; 79(7): 96-98. WHE 1817

Mathur, H.N. et al. The impact of training traditional birth attendants on the utilisation of maternal health services. *Journal of Epidemiology and Community Health,* 1979; 33: 142-144. WHE 1249

Miller, B.D. Prenatal and postnatal sex-selection in India: The patriarchal context, ethical questions and public policy. *Working Papers,* No. 107, Michigan State University, 1985. WHE 1366

Pratinidhi, A. at al. *Social custom of migration for delivery and perinatal mortality* (unpublished), 1989. WHE 2443

Raman, A.V. Traditional practices and nutritional taboos. *The Nursing Journal of India,* 1988; 74(6): 143-166. WHE 2228

Venkatramani, S.H. Female infanticide – Born to die. *India Today,* June 1986. WHE 1407

9. DATA SOURCES

WHE 0089   Bhasker Rao, K. Maternal mortality in a teaching hospital in southern India. A 13 year study. *Obstetrics and Gynaecology,* 1975; 46(4): 397-400.

WHE 0169   Datta, S.A. et al., Evaluation of maternal and infant care in a rural area. *Indian Journal of Medical Science,* 1973; 27(2): 120-128.

WHE 0172   Dawn, C.S. et al. Avoidable factors in maternal deaths. *Journal of the Indian Medical Association,* 1972; 59(3): 101-104.

WHE 0175   Deodhar, N.S. Primary health care in India. *Journal of Public Health Policy,* 1982; 3(1): 76-99.

WHE 0208   Engineer, A.D. and Lakshmi, M.S. Maternal mortality. *Journal of Obstetrics and Gynaecology of India,* 1976; 26(2): 186-192.

WHE 0247   Guha, M. Maternal mortality. *Journal of Obstetrics and Gynaecology of India,* 1972; 22(3): 254-261.

WHE 0256   Datta, K.K. et al. Morbidity patterns amongst rural pregnant women in Alwar, Rajasthan – a cohort study. *Health and Population Perspectives,* 1980; 3(4): 282-292.

WHE 0284   Bhasker Rao, K. *Report of the maternal mortality committee of the FOGSI,* 1978-81. (unpublished document), 1984.

WHE 0339   India, Ministry of Home Affairs, *Vital statistics of India 1976,* Office of Registrar General, New Delhi, 1981.

WHE 0395   Konar, M. et al. Abortion mortality: ten year's survey in Eden Hospital with critical analysis of last three years. *Journal of Obstetrics and Gynaecology of India,* 1973; 23(4): 436-422.

WHE 0403   Lahiri, D. and Konar, M. Abortion hazards. *Journal of the Indian Medical Association,* 1976; 66(11): 288-294.

WHE 0486   India, Government Planning Commission. Steering group report. Health and family planning welfare programme for the seventh 5-year plan. *Indian Journal of Pediatrics,* 1985; 52: 11-16.

WHE 0522   Patharajaiah, M.P. and Parvathamma, M. Study of maternal mortality in Cheluvamba Hospital, Mysore. *Journal of Obstetrics and Gynaecology of India,* 1975; 25(5): 665-670.

WHE 0577   Philips, F.S. and Grouse, N. Septic abortion – three year study 1971-73. Hazards of septic abortion as compared to medical termination of pregnancy at Government Erskine Hospital, Madurai. *Journal of Obstetrics and Gynaecology of India,* 1975; 652-656.

WHE 0605   Bhasker Rao, K. and Malika, P.E. A study of maternal mortality in Madras City. *Journal of Obstetrics and Gynaecology of India,* 1977; 27(6): 876-880.

WHE 0615   Roy Chowdhury, N.N. Maternal deaths due to haemorrhage. *Journal of the Indian Medical Association,* 1976; 67(7): 157-160.

WHE 0680   Sukthankar, D.M. Population health profile of the city of Bombay. In: *Joint UNICEF/ WHO Meeting on Primary Health Care in Urban Areas,* Geneva, 1983.

WHE 0813   World Health Organization. Eastern Mediterranean Regional Office. *Report of the EMR/SEAR meeting on the prevention of neonatal tetanus,* (WHO document no. EM/IMZ/27, EM/ BD/14, EM-SEA/MTG.PREV.NNL.TTN./8), Lahore, 1982.

WHE 0829   World Health Organization. Southeast Asia Regional Office. *Bulletin of Regional Health Information,* (unpublished WHO document no. SEA/VHS/165 Rev. 1), New Delhi, 1981

WHE 0834   World Health Organization *World health statistics annual – vital statistics and causes of death.* Geneva, various years.

WHE 0914   United Nations Children's Fund. *An analysis of the situation of children in India.* UNICEF, New Delhi, 1984.

WHE 0917   United Nations Economic and Social Commission for Asia and the Pacific. *The Asia and Pacific Atlas of Children in Development 1984,* UNICEF, Bangkok, 1984.

WHE 0918   World Health Organization. Southeast Asia Regional Office. Country papers. In: *Joint National/WHO/UNFPA Workshop,* New Delhi, 24-27 November 1984.

WHE 1098   Bhasker Rao, A. Maternal mortality in India. A review. *Paper presented to the Interregional Meeting on the Prevention of Maternal Mortality,* (WHO document no. FHE/PMM/85.9.4), Geneva, 11-15 November 1985.

WHE 1109   India, Ministry of Health and Family Welfare. *Family welfare programme in India 1982-83,* New Delhi, 1983.

WHE 1259   Bhatia, J.C. *A study of maternal mortality in Anantapur district, Andhra Pradesh.* Indian Institute of Management, Bangalore, 1982.

WHE 1375   Indian Council of Medical Research. Birth weight: a major determinant of child survival. *Future,* 1985; 17: 53-56.

WHE 1522   World Health Organization. Southeast Asia Regional Office. *Bulletin of Regional Health Information,* New Delhi, 1986.

WHE 1712   Mauldin W.P. and Segal, S.J., *Prevalence of contraceptive use in developing countries. A chart book.* Rockefeller Foundation, New York, 1986.

WHE 1812   Devi, Y.L. and Singh, J. Maternal mortality. A ten year study in R.M.C. Hospital, Imphal. *Journal of Obstetrics and Gynaecology of India,* 1987; 37(1): 90-94.

WHE 1844   Mehta, B. et al. Abortion and M.T.P. cases – a study of hospital admissions from 1971-1979. *Indian Journal of Public Health,* 1982; 24(1): 38-42.

WHE 1914   United Nations Children's Fund (UNICEF). *The state of the world's children,* Oxford, Oxford University Press, various years.

WHE 1915   United Nations. Department of International Economic and Social Affairs. *World population prospects: estimates and projections,* Population Studies, New York, various years.

WHE 1917   United Nations. Department of International Economic and Social Affairs. *Age structure of mortality in developing countries. A database for cross-sectional and time-series research.* New York, 1986.

WHE 1918   United Nations. Department of International Economic and Social Affairs. *First marriage: patterns and determinants.* New York, 1988.

WHE 1981   Pune Medical College. *Risk approach and intervention strategy in MCH care.* Project report, Sirur, 1984.

WHE 2007   Pandit, R.D. Changing trends in maternal mortality in developing countries. *Asia-Oceania Journal of Obstetrics and Gynaecology,* 1987; 13(4): 385-394.

WHE 2033   World Health Organization. *Global strategy for health for all by the year 2000. Second report on monitoring progress.* WHO document EB83/2 Add. 1, 1988.

WHE 2430   Karkal, M. *Health situation in India: can it be improved if neglect of women continues?* (unpublished) Bombay, 1989.

WHE 2482   Bhatt R.V. Professional responsibility in maternity care: role of the medical audit. *International Journal of Gynecology and Obstetrics,* 1989; 30: 47-50.

WHE 2630   Kumar, R. et al. Maternal mortality inquiry in a rural community of North India. *International Journal of Gynecology and Obstetrics,* 1989; 29: 313-319.

WHE 2732   Dyal Chand, A. and Khale, M. A community based surveillance system for perinatal and neonatal care. *Indian Pediatrics,* 1989; 26: 1115-1121.

INDONESIA

		Year	Source

1. BASIC INDICATORS

1.1 Demographic

1.1.1 Population

Size (millions)	180.5	1990	(1915)
Rate of growth	1.6	1985-90	(1915)

1.2 Life expectancy

Female	57	1985-90	(1915)
Male	55	1985-90	(1915)

1.1.3 Fertility

Crude Birth Rate	27	1985-90	(1915)
Total Fertility Rate	3.4	1985-90	(1915)

1.1.4 Mortality

Crude Death Rate	11	1985-90	(1915)
Infant Mortality Rate	84	1985-90	(1915)
Female	66	1977-87	(2718)
Male	84	1977-87	(2718)
1-4 years mortality rate			
Female	42	1977-87	(2718)
Male	37	1977-87	(2718)

1.2 Social and economic

1.2.1 Adult literacy rate (%)

Female	65	1985	(1914)
Male	83	1985	(1914)

1.2.2 Primary school enrolment rate (%)

Female	115	1986-88	(1914)
Male	120	1986-88	(1914)

1.2.3 Female mean age at first marriage

(years)	20	1980	(1918)

		Year	Source

1.2.4 GNP/capita

(US $)	450	1987	(1914)

1.2.5 Daily per capita calorie supply

(as % of requirements)	116	1984-86	(1914)

2. HEALTH SERVICES

2.1 Health expenditure

2.1.1 Expenditure on health

(as % of GNP)	2	1986-87	(2033)

2.1.2 Expenditure on PHC

(as % of total health expenditure)	7	1986-87	(2033)

2.2 Primary Health Care

(Percentage of population covered by):

2.2.1 Health services

National	64	1987	(2033)
Urban			
Rural			

2.2.2 Safe water

National	38	1987	(2033)
Urban	41	1987	(2033)
Rural	32	1987	(2033)

2.2.3 Adequate sanitary facilities

National	34	1987	(2033)
Urban	32	1987	(2033)
Rural	38	1987	(2033)

2.2.4 Contraceptive prevalence rate

(%)	48	1987	(2718)

2.3   Coverage of maternity care (%)

Area	Prenatal care	Trained attendant	Institutional deliveries	Postnatal care	Sample size	Year	Source
National	48-54		10			1983	(0641)
National	26	31				1983-84	(1489)
National	49	49				(1989)	(2033)
National:		36	20		8 176b	1982-87	(2718)
urban		69	48		2 217b	1982-87	(2718)
rural		24	9		5 959b	1982-87	(2718)
Bali		57	44		119b	1982-87	(2718)
Central Java		25	14		1 345b	1982-87	(2718)
East Java		30	15		1 252b	1982-87	(2718)
Jakarta		79	71		405b	1982-87	(2718)
S.Kalimantu		80	68	11	210	1982	(0808)
S.Sulawesi		43	70	8	210	1982	(0808)
S.Sumatra		72	50	1	210	1982	(0808)
West Java		21	13	1	1 618b	1982-87	(2718)
Yogyakarta		37	27		116	1982-87	(2718)

3.   COMMUNITY STUDIES

3.1   National, 1985-86 [2775, 2792]

A retrospective household health survey was undertaken. No further information is available on the survey design from the sources quoted.

3.2.1   Rate
MMR (per 100 000 live births)   450

3.2   Bali, 1980-82 [1260]

This reproductive age mortality (RAMOS) study covered a two year period 1980-82. Maternal deaths were located through family planning workers collaborating with village headmen, and surviving family members were interviewed. It is estimated that only 45%-50% of deaths were located. Rates have been adjusted accordingly.

3.2.1   Rate
Births	38 727
Maternal deaths	295
MMR (per 100 000 births)	761
MMR (per 100 000 women aged 15-44 years)	69

3.2.2   Causes of maternal deaths

	Number	%
Haemorrhage	135	46
Sepsis	31	10
Abortion	20	7
Hypertensive disorders of pregnancy	14	5
Embolisms	6	2
DIRECT CAUSES	206	70
Diseases of the circulatory system	19	6
Hepatitis	2	1
Other infections	23	8
Trauma	6	2
All other causes	19	6
Unknown causes	20	7
TOTAL	295	100

3.2.3   Avoidable factors

3.2.4 High risk groups
Age

	Births	Deaths*	MMR (per 100 000 births)	MMR (per 100 000 women)
15-19	1 545	17	1 100	82
20-24	12 752	62	486	83
25-29	12 550	68	542	83
30-34	6 748	47	696	70
35-39	3 753	61	1 625	89
40-44	1 030	15	1 456	29
45-49	349	8	2 292	21
Total	38 727	278	718	69

* non-obstetric deaths excluded

High parity women accounted for a large proportion of maternal deaths. Frequently, high age and high parity went together; 61% of the maternal deaths in Bali were to women who were above 30 years old and/or who were having their fourth or later child.

Maternal mortality rates were higher among women who lived in areas furthest from the main hospital.

3.3 Central Java, 1986-87 [(2494)]

A Maternal and Perinatal Mortality Study carried out by the Coordinating Board of Indonesian Fertility Research (BKS PENFIN) collected data through a retrospective, cross-sectional, community based survey conducted through household interviews. The survey was undertaken in three rural districts of Central Java. Maternal deaths are thought to be adequately registered due to the necessity of obtaining burial permits. For each maternal death identified during an interview, a follow-up investigation was conducted to determine the cause of death.

3.3.1 Rate
Live births	14 956
Maternal deaths	50
MMR (per 100 000 deliveries)	343

3.3.2 Cause of maternal deaths

	Number	%
Haemorrhage	23	46
Sepsis	10	20
Hypertensive disorders of pregnancy	8	16
DIRECT CAUSES	41	82
Hepatitis	2	4
Pneumonia	2	4
Tuberculosis	2	4
Renal failure	1	2
Other	2	4
INDIRECT CAUSES	9	18
TOTAL	50	100

3.3.3 Avoidable factors

Prenatal care

Women who died were less likely to have received prenatal care through the health services than those who survived.

	Maternal deaths	Survivors
	%	%
No prenatal care	17	38
Prenatal care from TBA only	0	0
Prenatal care from health services	83	63

3.4 Central Java, (1989) [(2565)]

A survey carried out by the National Family Planning Association used the "sisterhood method" to estimate maternal mortality. A total of 17,938 respondents were questioned about the deaths of ever married sisters. The life-time risk of dying from pregnancy related causes was calculated as 1 in 58.

3.4.1 Rate
Maternal deaths	208
MMR (per 100 000 live births)	385

3.4 West Java, (1989) [(2565)]

The Ministry of Health undertook a survey using the "sisterhood method" to estimate maternal mortality. Over 22,000 respondents participated and the life time risk of dying from pregnancy related causes was calculated as 1 in 39.

3.4.1 Rate
Maternal deaths	548
MMR (per 100 000 live births)	579

3.5 Mojokerto, East Java, (1989) [(2775)]

A community based survey was carried out using the "sisterhood method" to estimate maternal mortality. Interviews were conducted with 4,325 adults. 64 maternal deaths were identified and the lifetime risk of dying from pregnancy related causes was calculated as 1 in 63.

Maternal deaths	64
MMR (per 100 000 live births)	397

3.6 West Aceh, 1986-87 (3121)

An intervention project designed to implement mass distribution of vitamin A capsules and an expanded programme of childhood immunizations was used as a vehicle for assessing numbers of maternal deaths. The project covered a rural population of 150,000 divided into 422 villages. A complete population census was carried out in 1986 and a monthly birth and death reporting system established which included a list of causes and specified "childbirth" as a cause of death. In 1987, in conjunction with a survey of child mortality, attempts were made to examine the extent of accurate reporting of maternal deaths.

It was found that 19 deaths had been classified as maternal in the registration system. Cross matching of deaths of women of reproductive age with registered births located an additional 10 maternal deaths. However, this method depends on the coverage of birth reports which was found to be only 80% complete. During the survey, village heads were asked about any additional maternal deaths and a further 9 deaths were thus identified. After elimination of incorrectly reported maternal deaths and duplicates, there remained a total of 38 maternal deaths over the eighteen month period.

3.6.1 Rate

Births *	4 350
Maternal deaths **	25
MMR (per 100 000 births)	582

* Calculated on basis of estimated birth rate of 29.
** Annual average

4. HOSPITAL STUDIES

4.1 Twelve Teaching Hospitals, 1977-80 (0138)

4.1.1 Rate

Live births	34 647
Maternal deaths	135 *
MMR (per 100 000 live births)	390

* Deaths due to complications arising in early pregnancy such as ectopic pregnancy, molar pregnancy and abortion excluded.

There was considerable variation in maternal mortality rates among the participating hospitals; the highest rate was from Medan (1 164 per 100 000) and the lowest from Semrang (69 per 100 000). The study period was too short to permit an evaluation of the reasons for the differentials in mortality rates which might be due to a range of factors including the type of patients served, the availability of prenatal care, the referral mechanisms in the catchment area, accuracy in reporting mortality and hospital performance.

4.1.2 Causes of maternal deaths *(available for 108 cases)*

	Number	%
Haemorrhage	41	38
Sepsis	30	27
Hypertensive disorders of pregnancy	22	20
Complications of anaesthesia	4	4
Transfusion reaction	2	2
Other direct causes	3	3
DIRECT CAUSES	99	92
Indirect causes	5	5
Malignancy	1	1
TOTAL	108	100

4.1.3 Avoidable factors

4.1.4 High risk groups

Late referral

All but nine of the 108 women who died were admitted as emergency cases and 40 were moribund. Nineteen women presented with ruptured uterus and another nine with impending uterine rupture. Thirty women were admitted with various degrees of bleeding and 32 with malpresentations and prolonged labour. In all, 38 women were admitted in shock, coma or convulsions.

Age and parity

Age and parity specific analysis of maternal deaths shows that the highest rate was for women older than 35 who had more than four children. Women younger than than 20 years old and of parity two or more had higher rates than women of lower parity in the same age group. A somewhat higher rate was also detected for women above 30 years old who were delivering their first baby.

	MMR (per 100 000 maternity cases)				
Age	Parity				
	0	1	2-3	4+	Total
<20	408	(205)	(1667)	(0)	400
20-29	208	208	265	498	246
30-34	452	(410)	576	375	447
35+	(0)	(0)	624	907	815
Total	271	218	371	646	377 *

Figures in brackets indicate that the rates are based on fewer than 500 maternity cases.

* In the case of one maternal death and 532 maternity cases age and/or parity were unknown.

Urban/rural*

	Urban	Rural
MMR (per 100 000 maternity cases)	248	770

* Place of residence of the woman.

Anaemia

	Anaemic women	Non-anaemic women
MMR (per 100 000 maternity cases)	700	197

An interesting finding emerges when residence and anaemia are examined simultaneously. A greater proportion of the rural women than urban women was anaemic but this is thought to be due to the fact that the only haemoglobin determination recorded was the one made at admission. This "anaemic" condition reflected more the extent of haemorrhage at admission than the prenatal haemoglobin level for those patients admitted with haemorrhage. The difference in maternal mortality rates between the urban and rural women was much larger in the anaemic than in the non-anaemic group, strongly suggesting that late arrival (because of transportation difficulties) was one of the primary factors responsible for the higher mortality rate of the rural women.

	MMR (per 100 000 maternity cases)		
	Anaemic *	Non-anaemic *	Total
Urban	388	184	248
Rural	1348	228	762
Total	702	192	363

* Haemoglobin level determined at time of admission. Cases with a level of 9g or less classified as anaemic.

Prenatal care

	MMR (per 100 000 maternity cases)
No prenatal care	599
One or more prenatal visits	114

4.2 Hasan Sadikin Hospital, Bandung, 1970-72 [(0458)]

4.2.1 Rate
Deliveries	6 260
Maternal deaths	121
MMR (per 100 000 deliveries)	1 933

4.2.2 Causes of maternal deaths
Common causes of death were haemorrhage, trophoblastic disease, infection, toxaemia, and complications of anaesthesia, in that order.

4.3 Gunung Wenang Hospital, Manado, 1969-73 [(0461)]

4.3.1 Rate
Deliveries	13 704
Maternal deaths	26
MMR (per 100 000 deliveries)	190

4.3.2 Causes of maternal deaths

	Number
Hypertensive disorders of pregnancy	9
Haemorrhage	7
Sepsis	4
Ruptured uterus	2
Embolisms	2
Operative intervention	2
Total	26

4.3.3 Avoidable factors

Booking status

	Booked	Unbooked
Deliveries	11 786	1 923
Maternal deaths	10	16
MMR (per 100 000 deliveries)	85	832

4.4 Surabaya Hospital, East Java [(0641)]

4.4.1 Rate
Maternal mortality rates of 1 016 and 508 (per 100 000 live births) were reported for 1980 and 1981 respectively. The main cause of death was sepsis (30%). Most deaths occurred to women referred after prolonged and neglected labour.

5. CIVIL REGISTRATION DATA/GOVERNMENT ESTIMATES

6. OTHER SOURCES/ ESTIMATES

6.1 National, 1980 [(0918)]

6.1.1 Rate
A report presented at a joint national/WHO/UNFPA workshop quotes a household survey carried out in 1980 which estimated the maternal mortality rate to be 80 per 100 000 live births. No further information is given.

6.2 National, 1980 [0787]

6.2.1 Rate

A World Bank report quotes an institutional maternal mortality rate of 300 per 100 000 live births for 1980.

6.3 National, 1980 and 1984 [0829, 1522]

6.3.1 Rate

Regional Health Information Bulletins of the WHO quote maternal mortality rates of 300 and 80 per 100 000 live births for 1980 and 1985 respectively. Reference is made to a community survey which found a rate of 170 per 100 000 live births but no additional information is available.

6.4 National, 1987 [1784]

6.4.1 Rate

The Indonesian Midwives Association estimated the maternal mortality rate in Indonesia to be around 400 per 100 000 live births in 1987.

6.5 Kapupaten Jenponto, rural area, South Sulawesi, 1978-80 [2354]

A field enquiry was conducted among family heads.

6.5.1 Rate

Live births	836
Maternal deaths	9
MMR (per 100 000 live births)	1 076

All the deaths occurred among women of parity 4 or higher and all had been assisted by traditional birth attendants (dukun) only.

7. SELECTED ANNOTATED BIBLIOGRAPHY

8. FURTHER READING

Hull, T.H. Adapting the safe motherhood initiative to Indonesian society. *Child Survival Research Note*, The Australian National University, No. 20CS, 1988. WHE 2248

Indonesia, Central Bureau of Statistics, *An analysis of the situation of children and women in Indonesia*, UNICEF, 1984. WHE 1130

Leimena, S.L. Posyandu: a community based vehicle to improve child survival and development. *Asia-Pacific Journal of Public Health*, 1989; 3(4): 264-267. WHE 2719

Prajitno, A. et al. Traditional maternal health beliefs among married women in selected villages of East Java. *International Journal of Health Education*, 1979; 22(1): 30-37. WHE 0543

9. DATA SOURCES

WHE 0138   Chi, I.C. et al. Maternal mortality at twelve teaching hospitals in Indonesia: an epidemiological analysis. *International Journal of Gynecology and Obstetrics*, 1981; 19(4): 259-266.

WHE 0458   Mochtar, A. *Maternal mortality at the Hasan Sadikin Hospital, Bandung, Indonesia over a three-year period, 1970-72.* (unpublished document).

WHE 0461   Moningka, B.H. and Wowor, G.E. Influence of antenatal care on perinatal health at the Gunung Wenang Hospital, Manado, 1969-1973. In: *Proceedings of the 6th. Asian Congress of Obstetrics and Gynaecology*, Kuala Lumpur, Malaysia, 1974.

WHE 0641   Sebastian, E.V. *Report on maternal and child health in the context of family health* (unpublished WHO document no. SEA/MCH/159), 1982.

WHE 0787   International Bank for Reconstruction and Development, Staff appraisal report. *Indonesia provincial health project*. Population, Health and Nutrition Department, 1983.

WHE 0808   World Health Organization. *Sixth report on the world health situation 1973-77. Part II: review by country and area*. Geneva, 1980.

WHE 0829   World Health Organization, *Review of the expanded programme on immunization and selected primary health care activities in the Republic of Indonesia.* (unpublished WHO document no. SEA/EPI/42), 1983.

WHE 0918   World Health Organization, Southeast Asia Regional Office. Country papers. In: *Joint National/WHO/UNFPA Workshop*, New Delhi, 24-27 November 1984.

WHE 1260   Fortney, J.A. et al. Maternal mortality in Indonesia and Egypt. In: *Interregional Meeting on the prevention of maternal mortality*, Geneva, 11-15 November 1985.

WHE 1489   World Health Organization. Southeast Asia Regional Office. Evaluation of the strategy for Health for All by the year 2000. *Seventh report on the world health situation*, New Delhi, 1986.

WHE 1522   World Health Organization. Southeast Asia Regional Office. *Bulletin of regional health information*, Delhi, 1986.

WHE 1784   Martosewojo, S. Indonesian Midwives Association. *Personal communication,* 13 November 1987.

WHE 1914   United Nations Children's Fund (UNICEF). *The state of the world's children*, Oxford, Oxford University Press, various years.

WHE 1915   United Nations. Department of International Economic and Social Affairs. *World population prospects: estimates and projections*, Population Studies, New York, various years.

WHE 1918   United Nations. Department of International Economic and Social Affairs. *First marriage: patterns and determinants.* New York, 1988.

WHE 2033   World Health Organization. *Global strategy for health for all by the year 2000. Second report on monitoring progress.* WHO document EB83/2 Add. 1, 1988.

WHE 2354   Sopacua, A. et al. Some aspects of primary health care in obstetrics in South Sulawesi – a preliminary report. In: Walters, W.A.W. (ed.) *Seminar proceedings – Primary health care of mothers and infants with the aim of averting maternal and infant mortality in developing countries now and tomorrow.* VIII Asian and Oceanic Congress of Obstetrics and Gynaecology and First Congress of the Royal Australian College of Obstetricians and Gynaecologists, Melbourne, Australia, 1981.

WHE 2494   Agoestina, T. and Soejoenoes, A. *Technical report on the study of maternal and perinatal mortality, Central Java Province*, Republic of Indonesia, BKS PENFIN/Ministry of Health, 1989.

WHE 2565   Graham, W. *Results of the application of the sisterhood method for estimating maternal mortality*, (unpublished document), London School of Hygiene and Tropical Medicine, 1990.

WHE 2718   Demographic and Health Surveys, *National contraceptive prevalence survey 1987*, Central Bureau of Statistics/Institute for Resource Development/Westinghouse, 1989.

WHE 2775   Soemanti, S. Population based estimates of maternal mortality in Mojokerto, East Java. *Buletin Penelitian Kesehatan*, 1989; 17(4): 21-32.

WHE 2792   Soedarmo, S.P *Follow-up study on pregnancy and its outcome in West Java* (unpublished project proposal), 1991.

WHE 3121 Quinley, J. et al. *Preliminary report on maternal mortality double intervention project West Aceh, Indonesia*, (unpublished) 1988.

NOTES

IRAN
(ISLAMIC REPUBLIC OF)

		Year	Source

1. BASIC INDICATORS

1.1 Demographic

1.1.1 Population
		Year	Source
Size (millions)	56.6	1990	(1915)
Rate of growth (%)	3.5	1985-90	(1915)

1.1.2 Life expectancy
Female	66	1985-90	(1915)
Male	65	1985-90	(1915)

1.1.3 Fertility
Crude Birth Rate	42	1985-90	(1915)
Total Fertility Rate	5.6	1985-90	(1915)

1.1.4 Mortality
Crude Death Rate	8	1985-90	(1915)
Infant Mortality Rate	63	1985-90	(1915)
Female	142	1973-76	(1917)
Male	129	1973-76	(1917)
1-4 years mortality rate			
Female	19	1973-76	(1917)
Male	15	1973-76	(1917)

1.2 Social and economic

1.2.1 Adult literacy rate (%)
Female	39	1985	(1914)
Male	62	1985	(1914)

1.2.2 Primary school enrolment rate (%)
Female	105	1986-88	(1914)
Male	122	1986-88	(1914)

1.2.3 Female mean age at first marriage
(years)	19.7	1976	(1918)

		Year	Source

1.2.4 GNP/capita
(US $)

1.2.5 Daily per capita calorie supply
(as % of requirements)	138	1984-86	(1914)

2. HEALTH SERVICES

2.1 Health Expenditure

2.1.1 Expenditure on health
(as % of GNP)	7.5	1986	(2033)

2.1.2 Expenditure on PHC
(as % of total health
expenditure)	38	1986	(2033)

2.2 Primary Health Care
(Percentage of population covered by):

2.2.1 Health services
National	93	1987	(2033)
Urban			
Rural			

2.2.2 Safe water
National	75	1987	(2033)
Urban	90	1987	(2033)
Rural	60	1987	(2033)

2.2.3 Adequate sanitary facilities
National	60	1987	(2033)
Urban	90	1987	(2033)
Rural	24	1987	(2033)

2.2.4 Contraceptive prevalence rate
(%)	23	1978-79	(1712)

2.3   Coverage of maternity care (%)

Area	Prenatal care	Trained attendant	Institutional deliveries	Postnatal care	Sample size	Year	Source
National	5					1982	(0800)
National	11					1984	(1888)
National	47	69	69			1987	(2313)
Fars Province				40	2 655	1986	(1678)

3.   COMMUNITY STUDIES

3.1   Urban areas and all rural areas except Kurdistan, 1985 and 1987 [1320, 2702]

A 10% sample survey was undertaken covering urban areas and all rural areas except Kurdistan. The first survey was carried out between 1984 and 1985 and the second between 1986 and 1987. Both surveys covered periods between important calendar events in order to maximize recall among households interviewed.

3.1.1   Rate

	MMR (per 100 000 live births)	
	1984-85	1986-87
Rural areas	233	184
Urban areas	77	63
National	136	120

Rural provinces, 1984-85

	MMR (per 100 000 live births)
Semnan, Yazd, Tehran, Mazandaran, Markazi, Fars, Gilan, Boushehr, Khuzestan	114
Esfahan, Ilam, Kerman, Chaharmahal, Bakhtiyari, Lorestan, Kohkloayeh, Boyerahmad, Hormozgan, Hamedan	526
Sistan, Baluchestan, East Azarbayjan, West Azarbayjan, Khorasan, Bakhtaran, Zanjan	146
All provinces excluding Kurdistan	233

4.   HOSPITAL STUDIES

4.1   Saadi Hospital, Pahlavi University, Shiraz, 1963-76 [0099, 0168, 0523]

4.1.1   Rate

	Live births	Maternal deaths*	MMR (per 100 000 live births)
1963-69	–	–	392
1970-76	38 587	96	249

*   Includes deaths occurring up to 90 days after the termination of pregnancy.

4.1.2   Causes of maternal deaths

Sepsis (both puerperal and post-abortal) was the most important cause of death in both series, accounting for about 25% of all deaths. Infectious diseases claimed a large proportion of lives (about 20%). Deaths from hepatitis declined significantly in the second six year period, consistent with a decrease in the incidence of hepatitis in Southern Iran at that time.

	1963-69		1970-76	
	Number	%	Number	%
Sepsis	16	17	18	19
Embolisms	4	4	8	8
Haemorrhage	7	7	7	7
Abortions	8	8	7	7
Hypertensive disorders of pregnancy	4	4	6	6
Ruptured uterus	3	3	4	4
Complications of anaesthesia	1	1	1	1
DIRECT CAUSES	43	45	51	53
Hepatitis	16	17	2	2
Cardiac diseases	4	4	2	2
Other infections	19	20	17	18
Others	14	15	24	25
INDIRECT CAUSES	53	55	45	47
TOTAL	96	100	96	100

4.2 Amin Maternity Hospital, Isfahan, 1971-75 [0238]

4.2.1 Rate
Births	15 794
Maternal deaths	29
MMR (per 100 000 births)	184

4.2.2 Causes of maternal deaths

	Number
Sepsis	3
Haemorrhage	3
Hypertensive disorders of pregnancy	3
Renal failure	3
Embolisms	2
Ruptured uterus	2
Complications of anaesthesia	2
Cerebrovascular accident	2
DIRECT CAUSES	20
Hepatitis	4
Abortions	1
Other infections	2
Others	2
INDIRECT CAUSES	9
TOTAL	29

4.2.3 Avoidable factors
Avoidable factors were present in 14 of the 29 deaths. Patients usually came to the hospital too late, in most cases, after having travelled considerable distances. Of the 29 maternal deaths, 23 had developed complications prior to admission in the hospital, and ten died within 24 hours of admission. The lack of facilities in the hospital itself, including the unavailability of blood, also contributed to death in several cases.

5. CIVIL REGISTRATION DATA/GOVERNMENT ESTIMATES

5.1 National, 1985 [1962]

	MMR (per 100 000 live births)
Urban	63
Rural	184
National	120

5.2 Cities, 1985 and 1987 [2722]

	Maternal deaths	MMR (per 100 000 live births)
1985	48	9
1987	31	7

7. SELECTED ANNOTATED BIBLIOGRAPHY

8. FURTHER READING

Amidi, S. Family health by women's health corps (WHC) in Iran. *Journal of Tropical Pediatrics*, 1982; 28: 149-152. WHE 1866

9. DATA SOURCES

WHE 0099   Borazjani, G. et al. Maternal mortality in South Iran: a seven-year survey. *International Journal of Gynecology and Obstetrics*, 1979; 16(1): 65-69.

WHE 0168   Daneshbod, K. et al. Survey of maternal deaths in south Iran: analysis of 96 autopsies. *Journal of Obstetrics and Gynaecology of the British Commonwealth*, 1970; 77(12): 1103-1188.

WHE 0238   Ghanai, P. et al. Study of maternal deaths in Amin Hospital in Isfahan, Iran. *Iranian Journal of Public Health*, 1976; 5(3): 155-167.

WHE 0523   Paydar, M. and Hassanzadeh, A. Rupture of the uterus. *International Journal of Gynecology and Obstetrics*, 1978; 15: 405-409.

WHE 0800   World Health Organization. *Country reports to regional offices of the progress in implementing Health for All by the Year 2000.* (Unpublished documents) 1983.

WHE 1320   Malek-Afzali, H. and Rezali, P. *Survey of mortality indicators in Iran: Rural population, 1985* (unpublished), 1986.

WHE 1678   Sadeghi-Hasanbadi, A. Neonatal tetanus in Fars Province, Islamic Republic of Iran. *Eastern Mediterranean Region Health Services Journal*, 1987; 3: 14-21.

WHE 1712   Mauldin W.P. and Segal, S.J., *Prevalence of contraceptive use in developing countries. A chart book.* Rockefeller Foundation, New York, 1986.

WHE 1888   World Health Organization, Eastern Mediterranean Regional Office, *Evaluation of the strategy for Health for All by the year 2000. Seventh report of the world health situation.* EMRO, Alexandria, 1987.

WHE 1914   United Nations Children's Fund (UNICEF). *The state of the world's children,* Oxford, Oxford University Press, various years.

WHE 1915   United Nations. Department of International Economic and Social Affairs. *World population prospects: estimates and projections,* Population Studies, New York, various years.

WHE 1917   United Nations. Department of International Economic and Social Affairs. *Age structure of mortality in developing countries. A database for cross-sectional and time-series research.* New York, 1986.

WHE 1918   United Nations. Department of International Economic and Social Affairs. *First marriage: patterns and determinants.* New York, 1988.

WHE 1962   Baldo, M.H. *Improving managerial aspects of maternal and child health/family planning project,* assignment report (unpublished), 1987.

WHE 2033   World Health Organization. *Global strategy for health for all by the year 2000. Second report on monitoring progress.* WHO document EB83/2 Add. 1, 1988.

WHE 2313   World Health Organization, Eastern Mediterranean Regional Office. *Coverage of maternity care in the Islamic Republic of Iran* (personal communication), 1989.

WHE 2702   Malek-Afzali, H. Birth and death indicators in the Islamic Republic of Iran in 1984 and 1986. *Medical Journal of the Islamic Republic of Iran,* 1988; 2(4): 255-258.

WHE 2722   World Health Organization, *Maternal deaths and maternal mortality rates* (unpublished) 1990.

IRAQ

		Year	Source

1. BASIC INDICATORS

1.1 Demographic

1.1.1 Population

		Year	Source
Size (millions)	18.9	1990	(1915)
Rate of growth (%)	3.5	1985-90	(1915)

1.1.2 Life expectancy

Female	65	1985-90	(1915)
Male	63	1985-90	(1915)

1.1.3 Fertility

Crude Birth Rate	43	1985-90	(1915)
Total Fertility Rate	6.4	1985-90	(1915)

1.1.4 Mortality

Crude Death Rate	8	1985-90	(1915)
Infant Mortality Rate	69	1985-90	(1915)
Female			
Male			
1-4 years mortality rate			
Female			
Male			

1.2 Social and economic

1.2.1 Adult literacy rate (%)

Female	87	1985	(1914)
Male	90	1985	(1914)

1.2.2 Primary school enrolment rate (%)

Female	91	1985	(1914)
Male	105	1985	(1914)

1.2.3 Female mean age at first marriage
(years)

1.2.4 GNP/capita

(US$)	3 020	1987	(1914)

1.2.5 Daily per capita calorie supply

(as % of requirements)	124	1984-86	(1914)

2. HEALTH SERVICES

2.1 Health expenditure

2.1.1 Expenditure on health

(as % of GNP)	4.5	1983	(2033)

2.1.2 Expenditure on PHC
(as % of total health expenditure)

2.2 Primary Health Care
(Percentage of population covered by):

2.2.1 Health services

National1	93	1987	(2033)
Urban			
Rural			

2.2.2 Safe Water

National	90	1987	(2033)
Urban	95	1987	(2033)
Rural	85	1987	(2033)

2.2.3 Adequate sanitary facilities

National			
Urban	95	1987	(2033)
Rural	70	1987	(2033)

2.2.4 Contraceptive prevalence rate
(%)

2.3 Coverage of maternity care (%)

Area	Prenatal care	Trained attendant	Institutional deliveries	Postnatal care	Sample size	Year	Source
National	44	60				1985	(1888)
Abu-al-Khasib	54	73	75		178w	(1981)	(0702)
Baghdad		46	25		1 095w	1971	(0236)
Thiquar	44	5	2		123w	(1981)	(0702)

3. COMMUNITY STUDIES

3.1 National, 1977-89 [2728]

Maternal mortality was estimated using the "sisterhood method" in conjunction with a survey on immunization coverage and prevalence of diarrhoea among children. Interviews were conducted with over 8,100 ever married women of reproductive age who were questioned about deaths of sisters occurring since 1977. 420 deaths were identified of which 64 were classified, after analysis of the circumstances surrounding the death, as maternal. The maternal mortality rate was calculated on the basis of the total fertility rate of 6 as determined by the 1987 census. The lifetime risk of dying from pregnancy related causes was estimated as 1 in 143.

3.1.1 Rate

Maternal deaths	64
MMR (per 100 000 live births)	117

4. HOSPITAL STUDIES

5. CIVIL REGISTRATION DATA/GOVERNMENT ESTIMATES

6. OTHER SOURCES/ ESTIMATES

7. SELECTED ANNOTATED BIBLIOGRAPHY

8. FURTHER READING

9. DATA SOURCES

WHE 0236   Ghali, F. and Gadhalla, F. Fertility characteristics and family planning knowledge, attitudes and practices in Baghdad, Iraq. *Studies in Family Planning,* 1976; 4(6): 143-144

WHE 0702   Tikreeti, R.A.S. et al. A diagnostic study of pregnancy experiences of married women in Iraq. *International Journal of Health Education,* 1981; 4: 280-285

WHE 1888   World Health Organization, Eastern Mediterranean Regional Office, *Evaluation of the strategy for Health for All by the year 2000. Seventh report of the world health situation.* Alexandria, EMRO 1987

WHE 1914   United Nations Children's Fund (UNICEF). *The state of the world's children,* various years, Oxford, Oxford University Press

WHE 1915   United Nations. Department of International Economic and Social Affairs. *World population prospects: estimates and projections,* Population Studies, various years, New York 1986

WHE 2033   World Health Organization. *Global strategy for health for all by the year 2000. Second report on monitoring progress.* WHO document EB83/2 Add. 1, 1988

WHE 2728   United Nations Children's Fund *Iraq immunization, diarrhoeal disease, maternal and childhood mortality survey,* Evaluation series No. 9, UNICEF, Regional Office for the Middle East and North Africa, 1990.

ISRAEL

	Year	Source

1. BASIC INDICATORS

1.1 Demographic

1.1.1 Population

		Year	Source
Size (millions)	4.6	1990	(1915)
Rate of growth (%)	1.6	1985-90	(1915)

1.1.2 Life expectancy

		Year	Source
Female	77	1985-90	(1915)
Male	74	1985-90	(1915)

1.1.3 Fertility

		Year	Source
Crude Birth Rate	22	1985-90	(1915)
Total Fertility Rate	2.9	1985-90	(1915)

1.1.4 Mortality

		Year	Source
Crude Death Rate	7	1985-90	(1915)
Infant Mortality Rate	12	1985-90	(1915)
Female	13	1983	(0834)
Male	14	1983	(0834)
1-4 years mortality rate			
Female	1	1983	(0834)
Male	1	1983	(0834)

1.2 Social and economic

1.2.1 Adult literacy rate (%)

		Year	Source
Female	93	1985	(1914)
Male	97	1985	(1914)

1.2.2 Primary school enrolment rate (%)

		Year	Source
Female	97	1986-88	(1914)
Male	94	1986-88	(1914)

1.2.3 Female mean age at first marriage

		Year	Source
(years)	23.5	1983	(1918)

1.2.4 GNP/capita

		Year	Source
(US $)	6 800	1987	(1914)

1.2.5 Daily per capita calorie supply

		Year	Source
(as % of requirements)	118	1984-86	(1914)

2. HEALTH SERVICES

2.1 Health expenditure

2.1.1 Expenditure on health

		Year	Source
(as % of GNP)	7.5	1986	(2033)

2.1.2 Expenditure on PHC

		Year	Source
(as % of total health expenditure)	49	1987	(2033)

2.2 Primary Health Care
(Percentage of population covered by):

2.2.1 Health services

		Year	Source
National	100	1984	(0834)
Urban			
Rural			

2.2.2 Safe water

		Year	Source
National	98	1984	(0834)
Urban	100	1987	(2033)
Rural	97	1987	(2033)

2.2.3 Adequate sanitary facilities

		Year	Source
National	95	1984	(0834)
Urban	99	1987	(2033)
Rural	95	1987	(2033)

2.2.4 Contraceptive prevalence rate
(%)

2.3   Coverage of maternity care (%)

Area	Prenatal care	Trained attendant	Institutional deliveries	Postnatal care	Sample size	Year	Source
National			100			1980	(0357)
National	85	99				1984	(0834)
Refugee Camps:							
Gaza			60*		15 724d*	1986	(1628)
West Bank			53*		8 589d*	1986	(1628)

*   Percentages calculated on basis of expected deliveries as determined by birth rates.

3.   COMMUNITY STUDIES

4.   HOSPITAL STUDIES

4.1   Kaplan Hospital, Rehovot, 1954-76 [(0387)]

4.1.1   Rate

	Deliveries	Maternal deaths	MMR (per 100 000 births)
1954-61	19 090	10	52
1962-71	23 686	11	46
1972-76	21 221	6	28
1954-76	63 997	27	42

4.1.2   Causes of maternal deaths, 1954-76

	Number	%
Infection	5	19
Embolisms	5	19
Hypertensive disorders of pregnancy	4	15
Haemorrhage	3	11
Ruptured uterus	3	11
Complications of anaesthesia	3	11
Disseminated intravascular coagulation	2	7
DIRECT CAUSES	25	93
Cardiac diseases	2	7
TOTAL	27	100

5.   CIVIL REGISTRATION DATA/GOVERNMENT ESTIMATES

5.1   National, 1975-87 [(0753, 0834)]

5.1.1   Rate

Year	MMR (per 100 000 live births*)
1975	17
1976	9
1977	17
1978	10
1979	11
1980	5
1982	3
1983	2
1984	5
1985	8
1986	6
1987	3

*   Rates based on fewer than 30 maternal deaths

6. OTHER SOURCES/ ESTIMATES

6.1 National, 1962-71 [(0387)]

6.1.1 Rate

Year	MMR (per 100 000 deliveries)
1962	38
1963	44
1964	14
1965	41
1966	52
1967	30
1968	18
1969	36
1970	33
1971	16
1962-71	32

7. SELECTED ANNOTATED BIBLIOGRAPHY

8. FURTHER READING

Sabatello, E.F. Estimates of illegal abortions in Israel, 1980-83. *Israeli Journal of Medical Science,* 1990; 26: 204-209. WHE 2511

9. DATA SOURCES

WHE 0357   Israel, Central Bureau of Statistics. *Statistical abstract of Israel* 1982 No. 33. Jerusalem, 1982.

WHE 0387   Kessler, I. et al., Maternal mortality in an Israeli hospital: a review of 23 years. *International Journal of Gynaecology and Obstetrics,* 1979; 17(2): 154-158.

WHE 0753   United Nations, *Demographic Yearbook.* New York, various year

WHE 0834   World Health Organization *World health statistics annual – vital statistics and causes of death.* Geneva, various years.

WHE 1628   United Nations Relief and Works Agency for Pasestine refugees in the near East. *Annual report of the director of health 1986.* UNRWA, Vienna, 1987.

WHE 1914   United Nations Children's Fund (UNICEF). *The state of the world's children,* Oxford, Oxford University Press, various years.

WHE 1915   United Nations. Department of International Economic and Social Affairs. *World population prospects: estimates and projections,* Population Studies, New York, various years.

WHE 1918   United Nations. Department of International Economic and Social Affairs. *First marriage: patterns and determinants.* New York,1988.

WHE 2033   World Health Organization. *Global strategy for health for all by the year 2000. Second report on monitoring progress.* WHO document EB83/2 Add. 1, 1988.

NOTES

JORDAN

		Year	Source

1. BASIC INDICATORS

1.1 Demographic

1.1.1 Population

		Year	Source
Size (millions)	4.3	1990	(1915)
Rate of growth (%)	3.9	1985-90	(1915)

1.1.2 Life expectancy

Female	68	1985-90	(1915)
Male	64	1985-90	(1915)

1.1.3 Fertility

Crude Birth Rate	46	1985-90	(1915)
Total Fertility Rate	7.2	1985-90	(1915)

1.1.4 Mortality

Crude Death Rate	6.6	1985-90	(1915)
Infant Mortality Rate	44	1985-90	(1915)
Female*	62	1983	(1539)
Male*	40	1983	(1539)
1-5 years mortality rate			
Female*	17	1983	(1539)
Male*	6	1983	(1539)

* Squatter areas only.

1.2 Social and economic

1.2.1 Adult literacy rate (%)

Female	63	1985	(1914)
Male	87	1985	(1914)

1.2.2 Primary school enrolment rate (%)

Female	99	1986-88	(1914)
Male	98	1986-88	(1914)

1.2.3 Female mean age at first marriage

(years)	22.6	1981	(1918)

1.2.4 GNP/capita

		Year	Source
(US $)	1 560	1987	(1914)

1.2.5 Daily per capita calorie supply

(as % of requirements)	121	1984-86	(1914)

2. HEALTH SERVICES

2.1 Health Expenditure

2.1.1 Expenditure on health

(as % of GNP)	5.9	1987	(2033)

2.1.2 Expenditure on PHC

(as % of total health expenditure)	13	1985	(2033)

2.2 Primary Health Care
(Percentage of population covered by):

2.2.1 Health services

National	80	1983	(0834)
Urban			
Rural			

2.2.2 Safe water

National	97	1984	(0834)
Urban	100	1984	(0834)
Rural	90	1984	(0834)

2.2.3 Adequate sanitary facilities

National	98	1984	(0834)
Urban	100	1984	(0834)
Rural	95	1984	(0834)

2.2.4 Contraceptive prevalence rate

(%)	26	1983	(1712)

2.3   Coverage of maternity care (%)

Area	Prenatal care	Trained attendant	Institutional deliveries	Postnatal care	Sample size	Year	Source
National	58	75			–	1983	(1888)
National: urban	71	86			–	1983	(1888)
National: urban	81	90	82		210	1986	(1788)
National: rural	40	63			–	1983	(1888)
National: rural	68	69	61		212	1986	(1788)
Amman	80	89	71		215	1982	(0802)
Amman squatter areas		74	50		246w	1985	(1539)
Other than Amman	56	56	47		211w	1982	(0802)
Refugee Camps	80	98	45		209w	1982	(0802)
Refugee Camps	45*		27*		22 517d*	1986	(1628)

*   Percentages calculated on basis of expected deliveries as determined by birth rates.

3.   COMMUNITY STUDIES

4.   HOSPITAL STUDIES

4.1   26 hospitals throughout the country, 1979 (0704)

4.1.1   Rate

Deliveries	31 018
Maternal deaths	15
MMR (per 100 000 deliveries)	48

A morbidity study carried out in 1974 in the same hospitals revealed that there were 20 deaths among 19 327 admissions for abortions, pregnancy complications and deliveries, a death rate of 103 per 100 000 admissions.

7.   SELECTED ANNOTATED BIBLIOGRAPHY

Amr, M.F. Genito-urinary fistula in Jordan. Study of 72 cases. *Journal of the Kuwait Medical Association,* 1979; 13: 175-180. WHE 1044

Seventy-two cases of urinary fistulae were treated in the maternity departments of Bashir and Jordan University Hospitals, Amman, during a period of 8 years (1970-78). However, 52 of these cases (72%) occurred in the first four years of the study, indicating that in spite of the fact that most of the 8 000 annual deliveries are unbooked, intranatal care improved in the second part of the decade. Fifty-two cases (72%) of fistula were due to obstetric causes – operative or traumatic deliveries, with 17 due to prolonged labour with necrosis. Most of the women were multiparae (only 3 were primiparae), with the highest percentage (69%) being grand multiparae (5 children and over). Successful repair was achieved in 62 cases (86%). The study stresses the importance of nursing care particularly in relation to catheter problems, in improving results of repair.

Bisharat, L. and Zagha, H. *Health and population in squatter areas of Jordan: a reassessment after four years of upgrading.* Urban Development Department, The Hashemite Kingdom of Jordan, 1986. WHE 1539

In 1980 the Urban Development Department undertook interventions to upgrade housing in poor urban areas and to assist families to improve their own health status. The health of infants and children was selected as a sensitive indicator of overall progress. In 1985 follow-up surveys were conducted to determine to what extent the situation had changed since the baseline survey of 1980. It was found that while there had been a dramatic upgrading of certain facilities, in particular, of environmental sanitation and housing and while both infant and child mortality rates had fallen, there remained discrepancies in health indicators for boys and for girls. On the whole, boys benefitted more than girls from the improvements and sex differentials remained marked. Nutritional status of boys was markedly better than that of girls and girls were less likely to have been immunized than boys. However, three-quarters of the girls aged 15-19 years had completed secondary school and school attendance rates for those under 15 years were high and similar for both boys and girls.

Tekçe, B. and Shorter, F.C. Determinants of child mortality: a study of squatter settlements in Jordan. *Population Development Review,* 1984; suppl 10: 257-280. WHE 1332

The article examines in greater depth the results of the urban upgrading project described above and analyses some of the reasons for the continuance of sex differentials in childhood health indicators. It was found that parental education favours immunization and that more parental concern is shown for boys than for girls. Male children were brought to the local hospital substantially more often than female children and the latter were significantly more seriously ill than male children when brought for treatment. Girls were taken off breast milk earlier than boys though the authors point out that whether or not this is detrimental to their health will depend on the quality of the alternatives adopted which was not examined in this study. However, 29% of boys and 45% of girls were below the standard weight for age and 6% of boys and 13% of girls were malnourished.

8. FURTHER READING

Abbas, A.A. and Walker, G.J.A. Determinants of the utilization of maternal and child health services in Jordan. *International Journal of Epidemiology,* 1986; 15: 403-406. WHE 1490

Cook, R. and Hanslip, A. Nutrition and mortality of females under 5 years of age compared with males in the "Greater Syria" Region. *The Journal of Tropical Pediatrics,* 1964; 76-81. WHE 1273

Population Council, *A baseline health and population assessment for the upgrading of areas of Amman,* Giza, Egypt, 1982. WHE 1582

9. DATA SOURCES

WHE 0704   Tindall, V.R. *Report on the establishment of a system of confidential enquiries into maternal deaths in Jordan,* (unpublished WHO document), 1982.

WHE 0802   World Health Organization. Expanded Programme on Immunization. *Review of expanded programme on immunization, maternal and child health services,* (unpublished WHO document No. EM/MCH/168), 1982.

WHE 0834   World Health Organization *World health statistics annual – vital statistics and causes of death.* Geneva, various years.

WHE 1539   Bisharat, L. and Zagha, H. Health and population in squatter areas of Amman: a reassessment after four years of upgrading. (unpublished), 1986.

WHE 1628   United Nations Relief and Works Agency for Palestine refugees in the Near East. *Annual report of the director of health 1986.* UNRWA, Vienna, 1987.

WHE 1712   Mauldin W.P. and Segal, *Prevalence of contraceptive use in developing countries. A chart book.* Rockefeller Foundation, New York 1986.

WHE 1788   World Health Organization. Expanded Programme on Immunization. *Review of EPI and CDD programmes in the Hashemite Kingdom of Jordan.* (unpublished), September 15 – October 4 1986.

WHE 1888   World Health Organization, Eastern Mediterranean Regional Office, *Evaluation of the strategy for Health for All by the year 2000. Seventh report of the world health situation.* Alexandria, EMRO 1987.

WHE 1914   United Nations Children's Fund (UNICEF). *The state of the world's children,* Oxford, Oxford University Press, various years.

WHE 1915   United Nations. Department of International Economic and Social Affairs. *World population prospects: estimates and projections,* Population Studies, New York, various years.

WHE 1918   United Nations. Department of International Economic and Social Affairs. *First marriage: patterns and determinants.* New York, 1988.

WHE 2033   World Health Organization. *Global strategy for health for all by the year 2000. Second report on monitoring progress.* WHO document EB83/2 Add. 1, 1988.

KUWAIT

		Year	Source

1. BASIC INDICATORS

1.1 Demographic

1.1.1 Population

		Year	Source
Size (millions)	2.0	1990	(1915)
Rate of growth (%)	4.0	1985-90	(1915)

1.1.2 Life expectancy

Female	75	1985-90	(1915)
Male	71	1985-90	(1915)

1.1.3 Fertility

Crude Birth Rate	32	1985-90	(1915)
Total Fertility Rate	4.8	1985-90	(1915)

1.1.4 Mortality

Crude Death Rate	3	1985-90	(1915)
Infant Mortality Rate	19	1985-90	(1915)
Female	26	1979-81	(1917)
Male	31	1979-81	(1917)
1-4 years mortality rate			
Female	1	1979-81	(1917)
Male	1	1979-81	(1917)

1.2 Social and economic

1.2.1 Adult literacy rate (%)

Female	63	1985	(1914)
Male	76	1985	(1914)

1.2.2 Primary school enrolment rate (%)

Female	92	1986-88	(1914)
Male	95	1986-88	(1914)

1.2.3 Female mean age at first marriage

(years)	22.9	1985	(1918)

1.2.4 GNP/capita

		Year	Source
(US $)	14 610	1987	(1914)

1.2.5 Daily per capita calorie supply
(as % of requirements)

2. HEALTH SERVICES

2.1 Health Expenditure

2.1.1 Expenditure on health

(as % of GNP)	6	1983	(1888)

2.1.2 Expenditure on PHC
(as % of total health

expenditure)	20	1984-85	(2033)

2.2 Primary Health Care
(Percentage of population covered by):

2.2.1 Health services

National	100	1985	(0834)
Urban	100	1987	(2033)
Rural	99	1987	(2033)

2.2.2 Safe water

National	100	1985	(0834)
Urban	100	1985	(0834)
Rural	100	1985	(0834)

2.2.3 Adequate sanitary facilities

National	100	1985	(0834)
Urban	100	1985	(0834)
Rural	100	1985	(0834)

2.2.4 Contraceptive prevalence rate
(%)

2.3 Coverage of maternity care (%)

Area	Prenatal care	Trained attendant	Institutional deliveries	Postnatal care	Sample size	Year	Source
National	99	99				1985	(0834)

3. COMMUNITY STUDIES

4. HOSPITAL STUDIES

4.1 Kuwait Maternity Hospital, and MCH centres, 1969-80 [0424, 0556, 2250]

4.1.1 Rate

	Hospital	MCH centres	Total
Deliveries	226 772	218 729	445 501
Maternal deaths	82	11	93
MMR (per 100 000 deliveries)	36	5	21

4.1.2 Causes of maternal deaths *(for 50 deaths occurring over the period 1969-73)*

	Number	%
Hypertensive disorders of pregnancy	11	22
Complications of ceasarean section	10	14
Ruptured uterus	6	12
Abortions	2	4
Haemorrhage	2	8
Difficult labour and forceps delivery	2	4
Sepsis	1	6
Obstetric shock	1	2
DIRECT CAUSES	35	70
Chest and cerebral complications	10	20
Hepatitis	2	4
Cardiac diseases	1	2
Others	2	2
INDIRECT CAUSES	15	30
TOTAL	50	100

There was an increase in the rate of ceasarean section from 1.1% in 1960 to 4.3% during 1969-73 and 8.3% in 1980. Caesarean delivery had a mortality rate of 212 per 100 000 deliveries compared with 20 per 100 000 for vaginal deliveries.

4.1.3 Avoidable factors

4.1.4 High risk groups

4.1.5 Other findings

The report notes the almost total disappearance of the custom of vaginal packing with salt which was carried out to remedy supposed postpartum vaginal laxity. A not uncommon consequence was atresia of the cervix, the ensuing fibrosis leading to cervical dystocia during subsequent delivery.

4.2 National, 1980 [0715]

4.2.1 Rate

A WHO consultant assignment report found three maternal deaths in 1980 all of which occurred in Kuwait Maternity Hospital, an institutional maternal mortality rate of 10 per 100 000 live births.

5. CIVIL REGISTRATION DATA/GOVERNMENT ESTIMATES

5.1 National, 1976 [0424]

5.1.1 Rate

A government source gives a maternal mortality rate of 18 per 100 000 live births.

5.2 National, 1972-86 [0834, 2722]

5.2.1 Rate

	Live births	Maternal deaths	MMR (per 100 000 live births)
1972	–	–	13
1978	–	–	10
1980	–	–	7
1982	54 257	10	18
1983	55 617	7	13
1985	55 036	2	4
1986	53 786	3	6
1987	–	1	2

6. OTHER SOURCES/ ESTIMATES

7. SELECTED ANNOTATED BIBLIOGRAPHY

8. FURTHER READING

9. DATA SOURCES

WHE 0424   Mahran, M. The extent of the problem of eclampsia in Arab countries. In: *WHO meeting on hypertensive diseases of pregnancy, childbirth and the puerperium.* (unpublished WHO document no. MCH/TP/77.5), Geneva, 1977.

WHE 0556   Naim, A. and Hassan, H. Obstetric features in Kuwait: a reappraisal. *Journal of the Kuwait Medical Association,* 1974; 8(3): 125-134.

WHE 0715   Trussell, R.T. *Maternal health – Kuwait,* (unpublished WHO document no. EM/MCH/ 167), 1982

WHE 0834   World Health Organization *World health statistics annual – vital statistics and causes of death.* Geneva, various years.

WHE 1888   World Health Organization, Eastern Mediterranean Regional Office, *Evaluation of the strategy for Health for All by the year 2000. Seventh report of the world health situation.* EMRO,Alexandria, 1987.

WHE 1914   United Nations Children's Fund (UNICEF). *The state of the world's children,* Oxford, Oxford University Press, various years.

WHE 1915   United Nations. Department of International Economic and Social Affairs. *World population prospects: estimates and projections,* Population Studies, New York, various years.

WHE 1917   United Nations. Department of International Economic and Social Affairs. *Age structure of mortality in developing countries. A database for cross-sectional and time-series research.* New York, 1986.

WHE 1918   United Nations. Department of International Economic and Social Affairs. *First marriage: patterns and determinants.* NewYork,1988.

WHE 2033   World Health Organization. *Global strategy for health for all by the year 2000. Second report on monitoring progress.* WHO document EB83/2 Add. 1, 1988.

WHE 2250   Fahmy, K. Maternal mortality in Kuwait: a 12-year study (1969-80). Proceedings of an international conference, Cairo. In: Fayad, M.M. and Abdalla, M.I. (eds.) *Medical education in the field of primary maternal and child health,* 1983.

WHE 2722   World Health Organization, *Maternal deaths and maternal mortality rates* (unpublished) 1990.

NOTES

LAO PEOPLE'S DEMOCRATIC REPUBLIC

		Year	Source

1. BASIC INDICATORS

1.1 Demographic

1.1.1 Population

Size (millions)	4.1	1990	(1915)
Rate of growth (%)	2.5	1985-90	(1915)

1.1.2 Life expectancy

Female	50	1985-90	(1915)
Male	47	1985-90	(1915)

1.1.3 Fertility

Crude Birth Rate	41	1985-90	(1915)
Total Fertility Rate	5.7	1985-90	(1915)

1.1.4 Mortality

Crude Death Rate	16	1985-90	(1915)
Infant Mortality Rate	110	1985-90	(1915)
Female			
Male			
1-4 years mortality rate			
Female			
Male			

1.2 Social and economic

1.2.1 Adult literacy rate (%)

Female	76	1985	(1914)
Male	92	1985	(1914)

1.2.2 Primary school enrolment rate (%)

Female	85	1986-88	(1914)
Male	102	1986-88	(1914)

1.2.3 Female mean age at first marriage
(years)

1.2.4 GNP/capita

(US $)	170	1987	(1914)

1.2.5 Daily per capita calorie supply

(as % of requirements)	104	1984-86	(1914)

2. HEALTH SERVICES

2.1 Health expenditure

2.1.1 Expenditure on health

(as % of GNP)	2.0	1988	(3153)

2.1.2 Expenditure on PHC

(as % of total health expenditure)	50	1984	(1488)

2.2 Primary Health Care
(Percentage of population covered by):

2.2.1 Health services

National	67	1984	(0834)
Urban			
Rural			

2.2.2 Safe water

National	28	1990	(3153)
Urban	31	1990	(3153)
Rural	25	1990	(3153)

2.2.3 Adequate sanitary facilities

National	19	1990	(3153)
Urban	30	1990	(3153)
Rural	8	1990	(3153)

2.2.4 Contraceptive prevalence rate
(%)

2.3 Coverage of maternity care (%)

Area	Prenatal care	Trained attendant	Institutional deliveries	Postnatal care	Sample size	Year	Source
National		15				1974	(0796)
5 provinces and Vientiane	23*	71	69			1988	(2422)
5 provinces							
Municipality of Vientiane (rural areas):							
Hatxayphong	43		9		2 700b	1990	(2721)
Naxaythong	49		6		1 600b	1990	(2721)
Settatirath	16				9 900b	1990	(2721)
Xaythany	33		9		3 400b	1990	(2721)
Province of Vientiane (rural):							
Keo Oudom	17		6		740b**	1990	(2721)
Phone Hong	10				2 530b**	1990	(2721)
Toulakhoum	26		3		1 870b**	1990	(2721)
Province of Savannakhet:							
Champhone	42		1		3 420b**	1990	(2721)
Khanthaboury	36		26		5 040b**	1990	(2721)
Sonbouri	5		1		1 350b**	1990	(2721)
Xaiboury	3		1		1 600b**	1990	(2721)
Vientiane			50			(1987)	(1937)

*   Women receiving at least two prenatal visits
**   Estimated

3. COMMUNITY STUDIES

4. HOSPITAL STUDIES

4.6 Provincial Hospitals, 1986-87 [1948]

4.6.1 Rate

	Deliveries	Maternal deaths	MMR (per 100 000 deliveries)
1986	10 011	28	280
1987*	4 103	23	561

*   January-June

4.6.2 Causes of maternal deaths

Haemorrhage, anaemia, malaria, postpartum infections and eclampsia were reported as the most frequent causes of maternal deaths. Malaria was common among pregnant women, and was sometimes complicated by cerebral invasion.

5. CIVIL REGISTRATION DATA/GOVERNMENT ESTIMATES

5.1 Five provinces and Vientiane, 1988 and 1989 [2422]

5.1.1 Rate

	MMR (per 100 000 live births)
1988	282
1989	374

5.1.2 Causes of maternal deaths

The main causes of death were haemorrhage, malaria, anaemia and hypertensive disorders of pregnancy, in that order.

5.2 National, 1989 [2422]

5.2.1 Rate

MMR (per 100 000 live births)   460

5.3 National 1991 [3153]

5.3.1 Rate

MMR (per 100 000 live births)   300

6. OTHER SOURCES/ ESTIMATES

6.1 National, 1984 [1919]

6.1.1 Rate

A 1984 report for the World Health Organization quoted a maternal mortality rate of 200 per 100 000 live births.

6.2 National, 1990 [2721]

6.2.1 Rate

A consultant report quotes a maternal mortality rate of 350 per 100 000 live births for the country as a whole and up to 550 per 100 000 in some provinces.

6.2.2 Causes of maternal deaths

The major direct causes of maternal mortality were postpartum haemorrhage and retained placenta, obstructed labour and eclampsia. The main problems encountered during pregnancy were malaria leading to anaemia and abortion; poor diet and excessive labour during pregnancy leading to intrauterine malnutrition, foetal loss and low birth weight; frequent pregnancy and short birth intervals; and abortions, both spontaneous and induced.

6.2.3 Avoidable factors

The quality of prenatal care was sometimes inadequate and levels of utilization were low. Those who attended were more likely to be the better educated middle classes than the high risk families most in need. Transport difficulties, lack of understanding of the importance of health care during pregnancy and poor staff/patient communication are thought to be contributory factors. Facilities for safe hospital delivery were limited and few district level hospitals had the skills or equipment to deal with common obstetric emergencies.

7. SELECTED ANNOTATED BIBLIOGRAPHY

8. FURTHER READING

Leroy, O. *Mission report – Lao People's Democratic Republic*, Regional Office for the Western Pacific, Manila, 1988. WHE 2213

In 1983 six provinces were selected as pilot areas for maternal health activities. Using the 1985 population census data for these provinces, it was found that during 1986-87 only 25% of "expected" births were notified to MCH centres. Maternal deaths were also underreported.

Province	Expected/Notified maternal births*			Expected/Notified maternal deaths**		
	(1) No.	(2) No.	(2/1) %	(3) No.	(4) No.	(4/3) %
Municipal Vientiane	10 964	3 789	35	26	4	15
Vientiane	3 100	1 473	48	8	7	88
Khantouane	7 780	1 535	20	19	19	100
Savannakhet	15 528	1 088	7	39	3	8
Champassais	8 727	2 419	28	22	21	95
Luang Prabang	6 250	2 634	42	15	17	113
Total	52 349	12 938	25	130	71	55

*   Birth rate based on 1985 population census, 4.6%.

**   Assuming a maternal mortality rate of 240 per 100 000 births.

9. DATA SOURCES

WHE 0796   World Health Organization. *Global strategy for health for all by the year 2000*. Thirty-sixth World Health Assembly. (WHO document no. A36/INF.DOC/1), WHO, Geneva, 1983.

WHE 0834   World Health Organization *World health statistics annual – vital statistics and causes of death*. Geneva, various years.

WHE 1488   World Health Organization. Regional Office for the Western Pacific. *Evaluation of the strategy for health for all by the year 2000*. Seventh report on the world health situation, Manila, 1980.

WHE 1914   United Nations Children's Fund (UNICEF). *The state of the world's children*, Oxford, Oxford University Press, various years.

WHE 1915   United Nations. Department of International Economic and Social Affairs. *World population prospects: estimates and projections*, Population Studies, New York, various years.

WHE 1919   Kalicinski, K. *Assignment report – Laos*. Regional Office for the Western Pacific, Manila, 1987.

WHE 1948   Gallippi, G. *Assignment report – Laos*. Regional Office for the Western Pacific, Manila, 1988.

WHE 2422   Khamphong Khamoung and Douangdao Soukaloun, *Country report – Lao People's Democratic Republic*, Regional Office for the Western Pacific, Manila, 1989.

WHE2721   Hort, K.P *Mission report – Lao Peoples' Democratic Republic*. (unpublished document no. (WP)MCH/LAO/MCH/001-A), WPRO, 1991.

WHE 3153   World Health Organization. Western Pacific Regional Office. *Country data sheets*. (unpublished), 1991.

LEBANON

		Year	Source

1. BASIC INDICATORS

1.1 Demographic

1.1.1 Population

Size (millions)	3.0	1990	(1915)
Rate of growth (%)	2.1	1985-90	(1915)

1.1.2 Life expectancy

Female	69	1985-90	(1915)
Male	65	1985-90	(1915)

1.1.3 Fertility

Crude Birth Rate	29	1985-90	(1915)
Total Fertility Rate	3.4	1985-90	(1915)

1.1.4 Mortality

Crude Death Rate	7.8	1985-90	(1915)
Infant Mortality Rate	40	1985-90	(1915)
Female			
Male			
1-4 years mortality rate			
Female			
Male			

1.2 Social and economic

1.2.1 Adult literacy rate (%)

Female	69	1985	(1914)
Male	86	1985	(1914)

1.2.2 Primary school enrolment rate (%)

Female	95	1986-88	(1914)
Male	105	1986-88	(1914)

1.2.3 Female mean age at first marriage
(years)

1.2.4 GNP/capita
(US $)

1.2.5 Daily per capita calorie supply

(as % of requirements)	125	1984-86	(1914)

2. HEALTH SERVICES

2.1 Health expenditure

2.1.1 Expenditure on health

(as % of GNP)	10	1983	(2033)

2.1.2 Expenditure on PHC
(as % of total health expenditure)

2.2 Primary Health Care
(Percentage of population covered by):

2.2.1 Health services

National	95	1985	(0834)
Urban			
Rural			

2.2.2 Safe water

National	98	1985	(0834)
Urban	98	1985	(0834)
Rural	98	1985	(0834)

2.2.3 Adequate sanitary facilities

National	75	1985	(0834)
Urban	94	1985	(0834)
Rural	18	1985	(0834)

2.2.4 Contraceptive prevalence rate

(%)	55	1971	(1712)

2.3　Coverage of maternity care (%)

Area	Prenatal care	Trained attendant	Institutional deliveries	Postnatal care	Sample size	Year	Source
National		45				1976	(0834)
National	85					1985	(0834)
Refugee camps	50*		20*		7 069d*	1986	(1628)

* Percentages calculated on basis of expected deliveries as determined by birth rates.

3. COMMUNITY STUDIES

4. HOSPITAL STUDIES

4.1　American University of Beirut Medical Centre, 1971-82 [1110]

4.1.1　Rate

Live births	35 058
Maternal deaths	45
MMR (per 100 000 live births)	128

4.1.2　Causes of maternal deaths

	Number	%
Haemorrhage	11	24
Abortion	4	9
Sepsis	3	7
Hypertensive disorders of pregnancy	3	7
Ruptured uterus	2	4
Embolisms	2	4
Complications of anaesthesia	1	2
DIRECT CAUSES	26	58
Cerebrovascular accidents	5	12
Cardiac diseases	4	9
T.B. and tetanus	3	7
Hepatitis	1	2
Others	6	13
INDIRECT CAUSES	19	42
Total	45	100

4.1.3　Avoidable factors

	Booked	Unbooked
Maternal deaths	7	38
MMR (per 100 000 live births)	19	197

All the referred patients were admitted moribund and could have been saved had they had rapid access to a hospital with surgical and blood transfusion facilities.

4.1.4　High risk groups

5. CIVIL REGISTRATION DATA/GOVERNMENT ESTIMATES

6. OTHER SOURCES/ ESTIMATES

7. SELECTED ANNOTATED BIBLIOGRAPHY

8. FURTHER READING

9. DATA SOURCES

WHE 0834   World Health Organization *World health statistics annual – vital statistics and causes of death.* Geneva, various years.

WHE 1110   Mashini, I. et al. Maternal mortality in the American University of Beirut Medical Center (AUBMC) 1971-82.   *International Journal of Gynaecology and Obstetrics,* 1984; 22: 275-279.

WHE 1628   United Nations Relief and Works Agency for Palestine Refugees in the Near East. *Annual report of the director of health 1986,* Vienna, 1987.

WHE 1712   Mauldin W.P. and Segal, S.J., *Prevalence of contraceptive use in developing countries. A chart book.* Rockefeller Foundation, New York, 1986.

WHE 1914   United Nations Children's Fund (UNICEF). *The state of the world's children,* Oxford, Oxford University Press, various years.

WHE 1915   United Nations. Department of International Economic and Social Affairs. *World population prospects: estimates and projections,* Population Studies, New York, various years.

WHE 2033   World Health Organization. *Global strategy for health for all by the year 2000. Second report on monitoring progress.* WHO document EB83/2 Add. 1, 1988.

NOTES

MALAYSIA

	Year	Source

1. BASIC INDICATORS

1.1 Demographic

1.1.1 Population

		Year	Source
Size (millions)	17.9	1990	(1915)
Rate of growth (%)	2.6	1985-90	(1915)

1.1.2 Life expectancy

		Year	Source
Female	72	1985-90	(1915)
Male	68	1985-90	(1915)

1.1.3 Fertility

		Year	Source
Crude Birth Rate	32	1985-90	(1915)
Total Fertility Rate	4.0	1985-90	(1915)

1.1.4 Mortality

		Year	Source
Crude Death Rate	6	1985-90	(1915)
Infant Mortality Rate	24	195-90	(1915)
Female	38	1969-71	(1917)
Male	50	1969-71	(1917)
1-4 years mortality rate			
Female	5	1969-71	(1917)
Male	5	1969-71	(1917)

1.2 Social and economic

1.2.1 Adult literacy rate (%)

		Year	Source
Female	65	1985	(1914)
Male	83	1985	(1914)

1.2.2 Primary school enrolment rate (%)

		Year	Source
Female	102	1986-88	(1914)
Male	102	1986-88	(1914)

1.2.3 Female mean age at first marriage

		Year	Source
(years)	23.5	1980	(1918)

1.2.4 GNP/capita

		Year	Source
(US $)	1 940	1988	(1914)

1.2.5 Daily per capita calorie supply

		Year	Source
(as % of requirements)	121	1984-86	(1914)

2. HEALTH SERVICES

2.1 Health expenditure

2.1.1 Expenditure on health

		Year	Source
(as % of GNP)	1.6	1986	(2033)

2.1.2 Expenditure on PHC

		Year	Source
(as % of total health expenditure)	24	1986	(2033)

2.2 Primary Health Care

(Percentage of population covered by):

2.2.1 Health services

National
Urban
Rural

2.2.2 Safe water

		Year	Source
National	71	1983	(0834)
Urban	100	1986	(2033)
Rural	66	1986	(2033)

2.2.3 Adequate sanitary facilities

		Year	Source
National	75	1980	(0834)
Urban	100	1986	(2033)
Rural	67	1986	(2033)

2.2.4 Contraceptive prevalence rate

		Year	Source
(%)	51	1980-88	(1914)

2.3   Coverage of maternity care (%)

Area	Prenatal care	Trained attendant	Institutional deliveries	Postnatal care	Sample size	Year	Source
National	65	82				1983	(1488)
Peninsular	75	86	54	49		1984	(1211)
Kerian dist.	79	77	38	71	4 577	1982	(0380)

3.   COMMUNITY STUDIES

3.1   Kerian district, 1976-82 [0380, 0838, 2065]

3.1.1   Rate

	Deliveries	Maternal deaths	MMR (per 100 000 deliveries)
1976	4 699	9	192
1977	4 687	7	149
1978	4 485	9	200
1979	4 643	5	108
1980	4 463	5	112
1981	4 738	4	84
1982	4 577	0	–
1983	4 524	5	109

Following the adoption of the "Risk Approach" in maternal and child health care in the district, hospital deliveries increased from 29% of the total in 1976 to 38% in 1982. Home deliveries by government midwives increased from 23% to 37% over the same period while conversely, deliveries by TBAs fell from 47% to 23% of the total.

3.1.2   Causes of maternal deaths

	1976-79	1980-82
Haemorrhage	16	6
Hypertensive disorders of pregnancy	4	0
Sepsis	3	0
Obstetric shock	1	0
Associated with caesarean section	0	1
Associated medical complications	3	1
Cardiac arrest	3	1
Total	30	9

3.2   Kuala Lumpur and Selangor, 1982-83 [0173, 1099]

3.2.1   Rate

	Deliveries	Maternal deaths	MMR (per 100 000 deliveries)
Kuala Lumpur			
1982	43 662	6	14
1983	n.a.	3	7
Selangor			
1982	31 678	24	76
1983	n.a.	24	70

3.2.2   Causes of maternal deaths

	Number	%
Haemorrhage	23	40
Sepsis	10	18
Hypertensive disorders of pregnancy	6	11
Embolisms	6	11
Cardiac diseases	5	9
Others	7	11
Total	57	100

3.3   Kedah State, 1984 [2278]

3.3.1   Rate

Maternal deaths	38
MMR (per 100 000 live births)	120

4. HOSPITAL STUDIES

4.1 Government Hospitals, Western Malaysia, 1967-69 [0438]

4.1.1 Rate
Deliveries	269 574
Maternal deaths	683
MMR (per 100 000 deliveries)	253

4.1.2 Causes of maternal deaths

	Number	%
Haemorrhage	329	48
Hypertensive disorders of pregnancy	89	13
Sepsis	46	7
Pulmonary embolism	12	2
Anaemia	7	1
Other complications of pregnancy, childbirth and the puerperium	171	25
Other associated causes	29	5
Total	683	100

Deaths classified under "other complications of pregnancy, childbirth and the puerperium" include obstructed and prolonged labours due to cephalo-pelvic disproportion, and cases of abnormal lie or presentation and ruptured uterus referred from the rural areas to the hospitals.

4.2 University Hospital, Kuala Lumpur, 1968-73 [0397]

4.2.1 Rate
Deliveries	13 200
Maternal deaths	13
MMR (per 100 000 deliveries)	98

4.2.2 Causes of maternal deaths

	Number
Eclampsia	4
Abortion	3
Sepsis	3
Pulmonary embolism	2
Pulmonary tuberculosis	1
Total	13

5. CIVIL REGISTRATION DATA/GOVERNMENT ESTIMATES

5.1 National, 1970-1988 [0379, 2257, 2860]

5.1.1 Rate
Peninsular Malaysia

	Maternal deaths	MMR (per 100 000 births)
1970	n.a.	148
1975	n.a.	83
1980	208	63
1985	248	37
1988	158	26

By state

	MMR (per 100 000 live births)	
	1970	1980
Perlis	266	69
Kedah	248	82
Perak	150	74
Penang	72	40
Selangor	76	38
N.Sembilan	91	17
Malacca	159	50
Johore	118	41
Pahang	180	151
Trengganu	261	118
Kelantan	219	79

5.1.2 Causes of maternal deaths *(for 158 deaths during 1989)*

	Number	%
Haemorrhage	38	24
Embolisms	23	15
Sepsis	19	12
Hypertensive disorders of pregnancy	14	9
Abortion	2	1
Ectopic pregnancy	1	1
Associated medical complications	21	13
Cardiac diseases	17	11
Unknown	13	8
Other	10	6
TOTAL	158	100

5.1.3 Avoidable factors *(for 930 deaths between 1978 and 1981)*

Factor *	Number	%
Government midwife called too late by TBA or relatives	182	20
Handled by TBA alone, no medical aid	164	18
Refusal to go to hospital	95	10
Poor road/public transport facilities	73	8
Ambulance arrived too late	18	2
No government midwife available	11	1
Died en route from one hospital to another	7	1
Government midwife came too late	5	1

*   Factors not mutually exclusive

5.1.5 High risk groups

Over half the deaths occurred among women with one or more high risk factors such as grand multiparity, general ill health, anaemia, malnutrition, poor obstetric history.

6. OTHER ESTIMATES/ SOURCES

6.1 National, 1982 [1417]

6.1.1 Rate

The WHO data bank for the region gives a maternal mortality rate of 50 per 100 000 live births for Peninsular Malaysia.

6.2 National, 1985 [2608]

6.2.1 Rate

MMR (per 100 000 live births)	40

7. SELECTED ANNOTATED BIBLIOGRAPHY

Ng, K.H. and Sinnathuray, T.A. Maternal mortality from septic abortions in University Hospital, Kuala Lumpur, from March 1968 to February 1974. *Medical Journal of Malaysia*, 1975; 30(1): 52-54. WHE 0491.

Over a six year period, 1968-74, there were 1,699 admissions for complications of abortion at the University Hospital Kuala Lumpur which resulted in four maternal deaths, a case fatality rate of 0.23%. The number of abortion cases admitted steadily increased over the period while the numbers of deliveries increased only slightly. The four abortion-related deaths were all the consequence of induced abortion and were considered to have been avoidable given better provision of contraceptive services.

Teo Yu Keng, M. et al. Septic induced abortion – a report of 100 cases in Sarawak. *Medical Journal of Malaysia*, 1982; 37(4): 322-325. WHE 1838.

Over a 28 month period in the Sarawak General Hospital, Kuching, there were 100 "confirmed" cases of septic induced abortion and a further 75 "suspect" cases. There were two maternal deaths.

Wilson, C.S. Food taboos of childbirth: the Malay example. *Ecology of Food and Nutrition*, 1973; 2: 267-274. WHE 0976.

Food taboos observed by women during pregnancy and the puerperium are described. Fifty women, randomly selected from a fishing village were observed. A varied, normal diet was continued throughout pregnancy but changed after delivery when "cold" foods such as fruits and vegetables and "toxic" foods such as fish were avoided. The authors assert that intake of essential nutrients was considerably lowered during lactation as a result of such dietary restrictions.

8. FURTHER READING

Figa-Talamanca, I. et al. Illegal abortion: an attempt to assess its cost to the health services and its incidence in the community. *International Journal of Health Services*, 1986; 16(3): 375-389. WHE 1601.

Leigh, B. *Social deprivation an obstetric problem? A study of obstetric outcome in squatter settlements in Kuala Lumpur, Malaysia.* (unpublished), Institute of Child Health, University of London, 1982. WHE 1560.

Ong, H.C. Obstetrical data in Malaysian aborigine women. *Tropical and Geographical Medicine*, 1974; 26: 384-388. WHE 1841.

Sinnathuray, T.A. et al. *Report on maternal health and early pregnancy wastage in Peninsular Malaysia.* Federation of Family Planning Associations, Kuala Lumpur, 1977. WHE 0660.

9. DATA SOURCES

WHE 0173   Adeeb, N. Report on maternal mortality for Selangor and Kuala Lumpur in 1982 and 1983. (unpublished), 1984.

WHE 0379   Karim, R. *Overview of maternal mortality in Malaysia and the application of the risk approach strategy in maternal health.* Seminar on maternal health. Kemenlerian Kesthatan, 1982.

WHE 0380   Karim, R. *Priorities for MCH/FP/HSR in Malaysia: application of the risk approach.* Paper presented to the Meeting of the Steering Committee of the Task Force on the Risk Approach and Programme Research in MCH/FP Care, Geneva, 1983.

WHE 0397   Kong, H. et al. Maternal mortality in University Hospital, Kuala Lumpur, Malaysia. *Medical Journal of Malaysia*, 1974; 28(4): 226-228.

WHE 0438   Marzuki, A. and Thambu, J.A. Maternal mortality in the government hospitals, West Malaysia 1967-1969. *Medical Journal of Malaysia*, 1973; 27(3): 203-206.

WHE 0834   World Health Organization. *World health statistics annual – vital statistics and causes of death.* Geneva, various years.

WHE 0838   Yadav, H. Study of maternal deaths in Kerian (1976-1980). *Medical Journal of Malaysia*, 1982; 37(2): 165-169.

WHE 1099   Adeeb, N. *Prevention of maternal mortality in Malaysia.* In: Interregional Meeting for the Prevention of Maternal Mortality, Geneva, 11-15 November 1985.

WHE 1211   Hu Ching-Li. Report on a field visit to Malaysia. (unpublished WHO document No. WPR/MCH/FR/2), Regional Office for the Western Pacific, Manila, 1985.

WHE 1417   World Health Organization. Regional Office for the Western Pacific. *Databank on socioeconomic and health indicators.* WPRO, Manila, 1985.

WHE 1488   World Health Organization, Regional Office for the Western Pacific. *Evaluation of the strategy for health for all by the year 2000.* Seventh report of the world health situation, WPRO, Manila, 1980.

WHE 1914   United Nations Children's Fund (UNICEF). *The state of the world's children*, Oxford, Oxford University Press, various years.

WHE 1915   United Nations. Department of International Economic and Social Affairs. *World population prospects: estimates and projections*, Population Studies, New York, various years.

WHE 1917   United Nations. Department of International Economic and Social Affairs. *Age structure of mortality in developing countries. A database for cross-sectional and time-series research.* New York 1986.

WHE 1918   United Nations. Department of International Economic and Social Affairs. *First marriage: patterns and determinants.* New York 1988.

WHE 2033   World Health Organization. *Global strategy for health for all by the year 2000. Second report on monitoring progress.* WHO document EB83/2 Add. 1, 1988.

WHE 2065   Yadav, H. Utilization of traditional birth attendants in MCH care in rural Malaysia. *Singapore Medical Journal*, 1987; 28(6): 520-525.

WHE 2257   Asian Parasite Control/Family Planning Conference. *A strategy for maternal and child health*, Proceedings of the 14th Conference, Dhaka, Bangladesh, 1987.

WHE 2278   Desa, S.L.J. *A proposal for the improvement of management of high risk mothers in the District of Padang*. Management workshop for health managers: problem-solving through the team approach (unpublished), 1986.

WHE 2608   United Nations Children's Fund, *1988 Asian and Pacific atlas of children in national development*. UNICEF/ESCAP, Bangkok, 1987.

WHE 2860   Karim, R. et al. *Briefing on the Safe Motherhood Initiative*. Public Health Institute, 1991.

MALDIVES

	Year	Source

1. BASIC INDICATORS

1.1 Demographic

1.1.1 Population

Size (millions)	0.2	1989	(1914)
Rate of growth (%)	3.2	1985-88	(0753)

1.1.2 Life expectancy

Female	64	1987	(0753)
Male	60	1987	(0753)

1.1.3 Fertility

Crude Birth Rate	43	1987	(0753)
Total Fertility Rate			

1.1.4 Mortality

Crude Death Rate	8	1987	(0753)
Infant Mortality Rate	50	1987	(2068)
Female	45	1987	(2068)
Male	54	1987	(2068)
1-4 years mortality rate			
Female*	16	1987	(2068)
Male*	19	1987	(2068)

    *   Under 5 years mortality rate

1.2 Social and economic

1.2.1 Adult literacy rate (%)

Female	60	1985	(0753)
Male	80	1985	(0753)

1.2.2 Primary school enrolment rate (%)

Female	
Male	

1.2.3 Female mean age at first marriage
(years)

1.2.4 GNP/capita

(US $)	410	1988	(1914)

1.2.5 Daily per capita calorie supply
(as % of requirements)

2. HEALTH SERVICES

2.1 Health Expenditure

2.1.1 Expenditure on health

(as % of GNP)	5	1986-87	(2033)

2.1.2 Expenditure on PHC

(as % of total health expenditure)	100	1986-87	(2033)

2.2 Primary Health Care
(Percentage of population covered by):

2.2.1 Health services

National	75	1986-87	(2033)
Urban			
Rural			

2.2.2 Safe Water

National	63	1985	(2068)
Urban	91	1987	(2033)
Rural	17	1987	(2033)

2.2.3 Adequate sanitary facilities

National			
Urban	100	1987	(2033)
Rural	2	1987	(2033)

2.2.4 Contraceptive prevalence rate
(%)

2.3   Coverage of maternity care (%)

Area	Prenatal care	Trained attendant	Institutional deliveries	Postnatal care	Sample size	Year	Source
National	99	61				1988	(2033)
National:							
rural		38				1982	(1489)
19 atolls	46	39			445	1983	(1323)
Male'	47	42				1982	(1489)

3. COMMUNITY STUDIES

4. HOSPITAL STUDIES

5. CIVIL REGISTRATION DATA/GOVERNMENT ESTIMATES

5.1   National, Male' and Atolls 1978-87 [2068]

5.1.1   Rate

MMR (per 100 000 live births)

	National	Male'	Atolls
1978	600	300	600
1979	700	400	800
1980	500	300	500
1981	400	300	500
1982	500	300	500
1983	600	400	600
1984	400	100	400
1985	300	100	400
1986	400	300	400
1987	500	500	500

5.2   National, 1986-87 [0753]

5.2.1   Rate

MMR (per 100 000 live births)

1986	685
1987	646

6. OTHER SOURCES/ ESTIMATES

6.1   National, (1989) [2379]

6.1.1   Rate
MMR (per 100 000 live births)   480

7. SELECTED ANNOTATED BIBLIOGRAPHY

8. FURTHER READING

9. DATA SOURCES

WHE 0753   United Nations, *Demographic Yearbook*. New York, various years.

WHE 0834   World Health Organization *World health statistics annual – vital statistics and causes of death*. Geneva, various years.

WHE 1323   Maldives, Ministry of Health. *Preliminary report of the 1983 health survey*. Male', 1983.

WHE 1489   World Health Organization. Regional Office for South East Asia. *Evaluation of the strategy for health for all by the year 2000*. Seventh report on the world health situation, SEARO, New Delhi, 1986.

WHE 1914   United Nations Children's Fund (UNICEF). *The state of the world's children*, Oxford, Oxford University Press, various years.

WHE 2033   World Health Organization. *Global strategy for health for all by the year 2000. Second report on monitoring progress*. WHO document EB83/2 Add. 1, 1988.

WHE 2068   Maldives, Ministry of Health. *A decade of primary health care 1978-87*. Ministry of Health, 1988.

WHE 2379   Shareef, J.A. *Country presentation – Maldives*, Intercountry workshop on the Safe Motherhood Initiative, WHO/SEARO, New Delhi, 6-10 November 1989.

NOTES

MONGOLIA

		Year	Source

1. BASIC INDICATORS

1.1. Demographic

1.1.1 Population

Size (millions)	2.2	1990	(1915)
Rate of growth (%)	3.1	1985-90	(1915)

1.1.2 Life expectancy

Female	66	1985-90	(1915)
Male	62	1985-90	(1915)

1.1.3 Fertility

Crude Birth Rate	39	1985-90	(1915)
Total Fertility Rate	5.4	1985-90	(1915)

1.1.4 Mortality

Crude Death Rate	8	1985-90	(1915)
Infant Mortality Rate	45	1985-90	(1915)
Female			
Male			
1-4 years mortality rate			
Female			
Male			

1.2 Social and economic

1.2.1 Adult literacy rate

Female	90	1985	(1914)
Male	95	1985	(1914)

1.2.2 Primary school enrolment rate

Female	103	1986-88	(1914)
Male	100	1986-88	(1914)

1.2.3 Female mean age at first marriage
(years)

		Year	Source

1.2.4 GNP/capita
(US $)

1.2.5 Daily per capita calorie supply

(as % of requirements)	116	1984-86	(1914)

2. HEALTH SERVICES

2.1 Health expenditure

2.1.1 Expenditure on health

(as % of GNP)	10	1980-85	(2033)

2.1.2 Expenditure on PHC
(as % of total health expenditure)

2.2 Primary Health Care
(Percentage of population covered by):

2.2.1 Health services

National	100	1987	(2033)
Urban			
Rural			

2.2.2 Safe Water

National	100	1987	(2033)
Urban	100	1987	(2033)
Rural	100	1987	(2033)

2.2.3 Adequate sanitary facilities

National	100	1987	(2033)
Urban	100	1987	(2033)
Rural	100	1987	(2033)

2.2.4 Contraceptive prevalence rate
(%)

2.3 Coverage of maternity care (%)

Area	Prenatal care	Trained attendant	Institutional deliveries	Postnatal care	Sample size	Year	Source
National	100					1987	(2033)
National			99			(1989)	(2378)
Ulan Bator	25	51		24		1980-81	(1295)

3. COMMUNITY STUDIES

4. HOSPITAL STUDIES

5. CIVIL REGISTRATION DATA/GOVERNMENT ESTIMATES

5.1 Ulan Bator, (1985) [(1295)]

5.1.1 Rate
MMR (per 100 000 pregnancies)   60-80

5.2 National (1989) [(2378)]

5.2.1 Rate
MMR (per 100 000 live births)   140

6. OTHER SOURCE/ ESTIMATES

6.1 National, 1978 [(1231)]

6.1.1 Rate
MMR (per 100 000 live births)   140

6.2 National, 1970, 1975, 1981 [(1522)]

6.2.1 Rate

	MMR (per 100 000 live births)
1970	180
1975	150
1981	100

7. SELECTED ANNOTATED BIBLIOGRAPHY

8. FURTHER READING

9. DATA SOURCES

WHE 1231   Lazarenko, A.I. and Batsukh, L. *Epidemiological studies of population growth and strengthening of MCH services in Mongolia* (Second phase). Unpublished WHO document No. SEA/MCH/175, 1985.

WHE 1295   Stembera, Z. *Perinatal care in Mongolia.* Unpublished document No. SEA/MCH/179, SEARO, 1985.

WHE 1522   World Health Organization. Southeast Asia Regional Office. *Bulletin of regional health information,* WHO/SEARO, New Delhi, 1986.

WHE 1914   United Nations Children's Fund (UNICEF). *The state of the world's children,* Oxford, Oxford University Press, various years.

WHE 1915   United Nations. Department of International Economic and Social Affairs. *World population prospects: estimates and projections,* Population Studies, New York, various years.

WHE 2033   World Health Organization. *Global strategy for health for all by the year 2000. Second report on monitoring progress.* WHO document EB83/2 Add. 1, 1988.

WHE 2378   Mongolia, *Country presentation.* Paper presented at workshop on safe motherhood. New Delhi, 6-10 November 1989.

MYANMAR

		Year	Source

1. BASIC INDICATORS

1.1 Demographic

1.1.1 Population
Size (millions)	4.2	1990	(1915)
Rate of growth (%)	2.1	1985-90	(1915)

1.1.2 Life expectancy
Female	62	1985-90	(1915)
Male	58	1985-90	(1915)

1.1.3 Fertility
Crude Birth Rate	31	1985-90	(1915)
Total Fertility Rate	4.0	1985-90	(1915)

1.1.4 Mortality
Crude Death Rate	10	1985-90	(1915)
Infant Mortality Rate	70	1985-90	(1915)
Female			
Male			
1-4 years mortality rate			
Female			
Male			

1.2 Social and economic

1.2.1 Adult literacy rate (%)
Female	70	1985	(2608)
Male	86	1985	(2608)

1.2.2 Primary school enrolment rate (%)
Female			
Male			

1.2.3 Female mean age at first marriage
(years)	22.4	1983	(1918)

		Year	Source

1.2.4 GNP/capita
(US $)	200	1987	(1914)

1.2.5 Daily per capita calorie supply
(as % of requirements)	119	1984-86	(1914)

2. HEALTH SERVICES

2.1 Health expenditure

2.1.1 Expenditure on health
(as % of GNP)	1.1	1986-87	(2033)

2.1.2 Expenditure on PHC
(as % of total health expenditure)	35	1986-87	(2033)

2.2 Primary Health Care
(Percentage of population covered by):

2.2.1 Health services
National	45	1985	(0834)
Urban			
Rural			

2.2.2 Safe water
National	25	1983	(0834)
Urban	37	1987	(2033)
Rural	27	1987	(2033)

2.2.3 Adequate sanitary facilities
National	20	1983	(0834)
Urban	35	1987	(2033)
Rural	26	1987	(2033)

2.2.4 Contraceptive prevalence rate
(%)	5	1980	(1913)

2.3   Coverage of maternity care (%)

Area	Prenatal care	Trained attendant	Institutional deliveries	Postnatal care	Sample size	Year	Source
National*		50	23			1985	(1289)
National**		49	5			1985	(1289)
National	75	25				1988	(2033)
Irrawaddy	81	65	12			1983	(0901)
Mandalay	73	74	14			1983	(0901)
Rakhine	83	70	29			1983	(0901)
Rangoon	99	94	76			1983	(0901)
Rangoon		65	14		6 000	1985	(1533)
Shau	87	89	44			1983	(0901)
Shwe Taung: rural	84	75			18 217	1980	(0698)

*   Areas where an EPI programme was in operation.
**   Areas where there was no EPI programme.

3.   COMMUNITY STUDIES

3.1.   North Okkalapa Township - Five urban administrative wards and 91 rural villages, 1981* [(0703)]

3.1.1   Rate

	Rural	Urban
MMR (per 100 000 deliveries)	230	80

*   year of publication of study

3.1.2   Causes of maternal deaths

3.1.3   Avoidable factors

3.1.4   High risk groups

3.1.5   Other findings
Complications occurred in 5.8% of pregnancies. The majority of pregnant women were moderately or severely anaemic. Only 17% of the rural women and 25% of the urban women in the sample were not anaemic. Abortion was frequent especially in the urban sample, accounting for 231 (15%) of the 1 512 pregnancies studied.

3.2   Random sample of 33 000 households, 1985 [(1289)]

3.2.1   Rate
The Government of Myanmar, in collaboration with WHO, conducted a survey in connection with the Expanded Programme on Immunization (EPI) and compared rates in areas covered by the EPI Programme and those not so covered.

MMR (per 100 000 live births)

Areas with an EPI programme	170
Areas with no EPI programme	100

4.   HOSPITAL STUDIES

4.1   Central Women's Hospital, Rangoon, 1973-77 [(0681)]

4.1.1   Rate
Live births	89 611
Maternal deaths	306
MMR (per 100 000 live births)	341

4.2 Workers' Hospital, Rangoon, 1983-87 [2361]

4.2.1 Rate

Deliveries	7 446
Maternal deaths*	8
MMR (per 100 000 deliveries)	107

* Including abortion deaths

There were 3 101 abortion patients treated at the hospital over the period 1983-87, of which six died, a case fatality rate of 194 per 100 000.

4.2.2 Causes of maternal deaths

	Number
Abortion	6
Embolism	1
Malaria	1
Total	8

4.3 Women's and Children's Hospital, South Okkalapa, 1978-1982 [2259]

4.3.1 Rate

Deliveries	22 468
Maternal deaths*	44
MMR (per 100 000 deliveries)	196

* Including abortion deaths

During the period 1978-82 there were 10,623 abortion cases treated at the hospital, of which 22 died, a case fatality rate of 207 per 100 000.

4.3.2 Causes of maternal deaths

	Number	%
Abortion	22	50
Haemorrhage	9	21
Hypertensive disorders of pregnancy	5	11
Sepsis	1	3
Blood transfusion reaction	1	3
Trophoblastic disease	1	3
DIRECT CAUSES	39	89
Cardiovascular disease	4	9
Fortuitous	1	3
TOTAL	44	100

4.3.3 Avoidable factors

Many patients did not understand the importance of prenatal care; others were under the misconception that one prenatal visit was sufficient. Grand multiparae were too occupied with household chores and were unable to find the time to attend clinics. Among deaths due to causes other than abortion avoidable factors included lack of education, patient cooperation, efficient and prompt blood transfusion, efficient communications and adequate prenatal, intranatal and postnatal care as well as lack of responsibility on the part of some of the medical staff.

5. CIVIL REGISTRATION DATA/GOVERNMENT ESTIMATES

5.1 National, 1970 and 1980, [0116, 0830]

5.1.1 Rate

The maternal mortality rate calculated from civil registration figures in 1970 was 130 per 100 000 live births. In 1980, an estimate based on registration data in selected towns produced a rate of 120 per 100 000 live births.

6. OTHER SOURCES/ ESTIMATES

6.1 National, 1960-81 [1522]

6.1.1 Rate

A World Health Organization report of regional health information gave the following rates:

	MMR (per 100 000 live births)
1960	420
1965	310
1970	130
1975	100
1981	460 *

* The 1981 figure is not comparable to estimates for earlier years because it is based on a newly-introduced system of registration in rural areas. The comparable civil registration rate for 1981 was 70 per 100 000 live births.

6.2 National, 1978 [0167]

6.2.1 Rate

An article in a publication of the International Planned Parenthood Federation gave a maternal mortality rate of 120 per 100 000 live births.

6.3 National, urban areas only, 1965-77 [0832]

6.3.1 Rate

	MMR (per 100 000 live births)
1965	310
1966	290
1971	190
1972	170
1977	100

6.4 National, 1981-82 [(0829)]

6.4.1 Rate

A World Health Organization report of regional health information quotes a rate of 140 per 100 000 live births.

6.5 National, 1982 (2608)

6.5.1 Rate

MMR (per 100 000 live births)   150

7. SELECTED ANNOTATED BIBLIOGRAPHY

World Health Organization. International Collaborative Study of Hypertensive Disorders of Pregnancy. Geographic variation in the incidence of hypertension in pregnancy *American Journal of Obstetrics and Gynecology,* 1988; 158(1): 80-83. WHE 2552.

Prospectively collected information on blood pressure and proteinuria was available for primigravidas in a periurban area (North Okkalapa, 1398 subjects) and two rural areas (Hlegu, 890 subjects and Hmawbi, 477 subjects). Clinical diagnosis of hypertensive disorders of pregnancy was made in over 5% of the women in Burma. Proteinuric preeclampsia occurred in 4.4% of the women and eclampsia in 0.4% of the subjects (multigravidas and primigravidas). Similar studies were carried out in Viet Nam, Thailand and China. There were marked differences in the incidence of hypertensive disorders in the four countries under study (see relevant country profiles).

8. FURTHER READING

9. DATA SOURCES

WHE 0116   Burma, Ministry of Health. *Health report of the Director General,* Rangoon, 1971.

WHE 0167   Dalibor, G. Burma trains health volunteers. *People,* 1983; 10(4): 30-31.

WHE 0681   Sulaiman, S. *Strengthening of maternal and child health programmes in Burma* (unpublished WHO document no. SEA/MCH/133), 1980.

WHE 0698   Thwin, K.M. *Rural household survey on health and health care (Shwe Taung Township),* Health Information Service, Burma, 1981.

WHE 0703   Tin, U. and Kyaw-Myint, T.O. eds. *Report of the perinatal mortality and low birth weight study project* Burma, SEARO Inter-country collaborative project, Department of Medical Education/ Ministry of Health, 1981.

WHE 0829   World Health Organization. Southeast Asia Regional Office. *Bulletin of Regional Health Information,* (unpublished WHO document No. SEA/VHS/165 Rev.1), New Delhi, 1981.

WHE 0830   World Health Organization. Southeast Asia Regional Office. *Maternal mortality,* (WHO internal memorandum), 1979.

WHE 0832   World Health Organization. Expanded programme on immunization, Programme review Burma. *Weekly Epidemiological Record,* 1984; 59(36): 273-276.

WHE 0834   World Health Organization *World Health Statistics annual – vital statistics and causes of death.* Geneva, various years.

WHE 0901   World Health Organization. Expanded Programme on Immunization, Programme review. *Weekly Epidemiological Record,* 1984; 59: 273-280.

WHE 1289   World Health Organization. Expanded Programme on Immunization. Neonatal tetanus mortality survey, Burma *Weekly Epidemiological Record,* 1985; 60(49): 377-380.

WHE 1522   World Health Organization. Southeast Asia Regional Office. *Bulletin of regional health information,* 1986.

WHE 1533   Stroh, G. et al. *Surveys to measure mortality from neonatal tetanus in the People's Socialist Republic of the Union of Burma* (unpublished report), 1986.

WHE 1913   United Nations. Department of International Economic and Social Affairs. *World population policies.* Volume I, New York, 1987.

WHE 1914   United Nations Children's Fund (UNICEF). *The state of the world's children,* Oxford, Oxford University Press, various years.

WHE 1915   United Nations. Department of International Economic and Social Affairs. *World population prospects: estimates and projections,* Population Studies, New York, various years.

WHE 1918   United Nations. Department of International Economic and Social Affairs. *First marriage: patterns and determinants.* New York, 1988.

WHE 2033   World Health Organization. *Global strategy for health for all by the year 2000. Second report on monitoring progress.* WHO document EB83/2 Add. 1, 1988.

WHE 2259   Ma Khin Kyi Maternal mortality at the Women's and Children's Hospital, South Okkalapa (1978-1982). *Australia and New Zealand Journal of Obstetrics and Gynaecology,* 1988; 28(1): 36-40.

WHE 2361   Ma Khin Kyi, Maternal mortality at the Workers' Hospital, Rangoon (1983-1987) *Australia and New Zealand Journal of Obstetrics and Gynaecology,* 1988; 159(1): 80-83.

WHE 2608 United Nations Children's Fund, *1988 Asian and Pacific atlas of children in national development.* UNICEF/ESCAP, Bangkok, 1987.

NOTES

NEPAL

		Year	Source

1. BASIC INDICATORS

1.1 Demographic

1.1.1 Population

		Year	Source
Size (millions)	19.1	1990	(1915)
Rate of growth (%)	2.5	1985-90	(1915)

1.1.2 Life expectancy

		Year	Source
Female	50	1985-90	(1915)
Male	52	1985-90	(1915)

1.1.3 Fertility

		Year	Source
Crude Birth Rate	40	1985-90	(1915)
Total Fertility Rate	5.9	1985-90	(1915)

1.1.4 Mortality

		Year	Source
Crude Death Rate	15	1985-90	(1915)
Infant Mortality Rate	128	1985-90	(1915)
Female	164	1974-76	(1917)
Male	169	1974-76	(1917)
1-4 years mortality rate			
Female	30	1974-76	(1917)
Male	28	1974-76	(1917)

1.2 Social and economic

1.2.1 Adult literacy rate (%)

		Year	Source
Female	12	1985	(1914)
Male	39	1985	(1914)

1.2.2 Primary school enrolment rate (%)

		Year	Source
Female	47	1986-88	(1914)
Male	104	1986-88	(1914)

1.2.3 Female mean age at first marriage

		Year	Source
(years)	17.9	1981	(1918)

1.2.4 GNP/capita

		Year	Source
(US $)	160	1987	(1914)

1.2.5 Daily per capita calorie supply

		Year	Source
(as % of requirements)	102	1984-86	(1914)

2. HEALTH SERVICES

2.1 Health expenditure

2.1.1 Expenditure on health

		Year	Source
(as % of GNP)	1	1980-85	(2033)

2.1.2 Expenditure on PHC

		Year	Source
(as % of total health expenditure)	69	1984-85	(1489)

2.2 Primary Health Care

(Percentage of population covered by):

2.2.1 Health services

National
Urban
Rural

2.2.2 Safe water

		Year	Source
National	16	1983	(0834)
Urban	77	1987	(2033)
Rural	24	1987	(2033)

2.2.3 Adequate sanitary facilities

		Year	Source
National	2	1983	(0834)
Urban	54	1987	(2033)
Rural	1	1987	(2033)

2.2.4 Contraceptive prevalence rate

		Year	Source
(%)	7	1981	(1712)

2.3   Coverage of maternity care (%)

Area	Prenatal care	Trained attendant	Institutional deliveries	Postnatal care	Sample size	Year	Source
National			4			1981	(0813)
National	17	10				1983	(1489)
National	9	6				1988	(2033)
Dhantuta: rural	9	5		7	102	(1977)	(0649)
Tanahu	4	4		7	95	(1977)	(0649)

3. COMMUNITY STUDIES

3.1   Rupandehi, Kabhrepalanchowk, and Kathmandu district, 1975-78 [0634, 1369]

3.1.1   Rate
Live births	1 650
Maternal deaths	14
MMR (per 100 000 live births)	848

3.2   Dhankuta district, 1977 [0649]

A study carried out by the Institute of Medicine sought to assess health and family planning needs in local communities as well as patterns of health service utilization.

3.2.1   Rate
Deliveries	96
Maternal deaths	2
MMR (per 100 000 deliveries)	2 083
MMR (per 100 000 women aged 15-44 years)	319

3.3   Jumla, 1981 [1369]

3.3.1   Rate
Live births	724
Maternal deaths	12
MMR (per 100 000 live births)	1 657

4. HOSPITAL STUDIES

4.1   Maternity Hospital, Kathmandu, 1979-85 [1228, 1513, 1691]

4.1.1   Rate

	Live births	Maternal deaths	MMR (per 100 000 live births)
1979-80	5 848	12	205
1980-81	6 321	20	316
1981-82	6 952	18	259
1982-83	7 048	7	99
1983-84	7 633	13	170
1984-85	9 043	11	122
1979-85	42 845	81	189

4.1.2   Causes of maternal deaths, 1979-85

	Number	%
Haemorrhage	30	37
Sepsis	14	17
Obstructed labour	7	9
Hypertensive disorders of pregnancy	6	7
Ruptured uterus	5	6
Embolisms	5	6
Complications of anaesthesia	2	3
DIRECT CAUSES	69	85
Anaemia	5	6
Liver disorders	1	1
Other infections	2	3
Others	4	5
INDIRECT CAUSES	12	15
TOTAL	81	100

4.1.3 Avoidable factors

40% of the women who died were admitted in a very poor condition and 17% were unconscious. 45 deaths occurred on the day of admission with 38 occurring within the first eight hours.

4.2 Koshi Anchal Hospital, August 1985 [1228, 1513, 1691]

4.2.1 Rate

Live births	136
Maternal deaths	4
MMR (per 100 000 live births)	294

5. CIVIL REGISTRATION DATA/GOVERNMENT ESTIMATES

6. OTHER SOURCES/ ESTIMATES

6.1 National, 1986 [1522]

6.1.1 Rate

According to the WHO 1986 Regional Health Information Bulletin the maternal mortality rate in Nepal was 850 per 100 000 live births.

6.2 National, 1986 [2257]

6.2.1 Rate

MMR (per 100 000 live births)	833

7. SELECTED ANNOTATED BIBLIOGRAPHY

Dali, S.K. *Obstetric fistulae in Nepal.* (Personal communication), Kathmandu, 1989. WHE 2267

The incidence of obstetric fistula at the Tribhuvan University Teaching Hospital, Kathmandu, Nepal, is reported to vary from 0.5% to 1% of gynaecological admissions. The occurrence of obstetric fistula is described as being an indicator of poor obstetric services, and also due to lack of transport, high illiteracy rate, lack of prenatal care, low socio-economic status, local customs and traditions of keeping delivery secret. Most women are young primiparae who lose their firstborn child due to prolonged neglected labour. They become social outcasts and some have to leave their native village. Even after being cured, many are not accepted by their husbands.

Dali, S.M. et al. *Final report: study on the knowledge, attitudes and practices of mothers-in-law regarding the intraconceptual care of their daughters-in-law before and after educational sessions.* (unpublished), Kathmandu, 1990. WHE 2800

In Nepalese society, where the extended family is the norm, the mother-in-law is often the key person in the family and is responsible for making decisions related to family welfare. In rural communities most deliveries are conducted by mothers-in-law who will seek additional help only if she thinks it is needed. Little or no prenatal care is sought, deliveries are often conducted under unhygienic conditions and certain food taboos are observed. A study was undertaken to examine the extent to which education about pregnancy and delivery might result in changes in the knowledge and attitudes of the mothers-in-law in the anticipation that this would lead to increased attendance for prenatal care and improved delivery practices.

The study was carried out in Mahankal and Bhadrakali rural areas of Kathmandu District. In general, the educational sessions were highly successful in raising the awareness of the mothers-in-law and had a particularly beneficial effect on attitudes towards prenatal care, extra food and rest during pregnancy, tetanus toxoid immunization and awareness of danger signs and risk factors during pregnancy However, there remained considerable room for improvement in actual practices. In some aspects (place of delivery, hand washing, expulsion of the placenta) the change in knowledge was not consistent with the practice patterns reported. It was concluded that culturally inherent beliefs are resistant to behavioural changes and that educational sessions need to examine in depth the relationships between attitudes and practices.

Karki, Y.B. Sex preferences and the value of sons and daughters in Nepal. *Studies in Family Planning*, 1988; 19(3): 169-178. WHE 2012

Surveys were undertaken during 1979 in two areas of the West Central hills of Nepal, Gorkha, a rural district, and Pokhara, a town. The total fertility rate was 6.4 in the rural area and 4.3 in the town. Contraceptive prevalence was very low. Ideal family size among all respondents was, on average, five children, with three sons and two daughters being the preferred composition for 90% of all respondents. Sons are valued for the role they play in family life, particularly in providing support in old age, death rituals and continuing the family name. Family size preferences and the decision to practise contraception were both affected by son preference. The proportion of couples with at least one living son who desired additional children was very low compared to those with no sons. In both the urban and the rural samples, virtually none of the couples without sons were practising contraception. Among those who reported current contraceptive use, the mean number of living sons was higher than the mean number of living daughters.

Reissland, N. and Burghart, R. Active patients: the integration of modern and traditional obstetric practices in Nepal. *Social Science and Medicine*, 1989; 29(1): 43-52. WHE 2160

The integration of modern and traditional obstetric practices in a provincial hospital in the Maithili-speaking area of Southern Nepal is described. The doctors and nurses consciously distance themselves from the traditional practices of their obstetrical patients, who they view as "ignorant".

However, because hospital resources are insufficient to impose the normative form of modern medical organization, patients and their relatives assert a more active role in providing hospital-based care. In consequence, mothers are delivered according to both modern, clinical as well as local cultural practices. The authors conclude that in poor countries, the integration of traditional healing within the national health system may not lie exclusively with the medical professions. Patients and others in their social networks constrain and negotiate the terms on which modern medicine is integrated within traditional obstetric practices.

Scholz, S. and Norkyel, K. *A review of 10 cases of urinary fistulae treated at Patan Hospital.* (Unpublished paper) Nepal, 1989. WHE 2178

From August 1986 to January 1989, 40 cases of urinary fistulae were treated in Patan Hospital, Nepal. Obstetric causes accounted for 95% (38) of the cases, with 30 (79%) of these being caused by prolonged labour followed by vaginal delivery. The average age of the women was 31 years, the youngest being 15 and the oldest 55 years. The highest percentage (37% – 14 women) were primiparae. A description of various complicated fistulae is presented together with operative management. The repair success rate was 77.5% (31 women), with 12.5% (5) subsequently suffering unacceptable urinary incontinence.

8. FURTHER READING

Shah, K.P. *Enquiry on the epidemiology and surgical repair of obstetric related fistula in South-East Asia.* (Unpublished paper prepared for a Technical Working Group) WHO, Geneva, 1989. WHE 2122

9. DATA SOURCES

WHE 0634   Sangsingkeo, V. *Development of maternal and child health services in Nepal.* (unpublished WHO document no. SEA/MCH/156), SEARO, 1982.

WHE 0649   Shah, M. *Rural health needs: report of a study in the primary health care unit (district) of Dhankuta.* Tribhuvan University, Kathmandu, 1977.

WHE 0813   World Health Organization. Regional Office for the Eastern Mediterranean. *Report of the EMR/SEAR meeting on the prevention of neonatal tetanus,* (WHO document no. EM/IMZ/27, EM/BD/14, EM-SEA/MTG.PREV.NNL.TTN/8), Lahore, 1982.

WHE 0834   World Health Organization *World health statistics annual – vital statistics and causes of death.* Geneva, various years.

WHE 1228   Malla, D.S. Study of causes of maternal mortality in selected hospitals in Nepal. In: *Interregional meeting on the prevention of maternal mortality,* (unpublished WHO document no. FHE/PMM/85.9.9), Geneva, 1985.

WHE 1369   Wright, N. *Epidemiological review of data on primary health problems in Nepal: report.* (unpublished), 1986.

WHE 1489   World Health Organization. Regional Office for South East Asia. *Evaluation of the strategy of health for all by the year 2000.* Seventh report on the world health situation. SEARO, New Delhi, 1986.

WHE 1513   Malla, D.S. *Study on causes of maternal death in Nepal,* (unpublished), Government of Nepal, Kathmandu, 1986.

WHE 1522   World Health Organization, Regional Office for South-East Asia *Bulletin of regional health information,* New Delhi, 1986.

WHE 1691   Malla, D.S. *Study on causes of maternal death in Nepal: research findings* WHO/Government of Nepal, 1986.

WHE 1712   Mauldin W.P. and Segal, S.J., *Prevalence of contraceptive use in developing countries. A chart book.* Rockefeller Foundation, New York 1986.

WHE 1724   Malla, D.S. *Research protocol on prevention of maternal mortality in Nepal* (unpublished), 1987.

WHE 1914   United Nations Children's Fund (UNICEF). *The state of the world's children,* Oxford, Oxford University Press, various years.

WHE 1915   United Nations. Department of International Economic and Social Affairs. *World population prospects: estimates and projections,* Population Studies, New York, various years.

WHE 1917   United Nations. Department of International Economic and Social Affairs. *Age structure of mortality in developing countries. A database for cross-sectional and time-series research.* New York 1986.

WHE 1918   United Nations. Department of International Economic and Social Affairs. *First marriage: patterns and determinants.* New York 1988.

WHE 2033   World Health Organization. *Global strategy for health for all by the year 2000. Second report on monitoring progress.* WHO document EB83/2 Add. 1, 1988.

WHE 2257   Asian Parasite Control/Family Planning Conference, *IP – A strategy for maternal and child health,* Proceedings of the 14th Asian Parasite Control/Family Planning Conference,Dhaka, Bangladesh, 26-30 October 1987.

NOTES

OMAN

		Year	Source

1. BASIC INDICATORS

1.1 Demographic

1.1.1 Population

		Year	Source
Size (millions)	1.5	1990	(1915)
Rate of growth (%)	3.8	1985-90	(1915)

1.1.2 Life expectancy

		Year	Source
Female	66	1985-90	(1915)
Male	62	1985-90	(1915)

1.1.3 Fertility

		Year	Source
Crude Birth Rate	46	1985-90	(1915)
Total Fertility Rate	7.2	1985-90	(1915)

1.1.4 Mortality

		Year	Source
Crude Death Rate	8	1985-90	(1915)
Infant Mortality Rate	40	1985-90	(1915)
Female			
Male			
1-4 years mortality rate			
Female			
Male			

1.2 Social and economic

1.2.1 Adult literacy rate (%)

Female	
Male	

1.2.2 Primary school enrolment rate (%)

		Year	Source
Female	92	1986-88	(1914)
Male	103	1986-88	(1914)

1.2.3 Female mean age at first marriage
(years)

1.2.4 GNP/capita

		Year	Source
(US $)	5 000	1988	(1914)

1.2.5 Daily per capita calorie supply
(as % of requirements)

2. HEALTH SERVICES

2.1 Health Expenditure

2.1.1 Expenditure on health
(as % of GNP)

2.1.2 Expenditure on PHC

(as % of total health expenditure)	60	1981-85	(2033)

2.2 Primary Health Care
(Percentage of population covered by):

2.2.1 Health services

		Year	Source
National	92	1984	(2033)
Urban			
Rural			

2.2.2 Safe Water

		Year	Source
National			
Urban	90	1985	(2033)
Rural	55	1985	(2033)

2.2.3 Adequate sanitary facilities

		Year	Source
National			
Urban	88	1985	(2033)
Rural	25	1985	(2033)

2.2.4 Contraceptive prevalence rate
(%)

2.3   Coverage of maternity care (%)

Area	Prenatal care	Trained attendant	Institutional deliveries	Postnatal care	Sample size	Year	Source
National	79	60				1982-84	(2033)

3. COMMUNITY STUDIES

4. HOSPITAL STUDIES

5. CIVIL REGISTRATION DATA/GOVERNMENT ESTIMATES

6. OTHER SOURCES/ ESTIMATES

7. SELECTED ANNOTATED BIBLIOGRAPHY

8. FURTHER READING

9. DATA SOURCES

WHE 1914   United Nations Children's Fund (UNICEF). *The state of the world's children*, Oxford, Oxford University Press, various years.

WHE 1915   United Nations. Department of International Economic and Social Affairs. *World population prospects: estimates and projections*, Population Studies, New York, various years.

WHE 2033   World Health Organization. *Global strategy for health for all by the year 2000. Second report on monitoring progress.* WHO document EB83/2 Add. 1, 1988.

PAKISTAN

		Year	Source

1. BASIC INDICATORS

1.1 Demographic

1.1.1 Population

		Year	Source
Size (millions)	123	1990	(1915)
Rate of growth (%)	3.4	1985-90	(1915)

1.1.2 Life expectancy

Female	57	1985-90	(1915)
Male	57	1985-90	(1915)

1.1.3 Fertility

Crude Birth Rate	47	1985-90	(1915)
Total Fertility Rate	6.5	1985-90	(1915)

1.1.4 Mortality

Crude Death Rate	13	1985-90	(1915)
Infant Mortality Rate	109	1985-90	(1915)
Female	156	1968-71	(1917)
Male	156	1968-71	(1917)
1-4 years mortality rate			
Female	25	1968-71	(1917)
Male	17	1968-71	(1917)

1.2 Social and economic

1.2.1 Adult literacy rate (%)

Female	19	1985	(1914)
Male	40	1985	(1914)

1.2.2 Primary school enrolment rate (%)

Female	28	1986-88	(1914)
Male	51	1986-88	(1914)

1.2.3 Female mean age at first marriage

(years)	19.8	1981	(1918)

		Year	Source

1.2.4 GNP/capita

(US $)	350	1987	(1914)

1.2.5 Daily per capita calorie supply

(as % of requirements)	97	1984-86	(1914)

2. HEALTH SERVICES

2.1 Health Expenditure

2.1.1 Expenditure on health

(as % of GNP)	3.2	1984-85	(1888)

2.1.2 Expenditure on PHC

(as % of total health expenditure)	54	1984	(1888)

2.2 Primary Health Care
(Percentage of population covered by):

2.2.1 Health services

National	85	1987	(2033)
Urban			
Rural			

2.2.2 Safe water

National	44	1985	(0834)
Urban	84	1985	(0834)
Rural	28	1985	(0834)

2.2.3 Adequate sanitary facilities

National	19	1985	(0834)
Urban	56	1985	(0834)
Rural	5	1985	(0834)

2.2.4 Contraceptive prevalence rate

(%)	8	1981-85	(1914)

2.3   Coverage of maternity care (%)

Area	Prenatal care	Trained attendant	Institutional deliveries	Postnatal care	Sample size	Year	Source
National		24				1976	(1888)
National	26					1981	(1888)
National	60	60				1987	(2033)
Lahore:							
urban		77			1 117	1985-86	(1541)
rural		67			274	1985-86	(1541)
Punjab		13			13 858	1981	(0813)

3.   COMMUNITY STUDIES

3.1   National, (1988) [2565]

The "sisterhood method" was used to estimate maternal mortality in the context of a demographic survey carried out among men and women aged over 15 years. The unweighted sample size was 84,800 and there were 1,700 maternal deaths. The lifetime risk of dying from pregnancy related causes was calculated as one in 53.

MMR (per 100 000 live births)   270

3.2   Selected areas in Faisalabad District, 1977 and 1978-1987 [2365]

The study included equal numbers of patients from four areas: Department of Obstetrics and Gynaecology; Model Town, a heavily populated area in the centre of the city; Noorpur, a village five miles from the city; and Chak 30, a village 20 miles from the city. With the assistance of Family Planning Association workers a household survey was conducted and information collected on all pregnancies, abortions, births and maternal deaths.

3.2.1   Rate

Year	Pregnancies	Maternal deaths	MMR (per 100 000 pregnancies)
1977	n.a.	n.a.	1 007
1978-87	2 145	4	186

3.2.2   Causes of maternal deaths, 1978-87

	Number
Abortion	2
Sepsis	1
Postpartum haemorrhage	1

3.2.3   Avoidable factors

3.2.4   High risk groups

3.2.5   Other findings

The survey revealed that about 80% of the deliveries were conducted by TBAs who had undergone training courses.

3.3   Faisalabad City, 1989 [2710]

A survey was carried out to estimate the numbers of maternal deaths in the community. Hospital records were examined as were those of health centres and TBAs were questioned about deaths occurring during or after home deliveries. The municipal authorities recorded 34 maternal deaths. The community survey identified a further 14 deaths resulting from complications of pregnancy, delivery or the puerperium.

3.3.1   Rate

Births	55 560
Maternal deaths	48
MMR (per 100 000 births)	86

It is thought that the comparatively low rate was due to the fact that 1989 was designated as the "Year of the Mother and Child" and additional efforts were made to encourage women to deliver with the assistance of trained attendants.

3.3.2 Causes of maternal deaths

	Number	%
Haemorrhage	10	21
Hypertensive disorders of pregnancy	9	19
Ruptured uterus	6	13
Sepsis	5	10
Embolism	5	10
Hepatitis	4	8
Abortion	3	6
Complications of anaesthesia	2	4
Other	4	8
TOTAL	48	100

3.3.3 Avoidable factors

Avoidable factors were present in 33 (69%) deaths. There were considerable delays in referring women to hospital when complications arose. An obstetric flying squad has been set up in order to eliminate transportation problems for women in need.

4. HOSPITAL STUDIES

4.1 Eight city hospitals*, 1975 [1698]

4.1.1 Rate
Births	15 150
Maternal deaths	121
MMR (per 100 000 births)	799

* Shakut Haroon Hospital, Karachi; Civil Hospital, Unit II, Karachi; Jinnah Postgraduate Medical Centre, Karachi; Lady Willingdon Hospital, Lahore; United Christian Hospital, Lahore; Holy Family Hospital, Rawalpindi; Lady Reading Hospital, Peshawar; Federal Government Services Hospital, Islamabad.

4.2 Thirteen city hospitals*, 1977, [1698]

4.2.1 Rate
Births	17 891
Maternal deaths	124
MMR (per 100 000 births)	693

* Lady Dufferin Hospital, Karachi; Civil Hospital, Karachi; Sobraj Maternity Home, Karachi; Lady Willingdon Hospital, Lahore; United Christian Hospital, Lahore; Holy Family Hospital, Rawalpindi; Quaid-i-Azam Medical College, Bahawalpur; Lady Dufferin Hospital, Quetta; Hayat Shaheed Hospital, Peshawar; Pennel Memorial Hospital, Bannu; Military Hospital and Combined Military Hospital, Rawalpindi; Federal Government Services Hospital, Islamabad.

4.2.2 Causes of maternal deaths, *(for 118 cases)*

	Number	%
Sepsis	37	31
Haemorrhage	33	28
Hypertensive disorders of pregnancy	16	14
Ruptured uterus	9	8
Embolisms	2	2
Hepatitis	10	8
Cardiac arrest	7	6
Blood transfusion reaction	1	1
Other	3	3
Total	118	100

4.3 Ten city hospitals,* 1979, [1698]

4.3.1 Rate
Births	16 087
Maternal deaths	181
MMR (per 100 000 births)	1 125

* Sheikh Zayed Hospital, Larkana; Civil Hospital, Karachi; Sobraj Maternity Hospital, Karachi; Lady Dufferin Hospital, Karachi; Lady Willingdon Hospital, Lahore; District Headquarter Hospital, Faisalabad; Central Government Hospital, Rawalpindi; Lady Reading Hospital, Peshawar; Pannel Memorial Hospital, Bannu; Federal Government Services Hospital, Islamabad.

4.4 Ten city hospitals*, 1982 [1698]

4.4.1 Rate
Births	20 169
Maternal deaths	193
MMR (per 100 000 births)	957

* Naval Hospital and Jinnah Postgraduate Medical Centre, Karachi; Lady Willingdon Hospital and Services Hospital, Lahore; General Hospital, Rawalpindi; Federal Government Hospital, Islamabad; Lady Reading Hospital, Peshawar; Sandeman Civil Hospital, Quetta; Sheikh Zayed Hospital, Larkana; District Hospital, Faisalabad.

4.4.2 Causes of maternal deaths

	Number	%
Sepsis	54	28
Haemorrhage	44	23
Hypertensive disorders of pregnancy	25	13
Ruptured uterus	15	8
Embolisms	15	8
Complications of anaesthesia	8	4
Obstetric shock	3	2
DIRECT CAUSES	164	85
Anaemia	8	4
Cardiac arrest	5	2
Hepatitis	3	2
Other infections	5	2
Cardiac disease	2	1
Others	7	4
TOTAL	193	100

4.5 Liaquat Medical College Hospital, Hyderabad, 1961-65 [0051]

4.5.1 Rate

Deliveries	5 165
Maternal deaths	87
MMR (per 100 000 deliveries)	1 684

4.5.2 Causes of maternal deaths

	Number	%
Anaemia	34	39
Hypertensive disorders of pregnancy	15	17
Obstructed labour	9	10
Haemorrhage	8	9
Maternal injuries	8	9
Abortion	5	6
Other causes including cardiac diseases	8	9
Total	87	100

4.5.3 Avoidable factors

All the maternal deaths occurred among unbooked patients. Of the total obstetric admissions including abortions, only 15% were booked.

Avoidable factor	%
Patient factors	50
Dai and TBA factors	21
Delay in reaching hospital	20
Mismanagement by G.P.	5
Hospital factors	4
Total	100

4.6 Federal Government Hospital, Islamabad, 1975-84 [1226]

4.6.1 Rate

Live births	17 460
Maternal deaths*	30
MMR (per 100 000 live births)	171

*   Excluding abortions

4.6.2 Causes of maternal deaths

4.6.3 Avoidable factors

Prenatal care

In the majority of deaths (80%) the women had received no prenatal care by any trained medical personnel. Most of the patients were moribund on admission.

Mismanagement by TBAs

In seven women who died there was a history of mismanagement by the *Dai*. The women died due to uterine rupture, eclampsia or as a result of gas gangrene.

Delay in giving blood transfusion

Delays in providing blood transfusions were responsible for four deaths in 1979. Thereafter efforts were made to ensure rapid transfusion.

Avoidable factors within the hospital services

Six of the women who died in hospital had received inadequate treatment. Avoidable factors included failure to act in a case of prolonged obstructed labour, lack of aseptic techniques on the labour ward and inadequate monitoring of blood pressure in hypertensive patients.

4.7 Civil Hospital, Karachi, 1979-83 [1304]

4.7.1 Rate

Deliveries	4 641
Maternal deaths*	127
MMR (per 100 000 deliveries)	2 736

*   Including abortion deaths

4.7.2 Causes of maternal deaths

Haemorrhage from all causes and sepsis (including septic abortion) were the most important causes of death. Eleven of the 14 abortion deaths were from sepsis.

	Number	%
Haemorrhage	27	21
Sepsis	26	21
Hypertensive disorders of pregnancy	16	13
Abortion	14	11
Ruptured uterus	7	6
Embolisms	6	5
Complications of anaesthesia	4	3
DIRECT CAUSES	100	79
Hepatitis	12	9
Anaemia	9	7
Cardiac diseases	3	2
Others	3	2
INDIRECT CAUSES	27	21
TOTAL	127	100

4.7.3 Avoidable factors

120 of the 127 deaths were considered avoidable.

Avoidable factor	Number	%
Attitude of patient or relatives	85	71
Deficient management by GP and private nursing homes	20	17
Deficient management by TBA	4	3
Deficient management in the hospital	11	9
Total	120	100

4.8 Civil Hospital, Karachi, 1982-1983 [2369]

A retrospective analysis of 1 501 women who delivered at the hospital during the two year period was carried out in order to estimate the incidence of grand-multiparity and compare the incidence of obstetric and medical complications in the grandmultiparae (431 women) and in the less parous women (1 070 women).

4.8.1 Rate

	MMR (per 100 000 births)
Grandmultiparae (para 5 or higher)	800
Less parous women (para 1-4)	700

There was a higher incidence of anaemia, spontaneous abortion, abruptio placentae, postpartum haemorrhage, uterine rupture and stillbirths in the grand multiparae.

4.9 Lady Reading Hospital, Peshawar, 1982-86 [1916]

4.9.1 Rate

	Births	Maternal deaths	MMR (per 100 000 births)
1982	1 547	26	1 680
1983	1 490	17	1 149
1984	1 631	18	1 103
1985	1 664	23	1 382
1986	1 630	23	1 411
1982-86	7 962	107	1 343

Only six of the 107 women who died were booked patients. The remaining 101 patients were emergency admissions.

4.9.2 Causes of maternal deaths

	Number	%
Haemorrhage	36	34
Sepsis	18	17
Hypertensive disorders of pregnancy	16	15
Embolisms	9	8
Complications of anaesthesia	8	7
Ruptured uterus	6	6
Mismatched blood transfusion	2	2
DIRECT CAUSES	95	89
Hepatitis	2	2
Other infections	4	4
Others	6	5
INDIRECT CAUSES	12	11
TOTAL	107	100

4.10 Khyber Medical College, Northwest Frontier Province, (1985) [1234]

4.10.1 Rate

Maternity admission	10 000
Maternal deaths	501
MMR (per 100 000 maternity admissions)	5 010

4.10.2 Causes of maternal deaths

The main causes of death were haemorrhage, sepsis and ruptured uterus.

4.10.3 Avoidable factors

70% of the deaths were classified as avoidable.

4.10.4 High risk groups

Grand multiparae were at greatest risk of death.

5. CIVIL REGISTRATION DATA/GOVERNMENT ESTIMATES

6. OTHER SOURCES/ESTIMATES

6.1 National, 1985 [1310]

6.1.1 Rate

A 1985 publication estimated a maternal mortality rate of between 600 and 750 per 100 000 live births.

6.2   Lahore metropolitan area and two adjacent rural areas, 1984-88 [2894]

A comprehensive MCH care project was mounted in one urban and two rural areas near Lahore. The project started in 1984 and covers a total population of over 61,000 (urban 50, 600; rural 10,700) living in scattered communities. Each community has one MCH unit and the centres offer a comprehensive service to women and children. The authors assert that although the level of skills of MCH workers in the project area do not differ substantially from those in other areas, the administrative system, which fosters leadership, peer review and self appraisal, has resulted in an improvement in the quality of services. Contraceptive prevalence has increased substantially and there has been a decline in infant and maternal mortality rates which are now substantially lower than the national rates.

6.2.1   Rate

	MMR (per 100 000 live births)
Project area	
1984	560
1987	220
1988	260
National	
1988	430

7. SELECTED ANNOTATED BIBLIOGRAPHY

Ahmad, S. *Urinary fistulas in gynaecological practice in N.W.F.P.* Unpublished, Lahore, December 1988. WHE 2150

Urinary fistulae are described as being the outcome of a sequence of events starting with malnutrition and infections in childhood leading to poor pelvic development, followed by very early marriage, and inadequate management of pregnancy. This results in fistula in primiparous women. Multiparous women also suffer from fistula if they are malnourished: rapid childbearing and continuous lactation result in demineralization of the bones and subsequent osteomalacia causing secondary pelvic disproportion. Mismanagement of labour including manipulation, unskilled administration of oxytocic drugs and surgical intervention can also cause fistulae. Female literacy rate is below 26% and prenatal care is either not available or not accepted in rural areas.

A retrospective study of 325 women with urinary fistulae treated at the Lady Reading Hospital in Peshawar, Pakistan from 1979-1988 is presented.

The average age of patients was 32.2 years, with four women 16 years old and the oldest patient 65 years old. Grandmultiparae (over 5 previous births) accounted for 183 (56%) of the cases, and primiparae for 15%. The average height of patients was 147.5cm. There were 18 cases of recto-vaginal fistula, five of bladder calculus and three third degree perineal tears. Surgical repair was successful in 190 (61%) cases.

Ahmed, S. *Personal communication.* Peshawar, 1989. WHE 2266

The frequency of obstetric fistula in five hospitals in Peshawar, Pakistan, during the period from 1977 to 1989 was 3-4% of deliveries and between 0.36% and 0.8% of admissions.

Akhtar, A.Z. *Personal communication.* Karachi, 1989. WHE 2193

An analysis of 20 cases of obstetric fistulae admitted to the Abbassi-Shaheed Hospital in Karachi, Pakistan, from 1981-1988, showed that 19 women were primiparae and one para 4, with an average age of 25 years. Most women came from rural areas where there were no trained personnel or means of transport to a maternity hospital, and their fistulae were the result of prolonged, obstructed labour. Three cases of recto-vaginal fistulae were due to badly applied forceps in obstructed labour carried out in a small maternity home. There was one postoperative death after fistula repair.

Ansari, R.L. *Personal communication.* Karachi, 1989. WHE 2177

A tabulation of fistula cases referred to the Civil Hospital in Karachi, Pakistan, from 1983 to 1988, shows that there was a total of 38 cases of obstetric fistula. Twenty-eight percent of the women were aged 15-20, and 78% were aged 30 and under. Primiparous women accounted for 53% of cases. All the women were from poor families, and most from the rural areas. Seventeen women had successful repairs.

Awan, A.K. et al. Attitude of married women towards the current pregnancy. *Pakistan Journal of Medical Research*, 1990; 29(1): 8-10. WHE 2708

A community study of 1,274 pregnant women found that over 25% did not desire the current pregnancy. Lower income, lower educational status, higher parity and age were associated with higher incidence of unwanted pregnancy. Among the married women, 12% of those aged under 20 years did not desire the pregnancy and would have wished to start childbearing later. Over 63% of the women aged over 35 did not desire the pregnancy.

Aziz-Karim, S. et al. Anaemia in pregnancy – a study of 709 women in Karachi. *Tropical Doctor*, 1990; 20: 184-185. WHE 2709

A prospective study was carried out among 709 pregnant women in order to identify factors contributing to anaemia. It was found that 17% of the women were anaemic and that anaemia was commoner among women of high parity (7 and over) and in those presenting for prenatal care in the third trimester. Anaemia was strongly associated with inadequate diet. Low socioeconomic level was the main determinant of inadequate diet, high parity and anaemia.

Hanif, H. *Personal communication.* Lahore, 1989. WHE 2180

There were 95 cases of obstetric fistula admitted to the Sir Ganga Ram Hospital in Lahore, Pakistan, from 1978-1988. All women were in the age group 20-30 years, and 80% were primiparae. Seventy percent were from remote areas with poor medical coverage and low literacy rates, and all belonged to a poor socio-economic group. Out of the 72 women with vesico-vaginal fistulae, 67 (93%) were not living with their husbands, whereas only 28% of the women with recto-vaginal fistulae were separated. Of the 72 women who underwent repair, 62 (86%) had successful operations. It is estimated that there may be more than 500 unoperated cases in Pakistan.

Jafarey, S.N. *Personal communication.* Karachi. 1989. WHE 2172

At the Jinnah Postgraduate Medical Centre, Karachi, Pakistan, there are over 7,000 deliveries a year, more than half of which are unbooked, and about 15-20 cases of obstetric fistula (2-3 per thousand deliveries). From August 1985 to March 1989, 52 cases of obstetric fistula were admitted. The mean age of patients was 30 years, and 10 (19%) were primiparae. The women admitted with obstructed labour who delivered at the Medical Centre had travelled between 100-600 kilometres. Husbands of the younger women who had no live children tended to leave them as a result of the fistula.

Kazmi, S. *Safe motherhood: consumer viewpoints.* Preliminary results of a sample survey, (unpublished) Karachi, 1991. WHE 2992.

A survey of 1,200 women living in the Province of Sind, half of whom were illiterate found that the majority of women strongly preferred home delivery. This explains the pronounced preference for delivery with the assistance of Dais. Few of the Dais had received any formal training and most had learned their skills through their own mothers.

Lack of transport facilities, particularly acute in rural areas, and alternative child care arrangements mean that few women are able to go to hospital to deliver. Women living in urban areas who did use the hospitals expressed considerable dissatisfaction with the services offered. There were long delays at prenatal clinics. On admission to hospital women had to arrange for food to be brought in from home and for a friend or relative to buy medicines and blood (whether or not it is actually required during the delivery). They also had to be accompanied by at least one relative.

Within the hospitals themselves although modern equipment was available it was seldom in working order. Hospitals appeared to be overcrowded, this impression was reinforced by the large numbers of relatives in attendance and, in some cases, accompanying children. Record keeping was poor. Pressure on the medical personnel was severe, with a Lady Doctor able to spend only 12 minutes with each patient on average.

The local Health Centres and Basic Health Units exist in most areas and all are adequately linked to public transport systems. In rural areas, however, there was a shortage of Lady Doctors who are reluctant to work in isolated communities. Indeed, interviews with doctors of both sexes found that few were willing to be posted to a rural centre.

Sabir, N.I. and Ebrahim, G.J. Are daughters more at risk than sons in some societies? *Journal of Tropical Pediatrics*, 1984; 20: 237-239. WHE 0889

A household survey of 151 families in an urban slum near Lahore revealed a high preference for sons over daughters. Boys were better nourished than girls and had a lower prevalence of growth failure. During illness parents incurred expense to seek health care more often for boys than for girls. Mortality was higher among girls than boys, especially in the 1-2 year age group.

8. FURTHER READING

Janjua, S. National mortality in major city hospitals of Pakistan. *Journal of the Pakistan Medical Association*, 1979; 29(2): 31-35. WHE 0363

9. DATA SOURCES

WHE 0051   Aziz, S.A. Maternal mortality in non-booked patients in a teaching hospital in a southern region of Pakistan. *Pakistan Medical Review*, 1968; 3: 54-62.

WHE 0813   World Health Organization. Eastern Mediterranean Regional Office. *Report of the EMR/SEAR meeting on the prevention of neonatal tetanus.* (WHO document no. EM/IMZ/27, EM/BD/14, EM-SEA/MTG.PREV.NNL.TTN./8) Lahore, 1982.

WHE 0834   World Health Organization *World health statistics annual – vital statistics and causes of death.* Geneva, various years.

WHE 1226   Janjua, S. Ten years statistical survey of maternal mortality, 1975-1984. In: *Interregional Meeting on the Prevention of Maternal Mortality,* Geneva, 1985.

WHE 1234   Khattak, M.F. Paper presented to the 10th Asian congress of obstetrics and gynaecology. *IPPF Medical Bulletin*, 1985; 19(5): 1.

WHE 1304   Ahmad, Z. Maternal mortality in an obstetric unit. *Journal of the Pakistan Medical Association*, 1985; 35(8): 243-248.

WHE 1310   Awan, A.K. Mobilising TBAs for control of maternal and neonatal mortality in Pakistan. *Mother and Child*, 1985; 22(2): 4-7.

WHE 1541   Awan, A.H. et al. *Socioeconomic conditions as related to infant mortality.* Maternity and Child Welfare Association of Pakistan, Islamabad, 1987.

WHE 1698   Janjua, S. *Maternal mortality in Pakistan – a neglected tragedy.* (unpublished), 1987.

WHE 1888   World Health Organization, Eastern Mediterranean Regional Office, *Evaluation of the strategy for Health for All by the year 2000. Seventh report of the world health situation.* EMRO, Alexandria, 1987.

WHE 1914   United Nations Children's Fund (UNICEF). *The state of the world's children*, Oxford, Oxford University Press, various years.

WHE 1915   United Nations. Department of International Economic and Social Affairs. *World population prospects: estimates and projections,* Population Studies, New York, various years.

WHE 1916   Majid, S.S. *Maternal mortality report of Gynae B Unit,* (unpublished) Postgraduate Medical Institute, Lady Reading Hospital, Peshawar, 1986.

WHE 1917   United Nations. Department of International Economic and Social Affairs. *Age structure of mortality in developing countries. A database for cross-sectional and time-series research.* New York 1986.

WHE 1918   United Nations. Department of International Economic and Social Affairs. *First marriage: patterns and determinants.* New York 1988.

WHE 2033   World Health Organization. *Global strategy for health for all by the year 2000. Second report on monitoring progress.* WHO document EB83/2 Add. 1, 1988.

WHE 2365   Bashir, A. TBA training and maternal mortality in Faisalabad District. *Pakistan Journal of Medical Research*, 1989; 28(2): 81-83.

WHE 2369   Aziz-Karim, S. et al. Grandmultiparity: a continuing problem in developing countries. *Asia-Oceania Journal of Obstetrics and Gynaecology,* 1989; 15(2): 155-160.

WHE 2565   Graham, W. *Results of the application of the sisterhood method for estimating maternal mortality,* (unpublished document), London School of Hygiene and Tropical Medicine, 1990.

WHE 2710   Bashir, A. *Prevalence of maternal mortality in Faisalabad City in 1989.* (unpublished), 1990.

WHE 2894   International Association for Maternal and Neonatal Health. Pakistan – peer review and self-appraisal approach: a successful experience in contraceptive coverage. *MCI Mother and Child International Newsletter*, IAMANEH, 15, 1990.

PHILIPPINES

		Year	Source

1. BASIC INDICATORS

1.1 Demographic

1.1.1 Population
		Year	Source
Size (millions)	62.4	1990	(1915)
Rate of growth (%)	2.5	1985-90	(1915)

1.1.2 Life expectancy
		Year	Source
Female	65	1985-90	(1915)
Male	62	1985-90	(1915)

1.1.3 Fertility
		Year	Source
Crude Birth Rate	33	1985-90	(1915)
Total Fertility Rate	4.3	1985-90	(1915)

1.1.4 Mortality
		Year	Source
Crude Death Rate	8	1985-90	(1915)
Infant Mortality Rate	45	1985-90	(1915)
Female	52	1974-76	(1917)
Male	65	1974-76	(1917)
1-4 years mortality rate			
Female	10	1974-76	(1917)
Male	10	1974-76	(1917)

1.2 Social and economic

1.2.1 Adult literacy rate (%)
		Year	Source
Female	85	1985	(1914)
Male	86	1985	(1914)

1.2.2 Primary school enrolment rate (%)
		Year	Source
Female	107	1986-88	(1914)
Male	105	1986-88	(1914)

1.2.3 Female mean age at first marriage
		Year	Source
(years)	22.4	1980	(1918)

1.2.4 GNP/capita
		Year	Source
(US $)	590	1987	(1914)

1.2.5 Daily per capita calorie supply
		Year	Source
(as % of requirements)	104	1984-86	(1914)

2. HEALTH SERVICES

2.1 Health expenditure

2.1.1 Expenditure on health
		Year	Source
(as % of GNP)	5	1987	(2033)

2.1.2 Expenditure on PHC
		Year	Source
(as % of total health expenditure)	4	1985	(2033)

2.2 Primary Health Care
(Percentage of population covered by):

2.2.1 Health services
		Year	Source
National			
Urban			
Rural			

2.2.2 Safe water
		Year	Source
National	65	1985	(0834)
Urban	81	1987	(2033)
Rural	68	1987	(2033)

2.2.3 Adequate sanitary facilities
		Year	Source
National	57	1985	(0834)
Urban	76	1987	(2033)
Rural	66	1987	(2033)

2.2.4 Contraceptive prevalence rate
		Year	Source
(%)	32	1984	(1712)

2.3 Coverage of maternity care (%)

Area	Prenatal care	Trained attendant	Institutional deliveries	Postnatal care	Sample size	Year	Source
National		57	25			1983	(1540)
National	60	55				1987	(2636)
National	77	76				1987	(3153)
Bohol	85	42	10	80		1978	(0784)
Pakil district: Laguna	85	91				1985-86	(1894)

3. COMMUNITY STUDIES

3.1 Manila, 1972 [0432]

The study was designed to determine the leading causes of maternal and neonatal deaths and to identify some of the factors associated with them. Death certificates of Manila residents who died during 1972 were reviewed. All deaths of women of reproductive age (15-44 years) which occurred outside hospital were investigated by interviewing a responsible and immediate member of the family regarding the signs and symptoms observed during the terminal episode. An obstetrician evaluated the symptomatology and determined the most probable underlying cause of death. Investigation was conducted within three months of the death registration. Information on maternal variables not contained in the death certificate was gathered from hospital records and/or interviews with the family.

3.1.1 Rate
Live births	49 314
Maternal deaths	35
MMR (per 100 000 live births)	71

3.1.2 Causes of maternal deaths

	Number
Hypertensive disorders of pregnancy	13
Haemorrhage	12
Ectopic pregnancy	3
Sepsis	2
Other	5
Total	35

3.1.3 Avoidable factors

3.1.4 High risk groups

4. HOSPITAL STUDIES

4.1 78 Philippine Obstetrical and Gynaecological Society (POGS) accredited hospitals throughout the country, 1985-86 [1892]

4.1.1 Rate
Live births	126 064
Maternal deaths	306
MMR (per 100 000 live births)	242

4.1.2 Causes of maternal deaths

	Number	%
Haemorrhage	56	18
Sepsis	49	16
Hypertensive disorders of pregnancy	33	11
Embolisms	23	7
Congestive heart failure	20	7
Ruptured uterus	18	6
Abortion	17	5
Trophoblastic disease	9	3
Hepatitis	6	2
Complications of anaesthesia	4	1
Ectopic pregnancy	2	1
Other medical/surgical complications	20	7
Others	49	16
Total	306	100

4.1.3 Avoidable factors

4.1.4 High risk groups

65% of the women who died were admitted as emergency cases and had received no prenatal care. Only 12% had received at least three prenatal visits.

4.1.5 Other findings

Only 22% of the mothers had been tested for haemoglobin levels. 70% had a haemoglobin level of less than 9 g/l.

5. CIVIL REGISTRATION DATA/GOVERNMENT ESTIMATES

5.1 National, 1974 and 1975 (0535, 0536)

5.1.1 Rate

	1974	1975
Live births	1 081 073	1 223 837
Maternal deaths	1 690	1 753
MMR (per 100 000 live births)	156	143

5.1.2 Causes of maternal deaths

	1970-74*		1975	
	Number	%	Number	%
Haemorrhage	901	58	962	55
Hypertensive disorders of pregnancy	242	16	331	19
Abortion	102	7	124	7
Sepsis	73	5	106	6
Other complications	235	15	230	13
Total	1 554	100	1 753	100

* Annual average

5.1.3 Avoidable factors

5.1.4 High risk groups

Age

	Live births	Maternal deaths	MMR (per 100 000 live births)
15	337	0	0
15-19	95 669	95	99
20-24	320 461	307	96
25-29	281 540	306	109
30-34	191 711	329	172
35-39	126 037	388	308
40-44	44 729	201	449
45+	7 471	50	669
All ages	1 081 073	1 690	156

5.2 National, 1979-84 (1137, 1142, 1262, 2440)

5.2.1 Rate

	MMR (per 100 000 live births)
1979	114
1980	110
1981	110
1982	90
1984	80

5.3 National, 1984 (1890)

5.3.1 Rate

According to a spokesman of the Department of Health, the maternal mortality rate for Philippines was about 90 per 100 000 live births in 1984.

5.4 National, 1971 and 1977 (0834)

5.4.1 Rate

The World Health Statistics Annual quotes mortality rates of 131 and 142 per 100 000 live births in 1971 and 1977 respectively.

5.5 National, 1978 and 1981 (0753)

Figures quoted in the UN Demographic Yearbook are based on registration data which is less than 90% complete.

5.5.1 Rate

	MMR (per 100 000 live births)
1978	125
1981	106

5.6 National, 1989 (3153)

5.6.1 Rate

MMR (per 100 000 live births)	74

6. OTHER SOURCES/ ESTIMATES

6.1 National, 1980-1981 (2440)

6.1.1 Rate

MMR (per 100 000 live births)	110

6.2　National, by Province and by major cities, 1984 [(2257)]

6.2.1　Rate

	Live births	Maternal deaths	MMR (per 100 000 live births)
Province			
Cavite	18 084	17	94
Laguna	27 903	26	93
Camarines Sur	33 045	44	133
Iloilo	26 341	23	87
Cebu	33 620	28	83
Bukidnon	21 848	19	87
City			
Quezon City	40 865	20	49
Naga City	5 682	0	–
National	1 478 205	1 379	94

6.2.2　Causes of maternal deaths

	MMR (per 100 000 live births)	% of total deaths
Postpartum haemorrhage	30	31
Hypertensive disorders of pregnancy	30	28
Abortion	8	9
Other haemorrhage	6	7
Other	20	26
Total	94	100

6.3　National 1987 [(2636)]

6.3.1　Rate

MMR (per 100 000 live births)	100

6.3.2　Causes of maternal deaths

	Number	%
Haemorrhage	563	35
Hypertensive disorders of pregnancy	388	24
Abortion	159	10
Other	501	31

7.　SELECTED ANNOTATED BIBLIOGRAPHY

Fe Bacalzo, T. *Evaluation report of the home based mother's record*, Department of Health, Manila, 1987. WHE 2435

The home based mother's record is a tool for the provision of maternal care throughout a woman's reproductive years as well as a screening device for high risk pregnancies. The evaluation undertaken after field testing found that antepartum, postpartum and other health services coverage increased substantially. There was a significant increase in the percentage of mothers whose health was regularly checked and more women received advice on family planning, breastfeeding etc. The vast majority of those identified as high risk cases were successfully referred to local health centres. The home based mother's record was found to work most effectively where there was a well-functioning primary health care system and established supervisory mechanisms.

Raymundo, C.M. *Risks of motherhood among the urban poor.* Paper presented to the National Conference on Safe Motherhood, Manila, 1987. WHE 1891

A survey was conducted to estimate the extent of maternal morbidity among women living in squatter areas of urban Manila during 1987. 500 women with a child less than one year old were selected as respondents. (The survey design allowed only the currently living infants to be available as denominator). Overall the mothers perceived themselves to be generally in poor health. They were well able to articulate their problems and reported high levels of complications during their most recent pregnancies. Over 39% reported problems during the last delivery; 16% experienced profuse bleeding, 14% premature rupture of the membranes, 10% dyspnea and 8% infection or fever. Nearly half the women experienced problems after the delivery with 20% reporting painful urination and 14% fever. Women who received relatively less food than other members of the family were at greater risk of complications during pregnancy and delivery as were those who were recent migrants and those who had fewer than five prenatal visits.

Valenzuela, R.E. et al. Distribution of nutrients within the Filipino family. *Nutrition Reports International*, 1979; 19: 573-581. WHE 1286

Information on the distribution of nutrients within the family was gathered in a rural, rice-growing community in Laguna, Philippines. The dietary consumption of all respondents fell below recommended levels of all nutrients except iron. Parents had more adequate diets than their children. Fathers had slightly better diets than mothers and boys more adequate than girls. Of all sex-age groups, male preschoolers were the most adequately fed and female adolescents the least. These significant differences in nutritional adequacy persisted even when socioeconomic variables were accounted for.

Wong, E.L. et al. Accessibility, quality of care and prenatal care use in the Philippines. *Social Science and Medicine*, 1987; 24(11): 927-944. WHE 1588

The patterns and determinants of prenatal care were examined through the use of a randomly selected sample of 3,000 rural and urban women who were studied prospectively during pregnancy and at three or four days postpartum. The quality of care provided, accessibility to this care, and insurance available to the mother all had important effects on prenatal patterns. The provision of prenatal care insurance was associated with an increased likelihood of private care use, an increased number of visits and earlier recourse to prenatal care with lower use of traditional health care facilities. In urban areas, access to a doctor or nurse at the health facility, rather than a midwife, was an important determinant of public health care utilization, but this was not the case in rural areas where seeing the midwife had a positive effect on the number of public visits. In urban areas neither waiting time nor costs of health care had a major impact on the choice of public health care, but in rural areas, distance was an important determinant. The authors conclude that all women want better trained personnel located in nearby facilities but that the precise configuration of health care providers will be different in urban and rural areas.

8. FURTHER READING

Williamson, N.E. et al. Providing maternal and child health-family planning services to a large rural population: results of the Bohol Project, Philippines. *American Journal of Public Health*, 1983; 73(1): 62-71. WHE 1835

9. DATA SOURCES

WHE 0432   Manalo, C.Q. et al. A study of neonatal and maternal deaths. *Southeast Journal of Tropical Medicine and Public Health*, 1974; 5(2): 280-289.

WHE 0535   Philippines, Bureau of Health Services, *Report of the national consultation on maternal mortality and perinatal mortality*, Division of Maternal and Child Health, Manila, 1978.

WHE 0536   Philippines, National Economic and Development Authority, *Vital statistics report 1975: marriages, births and deaths in the Philippines*, National Census and Statistics Office, Manila, 1979.

WHE 0753   United Nations, *Demographic Yearbook*. New York, various years.

WHE 0784   Williamson, N.E. *The Bohol project: progress report on an experiment to improve rural; health and family planning in the Philippines*, The Population Council, New York, 1979.

WHE 0834   World Health Organization *World health statistics annual – vital statistics and causes of death*. Geneva, various years.

WHE 1137   Philippines, National Commission on the Role of Filipino Women, *Filipino women in health care and welfare services*, Manila, 1985.

WHE 1142   Philippines, National Commission on the Role of Filipino Women, *Filipino women. Facts and figures*, Manila, 1985.

WHE 1262   Cho, Hyong. *Health status of women in the western Pacific region*, (unpublished), 1984.

WHE 1540   Santos Ocampo, P.D. and David-Padilla, C. Child health in the Philippines. *Manila Philippine Pediatric Society*, 23rd annual convention, Manila, 1986.

WHE 1712   Mauldin W.P. and Segal, S.J., *Prevalence of contraceptive use in developing countries. A chart book*. Rockefeller Foundation, New York 1986.

WHE 1890   Roxas, M.G. *The Filipino mother and her health concerns*, Paper presented to the National Conference on Safe Motherhood, Department of Health, Manila, 1987.

WHE 1892   Sahagun, G. *Hospital maternal deaths: causes and implications.* Paper presented to the National Conference on Safe Motherhood, Department of Health, Manila, 1987.

WHE 1894   Fe Bacalzo, *Maternal health services: are they available?* Paper presented to the National Conference on Safe Motherhood, Department of Health, Manila, 1987.

WHE 1914   United Nations Children's Fund (UNICEF). *The state of the world's children*, Oxford, Oxford University Press, various years.

WHE 1915   United Nations. Department of International Economic and Social Affairs. *World population prospects: estimates and projections*, Population Studies, New York, various years.

WHE 1917   United Nations. Department of International Economic and Social Affairs. *Age structure of mortality in developing countries. A database for cross-sectional and time-series research.* New York 1986.

WHE 1918   United Nations. Department of International Economic and Social Affairs. *First marriage: patterns and determinants.* New York 1988.

WHE 2033   World Health Organization. *Global strategy for health for all by the year 2000. Second report on monitoring progress.* WHO document EB83/2 Add. 1, 1988.

WHE 2257   Asian Parasite Control/Family Planning Conference, *IP – A strategy for maternal and child health*, Proceedings of the 14th Asian Parasite Control/Family Planning Conference,Dhaka, Bangladesh, 26-30 October 1987.

WHE 2440   Briones, T.K. Philippines health indicators, *Bulletin of the International Pediatric Association*, 1985; 7(1): 53-55.

WHE 2636   Habacon, C.A. and Mora, V.E. *Country report – Philippines*, Paper presented to the regional workshop on the risk approach in mother and child health care (unpublished document no. WPR/MCH/MCH(1)/90.2n), Manila, 1990.

WHE 3153   World Health Organization. Western Pacific Regional Office. *Country data sheets.* (unpublished), 1991.

QATAR

		Year	Source

1. BASIC INDICATORS

1.1 Demographic

1.1.1 Population

Size (millions)	0.4	1990	(1915)
Rate of growth (%)	4.2	1985-90	(1915)

1.1.2 Life expectancy

Female	72	1985-90	(1915)
Male	67	1985-90	(1915)

1.1.3 Fertility

Crude Birth Rate	31	1985-90	(1915)
Total Fertility Rate	5.6	1985-90	(1915)

1.1.4 Mortality

Crude Death Rate	4	1985-90	(1915)
Infant Mortality Rate	31	1985-90	(1915)
Female			
Male			
1-4 years mortality rate			
Female			
Male			

1.2 Social and economic

1.2.1 Adult literacy rate (%)

Female	51	1985	(1914)
Male	51	1985	(1914)

1.2.2 Primary school enrolment rate (%)

Female	121	1983-86	(1914)
Male	120	1983-86	(1914)

1.2.3 Female mean age at first marriage
(years)

1.2.4 GNP/capita

(US $)	12 510	1987	(1914)

1.2.5 Daily per capita calorie supply
(as % of requirements)

2. HEALTH SERVICES

2.1 Health Expenditure

2.1.1 Expenditure on health

(as % of GNP)	5	1982-83	(1888)

2.1.2 Expenditure on PHC
(as % of total health expenditure)

2.2 Primary Health Care.
(Percentage of population covered by):

2.2.1 Health services

National	100	1987	(2033)
Urban			
Rural			

2.2.2 Safe water

National	100	1987	(2033)
Urban	100	1987	(2033)
Rural	100	1987	(2033)

2.2.3 Adequate sanitary facilities

National	100	1987	(2033)
Urban	100	1987	(2033)
Rural	100	1987	(2033)

2.2.4 Contraceptive prevalence rate
(%)

2.3　Coverage of maternity care (%)

Area	Prenatal care	Trained attendant	Institutional deliveries	Postnatal care	Sample size	Year	Source
National	100	100				1987	(2033)

3.　COMMUNITY STUDIES

4.　HOSPITAL STUDIES

4.1　Women's Hospital, Doha, 1977-85 [0206, 1538]

4.1.1　Rate

Deliveries	63 492
Maternal deaths	9
MMR (per 100 000 deliveries)	14

The maternal mortality rate fell from 18 per 100 000 deliveries in 1976-80 to 10 per 100 000 during 1981-85.

4.1.2　Causes of maternal deaths

	Number
Hypertensive disorders of pregnancy	6
Embolisms	2
Haemorrhage	1
Total	9

5.　CIVIL REGISTRATION DATA/GOVERNMENT ESTIMATES

6.　OTHER SOURCES/ ESTIMATES

7.　SELECTED ANNOTATED BIBLIOGRAPHY

8.　FURTHER READING

9.　DATA SOURCES

WHE 0206　Elnayal, Z.M. Maternal mortality at the Women's Hospital Doha, Qatar. *Arab Medical Bulletin*, 1982; 4(11,12): 29-33.

WHE 1538　Manoj, M. Maternal mortality – an avoidable catastrophe. *Middle East Journal of Anesthesiology*, 1986; 8(6): 453-462.

WHE 1888　World Health Organization, Eastern Mediterranean Regional Office, *Evaluation of the strategy for Health for All by the year 2000. Seventh report of the world health situation*. EMRO, Alexandria, 1987.

WHE 1914　United Nations Children's Fund (UNICEF). *The state of the world's children*, Oxford, Oxford University Press, various years.

WHE 1915　United Nations. Department of International Economic and Social Affairs. *World population prospects: estimates and projections*, Population Studies, New York, various years.

WHE 2033　World Health Organization. *Global strategy for health for all by the year 2000. Second report on monitoring progress*. WHO document EB83/2 Add. 1, 1988.

REPUBLIC OF KOREA

		Year	Source

1. BASIC INDICATORS

1.1 Demographic

1.1.1 Population

Size (millions)	43.6	1990	(1915)
Rate of growth (%)	1.0	1985-90	(1915)

1.1.2 Life expectancy

Female	73	1985-90	(1915)
Male	66	1985-90	(1915)

1.1.3 Fertility

Crude Birth Rate	17	1985-90	(1915)
Total Fertility Rate	1.7	1985-90	(1915)

1.1.4 Mortality

Crude Death Rate	6	1985-90	(1915)
Infant Mortality Rate	25	1985-90	(1915)
Female	37	1971-75	(1917)
Male	41	1971-75	(1917)
1-4 years mortality rate			
Female	3	1971-75	(1917)
Male	2	1971-75	(1917)

1.2 Social and economic

1.2.1 Adult literacy rate (%)

Female	88	1985	(1914)
Male	96	1985	(1914)

1.2.2 Primary school enrolment rate (%)

Female	104	1986-88	(1914)
Male	104	1986-88	(1914)

1.2.3 Female mean age at first marriage

(years)	24.1	1980	(1918)

		Year	Source

1.2.4 GNP/capita

(US $)	2 690	1987	(1914)

1.2.5 Daily per capita calorie supply

(as % of requirements)	122	1984-86	(1914)

2. HEALTH SERVICES

2.1 Health expenditure

2.1.1 Expenditure on health

(as % of GNP)	6	1988	(2033)

2.1.2 Expenditure on PHC

(as % of total health expenditure)	10	1988	(2033)

2.2 Primary Health Care

(Percentage of population covered by):

2.2.1 Health services

National	100	1986	(2033)
Urban			
Rural			

2.2.2 Safe water

National	83	1983	(0834)
Urban			
Rural			

2.2.3 Adequate sanitary facilities

National	100	1985	(2033)
Urban	100	1985	(2033)
Rural	100	1985	(2033)

2.2.4 Contraceptive prevalence rate

(%)	70	1985	(1712)

2.3   Coverage of maternity care (%)

Area	Prenatal care	Trained attendant	Institutional deliveries	Postnatal care	Sample size	Year	Source
National	70	70				1982	(1496)
National	78	65				1983	(0834)
National:	89	89	88			1988	(2432)
urban	92	94	93			1988	(2432)
rural	78	75	73			1988	(2432)
Gunee	18	14		6		1978-79	(1108)
Hongchou	20	17		13		1978-79	(1108)
Okgu	16	26		13		1978-79	(1108)

3.   COMMUNITY STUDIES

4.   HOSPITAL STUDIES

5.   CIVIL REGISTRATION DATA/GOVERNMENT ESTIMATES

5.1   National, 1970, 1975, 1980-84, 1985 and 1987, [0548, 1496, 2257]

5.1.1   Rate

Year	MMR (per 100 000 live births)
1970	83
1975	56
1980	42
1981	41
1982	40
1983	38
1984	36
1985	34
1987	26

5.1.2   Causes of maternal deaths 1985-87

	% of total
Hypertensive disorders of pregnancy	41
Haemorrhage	23
Sepsis	13
Other	23
Total	100

5.2   National, 1985-87 [0834, 2722]

5.2.1   Rate

	Maternal deaths	MMR (per 100 000 live births)
1985	114	17
1986	103	16
1987	63	9

5.2.2   Causes of maternal deaths, 1985

	Number	%
Hypertensive disorders of pregnancy	35	31
Haemorrhage	23	20
Abortion	3	3
Complications of the puerperium	43	38
Other direct obstetric causes	8	7
Indirect obstetric causes	2	1
Total	114	100

5.3 National, 1985-87 [0753]

The rates quoted in the UN Demographic Yearbook are described as being based on civil registration data which are less than 90% complete.

5.3.1 Rate

	MMR (per 100 000 live births)
1985	17
1986	16
1987	10

5.4 National, 1987 [2432]

5.4.1 Rate

MMR (per 100 000 live births)	32

6. OTHER SOURCES/ ESTIMATES

6.1 National, 1985 [1417]

6.1.1 Rate

A WHO report for the region quotes a maternal mortality rate of 34 per 100 000 births for the country in 1985.

7. SELECTED ANNOTATED BIBLIOGRAPHY

8. FURTHER READING

9. DATA SOURCES

WHE 0548 Republic of Korea, Ministry of Health and Social Affairs. *Yearbook of public health and social statistics*, Vol. 28, Seoul, 1982.

WHE 0753 United Nations, *Demographic Yearbook*. New York, various years.

WHE 0834 World Health Organization *World health statistics annual – vital statistics and causes of death*. Geneva, various years.

WHE 1108 Republic of Korea, *Korea Health Development Institute Report 1978-79*. Seoul, 1980.

WHE 1417 World Health Organization. Regional Office for the Western Pacific. *Databank on socioeconomic and health indicators*, 1985.

WHE 1496 Republic of Korea, *Major policies and programmes in health and social welfare services 1984*, Ministry of Health and Welfare, 1985

WHE 1712 Mauldin W.P. and Segal, S.J., *Prevalence of contraceptive use in developing countries. A chart book*. Rockefeller Foundation, New York 1986.

WHE 1914 United Nations Children's Fund (UNICEF). *The state of the world's children*, Oxford, Oxford University Press, various years.

WHE 1915 United Nations. Department of International Economic and Social Affairs. *World population prospects: estimates and projections*, Population Studies, New York, various years.

WHE 1917 United Nations. Department of International Economic and Social Affairs. *Age structure of mortality in developing countries. A database for cross-sectional and time-series research*. New York 1986.

WHE 1918 United Nations. Department of International Economic and Social Affairs. *First marriage: patterns and determinants*. New York 1988.

WHE 2033 World Health Organization. *Global strategy for health for all by the year 2000. Second report on monitoring progress*. WHO document EB83/2 Add. 1, 1988.

WHE 2257 Asian Parasite Control/Family Planning Conference, *IP – A strategy for maternal and child health*, Proceedings of the 14th Asian Parasite Control/Family Planning Conference, Dhaka, Bangladesh, 26-30 October 1987.

WHE 2432 Ok-Ju Chang, *Country report – Republic of Korea*. Paper presented to the regional workshop on the risk approach in mother and child health care, Manila, Philippines, 4-8 December 1989.

WHE 2722 World Health Organization, *Maternal deaths and maternal mortality rates* (unpublished) 1990.

NOTES

SAUDI ARABIA

		Year	Source

1. BASIC INDICATORS

1.1 Demographic

1.1.1 Population

		Year	Source
Size (millions)	14.1	1990	(1915)
Rate of growth (%)	4.0	1985-90	(1915)

1.1.2 Life expectancy

Female	65	1985-90	(1915)
Male	62	1985-90	(1915)

1.1.3 Fertility

Crude Birth Rate	42	1985-90	(1915)
Total Fertility Rate	7.2	1985-90	(1915)

1.1.4 Mortality

Crude Death Rate	8	1985-90	(1915)
Infant Mortality Rate	71	1985-90	(1915)
Female			
Male			
1-4 years mortality rate			
Female			
Male			

1.2 Social and economic

1.2.1 Adult literacy rate (%)

Female	31	1985	(1914)
Male	71	1985	(1914)

1.2.2 Primary school enrolment rate (%)

Female	65	1986-88	(1914)
Male	78	1986-88	(1914)

1.2.3 Female mean age at first marriage
(years)

1.2.4 GNP/capita

(US $)	6 200	1987	(1914)

1.2.5 Daily per capita calorie supply

(as % of requirements)	125	1984-86	(1914)

2. HEALTH SERVICES

2.1 Health Expenditure

2.1.1 Expenditure on health

(as % of GNP)	5	1986	(2033)

2.1.2 Expenditure on PHC

(as % of total health expenditure)	40	1982	(1888)

2.2 Primary Health Care
(Percentage of population covered by):

2.2.1 Health services

National	93	1987	(2033)
Urban			
Rural			

2.2.2 Safe water

National	93	1985	(2033)
Urban	100	1985	(2033)
Rural	68	1985	(2033)

2.2.3 Adequate sanitary facilities

National	86	1985	(2033)
Urban	100	1985	(2033)
Rural	33	1985	(2033)

2.2.4 Contraceptive prevalence rate
(%)

2.3   Coverage of maternity care (%)

Area	Prenatal care	Trained attendant	Institutional deliveries	Postnatal care	Sample size	Year	Source
National		74				1983	(1888)
National	61					1985	(1888)
Rural areas		14			23 700	1977-9	(0640)
Al-Jubail	60				1 000	1983	(0691)
Asir Province	51		100		7 000	1976-9	(0322)
Riyadh			70			1983	(0129)
Riyadh district: rural			16			1987	(2772)
Tarut Island	17	54	10		725b	1983	(0024)
Madinal							

3.   COMMUNITY STUDIES

4.   HOSPITAL STUDIES

4.1   Riyadh Government Hospital, 1969-72 [0424]

4.1.1   Rate
MMR (per 100 000 deliveries)   80

4.2   King Faisal Hospital, Asir Province, 1978-79 [0322]

4.2.1   Rate
This was a review of 1 000 obstetric deliveries in the hospital. Complications were present in 20% of the cases and there was 1 death, a maternal mortality rate of 100 per 100 000 deliveries.

4.2.2   Causes of maternal deaths.
The single maternal death during the study period was due to amniotic fluid embolism.

4.3   Maternity and Children Hospital, 1978-80 [0129]

4.3.1   Rate
Births   55 428
Maternal deaths   29
MMR (per 100 000 births)   52

4.3.2   Causes of maternal deaths

	Number	%
Haemorrhage	8	29
Embolisms	5	17
Abortion	3	10
Sepsis	2	7
Complications of anaesthesia	2	7
Ruptured uterus	1	3
Hypertensive disorders of pregnancy	1	3
DIRECT CAUSES	22	76
Hepatitis	2	7
Other infections	2	7
Others	3	10
INDIRECT CAUSES	7	24
TOTAL	29	100

4.3.3 Avoidable factors

Avoidable factors were present in 6 of the 8 haemorrhage deaths, and were due to a combination of factors involving the patient, clinical management and the administration. The women who died had not received prenatal care, there were difficulties in arranging for blood transfusion in the peripheral hospitals and the patients had to travel long distances to reach the referral hospital.

Mismatched blood transfusion was a factor in two deaths, one caused by haemorrhage and one resulting from septic abortion. Delays in decision-making by the health personnel occurred in two instances: in a case of uncontrollable haemorrhage during caesarean section, and in a patient with antepartum haemorrhage, where there was delay in deciding on definitive surgery. In one case the avoidable factor was clinical, combining major surgery with caesarean section in a peripheral hospital with limited facilities.

5. CIVIL REGISTRATION DATA/GOVERNMENT ESTIMATES

6. OTHER SOURCES/ESTIMATES

7. SELECTED ANNOTATED BIBLIOGRAPHY

8. FURTHER READING

Sebei, Z. and Reinke, W. Anthropometric measurements among pre-school children in Wadi Turaba, Saudi Arabia. *Journal of Tropical Pediatrics*, 1981; 27: 150-154. WHE 0965

Serenius, F. et al. Characteristics of the obstetric population in a Saudi maternity hospital. *Acta Paediatrica Scandinavia*, 1988 Suppl 346: 29-43. WHE 2325

9. DATA SOURCES

WHE 0024   Bhatty, A. et al. A survey of mother and child care in the Saudi community in Rabaiyah, Tarut Island. *Saudi Medical Journal*, 1983; 4(1): 37-43.

WHE 0129   Chattopadhyay, S.K. et al. Maternal mortality in Riyadh, Saudi Arabia. *British Journal of Obstetrics and Gynaecology*, 1983; 90: 809-814.

WHE 0322   Hartley, W. One thousand obstetric deliveries in the Asir Province, Kingdom of Saudi Arabia. *Saudi Medical Journal*, 1980; 1: 187-196.

WHE 0424   Mahran, M. The extent of the problem of eclampsia in Arab countries. In: *WHO meeting on hypertensive diseases of pregnancy, childbirth and the puerperium.* (unpublished WHO document no. MCH/TP/77.5), Geneva, 1977.

WHE 0640   Sebai, Z.A. et al. A study of three health centres in rural Saudi Arabia. *Saudi Medical Journal*, 1980; 1(4): 197-202.

WHE 0691   Thabet, M.A. and Rahman, S.A. Evaluation of the first 1000 deliveries in Saudi Arabia. *Arab Medical Bulletin* 1983; 5(1,2): 35-51.

WHE 1888   World Health Organization, Eastern Mediterranean Regional Office, *Evaluation of the strategy for Health for All by the year 2000. Seventh report of the world health situation.* EMRO, Alexandria, 1987.

WHE 1914   United Nations Children's Fund (UNICEF). *The state of the world's children*, Oxford, Oxford University Press, various years.

WHE 1915   United Nations. Department of International Economic and Social Affairs. *World population prospects: estimates and projections*, Population Studies, New York, various years.

WHE 2033   World Health Organization. *Global strategy for health for all by the year 2000. Second report on monitoring progress.* WHO document EB83/2 Add. 1, 1988.

WHE 2772   Al-Sekait, M.A. The traditional midwife in Saudian villages. *Journal of the Royal Society of Health*, 1989; 4: 137.

NOTES

SINGAPORE

		Year	Source

1. BASIC INDICATORS

1.1 Demographic

1.1.1. Population

		Year	Source
Size (millions)	2.7	1990	(1915)
Rate of growth (%)	1.3	1985-90	(1915)

1.1.2 Life expectancy

Female	76	1985-90	(1915)
Male	71	1985-90	(1915)

1.1.3 Fertility

Crude Birth Rate	18	1985-90	(1915)
Total Fertility Rate	1.8	1985-90	(1915)

1.1.4 Mortality

Crude Death Rate	5	1985-90	(1915)
Infant Mortality Rate	8	1985-90	(1915)
Female	11	1979-81	(1917)
Male	13	1979-81	(1917)
1-4 years mortality rate			
Female	1	1979-81	(1917)
Male	1	1979-81	(1917)

1.2 Social and economic

1.2.1 Adult literacy rate (%)

Female	79	1985	(1914)
Male	93	1985	(1914)

1.2.2 Primary school enrolment rate (%)

Female	113	1986-88	(1914)
Male	118	1986-88	(1914)

1.2.3 Female mean age at first marriage

(years)	26.2	1980	(1918)

1.2.4 GNP/capita

		Year	Source
(US $)	9 070	1988	(1914)

1.2.5 Daily per capita calorie supply

(as % of requirements)	124	1984-86	(1914)

2. HEALTH SERVICES

2.1 Health Expenditure

2.1.1 Expenditure on health

(as % of GNP)	1.2	1983	(1488)

2.1.2 Expenditure on PHC

(as % of total health expenditure)	10	1986	(2033)

2.2 Primary Health Care

(Percentage of population covered by):

2.2.1 Health services

National	100	1984	(0834)
Urban			
Rural			

2.2.2 Safe water

National	100	1982	(0834)
Urban			
Rural			

2.2.3 Adequate sanitary facilities

National	85	1984	(0834)
Urban			
Rural			

2.2.4 Contraceptive prevalence rate

(%)	71	1977	(1712)

2.3   Coverage of maternity care (%)

Area	Prenatal care	Trained attendant	Institutional deliveries	Postnatal care	Sample size	Year	Source
National		100	98			1981	(0659)
National	95	100		79		1984	(1488)
National			99			1987	(2434)

3.   COMMUNITY STUDIES

4.   HOSPITAL STUDIES

4.1   Kandang Kerabu Hospital and Thomson Road Hospital, 1964-70 [0137]

4.1.1   Rate

Deliveries	262 74
Maternal deaths*	126
MMR (per 100 000 deliveries)	48

*   Obstetric deaths

4.1.2   Causes of maternal deaths

Abortion accounted for 22% of the maternal deaths over the 7-year period.

4.2   Alexandra Hospital, Singapore 1978-88 [2445]

4.2.1   Rate

Maternal deaths	14
MMR (per 100 000 births)	30

4.2.2   Causes of maternal deaths

	Number
Hypertensive disorders of pregnancy	3
Haemorrhage	3
Embolism	3
Associated causes	4
Other	1
Total	14

4.2.3   Avoidable factors

The three women who died from hypertensive disorders all developed cardiac failure due to severe preeclampsia. All were unbooked cases and none had received any prenatal care. They were in severe congestive cardiac failure with uncontrolled hypertension on admission.

5.   CIVIL REGISTRATION DATA/GOVERNMENT ESTIMATES

5.1   National, 1957-75 and 1985-88 [0537, 2434, 2722]

5.1.1   Rate

	MMR (per 100 000 live births)
1957	90
1960	40
1965	40
1970	30
1975	30
1985	5
1986	13
1987	7
1988	10

6. OTHER SOURCES/ ESTIMATES

7. SELECTED ANNOTATED BIBLIOGRAPHY

8. FURTHER READING

Kurup, A. et al. Pregnancy outcome in unmarried teenage nulligravidae in Singapore. *International Journal of Gynecology and Obstetrics*, 1989; 30: 305-311. WHE 2870

Lee, S.T. et al. Obstetric outcome of the unwed adolescents. *Singapore Medical Journal*, 1990; 31: 553-557. WHE 2739.

9. DATA SOURCES

WHE 0137   Cheng, M.C.E. et al. Changing trends in mortality and morbidity from abortion in Singapore (1964 to 1970). *Singapore Medical Journal*, 1971; 12(5): 256-258.

WHE 0537   Phoon, W.O. The implications on behavioural patterns of health and social changes. *Tropical Doctor*, 1980; 10: 32-37.

WHE 0659   Singapore, Registrar General of Births and Deaths. *Report on registration of births and deaths 1981.* Singapore, 1981.

WHE 0834   World Health Organization *World health statistics annual – vital statistics and causes of death.* Geneva, various years.

WHE 1488   World Health Organization. Regional Office for the Western Pacific. *Evaluation of the strategy for health for all by the year 2000.* Seventh report on the world health situation. WHO/WPRO, Manila, 1980.

WHE 1712   Mauldin W.P. and Segal, S.J., *Prevalence of contraceptive use in developing countries. A chart book.* Rockefeller Foundation, New York 1986.

WHE 1914   United Nations Children's Fund (UNICEF). *The state of the world's children,* Oxford, Oxford University Press, various years.

WHE 1915   United Nations. Department of International Economic and Social Affairs. *World population prospects: estimates and projections,* Population Studies, New York, various years.

WHE 1917   United Nations. Department of International Economic and Social Affairs. *Age structure of mortality in developing countries. A database for cross-sectional and time-series research.* New York 1986.

WHE 1918   United Nations. Department of International Economic and Social Affairs. *First marriage: patterns and determinants.* New York 1988.

WHE 2033   World Health Organization. *Global strategy for health for all by the year 2000. Second report on monitoring progress.* WHO document EB83/2 Add. 1, 1988.

WHE 2434   Hwa Tay, V.L. *Singapore country report.* Paper presented at the Regional Workshop on risk approach in mother and child health care, Manila, December 1989.

WHE 2445   Vengadasalam, D. Maternal mortality – a review at the Department of Obstetrics and Gynaecology, Alexandra Hospital, Singapore. *Singapore Medical Journal*, 1989; 30(6): 561-564.

WHE 2722   World Health Organization, *Maternal deaths and maternal mortality rates* (unpublished) 1990.

NOTES

Sri Lanka

		Year	Source

1. Basic Indicators

1.1 Demographic

1.1.1 Population

Size (millions)	17.2	1990	(1915)
Rate of growth (%)	1.3	1985-90	(1915)

1.1.2 Life expectancy

Female	73	1985-90	(1915)
Male	68	1985-90	(1915)

1.1.3 Fertility

Crude Birth Rate	23	1985-90	(1915)
Total Fertility Rate	2.7	1985-90	(1915)

1.1.4 Mortality

Crude Death Rate	6	1985-90	(1915)
Infant Mortality Rate	28	1985-90	(1915)
Female	20	1982-87	(2873)
Male	31	1982-87	(2873)
1-4 years mortality rate			
Female	9	1982-87	(2873)
Male	10	1982-87	(2873)

1.2 Social and economic

1.2.1 Adult literacy rate (%)

Female	83	1985	(1914)
Male	91	1985	(1914)

1.2.2 Primary school enrolment rate (%)

Female	102	1986-88	(1914)
Male	105	1986-88	(1914)

1.2.3 Female mean age at first marriage

(years)	24.4	1981	(1918)

1.2.4 GNP/capita

(US $)	420	1988	(1914)

1.2.5 Daily per capita calorie supply

(as % of requirements)	110	1985	(1914)

2. Health Services

2.1 Health expenditure

2.1.1 Expenditure on health

(as % of GNP)	1.6	1986	(2033)

2.1.2 Expenditure on PHC

(as % of total health expenditure)	48	1986	(2033)

2.2 Primary Health Care
(Percentage of population covered by):

2.2.1 Health services

National	90	1987	(2033)
Urban			
Rural			

2.2.2 Safe water

National	37	1983	(0834)
Urban	82	1987	(2033)
Rural	35	1987	(2033)

2.2.3 Adequate sanitary facilities

National	66	1983	(0834)
Urban	69	1987	(2033)
Rural	41	1987	(2033)

2.2.4 Contraceptive prevalence rate

(%)	57	1982	(1712)

2.3 Coverage of maternity care (%)

Area	Prenatal care	Trained attendant	Institutional deliveries	Postnatal care	Sample size	Year	Source
National			76			1981-3	(1526)
National	68	87				1982-3	(1489)
National	97	94			3 906	1983-87	(2873)
National: urban rural			80 87 78			1987 1981-3 1981-3	(2317) (1526) (1526)
Colombo	96	99			307	1983-87	(2873)
Other urban	99	97			235	1983-87	(2873)
Rural	97	94			3 094	1983-87	(2873)
Estates	95	82			270	1983-87	(2873)

3. COMMUNITY STUDIES

4. HOSPITAL STUDIES

5. CIVIL REGISTRATION DATA/GOVERNMENT ESTIMATES

5.1 National, 1941-87 [0476, 0671, 0910, 0935, 1111, 1344, 1526, 2257, 2317, 2874]

5.1.1 Rate

	MMR (per 100 000 live births)
1941	1 530
1946	1 550
1951	580
1956	380
1961	260
1966	220
1971	120
1974	100
1975	100
1976	90
1977	100
1978	80
1979	80
1980	90
1985	60
1986	72
1987	80

5.1.2 Causes of maternal deaths, 1974-78, 1979 and 1983

	1974-78		1979		1983	
	No.	%	No.	%	No.	%
Haemorrhage	644	35	115	36	95	36
Hypertensive disorders of pregnancy	492	27	77	24	51	19
Abortion	142	8	35	11	21	8
Sepsis	122	7	10	3	6	2
Embolisms	31	2	–	–	–	–
Ruptured uterus	28	1	–	–	–	–
Obstructed labour	16	1	–	–	–	–
Ectopic pregnancy	15	1	–	–	–	–
Anaemia	60	3	–	–	–	–
Other	289	16	80	25	92	35
TOTAL	1 839	100	317	100	265	100

5.1.3 Avoidable factors

5.1.4 High risk groups
Age

	MMR (per 100 000 live births)		
	1973	1978	1979
15-19	80	90	80
20-24	100	60	70
25-29	100	70	60
30-34	120	90	70
35-39	210	170	120
40-44	300	140	180
45-49	520	520	780

5.2 All Districts, 1979 [(0910)]

5.2.1 Rate

	MMR (per 100 000 live births)
Nuwara Eliya	170
Mannar	140
Batticaloa	130
Amparai	120
Kandy	120
Moneragala	120
Vavuniya	120
Matara	110
Ratnapura	100
Badulla	90
Galle	90
Trincomalee	90
Polonnaruwa	70
Anuradhapura	60
Kegalle	60
Kurunegala	60
Matale	60
Puttalam	50
Colombo	50
Kalutara	50
Hambantota	40
Gempaha	30
Jaffna	20
Mullaitivu	0

5.3 National, 1985 [(0834)]

5.3.1 Rate

Live births	384 581
Maternal deaths	197
MMR (per 100 000 live births)	51

5.3.2 Causes of maternal deaths

	Number	%
Haemorrhage	63	32
Hypertensive disorders of pregnancy	45	23
Abortion	34	17
Complications of the puerperium	13	7
Other direct causes	30	15
DIRECT CAUSES	185	94
INDIRECT CAUSES	12	6
TOTAL	197	100

6. OTHER SOURCES/ ESTIMATES

6.1 Colombo, 1982 [(0527)]

6.1.1 Rate

According to a paper presented at a UNICEF/WHO meeting on Primary Health Care in urban areas, the maternal mortality rate in Colombo was 25 per 100 000 live births in 1982.

7. SELECTED ANNOTATED BIBLIOGRAPHY

8. FURTHER READING

Langford, C.M. Sex differentials in mortality in Sri Lanka: changes since the 1920s. *Journal of Biosocial Science*, 1984; 16: 399-410. WHE 1113.

Wanigasundara, M. Sri Lanka abortions cause concern. *People*, 1984; 11(2): 37. WHE 0887.

9. DATA SOURCES

WHE 0476   Nadarajah, T. The transition from higher female to higher male mortality in Sri Lanka. *Population and Development Review*, 1983; 9(2): 317-325.

WHE 0527   Peries, T. *Health services provided by the Colombo Medical Council.* In: Joint UNICEF/WHO Meeting on Primary Health Care in Urban Areas. (unpublished), Geneva, 1983.

WHE 0671   Sri Lanka, Ministry of Plan Implementation. *Bulletin of vital statistics, 1979.* Department of Census and Statistics, Colombo, 1981.

WHE 0834   World Health Organization *World health statistics annual – vital statistics and causes of death.* Geneva, various years.

WHE 0910   Sri Lanka, Ministry of Health. *Annual Health Bulletin Sri Lanka 1983.* Colombo, 1984.

WHE 0935   Sri Lanka, Ministry of Health. *Family health impact survey,* Family Health Bureau, Colombo, 1984.

WHE 1111   Pollack, M.P. *Health problems in Sri Lanka, Part II, an analysis of morbidity and mortality data.* US Agency for International Development, 1984.

WHE 1344   Sri Lanka, Ministry of Health. *Medium term plan. Family health programme 1985-89.* Family Health Bureau, Colombo, 1984.

WHE 1489   World Health Organization. Regional Office for Southeast Asia. *Evaluation of the strategy of Health for All by the year 2000.* Seventh Report on the World Health Situation. New Delhi, 1986.

WHE 1526   Vidyasagara, N.W. *Maternal services in Sri Lanka.* Paper presented to the Tenth Asian and Oceanic Congress of Obstetrics and Gynaecology, Colombo, 4-10 September 1985.

WHE 1712   Mauldin W.P. and Segal, S.J. *Prevalence of contraceptive use in developing countries. A chart book.* Rockefeller Foundation, New York 1986.

WHE 1914   United Nations Children's Fund (UNICEF). *The state of the world's children,* Oxford, Oxford University Press, various years.

WHE 1915   United Nations. Department of International Economic and Social Affairs. *World population prospects: estimates and projections,* Population Studies, New York, various years.

WHE 1918   United Nations. Department of International Economic and Social Affairs. *First marriage: patterns and determinants.* New York 1988.

WHE 2033   World Health Organization. *Global strategy for health for all by the year 2000. Second report on monitoring progress.* WHO document EB83/2 Add. 1, 1988.

WHE 2257   Asian Parasite Control/Family Planning Conference. *IP – A strategy for maternal and child health,* Proceedings of the 14th Asian Parasite Control/Family Planning Conference,Dhaka, Bangladesh, 26-30 October 1987.

WHE 2317   Sri Lanka, Ministry of Health. *Maternal mortality statistics 1987.*

WHE 2722   World Health Organization. *Maternal deaths and maternal mortality rates* (unpublished) 1990.

WHE 2873   Demographic and Health Surveys. *Sri Lanka demographic and health survey 1987.* Department of Census and Statistics/Institute for Resource Development/Westinghouse, 1988.

WHE 2874   Jayasena, K. *Assessment of needs for research in reproductive health in Sri Lanka.* Co-ordinating Committee for Research in Reproductive Health in Sri Lanka. Report of a WHO Special Programme of Research, Development and Research Training in Human Reproduction Workshop, Colombo, 15-16 November 1989.

SYRIAN ARAB REPUBLIC

		Year	Source

1. BASIC INDICATORS

1.1. Demographic

1.1.1 Population
		Year	Source
Size (millions)	12.5	1990	(1915)
Rate of growth (%)	3.6	1985-90	(1915)

1.1.2 Life expectancy
		Year	Source
Female	67	1985-90	(1915)
Male	63	1985-90	(1915)

1.1.3 Fertility
		Year	Source
Crude Birth Rate	44	1985-90	(1915)
Total Fertility Rate	6.8	1985-90	(1915)

1.1.4 Mortality
		Year	Source
Crude Death Rate	7	1985-90	(1915)
Infant Mortality Rate	48	1985-90	(1915)
Female	81	1976-78	(1917)
Male	91	1976-78	(1917)
1-4 years mortality rate			
Female	8	1976-78	(1917)
Male	8	1976-78	(1917)

1.2 Social and economic

1.2.1 Adult literacy rate (%)
		Year	Source
Female	43	1985	(1914)
Male	76	1985	(1914)

1.2.2 Primary school enrolment rate (%)
		Year	Source
Female	104	1986-88	(1914)
Male	115	1986-88	(1914)

1.2.3 Female mean age at first marriage
		Year	Source
(years)	20.7	1970	(1918)

1.2.4 GNP/capita
		Year	Source
(US $)	1 640	1987	(1914)

1.2.5 Daily per capita calorie supply
		Year	Source
(as % of requirements)	131	1985	(1914)

2. HEALTH SERVICES

2.1 Health Expenditure

2.1.1 Expenditure on health
		Year	Source
(as % of GNP)	4	1983	(1888)

2.1.2 Expenditure on PHC
		Year	Source
(as % of total health expenditure)	47	1986	(2033)

2.2 Primary Health Care
(Percentage of population covered by):

2.2.1 Health services
		Year	Source
National	83	1987	(2033)
Urban			
Rural			

2.2.2 Safe water
		Year	Source
National			
Urban	91	1987	(2033)
Rural	68	1987	(2033)

2.2.3 Adequate sanitary facilities
		Year	Source
National			
Urban	72	1987	(2033)
Rural	55	1987	(2033)

2.2.4 Contraceptive prevalence rate
		Year	Source
(%)	20	1978	(1712)

2.3   Coverage of maternity care (%)

Area	Prenatal care	Trained attendant	Institutional deliveries	Postnatal care	Sample size	Year	Source
National	21	37				1979	(1888)
National			43		6762	1981	(0813)
National	60	61				1987	(2033)
National:							
urban	35	63	17			1979	(0216)
rural	9	12	3			1979	(0216)
Refugee camps	62*		31*		6 758d*	1986	(1628)

*   Percentages calculated on basis of expected deliveries as determined by birth rates.

3. COMMUNITY STUDIES

3.1 National, (1990) [2781]

A sample survey was undertaken among 20,845 ever-married women of reproductive age (15-49 years), living in both urban and rural areas. The "sisterhood method" was used to derive estimates of maternal mortality. The respondents reported a total of 47,071 ever married sisters of which 698 had died. It was estimated that 183 of these deaths were maternity-related. The lifetime risk of dying from pregnancy-related causes was calculated as 1 in 110.

3.1.1 Rate
Maternal deaths	183
MMR (per 100 000 live births)	143

4. HOSPITAL STUDIES

4.1 Damascus University Maternity Hospital, Damascus, 1963, 1973 and 1981 [0216]

4.1.1 Rate
	1963	1973	1981
Deliveries	2356	3786	4345
Maternal deaths	7	21	6
MMR (per 100 000 deliveries)	297	555	138

4.1.2 Causes of maternal deaths *(1963 and 1973)*
	Number	%
Haemorrhage	7	25
Sepsis	6	21
Ruptured uterus	5	18
Hypertensive disorders of pregnancy	5	18
Abortion	2	7
Cardiac diseases	2	7
Others	1	4
Total	28	100

A study conducted in 1967-68 found an incidence of ruptured uterus of 1 in 106 deliveries with 10 deaths out of 49 cases.

4.2 Aleppo Maternity Hospital, 1977-78 and 1981 [0216]

4.2.1 Rate
	1977-78	1981
Deliveries	3 107	4 253
Maternal deaths	22	20
MMR (per 100 000 deliveries)	708	470

4.2.2 Causes of maternal deaths *(1977-78)*
	Number	%
Haemorrhage	7	32
Ruptured uterus	7	32
Sepsis	5	23
Hypertensive disorders of pregnancy	2	9
Cardiac diseases	1	4
Total	22	100

A study on ruptured uterus in Aleppo Hospital in 1976-78, found 112 cases of ruptured uterus out of a total of 9 689 deliveries, an incidence rate of 1 in 87. Twenty-two of the 112 died, a case fatality rate of 20%.

4.3 El-Zahrawy Hospital, Damascus, 1981[0216]

4.3.1 Rate

Deliveries	7 095
Maternal deaths	9
MMR (per 100 000 deliveries)	127

5. CIVIL REGISTRATION DATA/GOVERNMENT ESTIMATES

6. OTHER SOURCES/ESTIMATES

6.1 National, 1973, 1980 and 1985 [0834, 2722]

6.1.1 Rate

The maternal mortality as reported to WHO was as follows:

	MMR (per 100 000 live births)
1973	6
1980	7
1985*	6

* Reporting areas only

6.2 National, 1979 [0685]

6.2.1 Rate

A UNICEF and Government of Syria joint publication quotes a maternal mortality rate for the country of between 300-400 per 100 000 live births in 1979.

6.3 National [1414]

6.3.1 Rate

The report of Second Mission on Needs Assessment for Population Assistance published in 1984 gives a maternal mortality rate of 280 per 100 000 deliveries.

7. SELECTED ANNOTATED BIBLIOGRAPHY

8. FURTHER READING

9. DATA SOURCES

WHE 0216   Fathalla, M.F. *Maternal health – Syria.* (unpublished WHO document no. EM/MCH/171), 1982.

WHE 0685 Syrian Arab Republic, Central Bureau of Statistics and UNICEF. *Services for the child in the Syrian Arab Republic: a community study,* Arab Book Printers, Damascus, 1979.

WHE 0813   World Health Organization. Eastern Mediterranean Regional Office. *Report of the EMR/SEAR meeting on the prevention of neonatal tetanus.* (WHO document no. EM/IMZ/27, EM/BD/14, EM-SEA/MTG.PREV.NNL.TTN/8), Lahore, 1982.

WHE 0834   World Health Organization *World health statistics annual – vital statistics and causes of death.* Geneva, various years.

WHE 1414   United Nations Fund for Population Activities. *Syrian Arab Republic: report of second mission on needs assessment for population assistance.* UNFPA, New York, 1985.

WHE 1628   United Nations Relief and Works Agency for Palestine Refugees in the Near East. *Annual report of the director of health 1986,* Vienna, 1987.

WHE 1712   Mauldin W.P. and Segal, S.J., *Prevalence of contraceptive use in developing countries. A chart book.* Rockefeller Foundation, New York, 1986.

WHE 1888   World Health Organization, Eastern Mediterranean Regional Office, *Evaluation of the strategy for Health for All by the year 2000.* Seventh report of the world health situation. EMRO, Alexandria, 1987.

WHE 1914   United Nations Children's Fund (UNICEF). *The state of the world's children*, Oxford, Oxford University Press, various years.

WHE 1915   United Nations. Department of International Economic and Social Affairs. *World population prospects: estimates and projections*, Population Studies, New York, various years.

WHE 1917   United Nations. Department of International Economic and Social Affairs. *Age structure of mortality in developing countries. A database for cross-sectional and time-series research.* New York, 1986.

WHE 1918   United Nations. Department of International Economic and Social Affairs. *First marriage: patterns and determinants.* New York, 1988.

WHE 2033   World Health Organization. *Global strategy for health for all by the year 2000. Second report on monitoring progress.* WHO document EB83/2 Add. 1, 1988.

WHE 2722   World Health Organization, *Maternal deaths and maternal mortality rates* (unpublished), 1990.

WHE 2781 Alloush, K. *Maternal mortality in the Syrian Arab Republic, 1990.* Ministry of Health/UNICEF/WHO, 1990

THAILAND

	Year	Source

1. BASIC INDICATORS

1.1. Demographic

1.1.1 Population

		Year	Source
Size (millions)	55.7	1990	(1915)
Rate of growth (%)	1.5	1985-90	(1915)

1.1.2 Life expectancy

		Year	Source
Female	67	1985-90	(1915)
Male	63	1985-90	(1915)

1.1.3 Fertility

		Year	Source
Crude Birth Rate	22	1985-90	(1915)
Total Fertility Rate	2.6	1985-90	(1915)

1.1.4 Mortality

		Year	Source
Crude Death Rate	7	1985-90	(1915)
Infant Mortality Rate	39	1985-90	(1915)
Female	62	1969-71	(1917)
Male	86	1969-71	(1917)
1-4 years mortality rate			
Female	10	1969-71	(1917)
Male	9	1969-71	(1917)

1.2 Social and economic

1.2.1 Adult literacy rate (%)

		Year	Source
Female	88	1985	(1914)
Male	94	1985	(1914)

1.2.2 Primary school enrolment rate (%)

Female			
Male			

1.2.3 Female mean age at first marriage

		Year	Source
(years)	22.7	1980	(2799)

1.2.4 GNP/capita

		Year	Source
(US $)	850	1987	(1914)

1.2.5 Daily per capita calorie supply

		Year	Source
(as % of requirements)	105	1984-86	(1914)

2. HEALTH SERVICES

2.1 Health expenditure

2.1.1 Expenditure on health

		Year	Source
(as % of GNP)	5	1985	(2033)

2.1.2 Expenditure on PHC

		Year	Source
(as % of total health expenditure)	39	1985	(2033)

2.2 Primary Health Care
(Percentage of population covered by):

2.2.1 Health services

		Year	Source
National	93	1987	(2033)
Urban			
Rural			

2.2.2 Safe water

		Year	Source
National			
Urban	57	1987	(2033)
Rural	78	1987	(2033)

2.2.3 Adequate sanitary facilities

		Year	Source
National			
Urban	81	1987	(2033)
Rural	57	1987	(2033)

2.2.4 Contraceptive prevalence rate

		Year	Source
(%)	65	1984	(1712)

2.3   Coverage of maternity care (%)

Area	Prenatal care	Trained attendant	Institutional deliveries	Postnatal care	Sample size	Year	Source
National		40	40		13 659	1980	(0813)
National		33				1983	(0834)
National	57	52				1987	(2033)
National	65	71		84		1988	(2375)
Bang Pa-In	93	94	85		1 128w	1983-84	(1487)
Buriram Province	62	47	36			1982	(0803)
Chang Mai Province			40		263w	1974	(0472)
Chumporn Province	74	85	78			1982	(0803)
Lampang Province		75		10		1975	(0158)
Uthaithani Province	67	79	74		637w	1982	(0803)

3. COMMUNITY STUDIES

3.1 140 villages, Bang Pa-In district, Ayuthaya Province, 1977-83 [1487]

In 1981 the risk approach was adopted in maternal health care. The subsequent improvement in maternal health care provision resulted in the fall in the numbers of maternal deaths.

3.1.1 Rate

	Live Births	Maternal deaths	MMR (per 100 000 births)
1977-78	1 119	6	536
1979-80	996	2	201
1981-83	1 836	1	55

4. HOSPITAL STUDIES

4.1 Provincial hospitals, 1979 [0955]

4.1.1 Rate

Live births	155 975
Maternal deaths	240
MMR (per 100 000 live births)	154

4.1.2 Causes of maternal deaths

	Number	%
Abortion	65	28
Haemorrhage	45	19
Sepsis	25	11
Hypertensive disorders of pregnancy	20	8
Ectopic/molar pregnancy	15	6
Obstructed labour	10	4
Infective and parasitic conditions	20	8
Other	40	17
Total	240	100

4.2 Three regional MCH centres, 1968-71 [0614]

4.2.1 Rate

Deliveries	24 000
Maternal deaths	23
MMR (per 100 000 deliveries)	96

4.3 Ramathibodi Hospital, Bangkok, 1969-82 [1503]

4.3.1 Rate

	Live Births	Maternal deaths	MMR (per 100 000 births)
1969-75	27 628	12	43
1976-82	45 244	14	31
1969-82	72 872	26	36

4.3.2 Causes of maternal deaths

	Number
Abortion	10
Sepsis	3
Hypertensive disorders of pregnancy	3
Embolisms	3
Ruptured uterus	1
Hepatitis	3
Other	3
Total	26

4.3.3 Avoidable factors

4.3.4 High risk groups

Age

	MMR (per 100 000 live births)
< 19 years	80
20-34	20
35+	60

4.4 Siriraj, Rajvithi and Chulalongkorn Hospitals, Bangkok, 1973-77 [0602]

A case-control study was undertaken in three hospitals. Controls were unmatched apart from having delivered and survived over the same period of time as mothers who died.

4.4.1 Rate

	Siriraj Hospital	Rajvithi Hospital	Chulalongkorn Hospital
Deliveries	102 478	113 084	77 225
Maternal deaths	84	92	61
MMR (per 100 000 deliveries)	82	81	80

4.4.2 Causes of maternal deaths *(for 212 deaths)*

	Number	%
Abortion	62	30
Hypertensive disorders of pregnancy	32	15
Haemorrhage	28	13
Sepsis	20	9
Ruptured uterus	11	5
Embolisms	10	5
Ectopic/molar pregnancy	6	3
DIRECT CAUSES	169	80
Cardiovascular disease	17	8
Pulmonary disease	7	3
Anaemia/blood disease	5	2
Hepatitis	2	1
Malaria	2	1
INDIRECT CAUSES	33	16
Other	10	4
TOTAL	212	100

4.4.3 Avoidable factors

Prenatal care (for 212 deaths)

Number of prenatal visits	Maternal deaths (No.)	Controls (No.)	Relative risk (5+ visits = 1)
none	147	62	87
one	37	190	7
two	9	33	10
three	5	184	1
four	6	77	3
five and over	8	204	1

Women who commenced prenatal visits during the first or second trimesters of pregnancy had lower mortality rates than those who attended only during the last trimester.

Birth interval (for 132 deaths)

	Maternal deaths (No.)	Controls (No.)	Relative risk (24-35 months = 1)
<24 months	80	101	12
24-35 months	13	190	1
36-47 months	6	60	2
48-59 months	13	36	5
60-71 months	7	26	4
71+ months	13	43	4

4.4.4   High risk groups

Age

	Deliveries	Maternal deaths	MMR (per 100 000 births)
15-19	38 468	29	75
20-24	97 791	63	64
25-29	93 399	38	41
30-34	39 526	49	124
35-39	16 396	28	171
40+	7 027	30	427

Parity

	Deliveries	Maternal deaths	MMR (per 100 000 births)
0	118 286	89	75
1	76 125	42	55
2	42 942	27	63
3	20 690	20	97
4	15 615	21	134
5+	19 129	39	204

4.4.5   Other findings

Complications during previous pregnancies

Women who had experienced complications during previous pregnancies were significantly more at risk of death. The most frequent previous complications were abortion, haemorrhage, hypertensive disorders, heart disease and cervical dystocia. The relative risk of maternal death increased with the number of previous abortions. Women whose previous deliveries were not spontaneous vaginal deliveries were also at greater risk.

Abortion

Over 25% of all maternal deaths were due to illegal abortions mainly among nulliparous women aged under 20 years and those over 35 with four or more children.

5.   CIVIL REGISTRATION DATA/GOVERNMENT ESTIMATES

5.1   National, 1981 [0918]

5.1.1   Rate
MMR (per 100 000 live births)   110

5.2   National, 1986 [2375]

5.2.1   Rate
MMR (per 100 000 live births)   30

6.   OTHER SOURCES/ ESTIMATES

6.1   National, 1960-1981 [1522]

6.1.1   Rate

	MMR (per 100 000 live births)
1960	420
1965	310
1970	230
1975	170
1981	80*

*   A community survey found a maternal mortality rate of 540 per 100 000 live births. No further information is provided.

6.2   National, 1983 [1241]

6.2.1   Rate
A paper presented at an ASEAN workshop quoted a maternal mortality rate of 270 per 100 000 live births.

6.3   National, 1985-87 [2722]

6.3.1   Rate
Data provided to the World Health Organization databank indicated a maternal mortality rate of 37 per 100 000 live births in 1987.

	Maternal deaths	MMR (per 100 000 births)
1985	409	42
1986	326	35
1987	329	37

7. SELECTED ANNOTATED BIBLIOGRAPHY

Chamratrithirong, A. et al. The effect of reduced family size on maternal and child health: the case of Thailand. *World Health Statistics Quarterly*, 1987; 40: 54-62. WHE 2548

A study on the effect of reduced family size on maternal and child health was undertaken during 1985. Women with smaller families had a higher haematocrit level than those with larger families. However, health status as measured by parasitic infection, malnutrition (percentage underweight) and incidence of illness during the previous month, were not found to be any worse among women with large families. The percentage of last pregnancy with certain complications was found to be lower among women with smaller families. Pregnancy wastage, infant and child mortality were found to be less frequent among women with smaller families.

Chaturachinda, K. *Personal communication*. Bangkok, 1989. WHE 2179

From 1969-1989 there were 113,365 deliveries at the Ramathibodi Hospital, Bangkok, Thailand, no cases of vesico-vaginal fistula, and one case of recto-vaginal fistula. Additional information shows three cases of urinary fistula from Northeast Thailand caused by obstetric intervention, and two recto-vaginal fistulae from mismanaged labour at another hospital in Bangkok.

World Health Organization. International Collaborative Study of Hypertensive Disorders of Pregnancy. Geographic variation in the incidence of hypertension in pregnancy *American Journal of Obstetrics and Gynecology*, 1988; 158(1): 80-83. WHE 2552.

Prospectively collected information on blood pressure and proteinuria was available for 3,111 primigravidas in urban Ubon and 1,015 in rural Bang Pa-In. Clinical diagnosis of hypertensive disorders of pregnancy was made in 1.1% of the women and proteinuric preeclampsia occurred in 7.5% but only 0.93% developed eclampsia. There were marked differences in the incidence of hypertensive disorders and eclampsia in the different countries participating in the study, Burma, China, Thailand and Viet Nam but there is no satisfactory explanation for these variations (see relevant country profiles).

8. FURTHER READING

Chaturachinda, K. et al. Abortion: an epidemiological study at Ramathibodi Hospital, Bangkok. *Studies in Family Planning*, 1981; 12(6/7): 257-262. WHE 2229

Israngura Na Ayudhya, N. and Chaturachinda, K. The use of antenatal beds in Ramathibodi Hospital. *Journal of the Medical Association of Thailand*, 1988; 71(2): 78-81. WHE 2199

9. DATA SOURCES

WHE 0158   Coombs, P.H. *The Lamang Health Development Project*. Case study No. 8, International Council for Educational Development, Essex, Conn. U.S.A., 1979.

WHE 0472   Muecke, M.E. Health care systems as socializing agents: childbearing the North Thai and Western way. *Social Science and Medicine*, 1976; 10(7/8): 377-383.

WHE 0602   Rattanaporn, P. *The internal factors affecting maternal mortality*. Mahidol University (thesis), Bangkok, 1980.

WHE 0614   Rosenfield, A.G. and Asavasena, W. Rural-oriented maternity services. *American Journal of Obstetrics and Gynecology*, 1973; 115(7): 1013-1020.

WHE 0803   World Health Organization. Expanded Programme on Immunization. Programme review. *Weekly Epidemiological Record*, 1982; 57: 385-387.

WHE 0813   World Health Organization. Eastern Mediterranean Regional Office. *Report of the EMR/SEAR meeting on prevention of neonatal tetanus* (WHO document no. EM/IMZ/27, EM/BD/14, EM-SEA/MTG.PREV.NNL.TTN./8), Lahore, 1982.

WHE 0834   World Health Organization *World health statistics annual – vital statistics and causes of death*. Geneva, various years.

WHE 0918   World Health Organization. Southeast Asia Regional Office. *Country paper – Thailand*. In: Joint National/WHO/UNFPA Workshop, New Delhi, 1984.

WHE 0955   Thailand, Ministry of Public Health. *Statistical Report 1979*, Department of Medical Services, Bangkok, 1980.

WHE 1241   Pensri, K. Perinatal morbidity and mortality in Thailand. In: Abdul Kader, H. (ed.) *Proceedings of the ASEAN Pediatrics Federation Workshop on Perinatal Morbidity and Mortality: Asian perinatal health issues.*, Kuala Lumpur, 1983.

WHE 1487   Khanjanasthiti, P. et al. *Report on the risk approach strategy in MCH service research, Thailand May 1981 – January 1984,*, Ramathibodi Faculty of Medicine, Mahidol University, Bangkok, 1985.

WHE 1503   Winit, P. et al. Maternal mortality in Ramathibodi Hospital: a 14-year review. *Journal of the Medical Association of Thailand*, 1985; 68(12): 654-658.

WHE 1522   World Health Organization. Southeast Asia Regional Office. *Bulletin of regional health information*, WHO/SEARO, New Delhi, 1986.

WHE 1712   Mauldin W.P. and Segal, S.J., *Prevalence of contraceptive use in developing countries. A chart book.* Rockefeller Foundation, New York 1986.

WHE 1914   United Nations Children's Fund (UNICEF). *The state of the world's children*, Oxford, Oxford University Press, various years.

WHE 1915   United Nations. Department of International Economic and Social Affairs. *World population prospects: estimates and projections*, Population Studies, New York, various years.

WHE 1917   United Nations. Department of International Economic and Social Affairs. *Age structure of mortality in developing countries. A database for cross-sectional and time-series research.* New York 1986.

WHE 2033   World Health Organization. *Global strategy for health for all by the year 2000. Second report on monitoring progress.* WHO document EB83/2 Add. 1, 1988.

WHE 2375   Niyomwan, V. *Maternal care – mortality assessment process and its results in Thailand*, Paper presented at workshop on the Safe Motherhood Initiative, New Delhi, 6-10 November, 1989.

WHE 2722   World Health Organization, *Maternal deaths and maternal mortality rates* (unpublished) 1990.

WHE 2799   United Nations. Department of International Economic and Social Affairs. *Patterns of first marriage: timing and prevalence.* New York, 1990.

WHE 3122 Chongsuvivatwong, V. et al. Traditional society, health status and international migration of Muslim villagers in the lower part of Southern Thailand. *Southeast Asian Journal of Tropical Medicine and Public Health*, 1990; 21(3): 442-446.

TURKEY

		Year	Source

1. BASIC INDICATORS

1.1 Demographic

1.1.1 Population

Size (millions)	55.9	1990	(1915)
Rate of growth (%)	2.1	1985-90	(1915)

1.1.2 Life expectancy

Female	66	1985-90	(1915)
Male	63	1985-90	(1915)

1.1.3 Fertility

Crude Birth Rate	29	1985-90	(1915)
Total Fertility Rate	3.7	1985-90	(1915)

1.1.4 Mortality

Crude Death Rate	8	1985-90	(1915)
Infant Mortality Rate	76	1985-90	(1915)
Female			
Male			
1-4 years mortality rate			
Female			
Male			

1.2 Social and economic

1.2.1 Adult literacy rate (%)

Female	64	1985	(1914)
Male	88	1985	(1914)

1.2.2 Primary school enrolment rate (%)

Female	113	1986-88	(1914)
Male	121	1986-88	(1914)

1.2.3 Female mean age at first marriage

(years)	20.6	1980	(1918)

1.2.4 GNP/capita

(US $)	1 280	1985	(1914)

1.2.5 Daily per capita calorie supply

(as % of requirements)	125	1985	(1914)

2. HEALTH SERVICES

2.1 Health Expenditure

2.1.1 Expenditure on health

(as % of GNP)	2.7	1987	(2033)

2.1.2 Expenditure on PHC

(as % of total health expenditure)	27	1987	(2033)

2.2 Primary Health Care

(Percentage of population covered by):

2.2.1 Health services

National			
Urban			
Rural			

2.2.2 Safe water

National	67	1980	(0834)
Urban	100	1985	(2033)
Rural	70	1985	(2033)

2.2.3 Adequate sanitary facilities

National	90	1982	(0834)
Urban	95	1985	(2033)
Rural	90	1985	(2033)

2.2.4 Contraceptive prevalence rate

(%)	40	1978	(1712)

2.3   Coverage of maternity care (%)

Area	Prenatal care	Trained attendant	Institutional deliveries	Postnatal care	Sample size	Year	Source
National			50			1986	(1387)
National:	43	76	61			1983-88	(3144)
urban	56	86	72			1983-86	(3144)
rural	27	65	47			1983-86	(3144)
9 provinces		38	20		2 035	1985	(1524)
Centre	42	80	65			1983-86	(3144)
Cubuk district		61	47			1980	(0299)
Cubuk		80	67		1 313d	1984	(1265)
Eastern region			20			1986	(1387)
East	22	58	37			1983-86	(3144)
North	37	84	76			1983-86	(3144)
South	37	70	55			1983-86	(3144)
West	62	87	72			1983-86	(3144)

3.   COMMUNITY STUDIES

3.1   National, (1989) [2565]

The "sisterhood method" was used to estimate maternal mortality in the context of a demographic survey undertaken by the national government. The total sample size was 4,594 women of reproductive age who were asked about the deaths of ever married sisters. The life time risk of dying from pregnancy related causes was estimated as 1 in 159.

3.1.1   Rate

Maternal deaths	376
MMR (per 100 000 live births)	146

3.2   Adiyaman and K. Maras, Eastern Provinces, 1986 [1689]

3.2.1   Rate

	MMR (per 100 000 live births)
Adiyaman province	91
K. Maras province	284

A study done in the Eastern provinces of Turkey in 1986 found a maternal mortality rate of 284 per 100,000 live births.

3.3   Etimesgut and Cubuk rural areas, 1975-83 [1265, 1689]

3.3.1   Rate

Deliveries	31 051
Maternal deaths	37
MMR (per 100 000 deliveries)	119

3.3.2 Causes of maternal deaths

	Number	%
Haemorrhage	14	38
Hypertensive disorders of pregnancy	4	11
Embolism	4	11
Sepsis	2	5
DIRECT CAUSES	24	65
INDIRECT CAUSES	13	35
TOTAL	37	100

3.3.3 Avoidable factors

Over half of the deaths were considered preventable with existing local health care facilities and a further 24% could have been prevented given improved health facilities.

4. HOSPITAL STUDIES

4.1 Health centres in Cubuk area, 1977-83 [1265]

4.1.1 Rate

	MMR (per 100 000 live births)
Central health centre	163
Villages Group health centre*	207
Akyurt health centre	73
Yenice health centre	154
Y. Cav health centre	152
Kislacik health centre*	341

* Rural areas.

4.2 University of Hacettepe, Ankara, 1971-81 [2307]

4.2.1 Rate
Deliveries	20 291
Maternal deaths	13
MMR (per 100 000 deliveries)	64

4.3 All hospitals, 1986 [3144]

4.3.1 Rate
Admissions for pregnancy and childbirth	791 000
Maternal deaths	624
MMR (per 100 000 admissions)	79

4.3.2 Causes of maternal deaths,

	Number	%
Hypertensive disorders of pregnancy	256	41
Abortion	77	12
Normal delivery	53	8
Haemorrhage	47	8
Sepsis	13	2
Other infections	21	3
Complications of the puerperium	157	25
TOTAL	624	100

5. CIVIL REGISTRATION DATA/GOVERNMENT ESTIMATES

5.1 Urban areas, 1960-82 [1265]

5.1.1 Rate

	Maternal deaths	MMR (per 100 000 live births)
1960-66	3 299	145
1967-74	2 183	76
1975-82	735	22

There is thought to be considerable underreporting of maternal deaths.

6. OTHER SOURCES/ ESTIMATES

6.1 National [0934, 1265, 1387]

6.1.1 Rate

Several sources give a maternal mortality rate for the country as a whole of 208 per 100 000 live births.

7. SELECTED ANNOTATED BIBLIOGRAPHY

Kafkas, S.K. and Taner, C.E. Ruptured uterus. *International Journal of Gynecology and Obstetrics*, 1990; 34: 41-44. WHE 2738.

In a total of 3,962 deliveries at the Dicle University Medical School between 1983 and 1988, there were 41 cases of ruptured uterus, an incidence rate of 1 in 97 deliveries or 1%. All the cases occurred among poor uneducated women who had had no prenatal care. Delay in admission to hospital ranged from 9-72 hours and the uterus of each patient except one had ruptured prior to admission. There were no uterine ruptures in primigravidae and high parities of 5 and more accounted for over 60% of the cases. In 31 cases the rupture was due to cephalopelvic disproportion. Three of the patients died, a case fatality rate of 7.3%. Three patients developed vesico-vaginal fistulae and there were two cases of ruptured bladder.

8. FURTHER READING

9. DATA SOURCES

WHE 0299   Bertan, M. Integration of family planning in primary health care. *ICMR/WHO Workshop on Service and Psychosocial Research in Family Planning*, Trivandrum, December 1982.

WHE 0834   World Health Organization *World health statistics annual – vital statistics and causes of death*. Geneva, various years.

WHE 0934   Yener, S. *Women and health in Turkey.*Regional workshop in Women, Health and Development. Damascus, Syria, 11-15 November, 1984. (Unpublished).

WHE 1265   Dervisoglu, A.A. *Maternal mortality in Turkey*. (unpublished), Ankara, 1985.

WHE 1387   Fincancioglu, N. Turkey launches new drive. *People*, 1986; 13: 28-29.

WHE 1524   Dervisoglu, A.A. *Strengthening integrated FP/MCH services in 17 provinces*. Report of a baseline study carried out in 9 provinces. WHO/EURO Document no. TUR/MCH 501, 1985.

WHE 1689   Dervisoglu, A.A. *Maternal mortality in Turkey and its prevention*. (unpublished), 1988.

WHE 1712   Mauldin W.P. and Segal, S.J. *Prevalence of contraceptive use in developing countries. A chart book*. Rockefeller Foundation, New York, 1986.

WHE 1914   United Nations Children's Fund (UNICEF). *The state of the world's children*, Oxford, Oxford University Press, various years.

WHE 1915   United Nations. Department of International Economic and Social Affairs. *World population prospects: estimates and projections*, Population Studies, New York, various years.

WHE 1918   United Nations. Department of International Economic and Social Affairs. *First marriage: patterns and determinants*. New York, 1988.

WHE 2033   World Health Organization. *Global strategy for health for all by the year 2000. Second report on monitoring progress*. WHO document EB83/2 Add. 1, 1988.

WHE 2307   Ayhan, A. et al. Analysis of 20,291 deliveries in a Turkish institution. *International Journal of Gynecology and Obstetrics*, 1989; 29: 131-134.

WHE 2565   Graham, W. *Results of the application of the sisterhood method for estimating maternal mortality*. London School of Hygiene and Tropical Medicine (Unpublished) 1990

WHE 3144 Turkey, Government of, *The situation analysis of mothers and children in Turkey*. UNICEF/Government of Turkey, Ankara, 1991.

UNITED ARAB EMIRATES

		Year	Source

1. BASIC INDICATORS

1.1 Demographic

1.1.1 Population

Size (millions)	1.6	1990	(1915)
Rate of growth (%)	3.2	1985-90	(1915)

1.1.2 Life expectancy

Female	73	1985-90	(1915)
Male	69	1985-90	(1915)

1.1.3 Fertility

Crude Birth Rate	23	1985-90	(1915)
Total Fertility Rate	4.8	1985-90	(1915)

1.1.4 Mortality

Crude Death Rate	4	1985-90	(1915)
Infant Mortality Rate	26	1985-90	(1915)
Female			
Male			
1-4 years mortality rate			
Female			
Male			

1.2 Social and economic

1.2.1 Adult literacy rate (%)

Female	7	1970	(1914)
Male	24	1970	(1914)

1.2.2 Primary school enrolment rate (%)

Female	100	1986-88	(1914)
Male	98	1986-88	(1914)

1.2.3 Female mean age at first marriage

(years)	18.0	1975	(2799)

1.2.4 GNP/capita

(US $)	15 770	1988	(1914)

1.2.5 Daily per capita calorie supply
(as % of requirements)

2. HEALTH SERVICES

2.1 Health Expenditure

2.1.1 Expenditure on health

(as % of GNP)	9.0	1987	(2033)

2.1.2 Expenditure on PHC
(as % of total health expenditure)

2.2 Primary Health Care
(Percentage of population covered by):

2.2.1 Health services

National	100	1987	(2033)
Urban	100	1987	(2033)
Rural	100	1987	(2033)

2.2.2 Safe Water

National	100	1987	(2033)
Urban	100	1987	(2033)
Rural	100	1987	(2033)

2.2.3 Adequate sanitary facilities

National			
Urban	100	1987	(2033)
Rural	77	1987	(2033)

2.2.4 Contraceptive prevalence rate
(%)

2.3   Coverage of maternity care (%)

Area	Prenatal care	Trained attendant	Institutional deliveries	Postnatal care	Sample size	Year	Source
National			85			1980	(0807)
National	98	99				1987	(2033)

3. COMMUNITY STUDIES

4. HOSPITAL STUDIES

5. CIVIL REGISTRATION DATA/GOVERNMENT ESTIMATES

6. OTHER SOURCES/ ESTIMATES

7. SELECTED ANNOTATED BIBLIOGRAPHY

8. FURTHER READING

9. DATA SOURCES

WHE 0807   World Health Organization. Expanded Programme on Immunization. *Programme review, United Arab Emirates*, (unpublished WHO document no. EM/IMZ/18), 1981.

WHE 1914   United Nations Children's Fund (UNICEF). *The state of the world's children*, Oxford, Oxford University Press, various years.

WHE 1915   United Nations. Department of International Economic and Social Affairs. *World population prospects: estimates and projections*, Population Studies, New York, various years.

WHE 2033   World Health Organization. *Global strategy for health for all by the year 2000. Second report on monitoring progress.* WHO document EB83/2 Add. 1, 1988.

WHE 2799   United Nations. Department of International Economic and Social Affairs. *Patterns of first marriage: timing and prevalence.* New York, 1990.

VIET NAM

		Year	Source

1. BASIC INDICATORS

1.1 Demographic

1.1.1 Population

Size (millions)	67.1	1990	(1915)
Rate of growth (%)	2.2	1985-90	(1915)

1.1.2 Life expectancy

Female	64	1985-90	(1915)
Male	59	1985-90	(1915)

1.1.3 Fertility

Crude Birth Rate	32	1985-90	(1915)
Total Fertility Rate	4.1	1985-90	(1915)

1.1.4 Mortality

Crude Death Rate	10	1985-90	(1915)
Infant Mortality Rate	64	1985-90	(1915)
Female			
Male			
1-4 years mortality rate			
Female			
Male			

1.2 Social and economic

1.2.1 Adult literacy rate (%)

Female	80	1985	(1914)
Male	88	1985	(1914)

1.2.2 Primary school enrolment rate (%)

Female	94	1986-88	(1914)
Male	107	1986-88	(1914)

1.2.3 Female mean age at first marriage
(years)

1.2.4 GNP/capita
(US $)

1.2.5 Daily per capita calorie supply

(as % of requirements)	105	1984-86	(1914)

2. HEALTH SERVICES

2.1 Health Expenditure

2.1.1 Expenditure on health

(as % of GNP)	3.0	1990	(3153)

2.1.2 Expenditure on PHC

(as % of total health expenditure)	80	1988	(3153)

2.2 Primary Health Care
(Percentage of population covered by):

2.2.1 Health services

National	97	1987	(2033)
Urban			
Rural			

2.2.2 Safe water

National			
Urban	70	1987	(2033)
Rural	39	1987	(2033)

2.2.3 Adequate sanitary facilities

National	30	1983	(0834)
Urban			
Rural			

2.2.4 Contraceptive prevalence rate

(%)	20	1982	(1712)

2.3   Coverage of maternity care (%)

Area	Prenatal care	Trained attendant	Institutional deliveries	Postnatal care	Sample size	Year	Source
National	99		99			1982	(0900)
National		100				1982	(0834)
National	93	90				1987	(2033)
National	73					1990	(3153)

3.   COMMUNITY STUDIES

4.   HOSPITAL STUDIES

4.1   Six provincial and district hospitals and the Institute for the Protection of the Mothers and the Newborn, 1984-85 [(0997)]

4.1.1   Rate

Province	Deliveries	Maternal deaths	MMR (per 100 000 births)
Bac Thai	2 759	15	544
Ha Bac	2 255	18	798
Hai Hung	1 517	9	593
Ha Nam Ninh	2 662	18	676
Ha Son Binh	2 229	20	897
7 districts of Thai Binh	3 730	17	456
Vinh Phu	2 959	21	710
Institute	4 079	10	245
Total	22 190	128	576

4.1.2   Causes of maternal deaths*

	Number	%
Primary causes		
Haemorrhage	38	29
Sepsis	20	16
Ectopic pregnancy	8	6
Abortions	8	6
Ruptured uterus	8	6
Hypertensive disorders of pregnancy	5	4
Others	36	29
Associated causes		
Haemorrhage	31	24
Anaemia	20	16
Sepsis	16	13
Renal failure	8	6
Heart failure	8	6
Traditional herb	2	2
Other	27	21

*   categories not mutually exclusive.

4.1.3   Avoidable factors*

35% of the deaths were considered definitely preventable, 53% possibly preventable and 10% non-preventable.

	Number	%
Delay in treatment	80	63
Delay in referral	77	60
Delay in diagnosis	68	53
Wrong treatment	47	37
Lack of blood	46	36
Lack of transport	29	23
Wrong diagnosis	28	22
Lack of drugs	26	20
Patient not presented	22	17
Lack of equipment	14	11
Patient non compliance	13	10
Use of traditional medicine	6	5
Lack of staff	4	3
Wrong referral	1	8
Others	16	12

*   Categories not mutually exclusive.

4.1.4   High risk groups

For each maternal death identified during the study period the next five pregnant or delivered women were selected as controls for comparative purposes. Prior to the data analysis two of the five controls were matched to the cases for place of residence. No other matching criteria were used. It was found that women aged less than 20 years old and primiparous together with older women (over 30 years old) and those of para 4 and higher were at greatest risk of death. Women who had no prenatal care were also at greater risk of death. Only 34% of the women who died had received prenatal care compared with 74% of the women in the control group.

4.2 Provincial Hospital, Quang Ngai, South Vietnam, 1967-69 [(0862)]

4.2.1 Rate

Live births	5 371
Maternal deaths	51
MMR (per 100 000 live births)	1 060

4.2.2 Causes of maternal deaths

The number of deaths associated with caesarean sections was very high, constituting 35% of all maternal deaths. This high fatality rate was because caesarean section was performed as a last resort. The second most frequent cause of death was ruptured uterus, and the fact that no blood was available for transfusion no doubt greatly contributed to a number of deaths. Although severe anaemia was a direct cause of death in only eight cases, it was common among the pregnant women.

	Number	%
Associated with caesarean section	18	35
Ruptured uterus	8	16
Hypertensive disorders of pregnancy	7	14
Anaemia	7	14
Haemorrhage	7	14
Sepsis	3	5
Cardiac diseases	1	2
Total	51	100

4.2.3 Avoidable factors

4.2.4 High risk groups

4.2.5 Other findings

There were 284 admissions for complications of abortion during the three year period, of which slightly less than half were septic abortions. 25 women died.

5. CIVIL REGISTRATION DATA/GOVERNMENT ESTIMATES

5.1 National, 1985-87 [(1920, 2774)]

5.1.1 Rate

	MMR (per 100 000 live births)
1981	100
1983	110
1984	125
1985	140
1986	140
1987	130

6. OTHER SOURCES/ ESTIMATES

6.1 National, 1983 [(1417)]

6.1.1 Rate

According to the WHO regional data bank, the maternal mortality rate for the country in 1983 was 110 per 100,000 live births.

6.2 National, 1982 [(0917)]

6.2.1 Rate

A UNICEF publication quotes a maternal mortality rate of 100 per 100,000 live births in 1982.

6.3 National, 1989 [(3153)]

6.3.1 Rate

MMR (per 100 000 live births)	120

7. SELECTED ANNOTATED BIBLIOGRAPHY

Le Diem Huong and Hoang Kim Phung, *Country report – Viet Nam*. Paper presented at a regional workshop on the risk approach in mother and child health care. (unpublished) Regional Office for the Western Pacific, Manila, 1990. WHE 2774

A survey carried out to assess the health status of forestry workers and peasant women in two provinces, Ha Tuyen and Vinh Phu found that there were important differences in the utilization of prenatal care, trained assistance during delivery and institutional deliveries both between the two provinces and for the two groups of women.

	Prenatal visits %	Trained assistance at delivery %	Institutional delivery %
Ha Tuyen Province			
Forestry workers	67	88	43
Peasants	43	49	15
Ving Phu Province			
Forestry workers	86	87	62
Peasants	69	73	44

World Health Organization. International Collaborative Study of Hypertensive Disorders of Pregnancy. Geographic variation in the incidence of hypertension in pregnancy *American Journal of Obstetrics and Gynecology*, 1988; 158(1): 80-83. WHE 2552.

Prospectively collected information on blood pressure and proteinuria was available for 3 046 primigravidas in part of the city of Hanoi and 1 374 primigravidas in rural areas near Hanoi. Clinical diagnosis of hypertensive disorders of pregnancy

was made in 1.2% of the women and proteinuric preeclampsia occurred in 1.5% but only 0.34% developed eclampsia. There were marked differences in the incidence of hypertensive disorders and eclampsia in the different countries participating in the study, Burma, China, Thailand and Viet Nam but there is no satisfactory explanation for these variations (see relevant country profiles).

8. FURTHER READING

9. DATA SOURCES

WHE 0834   World Health Organization *World health statistics annual – vital statistics and causes of death.* Geneva, various years.

WHE 0862   Vennema, A. Perinatal mortality and maternal mortality at the Provincial Hospital, Quang Ngai, South Vietnam, 1967-70. *Tropical and Geographic Medicine*, 1975; 27: 34-38.

WHE 0900   United Nations. Secretariat of the Decade for Women. *Country response to the questionnaire on the review and appraisal of the UN decade for women: equality, development and peace*, Part II (B), Health and nutrition, (unpublished documents), 1984.

WHE 0917   United Nations Economic and Social Commission for Asia and the Pacific. *The Asian and Pacific atlas of children in national development.* UNICEF, 1984.

WHE 0997   Viet Nam, Institute for the protection of mother and newborn. Maternal mortality in selected areas of Viet Nam. In: *Interregional Meeting for the Prevention of Maternal Mortality*, Geneva, 11-15 November, 1985.

WHE 1417   World Health Organization. Regional Office for the Western Pacific, *Databank on socioeconomic and health indicators*, 1985.

WHE 1712   Mauldin W.P. and Segal, *Prevalence of contraceptive use in developing countries. A chart book.* Rockefeller Foundation, New York 1986.

WHE 1914   United Nations Children's Fund (UNICEF). *The state of the world's children*, Oxford, Oxford University Press, various years.

WHE 1915   United Nations. Department of International Economic and Social Affairs. *World population prospects: estimates and projections*, Population Studies, New York, various years.

WHE 1920   Deodato, G. *Report on a field visit to the Socialist Republic of Vietnam*, Manila, 10-24 July, 1987.

WHE 2033   World Health Organization. *Global strategy for health for all by the year 2000. Second report on monitoring progress.* WHO document EB83/2 Add. 1, 1988.

WHE 2774   Le Diem Huong and Hoang Kim Phung, *Country report – Vietnam.* Paper presented to the regional workshop on risk approach in mother and child health care, Manila, 1990.

WHE 3153   World Health Organization. Western Pacific Regional Office. *Country data sheets.* (unpublished), 1991.

YEMEN

		Year	Source

1. BASIC INDICATORS

1.1 Demographic

1.1.1 Population

Size (millions)	10.5	1990	(1915)
Rate of growth (%)	3.0	1985-90	(1915)

1.1.2 Life expectancy

Female	52	1985-90	(1915)
Male	49	1985-90	(1915)

1.1.3 Fertility

Crude Birth Rate	48	1985-90	(1915)
Total Fertility Rate	6.8	1985-90	(1915)

1.1.4 Mortality

Crude Death Rate	16	1985-90	(1915)
Infant Mortality Rate	117	1985-90	(1915)
Female			
Male			
1-4 years mortality rate			
Female			
Male			

1.2 Social and economic

1.2.1 Adult literacy rate* (%)

Female	11	1985	(1914)
Male	49	1985	(1914)

1.2.2 Primary school enrolment rate* (%)

Female	39	1986-88	(1914)
Male	130	1986-88	(1914)

1.2.3 Female mean age at first marriage
(years)

		Year	Source

1.2.4 GNP/capita*

(US $)	550	1987	(1914)

1.2.5 Daily per capita calorie supply

as % of requirements	94	1984-86	(1914)

2. HEALTH SERVICES

2.1 Health Expenditure

2.1.1 Expenditure on health
(as % of GNP)

2.1.2 Expenditure on PHC
(as % of total health expenditure)

2.2 Primary Health Care
(Percentage of population covered by):

2.2.1 Health services*

National	48	1985	(2033)
Urban			
Rural			

2.2.2 Safe water

National			
Urban	89	1985	(2033)
Rural	31	1985	(2033)

2.2.3 Adequate sanitary facilities

National			
Urban	67	1985	(2033)
Rural			

2.2.4 Contraceptive prevalence rate
(%)

* Estimated

2.3 Coverage of maternity care (%)

Area	Prenatal care	Trained attendant	Institutional deliveries	Postnatal care	Sample size	Year	Source
National	10	10				1982	(0834)
Aden			70			(1990)	(2712)

3. COMMUNITY STUDIES

3.1 North- eastern area, 1985 [(2711)]

A small retrospective community-based study found a maternal mortality rate of 1 040 per 100 000 live births.

4. HOSPITAL STUDIES

4.1 All institutions, 1985 [(2711)]

MMR (per 100 000 live births)   330

4.2 Abood Maternity Hospital, Aden, 1977-86 [(1676)]

4.2.1 Rate

	1977-81	1982-86
Live births	18 087	23 477
Maternal deaths	231	60
MMR (per 100 000 live births)	1 277	256

The rates dropped from 2 327 per 100 000 live births in 1977 to 632 per 100 000 live births in 1981, and to 268 in 1986.

4.2.2 Causes of maternal deaths, 1982-86

	Number	%
Haemorrhage	22	37
Sepsis	11	18
Hypertensive disorders of pregnancy	9	15
Embolisms	6	10
Abortion	4	7
Ectopic pregnancy	1	2
Other	2	3
DIRECT CAUSES	55	92
Malaria	2	3
Hepatitis	1	2
Other indirect causes	2	3
INDIRECT CAUSES	5	8
TOTAL	60	100

Sepsis accounted for 23% of deaths including abortion deaths and was present in 38% of the cases. Many of the women were severely anaemic with average haemoglobin levels ranging from 4-8 gms. Preeclampsia was a complication in a large number of the cases.

4.2.3 Avoidable factors

4.2.4 High risk groups

4.2.5 Other findings

Of the women who died, 10% were dead on admission and another 15% died within an hour.

5. CIVIL REGISTRATION DATA/GOVERNMENT ESTIMATES

5.1 National (1984) [(0303)]

5.1.1 Rate

A report by the Ministry of Public Health to a regional workshop held in 1984 quotes a maternal mortality rate of 100 per 100 000 births.

6. OTHER SOURCES/ ESTIMATES

6.1 National (1979) [(0650)]

6.1.1 Rate

A WHO assignment report published in 1979 quotes a maternal mortality rate of 1 000 per 100 000 births.

7. SELECTED ANNOTATED BIBLIOGRAPHY

8. FURTHER READING

9. DATA SOURCES

WHE 0303   Democratic Yemen, Ministry of Public Health. Aden country study on women health and development. *Paper presented to the regional workshop*, (unpublished document) Damascus, 1984.

WHE 0650   Shakir, A. *Child health, Democratic Yemen*, (unpublished assignment report), April 1979.

WHE 0834   World Health Organization *World health statistics annual – vital statistics and causes of death.* Geneva, various years.

WHE 1676   Ahmed Ali, A. *A review of maternal mortality at Abood Maternity Hospital (Aden) from 1982-86.* (unpublished document), 1987.

WHE 1914   United Nations Children's Fund (UNICEF). *The state of the world's children*, Oxford, Oxford University Press, various years.

WHE 1915   United Nations. Department of International Economic and Social Affairs. *World population prospects: estimates and projections*, Population Studies, New York, various years.

WHE 2033   World Health Organization. *Global strategy for health for all by the year 2000. Second report on monitoring progress.* WHO document EB83/2 Add. 1, 1988.

WHE 2711   Abdulghani, N.A. *Risk factors for maternal mortality among women using hospitals in Yemen Arab Republic.* (unpublished), 1990.

WHE 2712   El Serour, G.A. *Infant mortality rate and maternal mortality rate survey.* WHO consultant assignment report, 1990.

NOTES

Oceania

Fiji

	Year	Source

1. Basic Indicators

1.1 Demographic

1.1.1 Population

		Year	Source
Size (millions)	0.7	1988	(1914)
Rate of growth (%)	1.9	1985-90	(1915)

1.1.2 Life expectancy

		Year	Source
Female	73	1989-90	(1915)
Male	68	1985-90	(1915)

1.1.3 Fertility

		Year	Source
Crude Birth Rate	27	1985-90	(1915)
Total Fertility Rate	3.2	1985-90	(1915)

1.1.4 Mortality

		Year	Source
Crude Death Rate	5	1985-90	(1915)
Infant Mortality Rate	27	1985-90	(1915)
Female			
Male			
1-4 years mortality rate			
Female			
Male			

1.2 Social and economic

1.2.1 Adult literacy rate (%)

		Year	Source
Female	81	1985	(1914)
Male	90	1985	(1914)

1.2.2 Primary school enrolment rate (%)

		Year	Source
Female	129	1983-86	(1914)
Male	129	1983-86	(1914)

1.2.3 Female mean age at first marriage

		Year	Source
(years)	21.6	1976	(1918)

1.2.4 GNP/capita

		Year	Source
(US $)	1 570	1985	(1914)

1.2.5 Daily per capita calorie supply
(as % of requirements)

2. Health Services

2.1 Health Expenditure

2.1.1 Expenditure on health

		Year	Source
(as % of GNP)	10	1987	(2033)

2.1.2 Expenditure on PHC

		Year	Source
(as % of total health expenditure)	25	1987	(2033)

2.2 Primary Health Care
(Percentage of population covered by):

2.2.1 Health services

		Year	Source
National	100	1986	(2033)
Urban			
Rural			

2.2.2 Safe water

		Year	Source
National	83	1980	(0834)
Urban			
Rural			

2.2.3 Adequate sanitary facilities

		Year	Source
National			
Urban			
Rural			

2.2.4 Contraceptive prevalence rate
(%)

2.3   Coverage of maternity care (%)

Area	Prenatal care	Trained attendant	Institutional deliveries	Postnatal care	Sample size	Year	Source
National			90			1977	(0222)
National			92			1981	(0917)
National	97	98				1982	(0834)
National		96				1989	(2431)

3. COMMUNITY STUDIES

4. HOSPITAL STUDIES

5. CIVIL REGISTRATION DATA/GOVERNMENT ESTIMATES

5.1 National, 1970-77, 1982-86 [(0072, 0223, 2096)]

5.1.1 Rate.

	Live Births	Maternal deaths	MMR (per 100 000 births)
1970	15 339	24	156
1971	15 722	15	100
1972	15 825	10	63
1973	16 131	21	130
1974	17 048	21	123
1975	16 794	24	143
1976	17 706	21	119
1977	18 295	11	60
1982	–	10	47
1983	–	7	33
1984	–	9	44
1985	–	9	43
1986	–	14	69

By administrative division, 1976 and 1986

	Live Births	Maternal deaths	MMR (per 100 000 births)
1976			
Central	6 662	5	75
Western	7 098	8	113
Northern	3 040	7	230
Eastern	906	1	110
Total	17 706	21	119

	Births	Maternal deaths	MMR (per 100 000 births)
1986			
Central	–	–	26
Western	–	–	91
Northern	–	–	103
Eastern	–	–	100
Total	–	–	69

5.1.2 Causes of maternal deaths, 1969-76 and 1982-86.

Haemorrhage, both post and antepartum, was the commonest cause of death during the two periods, accounting for 38% of all maternal deaths during 1969-76 and 25% during 1982-86. Anaemia, which is the most common complication of pregnancy in Fiji (24% of all pregnant women suffer from anaemia), was a direct cause of death during the earlier period and it is likely that anaemia was an underlying cause of several other maternal deaths, especially those from haemorrhage.

	1969-76 No.	1969-76 %	1982-86 No.	1982-86 %
Haemorrhage	61	38	12	25
Heart failure	18	11	8	16
Sepsis	8	5	5	10
Hypertensive disorders of pregnancy	21	13	4	8
Ectopic pregnancy	5	3	3	6
Abortions	22	13	2	4
Ruptured uterus	7	4	2	4
Complications of anaesthesia	6	4	0	0
Anaemia	7	4	0	0
Embolisms	–	–	2	4
Hepatitis	–	–	1	2
Others	9	5	10	20
Total	164	100	49	100

5.1.3 Avoidable factors

5.1.4 High risk groups

5.1.5 Other findings

There were ethnic differences in maternal mortality rates. The rate for the Fijian population was 102 per 100 000 live births in 1976 compared with 142 per 100 000 for the Indian population.

5.2 National, 1978 [0900]

5.2.1 Rate

Government estimates provided for the review and appraisal of the UN Decade for the Advancement of Women gave a rate of 86 per 100 000 live births in 1978.

5.3 National, 1982 [0876]

5.3.1 Rate

A 1982 Government report on the health status of women gave a maternal mortality rate of 47 per 100 000 live births.

5.4 National, 1989 [3153]

5.4.1 Rate

MMR (per 100 000 live births)   90

6. OTHER SOURCES/ ESTIMATES

6.1 National, 1978 [0834]

6.1.1 Rate

MMR (per 100 000 live births)   53

6.2 National 1985 [2608]

6.2.1 Rate

MMR (per 100 000 live births   40

7. SELECTED ANNOTATED BIBLIOGRAPHY

8. FURTHER READING

9. DATA SOURCES

WHE 0072   Bavadra, T.V. et al. Maternal mortality in Fiji. *Fiji Medical Journal,* 1978: 61(1); 4-11.

WHE 0222   Fiji, Bureau of Statistics. *Social indicators for Fiji* Issue no. 4. Suva, 1979.

WHE 0223   Fiji, Ministry of Health, *Annual Report for the year 1975,* Issue no. 4, Bureau of Statistics, Suva, 1976.

WHE 0834   World Health Organization *World Health Statistics annual – vital statistics and causes of death.* Geneva, various years.

WHE 0876   World Health Organization Western Pacific Regional Office. *Fiji, women and health questionnaire* (unpublished document) 1984.

WHE 0900   United Nations, Secretariat of the Decade for Women. *Country responses to the questionnaire on the review and appraisal of the UN Decade for Women* Part II, Health and Nutrition (unpublished documents), 1984.

WHE 0917   United Nations Economic and Social Commission for Asia and the Pacific. *The Asian and Pacific atlas of children in national development, 1984,* UNICEF/ESCAP, 1984.

WHE 1914   United Nations Children's Fund (UNICEF). *The state of the world's children*, Oxford, Oxford University Press, various years.

WHE 1915   United Nations. Department of International Economic and Social Affairs. *World population prospects: estimates and projections,* Population Studies, New York, various years.

WHE 1918   United Nations. Department of International Economic and Social Affairs. *First marriage: patterns and determinants.* New York, 1988.

WHE 2033   World Health Organization. *Global strategy for health for all by the year 2000. Second report on monitoring progress.* WHO document EB83/2 Add. 1, 1988.

WHE 2096   World Health Organization. *Report of a visit to Fiji,* WPRO, WPR/MCH(FP)/FR/19. 1989.

WHE 2431   Tamani, M. *Country Report Fiji* , (unpublished document no. WPR/MCH/MCH(1)/89.8a), Regional Office for the Western Pacific/WHO, 1989.

WHE 2608 United Nations Children's Fund, *1988 Asian and Pacific atlas of children in national development.* UNICEF/ESCAP, Bangkok, 1987.

WHE 3153   World Health Organization. Western Pacific Regional Office. *Country data sheets.* (unpublished), 1991.

NOTES

PAPUA NEW GUINEA

		Year	Source

1. BASIC INDICATORS

1.1 Demographic

1.1.1 Population

		Year	Source
Size (millions)	3.8	1988	(1914)
Rate of growth (%)	2.6	1980-87	(1914)

1.1.2 Life expectancy

Female	55	1985-90	(1915)
Male	53	1985-90	(1915)

1.1.3 Fertility

Crude Birth Rate	39	1988	(1914)
Total Fertility Rate	5.7	1988	(1914)

1.1.4 Mortality

Crude Death Rate	12	1988	(1914)
Infant Mortality Rate	57	1988	(1914)
Female			
Male			
1-4 years mortality rate			
Female			
Male			

1.2 Social and economic

1.2.1 Adult literacy rate (%)

Female	35	1985	(1914)
Male	55	1985	(1914)

1.2.2 Primary school enrolment rate (%)

Female	64	1986-88	(1914)
Male	75	1986-88	(1914)

1.2.3 Female mean age at first marriage
(years)

1.2.4 GNP/capita

		Year	Source
(US $)	799	1987	(1914)

1.2.5 Daily per capita calorie supply

(as % of requirements)	96	1984-86	(1914)

2. HEALTH SERVICES

2.1 Health Expenditure

2.1.1 Expenditure on health

(as % of GNP)	3	1987	(2033)

2.1.2 Expenditure on PHC

(as % of total health expenditure)	55	1987	(2033)

2.2 Primary Health Care
(Percentage of population covered by):

2.2.1 Health services

National	96	1987	(2033)
Urban			
Rural			

2.2.2 Safe water

National			
Urban	54	1983	(0834)
Rural	10	1983	(0834)

2.2.3 Adequate sanitary facilities

National	57	1985	(0834)
Urban			
Rural			

2.2.4 Contraceptive prevalence rate
(%)

2.3 Coverage of maternity care (%)

Area	Prenatal care	Trained attendant	Institutional deliveries	Postnatal care	Sample size	Year	Source
National	54	34				1983	(1488)
National	62					1986	(2424)
National	68	20				1989	(3153)
National: urban	50		90			1984	(1230)
Lae urban			83			1968-79	(1868)

3. Community Studies

3.1 Sepik district, 1963-69 [(0677)]

This was a longitudinal study of natality and fertility patterns in a population of 3 500 living in 16 villages. The population was surveyed at approximately six-monthly intervals and every person was either seen or accounted for. Records kept on individual cards included births, deaths, marriages, adoptions, morbidity, immunizations, tests, physical measurements and causes of death. Each survey was conducted by a doctor, accompanied by a nurse who examined the children and also all women for evidence of pregnancy.

3.1.1 Rate

Live births	877
Maternal deaths	14
MMR (per 100 000 live births)	1 596

3.2 Tari, Southern Highlands, 1977-83, [(1309)]

This is an area with well-established obstetric services. Since the number of births is known it is possible to make population-based estimates of maternal mortality.

3.2.1 Rate

MMR (per 100 000 live births)	460

4. Hospital Studies

4.1 Goroka Base Hospital, Eastern Highlands 1964-73 [(0121)]

4.1.1 Rate

Deliveries	6 031
Maternal deaths	142
MMR (per 100 000 deliveries)	2 355

4.1.2 Causes of maternal deaths

	Number	%
Sepsis	44	31
Obstructed labour	29	20
Abortion	14	10
Ruptured uterus	13	9
Haemorrhage	9	6
Hypertensive disorders of pregnancy	4	3
Ectopic pregnancy	1	1
Embolism	1	1
DIRECT CAUSES	115	81
Hepatitis	7	5
Cardiac diseases	3	2
Anaemia	1	1
Malaria	1	1
Other infections	10	7
Others	5	3
INDIRECT CAUSES	27	19
TOTAL	142	100

4.2 Simbu Province hospitals and health centres, 1982-86 [(2335)]

4.2.1 Rate

Supervised births	9 429
Maternal deaths	20
MMR (per 100 000 births)	212

5. CIVIL REGISTRATION DATA/GOVERNMENT ESTIMATES

5.1 National, 1970-83 [0053, 0367, 0761, 1309]

5.1.1 Rate

It is not possible to calculate maternal mortality rates because not all maternal deaths are reported and not all births are notified.

5.1.2 Causes of maternal deaths

Causes of death are available for the deaths reported to the Death Registry, for various years between 1970 and 1983.

	1970 %	1971-72 %	1973-75 %	1976-83 % *
Haemorrhage	51	49	49	29
Sepsis	21	19	22	27
Obstructed labour	–	4	5	5
Hypertensive disorders of pregnancy	1	–	1	4
Abortion	–	3	3	4
Ruptured uterus	9	4	4	4
Embolisms	–	–	–	3
Ectopic pregnancy	–	–	–	2
Complications of anaesthesia	–	–	–	2
Associated with caesarean section	9	–	–	–
Others	9	21	16	20
Total	100	100	100	100

* As a percentage of known causes.

The pattern of causes of death differed in the coastal and highlands districts. Maternal anaemia was much more common in the coastal districts, whereas contracted pelvis was more common in the highlands. As a result, haemorrhage was a major killer in the coastal districts whereas puerperal sepsis following prolonged and difficult labour was predominant in the highlands.

5.2 National, 1980 [0873]

5.2.1 Rate.

According to the Government report to the WHO regional office, the maternal mortality rate was 900 per 100,000 live births in 1980.

6. OTHER SOURCES/ ESTIMATES

6.1 National, 1976-83 [1230]

Death certification in Papua New Guinea is only compulsory for those deaths which occur in health facilities. In April 1970 a Maternal Mortality Register was set up in an attempt to record in more detail deaths occurring both at home and in health care facilities. Between 10 January 1976 and 31 December 1983, 628 maternal deaths were recorded on death certificates and 385 deaths reported to the Maternal Mortality Register. Over the eight-year period the number of deaths being notified to the Death Register remained relatively stable. By contrast, the numbers of deaths notified to the Maternal Mortality Register declined considerably. The author estimates that while the percentage of hospital and health centre deaths reported is high (78-96%), reporting to the Maternal Mortality Register is erratic and considerably less complete (18-55%).

6.1.1 Rate

After examining all death certificates and eliminating double counting, the author estimates that there were a total of 895 maternal deaths over the period. As the number of births is not known the maternal mortality rate cannot be calculated. However, the author estimates maternal mortality rates for urban and rural areas.

	MMR (per 100 000) live births *
Urban areas	200
Rural areas	2 000
National	800

* Estimate

6.1.2 Causes of maternal deaths

	Coast No.	Coast %	Highlands No.	Highlands %	Total No.	Total %
Haemorrhage	182	33	67	19	249	28
Sepsis	110	20	123	36	233	26
Medical and surgical conditions	98	18	42	12	140	16
Obstructed labour	21	4	24	7	45	5
Ruptured uterus	24	4	14	4	38	4
Abortion	24	4	14	4	38	4
Hypertensive disorders of pregnancy	15	3	15	4	30	3
Trophoblastic disease	18	3	7	2	25	3
Pulmonary embolism	14	3	11	3	25	3
Ectopic pregnancy	16	3	4	1	20	2
Operative and anaesthetic death	11	2	3	1	14	2
Other	5	1	5	1	10	1
Unknown	12	2	16	5	28	3
TOTAL	550	100	345	100	895	100

6.2   National, 1984-86 [2335]

An examination of death certificates sent to the Registrar General's office and of deaths reported to the Maternal Mortality Register found a total of 304 maternal deaths, of which only 134 were reported to the Maternal Mortality Register.

6.2.1   Rate

In view of the absence of data on the numbers of births the maternal mortality rates were not calculated.

6.2.2   Causes of maternal deaths

	Number	%
Haemorrhage	83	27
Sepsis	77	25
Associated medical/surgical conditions	31	10
Abortion	20	7
Obstructed labour	13	4
Trophoblastic disease	10	3
Ruptured uterus	8	3
Hypertensive disorders of pregnancy	6	2
Ectopic pregnancy	6	2
Operative and anaesthetic deaths	3	1
DIRECT CAUSES	257	85
Malaria	15	5
Typhoid fever	6	2
Anaemia	5	2
Hepatitis	3	1
Other	8	3
INDIRECT CAUSES	37	12
Unknown	10	3
TOTAL	304	100

6.3   National [0189]

6.3.1   Rate

A report of the Economic Commission of Asia and the Pacific published in 1982 estimated the maternal mortality rate to be between 700 and 1000 per 100 000 live births.

6.4   Simbu Province, 1982-86 [2335]

Simbu Province has a provincial health team which has been diligent in obtaining health statistics from aid posts and health centres. The numbers of unsupervised births have been estimated using 1986 national census figures and crude birth rates from the Department of Health.

6.4.1   Rate

Total unsupervised births	14 071
Maternal deaths	105
MMR (per 100 000 births)	746

6.5   National, 1989 [2604]

6.5.1   Rate

Rates calculated on the basis of estimated numbers of births.

	MMR (per 100 000 live births)	Lifetime chance of pregnancy-related death***
Rural areas with services*	500	1:37
Rural areas without services**	1 200	1:15
Urban areas	200	1:98
National	700	1:26

*   Rural villages with well-established obstetric services.
**   Rural areas where obstetric services are limited or nonexistent.
*** MMR x TFR

7.   SELECTED ANNOTATED BIBLIOGRAPHY

Barss, P. and Misch, K.A. Endemic placenta accreta in a population of remote villagers in Papua New Guinea *British Journal of Obstetrics and Gynaecology,* 1989: 97; 167-174. WHE 2607

In Papua New Guinea, retained placenta, including placenta accreta, has long been recognised as an important cause of maternal mortality and morbidity. Using a combination of prospective registration of definite cases and retrospective identification of probable cases over a 6.5 year period, the incidence rate was estimated to be in excess of 2.3 per 1000 births. The true rate is probably much higher as most deliveries take place outside hospital. A number of factors appear to be important in the aetiology of the condition, including infection associated with previous childbirth and abortion. Over three quarters of the cases would have been avoided if all women of para 4 and over with a history of retained placenta had used effective contraception. Better obstetric care, including early treatment of postpartum sepsis and incomplete abortion, may also help reduce the frequency of placenta accreta.

Mola, G. Personal communication. Port Moresby, 1989. WHE 2293

Reasonable access to provincial hospitals for the great majority of the obstetric population of Papua New Guinea means that obstetric fistulae are not common. At Port Moresby approximately 10 obstetric fistulae are repaired annually, at least half of which are referred from other parts of the country. It is estimated that another 10 fistulae would present to provincial centres annually. Cephalopelvic disproportion, which is usually the cause of obstetric fistulae, is only a common problem in the highlands.

8. FURTHER READING

Barss, P. and Blackford, C. Grand multiparity: Benefits of a referral programme for hospital delivery and postpartum tubal ligation. *Papua New Guinea Medical Journal,* 1985: 28(1); 35-39. WHE 1276

Brabin, B.J. et al. Consequences of maternal anaemia on outcome of pregnancy in a malaria endemic area in Papua New Guinea. *Annals of Tropical Medicine and Parasitology,* 1990; 84(1): 11-24. WHE 2605

Brabin, B.J. et al. Failure of chloroquine prophylaxis for falciparum malaria in pregnant women in Madang, Papua New Guinea. *Annals of Tropical Medicine and Parasitology,* 1990: 84(1); 1-9. WHE 2606

McGoldrick, I.A. Termination of pregnancy in Papua New Guinea: The traditional and contemporary position. *Papua New Guinea Medical Journal,* 1981: 24(2). WHE 1867

McGoldrick, I.A. Pelvic inflammatory disease. *Papua New Guinea Medical Journal,* 1982: 25(1); 37-42. WHE 1185

Rooke, P.W. Pelvic inflammatory disease in Port Moresby General Hospital *Papua New Guinea Medical Journal,* 1982: 25(1); 29-32. WHE 0940

Vacca, A. and Henderson, A. Puerperal sepsis in Port Moresby, Papua New Guinea *Papua New Guinea Medical Journal,* 1980: 23(3); 120-125. WHE 0958

9. DATA SOURCES

WHE 0053   Babona, G. et al. Maternal mortality in Papua New Guinea 1971 and 1972 *Papua New Guinea Medical Journal,* 1974: 17(4); 331-334.

WHE 0121   Campbell, G.R. Maternal mortality at Gonka Base Hospital. *Papua New Guinea Medical Journal,* 1974: 17(4); 335-341.

WHE 0189   Economic and Social Commission for Asia and the Pacific: South Pacific Commission. *Population of Papua New Guinea.* Country monograph no.72, 1982.

WHE 0367   Johnson, D.G. Maternal mortality in Papua New Guinea *Papua New Guinea Medical Journal* 1971: 14(4); 133-135.

WHE 0677   Sturt, R.J. and Sturt, A.E. Natality, fertility and marriage status in a Sepik River population of New Guinea. *Tropical and Geographic Medicine* 1974: 26; 399-413.

WHE 0761   Vacca, A. et al. Maternal mortality in Papua New Guinea. *Papua New Guinea Medical Journal* 1977: 20(4); 180-186.

WHE 0834   World Health Organization *World Health Statistics annual – vital statistics and causes of death.* Geneva, various years.

WHE 0873   World Health Organization. Western Pacific Regional Office. *Papua New Guinea: women and health questionnaire* (unpublished document) 1984.

WHE 1230   Mola, G. and Aitken, I. Maternal mortality in Papua New Guinea, 1976-1983 *Papua New Guinea Medical Journal,* 1984: 27(2); 65-71.

WHE 1309   Aitken, I. *Obstetric care in Papua New Guinea. An assessment of some aspects of the current situation, 1985.* (unpublished paper), 1985.

WHE 1488   World Health Organization. Western Pacific Regional Office. *Evaluation of the strategy for Health for All by the year 2000.* Seventh Report on the World Health Situation. Manila, 1985.

WHE 1868   Marshall, L.B. and Lakin, J.A. Antenatal health care policy, services and clients in urban Papua New Guinea. *International Journal of Nursing Studies,* 1984: 21(1); 19-34.

WHE 1914   United Nations Children's Fund (UNICEF). *The state of the world's children,* Oxford, Oxford University Press, various years.

WHE 1915   United Nations. Department of International Economic and Social Affairs. *World population prospects: estimates and projections,* Population Studies, New York, various years.

WHE 2033   World Health Organization. *Global strategy for health for all by the year 2000. Second report on monitoring progress.* WHO document EB83/2 Add. 1, 1988.

WHE 2335   Mola, G. Maternal death in Papua New Guinea, 1984-86. *Papua New Guinea Medical Journal,* 1989: 32; 27-31.

WHE 2424   Vagi, E. *Country Report Papua New Guinea,* Paper presented at the Workshop on the risk approach in mother and child care. World Health Organization. Regional Office for the Western Pacific, 1989.

WHE 2604   Gillet, J.E. *The health of women in Papua New Guinea,* New Guinea Institute of Medical Research, 1990.

WHE 3153   World Health Organization. Western Pacific Regional Office. *Country data sheets.* (unpublished), 1991.

SAMOA

		Year	Source

1. BASIC INDICATORS

1.1 Demographic

1.1.1 Population
Size Millions)	0.2	1988	(1914)
Rate of growth (%)	0.6	1976-81	(1262)

1.1.2 Life expectancy
Female	64	1976	(1262)
Male	61	1976	(1262)

1.1.3 Fertility
Crude Birth Rate			
Total Fertility Rate	5.8	1975-80	(1262)

1.1.4 Mortality
Crude Death Rate			
Infant Mortality Rate	33	1988	(1914)
Female			
Male			
1-4 years mortality rate			
Female			
Male			

1.2 Social and Economic

1.2.1 Adult literacy rate
(%)	98	1982	(1262)
Female			
Male			

1.2.2 Primary school enrolment rate (%)
Female	
Male	

1.2.3 Female mean age at first marriage
(years)

1.2.4 GNP/capita
(US $)	550	1987	(1914)

1.2.5 Daily per capita calorie supply
(as % requirements)

2. HEALTH SERVICES

2.1 Health Expenditure

2.1.1 Expenditure on health
(as % of GNP)

2.1.1 Expenditure on PHC
(as % of total health			
expenditure)	28	1988	(2033)

2.2 Primary Health Care
(Percentage of population covered by):

2.2.1 Health services
National	100	1987	(2033)
Urban			
Rural			

2.2.2 Safe water
National			
Urban	97	1980	(1262)
Rural	94	1980	(1262)

2.2.3 Adequate sanitary facilities
National			
Urban	86	1980	(1262)
Rural	83	1980	(1262)

2.2.4 Contraceptive prevalence rate
(%)	12	1975	(1262)

2.3 Coverage of maternity care (%)

Area	Prenatal care	Trained attendant	Institutional deliveries	Postnatal care	Sample size	Year	Source
National	50	95				1987	(2033)

3. COMMUNITY STUDIES

4. HOSPITAL STUDIES

5. CIVIL REGISTRATION DATA/GOVERNMENT ESTIMATES

5.1 National, 1986 [3153]

5.1.1 Rate
MMR (per 100 000 live births)   400

6. OTHER SOURCES/ ESTIMATES

6.1 National, 1982 [1262]

6.1.1 Rate
MMR (per 100 000 live births)   200

7. SELECTED ANNOTATED BIBLIOGRAPHY

8. FURTHER READING

9. DATA SOURCES

WHE 1262   Cho, Hyoung, *The health status of women in the Western Pacific Region,* Seoul, Korea, 1984.

WHE 1914   United Nations Children's Fund (UNICEF). *The state of the world's children,* Oxford, Oxford University Press, various years.

WHE 2033   World Health Organization. *Global strategy for health for all by the year 2000. Second report on monitoring progress.* WHO document EB83/2 Add. 1, 1988.

WHE 3153   World Health Organization. Western Pacific Regional Office. *Country data sheets.* (unpublished), 1991.

DEVELOPED COUNTRIES

With the notable exception of Romania and Albania, maternal mortality in the developed countries is uniformly low and reasonably well documented. Information relating to the developed countries is thus given here mainly to serve as a yardstick.

Data are presented in summary form. The table on the next two pages gives, for 33 developed countries, the latest available maternal mortality rates, derived from the civil registration system, together with the indicators appearing in sections 1 and 2 of the other country profiles.

Country	Demographic								Social and economic			
	Population		Life expectancy (years)		Fertility		Mortality		Adult literacy rate (%)		Female age at first marriage (years)	GNP per capita US$
	Size (millions)	Rate of growth (%)	Female	Male	Crude birth rate	Total fertility rate	Crude death rate	Infant mortality rate	Female	Male		
	1980-85	1980-85	1980-85	1980-85	1980-85	1980-85	1980-85	1980-85	1985	1985	1980-85	1987
Albania	3.2	1.8	74.2	69.2	24	3.0	6	39	n.a.	n.a.	n.a.	790
Australia	16.9	1.4	79.5	72.9	15	1.9	8	8	n.a.	n.a.	23.5	12 340
Austria	7.6	0.1	77.8	70.6	12	1.5	12	11	n.a.	n.a.	23.5	15 470
Belgium	10.0	0.0	78.1	71.5	12	1.6	12	10	99	99	22.4	14 490
Bulgaria	9.0	0.1	75.0	69.2	13	1.9	12	16	89	94	21.7	4 150
Canada	26.5	1.0	80.3	73.3	14	1.7	8	7	n.a.	n.a.	23.1	16 960
Czechoslovakia	15.7	0.2	75.0	67.5	14	2.0	12	15	n.a.	n.a.	21.7	5 820
Denmark	5.1	0.1	78.3	72.6	11	1.5	11	7	n.a.	n.a.	25.6	18 450
Finland	5.0	0.3	75.0	78.8	13	1.7	10	6	n.a.	n.a.	24.6	18 590
France	56.1	0.4	80.0	71.9	14	1.8	10	8	98	99	24.5	16 090
Germany: DDR	16.2	-0.5	76.2	70.4	13	1.7	13	9	n.a.	n.a.	21.7	7 180
Germany: RDF	61.3	0.1	78.2	71.6	11	1.4	12	9	n.a.	n.a.	23.6	18 480
Greece	10.0	0.2	77.9	73.5	12	1.7	10	17	86	97	22.5	4 800
Hungary	10.6	-0.2	74.0	66.5	12	1.8	13	20	98	98	21.0	2 460
Iceland	0.3	1.0	80.4	74.8	17	2.1	7	5	n.a.	n.a.	n.a.	n.a.
Ireland	3.7	0.9	76.9	71.5	18	2.5	9	9	n.a.	n.a.	23.4	7 750
Italy	57.0	0.0	78.9	72.4	10	1.3	10	11	96	97	23.2	13 330
Japan	123.4	0.4	81.1	75.4	11	1.7	7	5	99	99	25.8	21 020
Luxembourg	0.4	0.3	77.7	71.0	12	1.5	12	10	n.a.	n.a.	23.1	n.a.
Malta	0.4	0.5	74.6	71.0	15	1.9	10	10	n.a.	n.a.	n.a.	n.a.
Netherlands	15.0	0.6	80.2	73.5	13	1.6	9	8	n.a.	n.a.	23.2	14 520
New Zealand	3.4	0.9	7.9	71.8	16	2.0	8	11	n.a.	n.a.	22.8	10 000
Norway	4.2	0.3	80.2	73.5	12	1.7	11	7	n.a.	n.a.	24.0	19 990
Poland	38.4	0.7	75.5	67.5	16	2.2	10	18	97	98	22.8	1 860
Portugal	10.3	0.3	76.8	70.0	14	1.8	10	15	77	86	22.1	3 650
Romania	23.3	0.5	73.0	67.5	16	2.1	11	22	91	96	21.1	2 560
Spain	39.2	0.3	79.7	73.6	12	1.6	9	10	92	97	23.1	7 740
Sweden	8.4	0.2	80.1	74.2	13	1.9	12	6	n.a.	n.a.	27.6	19 300
Switzerland	6.6	0.4	80.4	73.8	12	1.5	10	7	n.a.	n.a.	25.0	27 500
United Kingdom	57.2	0.2	78.1	72.4	14	1.8	12	9	n.a.	n.a.	22.7	12 810
United States	249.2	0.8	79.0	71.9	15	1.8	9	10	99	99	23.3	19 840
USSR	288.6	0.8	74.2	65.0	18	2.4	11	24	97	98	21.8	4 550
Yugoslavia	23.8	0.6	75.0	69.1	15	2.0	9	25	85	97	22.2	2 520

Health expenditure		Primary Health Care (% of population covered)					Coverage of maternity care			Maternal mortality		Country
Expenditure on health (as % of GNP)	Expenditure on PHC (as % of total health expenditure)	Safe water		Adequate sanitary facilities		Contra-ceptive prevalence (%)	Prenatal care (%)	Trained attendant (%)	Institu-tional deliveries (%)	Number of maternal deaths	Maternal deaths per 100 000 live births	
		Urban	Rural	Urban	Rural							
1980-87	1980-87	1985-87	1985-87	1985-87	1985-87	1975-84	1982-87	1982-87	(latest)	(latest)	(latest)	
6.9	n.a.	100	95	100	100	n.a.	n.a.	99	n.a.	n.a.	n.a.	**Albania**
7.7	34	n.a.	n.a.	n.a.	n.a.	n.a.	100	99	n.a.	8	3	**Australia**
10.0	n.a.	100	100	100	100	71	n.a.	n.a.	85	7	8	**Austria**
9.1	n.a.	100	100	100	100	81	90	100	98	4	3	**Belgium**
6.3	80	100	96	100	100	76	100	100	100	11	9	**Bulgaria**
8.6	n.a.	100	100	n.a.	n.a.	73	100	100	99	18	5	**Canada**
4.2	43	100	100	100	100	95	100	100	100	20	10	**Czechoslovakia**
6.0	28	100	100	100	100	63	99	99	99	2	3	**Denmark**
7.0	26	99	90	100	100	80	100	100	100	7	11	**Finland**
8.0	n.a.	100	100	100	100	79	99	n.a.	99	72	9	**France**
5.2	20	100	100	100	100	n.a.	100	100	100	10	5	**Germany: DDR**
9.6	17	100	100	95	83	78	98	100	n.a.	36	5	**Germany: RDF**
3.0	17	100	95	100	95	n.a.	n.a.	97	94	5	5	**Greece**
7.1	40	100	95	100	100	73	100	99	99	19	15	**Hungary**
10.0	25	100	100	100	100	n.a.	100	100	98	0	0	**Iceland**
7.4	n.a	100	100	100	100	n.a.	n.a.	n.a.	n.a.	1	2	**Ireland**
6.4	31	100	100	100	100	78	100	100	100	25	4	**Italy**
5.2	n.a.	100	100	100	100	64	99	100	100	135	11	**Japan**
4.9	n.a.	100	100	100	100	n.a.	98	100	100	0	0	**Luxembourg**
8.1	21	100	100	100	100	n.a.	100	98	n.a.	0	0	**Malta**
8.3	30	100	100	100	100	76	95	100	64	18	10	**Netherlands**
7.0	23	n.a.	n.a.	100	n.a.	70	95	100	100	7	13	**New Zealand**
7.1	10	100	100	100	100	71	95	100	99	2	3	**Norway**
5.0	15	94	82	100	100	75	99	99	92	60	11	**Poland**
3.5	50	97	90	100	95	66	96	87	80	12	10	**Portugal**
5.4	n.a.	100	90	100	95	58	100	99	98	522	149	**Romania**
4.3	n.a.	100	100	100	100	59	96	96	90	24	5	**Spain**
9.1	15	100	100	100	100	78	100	100	n.a.	5	5	**Sweden**
7.3	n.a.	100	100	100	100	71	n.a.	99	n.a.	3	4	**Switzerland**
6.1	30	100	100	100	100	83	98	98	98	60	8	**United Kingdom**
10.9	n.a.	n.a.	n.a.	n.a.	n.a.	68	94	99	99	330	8	**United States**
4.1	n.a.	100	100	100	100	n.a.	100	100	n.a.	1 151	21	**USSR**
4.5	35	100	65	78	46	55	100	86	83	28	8	**Yugoslavia**

DATA SOURCES

Indicator	Source
Demographic	WHE 1915
Social and economic	WHE 1914, WHE 2799
Health expenditure	WHE 2033
Primary health care	WHE 2033
Contraceptive prevalence	WHE 1712, WHE 3148
Coverage of maternity care	WHE 2033, WHE 3139
Maternal mortality	WHE 0834

WHE 0834   World Health Organization. *World health statistics annual: vital statistics and causes of death.* Geneva, various years.

WHE 1712   Mauldin, W.P. and Segal, S.J. *Prevalence of contraceptive use in developing countries. A short book.* Rockefeller Foundation, New York, 1986.

WHE 1914   United Nations Children's Fund. (UNICEF). *The state of the world's children.* Oxford University Press, Oxford, various years.

WHE 1915   United Nations. Department of International Economic and Social Affairs. *World population prospects: estimates and projections.* Population Studies. New York, various years.

WHE 2033   World Health Organization. *Global strategy for health for all by the year 2000. Second report on monitoring progress.* WHO document no. EB83/2 Add 1, 1988.

WHE 2799   United Nations. Department of International Economic and Social Affairs. *Patterns of first marriage: timing and prevalence.* New York, 1990.

WHE 3148   United Nations. Department of International Economics and Social Affairs. *Level and trends of contraceptive use as assessed in 1988.* Population Studies No. 110. New York, 1989.

WHE 3139   World Health Organization. *Coverage of maternity care: a tabulation of available information.* Second Edition. FHE/89.2. Geneva, 1989.